PSYCHOLOGY OF WOMEN

Psychology
of
Women

A HANDBOOK
OF ISSUES AND THEORIES

Edited by FLORENCE L. DENMARK
and MICHELE A. PALUDI

Foreword by Leonore Loeb Adler

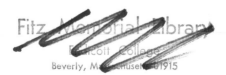

Greenwood Press
Westport, Connecticut • London

Library of Congress Cataloging-in-Publication Data

Psychology of women : a handbook of issues and theories / edited by
   Florence L. Denmark and Michele A. Paludi ; foreword by Leonore Loeb Adler.
      p.   cm.
   Includes bibliographical references and index.
   ISBN 0–313–26295–0 (alk. paper)
      1. Women—Psychology.   2. Feminist psychology.   I. Denmark,
   Florence.   II. Paludi, Michele Antoinette.
   HQ1206.P747   1993
   155.3′33—dc20   92–8642

British Library Cataloguing in Publication Data is available.

Library of Congress Catalog Card Number: 92–8642
ISBN: 0–313–26295–0

First published in 1993

Greenwood Press, 88 Post Road West, Westport, CT 06881
An imprint of Greenwood Publishing Group, Inc.

Printed in the United States of America

The paper used in this book complies with the
Permanent Paper Standard issued by the National
Information Standards Organization (Z39.48–1984).

10 9 8 7 6 5 4 3 2 1

In memory of the first generation of women psychologists,
we dedicate this handbook to future scholars
in the psychology of women

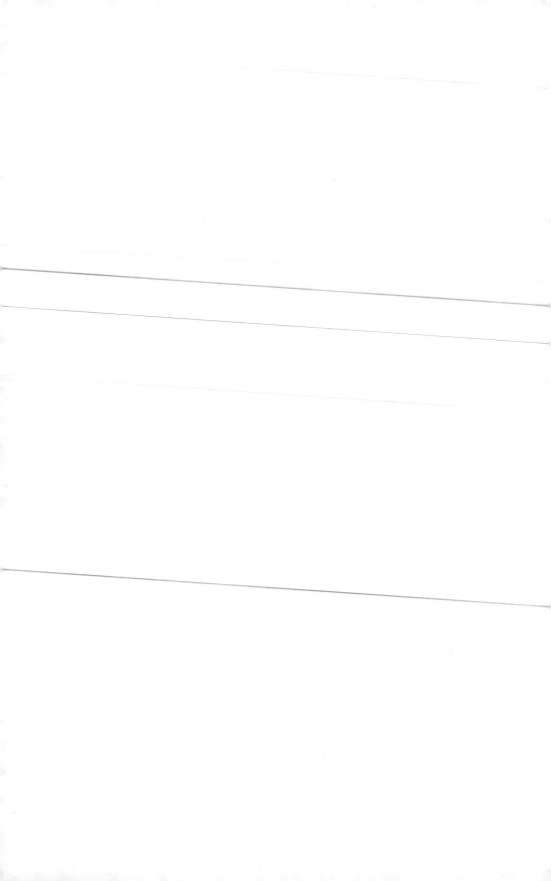

Contents

Foreword

Leonore Loeb Adler

Concern about women's worlds—their realities, roles, and choices—has now become part of the international consciousness. Increasing interest in women and gender is taking place in the context of the changing and expanding roles for women and a growing feminist awareness throughout the world. Over the last decade several international conferences and congresses on women have been held in different parts of the developed and developing world. For example, the International Interdisciplinary Congress on Women will hold its Fifth triennial meeting in Costa Rica in 1993. Professional societies like the American Psychological Association and the American Psychological Society now have thriving women's divisions which have begun to play an important role in setting the goals and agendas of their organizations. The past two decades have witnessed the emergence of several major journals focussing on women and gender.

This concern has also been reflected in the increasing number of educational programs that now include courses on the psychology of women. In the results of her 1989 survey, Margaret Matlin reported that such courses were being taught, not only throughout the United States, but also in Argentina, Ireland, Israel, and the Netherlands. A more recent survey shows that this trend has continued to accelerate in many other countries. These international efforts concomitant with trends of cities and communities across the world to become increasingly multicultural in the composition of their residents are contributing to diverse perspectives on sex and gender. They are also highlighting the importance of making cross-cultural and cross-ethnic comparisons in social and scientific analyses. The convention of treating ''women'' as a single universe is slowly giving way to a richer, more complex way of conceptualizing women and gender. This reference work is a reflection of this increasing concern and the new wealth of scholarship on women.

Editors Florence Denmark and Michele Paludi have indeed assembled an elegant series of papers by a group of diverse psychologists, each of outstanding expertise in the topic they address. The collection consists of eighteen chapters, two appendices of important resources, a bibliographical essay and a section on the eminent contributors to this volume which reads like a ''Who's Who of Women in Psychology.'' While not exhausting every issue pertaining to the psychology of women, this reference work goes far beyond providing a mere compendium of research findings relevant to women. Instead, this volume tells the story of the beginning of the psychological study of women, offers feminist perspectives on research methodology, considers society's views of women, discusses social, personality, and cognitive development across the lifespan, probes women's bodies and women's minds, traces their career development and working lives, and finally explores their victimization.

As I read through this handbook I came to realize that this was not just a series of papers written by psychologists concerned about women, but a collection of unique perspectives on the psychology of women. When I finished one chapter in a particular section and began the next, it was as if I were looking through a different set of optical lenses. In bringing her own special expertise, viewpoint, and background to the psychology of women, each author came to focus on a distinct aspect of her image of women. Some of these images were tinted with hues of hope, and some with despair. For instance, the chapters on work and achievement emphasize how much progress has been made, but those focusing on the victimization of women remind us of how much work society and science have yet to do.

It is unusual to find such shifting yet remarkably coherent perspectives on the psychology of women reflected in a single collection as Florence Denmark and Michele Paludi have provided. I know the enjoyment and satisfaction I derived from reading this book and how much I valued the fund of knowledge contained therein. I am certain that others, regardless of their background or discipline, will have a similar experience. This handbook is a collection that I will read and refer to again and again in the coming years, and it is one that I will be proud to display on my bookshelf. This volume will serve as a major resource internationally for scientists, mental and physical health practitioners, graduate and undergraduate students interested in sex and gender issues, and also for educators, counselors, and advocates for women.

It is my sense that this reference work is itself a landmark in the psychological study of women and will be of still increasing significance as time goes on. Surely the topics that are treated here are of enduring importance and the perspectives represented are all inclusive. This volume makes original contributions to theory, research methodology, and clinical and social practice, and it exposes a timeless truth—all women are in some ways universal, in some ways particular, and in some ways unique. The publication of this handbook occurs at a very special and exciting moment in the history of the psychology of women: women around the world look to American scholars for support and validation in their diverse roles as women as they prepare to take their place in the coming century. At the same time, we recognize, more than ever before, our interdependence with other women around the world and the transformative power of feminist thought and their impending contributions to science and society.

Acknowledgments

We wish to express our appreciation to the contributors to this volume for their participation, their collaboration, and their patience with the production of this handbook. We thank Robert Wesner for his comments on the chapters and for his support. The library staff at Pace University and Hunter College deserves our recognition. We wish to thank our colleagues at Pace University and Hunter College for sharing their ideas with us and supporting us through this process: Fina Bathrick, June Chisholm, Nancy Dean, Dorothy O. Helly, Barbara Mowder, Joan Tronto, and Sue Rosenberg Zalk. We apppreciate the valuable editorial contributions of George Butler, Associate Editor, Acquisitions, of Greenwood Press. We especially thank Karen Nielson and Kristin Scholl, graduate student assistants, who worked on finding and clarifying references, and who performed numerous other endless chores. Justine Adam and Angelynn Pinto should also be thanked for their assistance on this project. We acknowledge the researchers and instructors in the field of the psychology of women who have made this handbook possible.

Florence L. Denmark
Michele A. Paludi

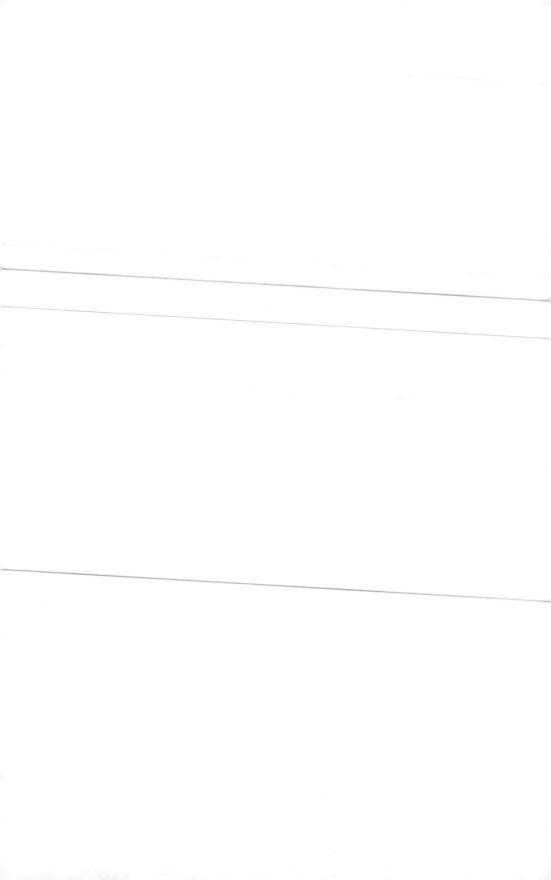

Introduction

Florence L. Denmark and Michele A. Paludi

As women have become more prominent in psychology, psychology has become more concerned with women. This reference work reflects the changes that have taken place in psychology, and it systematically overviews the most important issues and theories related to the psychology of women. Scholars, practitioners, and students will find it a valuable repository of current information on virtually every aspect of the intellectual and emotional lives of women, and will turn to it as an introduction to many of the most significant psychological issues of our day. Because each chapter offers a needed synthesis of recent research, this handbook is the first resource the reader should consult for information on the psychology of women. Because each chapter contains extensive reference lists, the reader will have no trouble identifying additional works for further reading.

This handbook on the psychology of women reflects the changes occurring in psychology. The topics in this handbook represent much of the recent research foci in the field, as evidenced by information published in the last four to five years in such sources as the *Psychology of Women Quarterly* and *Sex Roles*. In addition, one of the most important aspects is its timelessness. While providing specific information, the reader will not find it restricted to the present era but reflecting a broad and flexible outlook. Each chapter reviews relevant issues and anticipates coming trends in its area. Thus, this handbook will surely encompass future developments in the psychology of women; its themes and contents will endure over the next generation as our knowledge about women continues to unfold.

The contributors to this handbook have all conducted research in various topics in the psychology of women; several have been founding members and presidents of the American Psychological Association's Division 35 (Division of Women) and founding members of the Association for Women in Psychology. Several have authored and/or edited textbooks on the psychology of women.

There are six major sections to this handbook. In each of the chapters, contributors have integrated global feminist research and theories. In addition, the chapters are all balanced for sexual orientation, class, and ethnicity. In the first section, "Foundations," three chapters are devoted to women's heritage in psychology and research methodologies feminist scholars use in studying women's lives and realities. In this section, feminist researchers examine sources of biases that have influenced individuals' views of women and feminist methods to correct these biases, methods that include guidelines for conducting nonsexist psychological research and literature reviews.

In the second section of this handbook, "Society's View of Women," the theme of sexism is illustrated in stereotypes of women and women's work, including discrimination against women's performance, assumptions about attractiveness and gender, affirmative action, and cultural sexism.

The third section, "Social, Personality, and Cognitive Development Across the Life Span," surveys the developmental psychology of women from conception to older adulthood, with special emphasis on personality development, friendship patterns, and physical changes accompanying pubescence and menopause.

In "Women's Bodies and Minds," the research on women's mental health and physical health is reviewed, with special attention to women's health status and quality of care, gender differences, emotional disorders, utilization services, the psychology of the menstrual cycle and premenstrual syndrome, pregnancy, acquired immune deficiency syndrome (AIDS), and health issues of women in developing countries (pregnancy and birth, infections and parasitic disease, and toxic substances).

In the fifth section, "Victimization of Women," the incidence and dimensions of several kinds of sexual victimization are reported, including gender and sexual harassment in the workplace and academia, battering, and rape.

In the last section, "Achievement Motivation, Career Development, and Work," sociopsychological and structural factors affecting women's career choices and career pathways are addressed. Topics include trends in the extent of women's labor force participation, bias in career counseling and testing, mathematics as the critical filter for women, gender bias in education, and power issues in mentoring relationships for women.

The chapters in this handbook were guided by the following feminist frameworks:

- The psychology of women should treat women as the norm. A non-Euro-centric perspective on women should be presented.
- The psychology of women should identify the women of psychology; contributions by historical and contemporary women psychologists should be noted.

- The information in the psychology of women should encourage individuals to critically analyze all subareas in psychology for the portrayal of women. (adapted from Lord, 1982)

The psychology of women, as Walsh (1985) suggests, serves as a "catalyst for change," through its revealing serious deficiencies in psychological research and theories relevant to gender, cultural, and ethnic issues. Our goal is to have this handbook be a catalyst for change and to stimulate further research on the psychology of women. We hope this handbook continues to realize the goal first articulated by the Task Force Report on the Status of Women in Psychology in 1973: to expand knowledge about women.

REFERENCES

Lord, S. B. (1982). Research on teaching the psychology of women. *Psychology of Women Quarterly, 7,* 96–104.

Task force report on the status of women in psychology. (1973). *American Psychologist, 28,* 611–616.

Walsh, M. R. (1985). The psychology of women course: A continuing catalyst for change. *Teaching of Psychology, 12,* 198–203.

Part I
Foundations

1

Historical Development of the Psychology of Women

Florence L. Denmark and Linda C. Fernandez

Just as most disciplines have traditionally been male-dominated, so too has the discipline of psychology. Historically, women and psychology have been kept separate from one another. As O'Connell and Russo (1991) note, psychology's history has been a social construction by and for male psychologists. While women have made significant contributions to psychology, they largely remained invisible (Russo & Denmark, 1987; O'Connell & Russo, 1991). It has only been within the last few decades that psychology has begun to accept women as psychologists, as research participants, and as valued researchers.

When one examines the psychological research from Wundt's 1874 establishment of the domain of psychology up to recent times, psychology appeared to focus almost exclusively on the behavior of men or male animals. If females were included in the sample, neither sex nor gender differences were reported. In fact, most early research never investigated comparisons between women and men (Schwabacher, 1972). McKenna and Kessler (1976) reported that over 95% of all early research did not examine female-male comparisons. Prior to the 1970s almost all research on women had been relegated to the periphery of psychology rather than being integrated into its main body. Although the definition of psychology has undergone a metamorphosis over time, one fact remains increasingly clear—women and women's issues have not been adequately examined. The knowledge that theories derived from studies that included only male subjects are not based on representative samples and, therefore, not generalizable to the female 52% of the population called for the reevaluation of many topics, such as the concept of achievement and leadership styles.

As one of the authors of this paper noted (Denmark, 1977), during the 1970s an increase in the research on women reflected a rapidly growing interest in them, their psychology, and their issues. This occurred concurrently with the women's liberation movement. However, rather than a political movement, the psychology of women represents a legitimate area of scientific investigation that can be traced back to the early 1900s. Some male researchers studied sex differences and largely interpreted them to demonstrate female inferiority (Shields, 1975). In contrast, Hollingworth's work in the early 1900s revealed no evidence of female-male differences in variability.

While the psychology of women is an area of scientific investigation that can trace its roots back to early studies of so-called sex differences, the field encompasses much more than variation. Indeed, the emphasis on difference has an implicit assumption of a more global lack of similarity and erroneously implies a myriad of differences other than gender. While the psychology of gender comparisons is more apt a title, it still leaves out the many topics of investigation that encompass experiences unique to women, such as pregnancy, breast-feeding, and menstruation. The term *feminist psychology* seems to invoke too many connotations and has a varied meaning among different feminists. How, then, can we best define the psychology of women? Mednick (1976) defines the field as "the study of variations within a group and across time of the female experience." Henley (1974) favors "psychology and women" as a descriptive term. However, Mednick believes this is too broad.

We believe that Russo's (1975) definition of the psychology of women, as the study of behavior (not excluding male gender-role behavior) mediated by the variable of female sex, is one of the most useful. In the past, psychology studied behavior, but it was not mediated by the variable of female sex. Thus, the psychology of women is also defined as that which includes all psychological issues pertaining to women and their experiences (Denmark, 1977).

Prior to the early 1970s, any mention of the psychology of women was usually a reference to the title of Deutsch's 1946 book and did not refer to a separate area of scientific investigation. In short, the psychology of women did not yet exist as a field. Words such as *sexism* or *feminisim* could be found in Merriam Webster's 1969 dictionary but were not widely used and were not a part of people's vernacular. Gender was primarily a grammatical term.

Psychology was often defined as the science of behavior. Yet it was a common practice of researchers to include only white male humans or male animals in their sample. It is especially ironic because even then every undergraduate statistics book stressed the basic premise that for any study to be generalizable, it had to have a representative, not a skewed, sample. Nevertheless, the idea of "male as representative of the norm" was so strong that even well-trained psychologists did not realize that they were excluding at least 50% of the population. What they fostered was not psychology, the science of behavior, but psychology, the science of white male behavior.

Although no such separate field as the psychology of women existed prior to the 1970s, there were early scientists whose research impacted on the field. Leta

Hollingworth was a leading harbinger of the psychology of women; she was adamant that psychology apply vigorous scientific stringency to research on women. She was one of many early scholars, along with Helen Thompson, Mary Calkins, and Mary Putnam Jacobi, who responded to the trends of social Darwinism of her time with myth-refuting, solid empirical evidence.

MYTHS OF SOCIAL DARWINISM

Social Darwinism was based on the social theories that arose as a result of the publication of Darwin's *On the Origin of the Species* in 1859. In an attempt to explain individual variability and variability among different species, Darwin posited theories of natural and sexual selection. Darwin noted that while all members of a species had the possibility of producing many progeny, the population of any species remained fairly constant over time. Thus, he concluded that individuals within a species compete with each other in their "struggle for existence." In addition, he also observed that all organisms vary. Combining these thoughts, he posited the theory of natural selection, popularly known as "the survival of the fittest." Individuals who had favorable variations survived and reproduced, thus transmitting the favorable traits to their offspring. In this manner, "genetic housecleaning" was performed in that natural selection eliminated unfavorable traits, since those who had them did not survive long enough to reproduce and pass the unfavorable traits to their offspring.

Darwin also observed that not all variability seemed essential to individual survival. He attempted to account for this nonessential individual variability with his theory of sexual selection. Briefly, sexual selection was similar to natural selection in that it depended on a struggle, this one "not a struggle for existence but on a struggle between males for possession of the females" (Darwin, 1871, p. 575). Unsuccessful traits resulted not in "death to the unsuccessful competitor, but in few or no offspring" (Darwin, 1859, p. 100).

Darwin also believed that most traits were inherited, but he did differentiate between "transmission of character" and the "development of character." This differentiation was important in the development of sexual differences. Sexual selection theory encompassed an associated law of partial inheritance, which stated that the law of equal transmission (that is, the transmission of certain characteristics to both sexes) was not always equal; sometimes transmission was only to the same-sex offspring. Darwin stated that he was unsure as to why the inheritability of some traits seemed to be governed by the law of equal transmission, while other traits' inheritability seemed to be governed by the law of partial inheritance. Darwin's further observations led him to believe that physical traits such as size were inherited via natural selection and equally transmitted to both sexes, but not always developed in both sexes. Other traits, such as intelligence and reason, he believed, were acquired through sexual selection and seemed to be governed by the law of partial inheritance and same-sex transmission. Now, here's the rub. It appeared to Darwin that since females did not compete for males, they did not have the same evolutionary opportunity to develop the same intelligence, perseverance, and courage as males. Thus for Darwin, the result of natural and sexual selection was that men were "superior" to women. This is the central myth of social Darwinism.

Spencer based his theories on Darwin's views and expanded them to include the interaction effects of function on biological modification. According to Spencer, since women were the primary childrearers in society, such traits as maternal instinct and nurturing ability would have been acquired as a result of their function, that is, daily care of children. Over time, according to Spencer, these traits became fixed in biological structures, that is, there would be a "constitutional modification produced by excess of function" (Spencer, 1864, p. 252). In addition, in his book, *The Principles of Biology*, Spencer also applied Hermann Helmholtz's conservation of energy theory to human growth. Spencer believed that human beings had a finite fund of energy ("vital force") that could be applied to one's individual growth or to reproduction. He also believed that the female reproductive system obviously required more "vital force" than the male's reproductive system. So, simply put, women had less available "vital force" or energy for their individual mental and physical growth than men. Thus, women's reproductive systems demanded a great supply of energy, and any requirement of energy demand for mental activity or "brain-work," particularly during adolescence, was thought by Spencer to lead to reproductive disorders, inability to breast-feed, or even infertility.

REFUTATION OF THE MYTH

Mary Putnam Jacobi and Mary Bissell

Mary Putnam Jacobi (1877) in her book, *The Question of Rest for Women During Menstruation*, argued against the widespread belief of her time that menstruation was so debilitating that women should refrain from physical activity. In addition, mental activity did not lead to a greater incidence or probability of pain or infertility. Jacobi's research found that exercise and higher level of education correlated with less discomfort during menstruation.

Another early researcher was Mary Bissell, who argued against the popular notion that in females, emotional fragility was the norm and therefore part of femininity. She was one of the early researchers who also pointed out the social factors that accounted for some of the emotional "fragility" of women. She recommended young women be allowed to develop their physical, as well as their intellectual, potential strength by outdoor play and the pursuit of mentally stimulating activities to eliminate boredom.

Leta Hollingworth

Leta Stetter Hollingworth was one of the early researchers who concentrated on research issues that would later become relevant to the psychology of women.

She investigated areas of well-established bias in psychology, such as women's social role, the mental and physical performance during the menstrual cycle, and the variability hypothesis. While a graduate student at Columbia Teachers College, she was under the tutelage of Edward Thorndike, who was himself a strong supporter of the variability hypothesis.

One of Hollingworth's contributions was her research on physical and mental performance during the menstrual cycle, research that demonstrated that changes in performance were unrelated to cyclical phases. Her doctoral dissertation was titled "Functional Periodicity: An Experimental Study of the Mental and Motor Abilities of Women During Menstruation" (Hollingworth, 1914). Through her research she found no evidence to support the variability hypothesis, which mistakenly concluded that the higher status of males was based upon their greater variability. In 1914, with Helen Montague, Hollingworth examined the birth records of 1,000 male and 1,000 female neonates. When birth weight and length were noted, the researchers found that if variability "favored" any sex, it was the female sex (Montague & Hollingworth, 1914).

Also in 1914, Hollingworth responded to social Darwinist myths by critiquing the incorrect assumptions on which they were based. For example, greater (male, of course) variability was considered to suggest greater range also. This inference is appropriate only if the distribution is Gaussian, which had not been proven. In short, Darwin may have had some romantic notion of greater male variability due to the "noble and intellectually enriching" male competition for females. However, in reality, no greater male variability had been demonstrated. Further, even if there had been greater physical male variability, it would indicate nothing about greater male intellectual variability. Greater male intellectual variability had also not been proven, and, even if it had been, it would not mean an innately greater intellectual variability among males. Rather, Hollingworth suggested that in order for the social sciences to examine adequately the cause of seemingly lesser female achievement, social scientists also needed to examine the interaction of social constraints and cultural barriers to female achievement.

To Hollingworth and to many later feminists, the essence of the problem was that throughout history, women bore children and were their caretakers. She stated that she did not intend this issue to be interpreted as an attack on motherhood, but rather a more plausible explanation than lack of "vital force" or "lack of variability." Hollingworth fostered the examination of social and cultural factors that mediate female achievement.

It is important to note that Hollingworth refuted myth with research. In 1916, she and an eminent anthropologist, Robert Lowie, reviewed the scientific literature of their day. They found when cross-cultural, biological, and psychological studies were examined, the objective evidence did not support the notion of innate female inferiority (Lowie & Hollingworth, 1916). Lowie and Hollingworth were quick to note that "every sex difference that has been discovered or alleged has been interpreted to show the superiority of males" (p. 284). For example, the higher number of males who were institutionalized was often interpreted as proof of greater male variability. If there had been a greater number of females in prisons and asylums, they wondered, would not that fact have been interpreted as evidence of general female inferiority? In summary, Hollingworth was one of the most prolific early feminist researchers whose myth-refuting empirical evidence and logical mind did much to pave the way for what was later to become the psychology of women.

Helen Thompson and Mary Calkins

Other early researchers who responded to social Darwinism were Helen Thompson and Mary Calkins. Helen Thompson's psychological research challenged the social mores and cultural assumptions of her time. For her doctoral thesis, H. Thompson (1903) studied sex differences in mental ability. Often she found similarities rather than differences between male and female subjects. When differences did occur, she also was able to show how experience and environment, rather than biology alone, would account for them. Like Hollingworth, Mary Calkins also disputed the popular social Darwinist myth that women's mental capabilities were less varied than men's (1896).

FREUD AND OTHER PSYCHOANALYTIC INFLUENCES ON THE PSYCHOLOGY OF WOMEN

In addition to the reaction to social Darwinism, another thread in the development of the psychology of women was based on reaction to Sigmund Freud. Freud, a 19th-century Viennese medical doctor who practiced neurology, founded the psychoanalytic school of psychology. Freud constructed his personality theory based on his own self-analysis and his analysis of individual case studies. When evaluating the validity and generalizability of Freudian results, one must take into account the limitations of his methodology.

Freud believed sexual drives were very important in the personality growth of both men and women. Successful satisfaction of sexual drives resulted in healthy development, whereas failure to obtain drive satisfaction would result in neurosis. Thus, a healthy individual is one who manages to obtain gratification of drives while remaining within societal norms and physiological capability. The disturbed individual would be someone who is unable to obtain gratification within the bounds of social and biological reality.

According to Freud's theory of psychosexual development, at birth there is little psychological difference between the male and female, with infants of both sexes viewing the mother as their primary love object. (In 19th-century Vienna, the mother was the expected caretaker. So in fairness to Freud, we must take into account limitations of 19th-century Viennese cultural norms.) Psychosexual development is similar for boys and girls in the "oral" and "anal" stages up until the "phallic" stage. At approximately three years of age, the boy's sexual impulses are centered around the penis and the girl's sexual impulses are centered around the clitoris. Both boys and girls are said to have "active" or "masculine" sexual aims. By labeling these sexual aims, which occur in both sexes, as "masculine," rather than bisexual, Freud implies such active sexual aims are somehow not appropriate for females and begins to focus on males. Just as early experimental psychology had used mostly male subjects and had focused on male behavior, the earliest psychoanalytic writings focused on male psychic development. Very briefly, one cornerstone of Freudian theory is that of the Oedipus complex, in which the boy feels rivalry and hostility toward the father and desires his mother for himself. He fears his father's retaliation and thus fears castration by the father. His fears of castration are made worse when, according to Freudian theory, he observes females and concludes that they have been castrated and the same thing could happen to him. This complex is resolved by identifying with the father (identification with the aggressor). By identifying with the aggressor (the father), the boy gives up his mother as his love object with the expectation that he will later find a substitute who will not arouse the wrath of his father. At this time, the boy identifies with the father and incorporates his moral values and also those of society for which the male moral value is seen as representative. This internalization of paternal/societal male moral standards results in the formation of a superego, or what is often called the conscience. Male psychosexual development contains both conflict and compromise. However, in males, the conflict resolution manages to preserve the "active" sexual aims present during the phallic period, thus leaving the males active in attaining their satisfaction.

Females, according to Freud, do not have the same constellation, because when they discover they do not have a penis, they envy little boys and blame their mothers for what they are lacking (a penis). Little girls switch their affectional cathexis from the mother to the father, hoping to obtain a penis, but there is no identification with the aggressor and thus no internalization of that parent's moral code. Thus, in females, according to Freud, superego development is stunted. The girl perceives her anatomical inferiority and blames her mother but does not identify with her "fellow castrati." Curiously, she does not identify with her father either. According to Freudian theory, in time the "normal" female realizes that she cannot have a penis, so she wishes instead for a baby. Her sexual aims, which were "active, masculine" aims during the phallic stage, are now transformed. Freudian theory posits that in "normal" development, the girl accepts the lack of a penis and also renounces the clitoris as the seat of sexual satisfaction. She transforms her active masculine sexuality into passive feminine receptivity.

For Freud a "masculine" woman has not adjusted to her anatomy. Then a tripartite bridge is formed in Freudian theory among anatomy, active versus passive sexuality, and feminine personality. The anatomical differences are perceived as causal factors in psychological and social differences. Thus, for Freud, the healthy woman renounces the active sexual satisfaction of the clitoris, has passive sexual aims, with her primary motivation being her wish for a baby, and does not socially engage in aggressive or achievement-oriented behaviors. Narcissism and vanity are essentially the "feminine" compensatory consequences of castration. In addition, jealousy, feelings of inferiority, and shame are more direct expressions of female genital dissatisfaction, since the female is less motivated to identify with the same-sexed parent during the Oedipal conflict. The boy is motivated because he still has a penis and fears castration; the girl feels that she is already castrated and is not motivated. Therefore, women are less likely to internalize the moral codes and cultural ideals than men.

The social and political implications of Freudian theory are vast. Quite simply, by virtue of their anatomy, women are destined to be less morally mature and less acculturated than men. They are also destined to exhibit more unsatisfactory personality characteristics.

According to Freudian theory, anatomical differences and the resulting differences in sexual functions are viewed as being the causal factors in the development of psychological differences. Here, body creates psyche, and the phrase "biology is destiny" is formed. The biologically "healthy" woman has passive sexual aims, is motivated by motherhood, and spurns achievement-related behaviors. Thus, biological differences are instrumental in the creation of psychological differences, which, in turn, explain social behavior and serve to maintain the status quo.

Helene Deutsch

Helene Deutsch, a psychoanalyst who was trained by Freud, extended Freudian theory in her 1946 book, ironically titled *The Psychology of Women*. In her book, Deutsch posited that personality traits such as narcissism, passivity, and masochism are the result of "feminine" biology. In response to Freudian theory, Deutsch views women as being masochistic since they are biologically bound to childbirth and menstruation, which contain both pleasure and pain. The fact that all living organisms (including men) experience both pleasure and pain is overlooked by Deutsch, who goes on to posit that masochism is therefore an adaptive formation for females. The "healthy" female is not masochistic to the point of total self-annihilation, but she does renounce her "self" in that she denies her own needs in order to obtain "love," that is, by becoming a wife and mother. Both clitoral sexuality and active vaginal pleasure are viewed by Deutsch as deviating from "normal" femininity. "Normal" female sexuality is operationally defined as female passivity, which Deutsch refers to as "receptive readiness." In addition, she also posits the circular logic that women possess a predisposition for compensatory narcissism that attempts to make up for their lack of a penis and to balance out their masochism, which is also the result of not having a penis.

Pleasure and pain, childbirth, and menstruation are facts of life. At the present time, a biological fact is that women have greater life expectancy than men, and behaviorally men tend to exhibit greater alcohol and narcotic abuse than do women. However, present-day Freudians would not conclude that man's lack of a vagina leads to greater self-destructive tendencies and earlier death. It is interesting to note that when this "biology is destiny" thinking is applied to men, the leaps in logic are glaring, yet the same leaps have long gone unnoticed as they apply to women.

Alfred Adler and Carl Jung

Two of the early defectors from Freud's inner circle who served to broaden the base of the biologically centered psychoanalytic theory were Alfred Adler and Carl Jung. Adler recognized sociocultural factors in psychic development and noted the constraining contradictions of a culture that simultaneously encouraged women to adopt "feminine" characteristics while admiring and placing a higher value (economic and social) on actions and attributes characterized as "masculine." Thus, Adler was a harbinger of social psychological theories that emphasize the social context as an underlying determinant of behavior.

Rather than Freud's emphasis upon sexual motivations, Carl Jung stressed the individual's struggle to achieve psychic harmony via the reconciliation of what is masculine and feminine in each individual. Jung believed that the experience of each individual was influenced by the experience of all of humanity, which is transmitted to each successive generation and constitutes what he termed the "collective unconscious." These memories of all of human experience, so-called racial memories, take the form of "archetypes" that unconsciously influence each individual. Two archetypes that Jung used to explain masculinity and femininity are the animus and anima. The animus is the masculine archetype, which Jung believed was present in the female's unconscious, and the anima is the feminine archetype in the male's unconscious. While the Jungian ideal of psychic harmony would encompass the integration of one's masculine and feminine traits (which is consistent with some modern feminist thinking), he still believed that personality was formed not only from one's individual socialization experience, which is subject to change, but also by a collective historical experience, which cannot be changed. Thus for Jung, gender-role differentiation is the inevitable result of sex-linked masculine and feminine polarities. Females were seen only from a male point of view.

Karen Horney

Karen Horney (1926) in her book *Flight from Womanhood* was the first to question this bias in the psychoanalytic literature:

Until quite recently the minds of boys and men only were taken as the objects of investigation. The reason for this is obvious. Psychoanalysis was the creation of a male genius, and almost all of those who have developed his ideas have been men. It is only right and reasonable that they should evolve more easily a masculine psychology and understand more of the development of men than of women. (p. 59)

After years of analyzing male and female patients, Horney was struck by strong male "envy of pregnancy, childbirth and motherhood, as well as breasts and the act of sucking" (p. 60). Horney believes that little boys encounter "womb envy" and states that there is an unconscious male desire to deprecate women and their ability to give birth. Penis envy is a way to shift the focus away from women's childbearing ability and focus instead on male anatomy. According to Horney, "this (male) depreciation would run as follows: In reality woman do simply desire the penis, when all is said and done motherhood is only a burden that makes the struggle for existence harder, and men may be glad that they have not to bear it" (p. 61). In a paper titled "Inhibited Femininity," Horney (1926, 1967) regarded "frigidity as an illness" and not "the normal sexual attitude of civilized woman." She was also first to point out the social and cultural factors that impact on psychic development.

Horney was the first of Freud's students to break from him on the issue of preoedipal injury resulting in neurosis. Horney believed in the possibility of preoedipal injury and was also the first psychoanalyst to speak about the "real self." Preoedipal injury, according to Horney, results when a child perceives himself or herself as helpless in a hostile environment; "instead of developing a basic confidence in self and others the child develops basic anxiety" (Horney, 1950, p. 366). The child puts a check on spontaneous feelings because of a need to relieve basic anxiety. Above all, there exists a need to feel safe. This is the beginning of what Horney calls the alienation from self. "Not only is his *real self* prevented from a straight growth, but in addition his need to evolve artificial strategic ways to cope with others has forced him to override his genuine feelings. . . . It does not matter what he feels if only he feels safe" (Horney, 1950, p. 21).

The child seeks to feel safe in a hostile environment. Solutions may be based on the appeal of love (moving toward), the appeal of mastery (moving against), or the appeal of freedom (moving away). In short, the child will attempt to change the environment by loving it, by fighting it, or by leaving it (Horney, 1950).

Healthy people love, fight, and leave at appropriate times. Since the neurotic puts a check on spontaneous feelings, he or she does not know which solution is appropriate at different times. "The three moves toward, against, and away from others therefore constitute a conflict, his *basic conflict*. In time, he tries to solve it by making one of these moves consistently predominant—(he) tries to make his prevailing attitude one of compliance, or aggressiveness, or aloofness" (Horney, 1950, p. 19).

Horney's reaction to Freud influenced others and is part of one of the threads to what would later become the psychology of women. As Hollingworth and others were able to do in the area of experimental psychology, Horney was able to apply strict scrutiny to psychoanalytic theory and to refute androcentrism and sexist bias. By taking the focus of psychoanalysis away from the androcentric Oedipus complex, she was able to pave the way for the "psychology of the self," so crucial to our present understanding of borderline and narcissistic personality disorders.

Horney suggests that Freud's observation of the female's wish for a penis may be no more important than the young male's frequently observed wish for breasts. Attributes with which Freud composed the constellation of the "masculinity complex," that is, desire for power, envy, and egocentric ambition and which he ascribed to penis envy were noted by Horney as characteristics exhibited by neurotic men as well as neurotic women. Horney posits that the characteristics of the "masculinity complex" are the result of feelings of inferiority that are present in both neurotic men and neurotic women and are multiply determined. She also looks at the social and cultural factors involved in the development of feelings of inferiority, such as the cultural restrictions of women's potential.

Horney (1939) differs from Deutsch in her interpretation of masochism in that she views masochism as an empowering device used to promote well-being in life through influencing others by emphasizing one's frailty and pain. Masochism is not viewed by Horney as a biologically based adaptive behavior incorporating pleasure and pain as bound to feminine physiology, but rather, as a social, often economically based attitude. Our society tends to idealize the maternal woman who puts the needs of others before her own, and it tends to pay women less than men. Horney posits that these factors better account for masochistic tendencies in women than do physiological differences. Horney believes that rather than being fueled by a symbolic desire to possess a penis, both normal and neurotic women tend to "overvalue love" as the result of their economic and social dependence on men due to cultural constraints on women's direct access to security, prestige, and power. By stressing the social and cultural factors as determinants of "feminine" psychology, Horney leaves room for the possibility of remediation of undesirable personality traits via the process of social change. Changes in economic opportunity as well as changes in socialization of women are presumed to impact on the female personality constellation. Conversely, when "feminine" psychology is attributed to penis envy and pain inherent in childbirth, societal changes are presumed to be psychologically inconsequential and psychological changes in personality are deemed to be impossible.

Clara Thompson

Another psychologist who responded to Freudian orthodoxy by walking out of the New York Psychoanalytic Institute with Horney was Clara Thompson. Both Horney and Thompson stressed the importance of experience, environment, and social influences that impact on personality development. Like Horney, Thompson responded to androcentric Freudian psychosexual etiology of female personality development (1941, 1942, 1943, 1964a, 1964b). Her alternative theory also stresses the impact of social and cultural factors on personality development. Thompson posits that the discovery of the vagina, rather than the penis, in and of itself need not necessarily represent psychic trauma for a female. However, it can be traumatic if the presence of a vagina, rather than a penis, is associated with lower status (both social and economic) within the family constellation. Our historical obsession with primogenesis, a system that confers the highest status on the eldest male, serves to reinforce the association of "feminine" with lower status. As children reach the "phallic" stage of development (at approximately three to five years of age), both sexes struggle for autonomy and seek independence from their primary caretaker. If one assumes the primary caretaker is the mother, Thompson posits that the mother often will respond differently to her son's and daughter's attempts at autonomy, with female children being given less overt encouragement to express independence and instead given more rewards for remaining within the confines of the home. Often with the onset of puberty, previously tolerated tomboyish activities are not accepted in the adolescent girl. She is pressured by society to become "attractive" and rewarded with marriage and motherhood. Rather than the renunciation of active aims for passivity, Thompson views behavioral changes in teenage girls and differences in sexual experimentation as the result of multiple societal pressures. Thompson views female psychology as an attempt to adjust to the existing social realities; she finds women who choose to find pleasure in a life of self-sacrifice not so much seeking pain (masochistic), but rather seeking a positive adaptation to a limiting status quo.

Freudian theory also viewed women as morally inferior to men, since they did not benefit from the internalization of a superego as a result of the resolution of the Oedipus complex via identification with the aggressor and since they did not have a penis and were "already castrated." Freud also observed that many women simply mimic the views of their male companions. Thompson posits that if this view is true, it is a function of females' lower status rather than female failure to develop a conscience. People who are in a lowered status situation, one in which they are dependent upon, and subject to, the moods and authority of a more powerful other, do "try harder" to get along with the more powerful other even to the extent of entertaining the same opinions. Social psychological research on the behavior of blacks and whites, that is, "integration" behavior (Jones, 1964), provides empirical support for Thompson's position in that the higher the status of an individual, the more successful such an individual would be in influencing others and the less vulnerable to being influenced by a lower-status individual. Social psychological data indicate that gender differences in interactional behavior follow status differences; males are more successful than females in their influence on others and less apt to change their positions than females. Within gender, status differences simply cannot be attributed to penis envy, castration anxiety, or the failure to identify with the aggressor and internalize a superego. The real differences between men's and women's power and status appear to be a more parsimonious explanation of the behavioral differences that Freud observed.

The work of Horney and Thompson has had somewhat limited impact on psychoanalytic theory, and, ironically, until recently, Deutsch's book *The Psychology of Women* was viewed as the classic psychoanalytic view of female personality development. However, the development of the psychology of women brought other work into the forefront. Horney and Thompson have now been recognized for their contributions.

THE 1950s AND THE 1960s

Questions regarding inherited versus environmentally induced behaviors as the causal factors of gender differences began to be raised. Ethical considerations conflict with, and ultimately override, the spirit of strict scientific stringency in that we can never conduct the ultimate experiment, that is, take a group of different-sex twins and place them in different environments. Another methodological problem arises because no environment impacts on organisms of different sexes in the same way.

After responding to Darwin and to Freud, the development of the psychology of women proceeded to examine the nature-nurture controversy as it applied to gender differences. Prior to the development of the psychology of women and of psychology overall, Judeo-Christian tradition designated quite rigid gender-role specific behaviors. Both Darwinian and Freudian theories aligned with the Judeo-Christian tradition and served the evolution of clear-cut gender stereotypes.

Viola Klein

Viola Klein (1950) contributed to the field's growth with her description of the female stereotype. In short, she pointed out our cultural tendency to note a wide variety of differences in male ability, character, and disposition while trying to summarize women as a homogeneous psychological type. Overall, a stereotype is a false, quick-fix oversimplification of a complex social reality that tends to evoke a strong, negative emotional response. Since they typically embody a negative emotional response, it is indicative of stereotypes that they be projected outward, that is, applied not to "us" but to "them." Klein finds it no surprise that within a largely man-made system, male researchers tend to note the individual differences of men ("us") but tend to view women as a distinct psychological type ("them"). Thus, stereotypes function to provide a quick explanation of a potpourri of individual woman's behavior: "Whether she is strong-willed or meek, single-minded or hesitant, gentle or quarrelsome—she is supposed to possess a particular version of whatever trait she manifests and her stubbornness or submissiveness, her capriciousness or lack of humor will be found 'typically feminine' " (Klein, 1950, p. 4).

In addition, stereotypes serve to reflect back to oneself a view of how "one is seen by others,'' thus contributing to an internalization of societal values. Traditionally, women were viewed as either of two feminine types, that is, ''good women'' or ''bad women,'' ''madonnas'' or ''courtesans.'' Both types were viewed solely in terms of their sexual relations with men. For the ''madonna,'' sex is primarily a means of reproduction; the ''courtesan'' engages in sex primarily for her own pleasure. However, both types revolve around men.

Helen Hacker

Helen Hacker (1951) was one of the first feminist researchers to point out the status of women as a minority group. Ironically, women are a majority (52%) of the population but have been the recipients of unequal treatment and societal discrimination. Hacker helped to advance what would later become the psychology of women, since in the early part of the 1950s, the implications of the female stereotype were largely unnoticed. The comic genius of Lucille Ball and Gracie Allen rose above the media's stereotype of women of their day, but they were the exceptions in the days of traditional TV shows such as ''Father Knows Best,'' ''Leave It to Beaver,'' and ''Ozzie and Harriet.'' On other shows, the Andersons', the Cleavers', and the Nelsons' households all depicted the 1950s ''shirtwaist and pearls,'' ''yes, dear'' stereotypical housewife. Hacker was ahead of her time in pointing out that females were not only being stereotyped but reduced to minority group status as well. In her 1951 paper, Hacker discussed the similarities in the status of women and blacks. Psychologically, women often exhibit similar traits ascribed to other minority groups. For example, Hacker described the ''marginal woman,'' who is deeply conflicted as to whether or not to maintain or to change her traditional role. Women are also like minority group members in that they often exhibit self-deprecation, feelings of inferiority, and being out of the cultural mainstream. In a paper written 20 years later, Hacker cited evidence that the similarities in status between blacks and women still existed and called for the emotional reeducation of men and women to expand the traditional status quo (1975). During the 1960s many traditions were reexamined, and the status quo has never been quite the same.

Although some articles in the 1950s appeared relevant to the psychology of women, they were few and far between. During the 1960s one of the authors of this chapter continued a study on women and leadership that she began while an undergraduate and later completed and published (Denmark & Diggory, 1966). This study found that women were less authoritarian than male leaders but that women followers did not conform more than their male counterparts to their leaders' viewpoints. During the mid-1960s these findings were unexpected and contrary to the predicted outcome.

Also, in 1966 and 1967, Florence Denmark and Marcia Guttentag examined the effect of college attendance on mature women by measuring changes in their self-concept and their evaluation of the student role. Denmark and Guttentag found that college attendance resulted in a decrease in the perception of the ideal self along with a decrease in the discrepancy between present self and ideal self. A possible explanation offered was that perhaps the rigors of college work served to reduce dissonance by releasing the student from the need to strive for unrealistically lofty aims and permitting the student to be more accepting of her present self. These results contrasted with the warning of G. Stanley Hall, the founder of the American Psychological Association, in the early 1900s, of the dangers to females if they became too educated.

Although Hacker, Klein, Denmark, Diggory, and Guttentag did contribute research during the 1950s and 1960s that would be relevant to the psychology of women, it was not until the late 1960s that the women's liberation movement brought its issues to the forefront of psychology. College campuses witnessed the presence of feminists who worked to give rise to women's centers and women studies programs and courses in the psychology of women.

INDICATORS OF THE GROWTH AND IMPACT OF THE PSYCHOLOGY OF WOMEN

The increasing interest in the psychology of women beginning during the late 1960s and continuing to the present time can be shown by many indicators of growth, such as papers presented at regional meetings, dissertation topics, journal articles, and books published.

Papers

The 1969 program of the American Psychological Association (APA) listed one symposium that specifically pertained to women. The total portion of the 1969 program that dealt with women amounted to 7 papers, 4 participants, and 2 discussants. To measure our growth, contrast this with the 1991 convention, in which Division 35 sponsored 42 papers and poster sessions, 27 symposia, 5 invited addresses, 4 roundtable sessions, 2 workshops, and 5 conversation hours and cosponsored nearly 200 other activities.

Books

By the 1970s the psychology of women finally emerged as a field of psychology. Bardwick (1970) published the first book titled *The Psychology of Women*, soon followed by Sherman's (1971) in-depth analysis, *On the Psychology of Women*, and Baer and Sherif's (1974) *A Topical Bibliography on the Psychology of Women*. In 1975 Unger and Denmark edited the first issue-oriented reader in the field, containing original as well as reprinted articles. Also, in 1975, Mednick and Weissman noted the growth of the psychology of women by reviewing pertinent topics in the *Annual Review of Psychology*. In 1976, a volume of reprinted articles that was totally focused on women appeared (Denmark). In 1978 Sherman and Denmark coedited a book based on a 1975 conference, "New Directions in Research," the first research conference on the psychology of women.

Journals

The appearance of several new journals, such as *Sex Roles* and *Signs* in 1975 and *The Psychology of Women Quarterly* in 1976, indicated further growth of the field. These journals continue to flourish. Overall, the percentage of articles related to the psychology of women in APA journals has increased significantly and continues to grow.

Dissertations

There has been a great increase in the number of dissertations in the field. In the July 1970 *Dissertation Abstracts International* there were only 11 dissertations that even contained the word *woman* or *women* in the title. By 1990 the total number of citations that included these key words had grown to many hundreds. In spite of the crudeness of this indicator, the rise in the number of dissertations with topics relevant to the psychology of women is still another sign of growth of the field.

Division 35

Official indication of the acceptance of the psychology of women as a legitimate field of study within psychology came in 1973, when the Division of the Psychology of Women was established as Division 35 of the American Psychological Association.

The origins of Division 35 can be traced back to the 1969 APA convention, at which members of the Association for Women in Psychology (AWP) overtly attacked the discriminatory hiring practices of APA's own employment center. At that time women, but not men, were routinely asked their marital status, spousal employment status, and their intention to have children. AWP members protested these unfair procedures, and the APA Council of Representatives responded in 1970 by creating an active task force to study the status of women in psychology. The goal of the task force was "furthering the major purpose of APA, to advance psychology as a science and as a means of promoting human welfare—by making recommendations to insure that women be accepted as fully enfranchised members of the profession" (Task Force Report, 1973). The task force examined the status of female faculty and students in graduate psychology departments and gave recommendations to APA. In particular, the task force had concerns about graduate curricula: "Colleges and universities should offer general education courses and programs that inquire into the psychology of women, and an opportunity for in-depth study at both undergraduate and graduate levels of the psychology of women" (Task Force Report, 1973). The task force realized that knowledge of women needed to be expanded and that the generalizability of much research was questionable, since women were not included in the sample. Many people believed that a new division within APA would better meet the needs of women in psychology. The APA Council of Representatives responded by approving the Division 35 petition, signed by 800 members who indicated interest in joining the new division in September 1973. The purpose of Division 35 was "to promote the research and study of women . . . to encourage the integration of this information about women with the current psychological knowledge and beliefs in order to apply the gained knowledge to the society and its institutions" (Article 1.2, Division 35 Bylaws). Mednick (1978) reports that in a 1973 APA *Monitor* article she was quoted as saying, "The new division would not be a political organization." Rather than being a political organization, Mednick stressed the division's role of expanding knowledge about women. One of the ways in which knowledge about women has been expanded is through Division 35's journal, *The Psychology of Women Quarterly*.

By 1977, Division 35 had grown to be one of the larger APA divisions, with close to 1,500 members and affiliates. By 1992 Division 35 had 2,526 members, with 96.5% of the members being women. Division 35 membership is diverse, with members in every other division of APA. Most of its members have doctorates in counseling, clinical, developmental, and social psychology.

As one of the 47 divisions of APA, Division 35 has representation on the Council of Representatives, which is the decision-making body of APA. Since Division 35 was formed, three of its fellows have served as president of the APA: Florence L. Denmark in 1980, Janet T. Spence in 1984, and Bonnie R. Strickland in 1987. George Albee, another Division 35 fellow, was APA president in 1970. The psychology of women therefore has a recognized voice in the formal and informal decision making of APA.

The impact of the growth of the psychology of women is evidenced in the United States and internationally as well. In 1975, the APA task force provided *Guidelines for the Non-sexist Use of Language*, and in 1977 the APA, in the third edition of the *Publication Manual*, set guidelines to avoid sexist language specific to journal articles. In 1988 the APA Council of Representatives unanimously endorsed *Guidelines for Avoiding Sexism in Psychological Research* (Denmark, Russo, Frieze, & Sechzer, 1988). APA's nonsexist guidelines have opened the way for nonsexist guidelines in other countries as well as the preparation of nonracist, nonageist, and nonheterosexist guidelines.

As Division 35 grew, it functioned to provide a forum for the development of an in-depth focus on understanding both the psychological and the social realities of women. The Committee on Black Women's Concerns was formed in 1977 as part of the division. This group became a section of the division in 1984. Committees on Hispanic women and Asian American women were also established by Division 35. Thus the growth of the psychology of women has fostered growth in the areas of minority concerns.

Growth is also evident internationally. Courses in the psychology of women are taught in many countries, including Israel, Ireland, the Netherlands, and Argentina as well as the United States.

Overall, the psychology of women impacts on all of psychology by highlighting the former methodological biases and by reexamining issues with representative samples to yield generalizable data. The psychology of women should be integrated into general psychology as well as specific content areas such as abnormal, developmental, and social psychology courses (Denmark & Fernandez, 1984). In addition, the psychology of women should continue to examine issues unique to women, such as menstruation, pregnancy, and breast-feeding.

The psychology of women or gender has also blossomed into an interdisciplinary field—women's studies. The cross-fertilization of women's studies and psychology has resulted in an increased awareness of class and racial issues, as well as gender issues. Paludi (1987) noted that our model of female development has grown from that of white, middle-class women to encompassing women of color. The psychology of women continues to give rise to feminist pedagogy that fosters the development of feminist identity, shared leadership during the learning process, and integration of emotional and factual learning, resulting in greater overall congruence and enhanced self-esteem. Thus, feminist pedagogy based on the psychology of women will make an invaluable contribution to the teaching of any subject.

REFERENCES

American Psychological Association. (1983). Guidelines for nonsexist language in APA journals. In *Publication Manual of the American Psychological Association* (3rd ed.) (pp. 45-49). Washington, D.C.: American Psychological Association.

Baer, H., & Sherif, C. (1974). A topical bibliography (selectively annotated) on the psychology of women. *Catalogue of Selected Documents in Psychology, 4,* 42.

Bardwick, J. (1970). *The psychology of women: A study of bio-cultural conflicts.* New York: Harper & Row.

Bissell, M. T. (1985). Emotions versus health in women. In L. M. Newman (Ed.), *Men's ideas/women's realities* (pp. 48–53). Elmsford, NY: Pergamon Press. (Original work published in 1888.)

Calkins, M. W. (1896). Community of ideas of men and women. *Psychological Review, 3,* 426–430.

Darwin, C. (1859). *On the origin of the species by means of natural selection.* London: John Murray.

Darwin, C. (1871). *Descent of man.* London: John Murray.

Denmark, F. L. (Ed.). (1976). *Women: Volume I.* New York: Psychological Dimensions.

Denmark, F. L. (1977). The psychology of women: An overview of an emerging field. *Personality and Social Psychology Bulletin, 3,* 356–367.

Denmark, F. L., & Diggory, J. (1966). Sex differences in attitudes toward leaders' display of authoritarian behavior. *Psychological Reports, 18,* 863–872.

Denmark, F. L., & Fernandez, L. (1984). Integrating information about the psychology of women into social psychology. In F. L. Denmark (Ed.), *Social/ecological psychology and the psychology of women* (pp. 355–368). Proceedings of the 23rd International Congress of Psychology. North Holland: Elsevier Science.

Denmark, F. L., & Guttentag, M. (1966). The effect of college attendance on mature women: Changes in self-concept and evaluation of student role. *Journal of Social Psychology, 69,* 155–158.

Denmark, F. L., & Guttentag, M. (1967). Dissonance in the self and educational concepts of college and non-college oriented women. *Journal of Counseling Psychology, 14,* 113–115.

Denmark, F. L., Russo, N., Frieze, I., & Sechzer, J. A. (1988). Guidelines for avoiding sexism in psychological research. *American Psychologist, 43* (7), 582–585.

Deutsch, H. (1946). *The psychology of women.* New York: Grune & Stratton.

Hacker, H. M. (1951). Women as a minority group. *Social Forces, 30,* 60–69.

Hacker, H. M. (1975). Women as a minority group: Some twenty years later. In R. K. Unger & F. L. Denmark (Eds.), *Woman: Dependent or independent variable?* (pp. 103–112). New York: Psychological Dimensions.

Hebb, D. O. (1953). Heredity and environment in mammalian behavior. *British Journal of Animal Behavior, 1,* 43–47.

Henley, N. (1974). Resources for the study of psychology and women. *Journal of Radical Therapy, 4,* 20–21.

Hollingworth, L. S. (1914). Functional periodicity: An experimental study of the mental and motor abilities of women during menstruation. *Teachers College Contributions to Education, 69.*

Horney, K. (1926). The flight from womanhood: The masculinity complex in women as viewed by men and by women. *International Journal of Psychoanalysis, 7,* 324–339.

Horney, K. (1939). *New ways in psychoanalysis.* New York: W. W. Norton.

Horney, K. (1950). *Neurosis and human growth: The struggle toward self realization.* New York: W. W. Norton.

Horney, K. (1967). Inhibited femininity: Psychoanalytical contribution to the problem of frigidity. In H. Kelman (Ed.), *Feminine psychology* (pp. 71–83). New York: W. W. Norton. (Original work published in 1926.)

Jacobi, M. (1877). *The question of rest for women during menstruation.* New York: G. P. Putnam & Sons.

Jones, E. (1964). *Ingratiation: A social psychological analysis.* New York: Appleton-Century-Crofts.

Klein, V. (1950). The stereotype of femininity. *Journal of Social Issues, 6,* 3–12.

Lowie, R., & Hollingworth, L. S. (1916). Science and feminism. *Scientific Monthly, 3,* 277–284.

McKenna, W., & Kessler, S. (1976). Experimental design as a source of sex bias in social psychology. *Sex Roles: A Journal of Research.*

Mednick, M. (1976). Some thoughts on the psychology of women. *Signs, 1,* 774.

Mednick, M. (1978.) Now we are four: What should we be when we grow up? *Psychology of Women Quarterly, 3,* 123–138.

Mednick, M., & Weissman, H. (1975). The psychology of women: Selected topics. *Annual Review of Psychology, 26,* 1–18.

Montague, H., & Hollingworth, L. S. (1914). The comparative variability of the sexes at birth. *American Journal of Sociology, 20,* 335–370.

O'Connell, A., & Russo, N. (1991). Overview: Women's heritage in psychology: Origins, development, and future directions. *Psychology of Women Quarterly, 15*, 495–504.

Paludi, M. A. (1987). *Teaching the psychology of women: Developmental considerations.* Paper presented at the meeting of the Association for Women in Psychology, Denver, CO.

Russo, N. F., & Denmark, F. L. (1987). Contributions of women in psychology. *Annual Review of Psychology, 38*, 279–298.

Schwabacher, S. (1972). Male vs. female representation in psychological research: An examination of the *Journal of Personality and Social Psychology. JSAS Catalogues of Selected Documents in Psychology, 2*, 20.

Sherman, J. (1971). *On the psychology of women.* Springfield, Ill.: Charles C. Thomas.

Sherman, J., & Denmark, F. L. (1978). *The psychology of women: Future directions of research.* New York: Psychological Dimensions.

Shields, S. (1975). Functionalism, Darwinism and the psychology of women. A study in social myth. *American Psychologist, 30*, 739–754.

Spencer, H. (1864). *The principles of biology.* New York: Appleton.

Task force report on the status of women in psychology. (1973). *American Psychologist, 28*, 611–616.

Thompson, C. (1941). The role of women in this culture. *Psychiatry, 4*, 1–8.

Thompson, C. (1942). Cultural pressures in the psychology of women. *Psychiatry, 5*, 331–339.

Thompson, C. (1943). Penis envy in women. *Psychiatry, 6*, 123–125.

Thompson, C. (1964a). *Interpersonal psychoanalysis.* M. R. Green (Ed.). New York: Basic Books.

Thompson, C. (1964b). *On women.* New York: New American Library.

Thompson, H. (1903). *The mental traits of sex.* Chicago: University of Chicago Press.

Unger, R., & Denmark, F. L. (1975). *Woman: Dependent or independent variable?* New York: Psychological Dimensions.

2

Feminist Perspectives on Research Methods

Vita Carulli Rabinowitz and Jeri A. Sechzer

INTRODUCTION

The major goal of this chapter is to offer a feminist perspective on the research process from its inception to its completion—from problem selection to the analysis and interpretation of results. We begin our analysis with a brief review of past feminist critiques of scientific psychology, focusing in particular on three interdependent areas of special concern to feminists: the role of values in science, issues embedded in the language and conduct of science, and a general comparison of qualitative and quantitative modes of research.

Next, we use the stages of the research process to organize feminist scholarship and perspectives on such methodological issues as question formulation, integrative reviews of previous research, descriptions of researchers, sample selection, research designs, operationalizations of independent and dependent variables, and data analysis and interpretation. We conclude by considering the implications of our analyses for the teaching of research methods in psychology.

Our general view of research methods, expressed in various forms throughout the chapter, is that no research method is inherently feminist or sexist and that no scientific research method is inherently superior or inferior to another. There are, of course, highly biased research questions and applications of methods, inappropriate matches between research questions and the designs, materials, research participants, and operations used to probe them, and biased or otherwise mistaken analyses, interpretations, and uses of research data. We hope to make the point that the careful consideration of the research question—not preconceived notions of what constitutes accepted practice in one's area—should be the ultimate arbiter of which research strategies are used.

FEMINIST ASSESSMENTS OF MAINSTREAM PSYCHOLOGY

The past two decades have witnessed several fundamental challenges to traditional psychological research. Scientific psychology has been criticized repeatedly for theories and research practices that are fraught with biases of many types (Bronfenbrenner, 1977; Ellsworth, 1977) and are now considered essentially faddish, dated, trivial, or meaningless (cf. Gergen, 1973; Koch, 1981). Disenchantment with certain subfields of psychology, particularly the social, personality, and developmental areas, has reached "crisis" proportions, according to some observers (Gergen, 1973).

Some of the most pervasive and persistent attacks on mainstream psychology have been written by feminist psychologists, who have long documented the existence of blatantly sexist (and racist, ethnocentric, ageist, and classist) assumptions, theories, research methods, and interpretations (Shields, 1975a, 1975b; Grady, 1981; Jacklin, 1983; McHugh, Koeske, & Frieze, 1986; Sherif, 1987). Indeed, feminists have been criticizing academic psychology in so many outlets on so many grounds for so long, that recent reviews have commenced by considering why these earlier messages have gone unheeded (Sherif, 1987; Unger, 1981; Wallston & Grady, 1985). As a group, feminist critics argue that the quality and integrity of psychology's contribution to science and society are at stake.

Feminist critiques of psychological research can be roughly divided into two overlapping categories. In the first category are those that essentially argue that the pervasive male bias in psychology has created bodies of knowledge that are scientifically flawed—that are inaccurate for, or irrelevant to, half the human race. Within this category, the reviews vary widely in the depth and extent of their criticisms. On one end of the continuum are relatively early reviews that call on psychology to "add women" to existing, male-dominated research. Examples of such reviews are those that note the preponderance of men as subjects in single-sex designs (Carlson & Carlson, 1960), the effects of sex of the experimenter on the respondents' performance (Harris, 1971), and the fallacy of generalizing from male samples to people generally (Denmark, Russo, Frieze & Sechzer, 1988; Gannon et al., 1992). At the other end of this spectrum are those that locate the operation of white, middle-class male bias at virtually every decision point in the research process, from the identification of what topics are worthy of study, through the choice of a research design, the selection of research participants, the operationalization of independent variables, the choice of dependent measures, the types of analyses performed, to the interpretation and generalization of results (Grady, 1981; Wallston, 1983; Lott, 1985; Wallston & Grady, 1985; Denmark et al., 1988). The more sweeping of these criticisms call for more sensitivity to the ways in which a sexist society generally and a sexist profession specifically distort the research process and the products of research. They take academic psychology to task for failing on its own terms—for not following the scientific method—and for using data-gathering techniques, research materials, and designs in ways that have compromised the interpretability of data.

The second, more radical, type of critique challenges the use or overuse of the scientific method in psychology (Keller, 1974; Sherif, 1987; Unger, 1983; Fine & Gordon, 1989). One of the central themes in this view is that science has historically been inhospitable to women and may be inherently so. One of the most prominent proponents of this viewpoint, physicist Keller (1974) wrote: "To the extent that analytic thought is conceived as 'male' thought, to the extent that we characterize the natural sciences as the 'hard sciences,' to the extent that the procedure of science is to 'attack' problems, and its goal, since Bacon, has been to 'conquer' or 'master' nature, a woman in science must in some way feel alien" (p. 18).

This view sees as intrinsically masculine and distorted the emphasis in science of studying events out of context, separating and compartmentalizing processes into their most basic elements. It argues for a more "feminine" approach of studying events as they occur naturally in their historical, cultural, and organizational contexts. Within psychology, Sherif (1987) and Unger (1983) have forcefully articulated this view. Sherif (1987) noted that psychology from its earliest days aped the forms and procedures of the natural sciences to gain prestige and respectability, even though the subject matter of psychology did not lend itself to these modes of inquiry. She (1987) wrote: "Psychologists, in their strivings to gain status with other scientists did not pause long on issues raised by the differences between studying a rock, a chemical compound, or an animal, on [the] one hand, and a human individual, on the other" (p. 43).

The most severe judgments are often reserved for the laboratory experiment and its characteristic features of manipulation of variables, high experimenter control, contrived contexts, deception of respondents, and so on. On the topic of experimental methods, Unger (1983) said: "The logic of these methods (and even their language) prescribes prediction and control. It is difficult for one who is trained in such a conceptual framework to step beyond it and ask what kind of person such a methodology presupposes" (p. 11).

Rarely do feminists who challenge the dominance of the scientific method in psychology actually call for its wholesale abandonment; but most do argue for a vastly increased use of already existing nonexperimental, naturalistic research methods in psychology and the development of new unobtrusive methods to be used along with "sex-fair" experimental techniques (McHugh et al., 1986; Wallston & Grady, 1985; Wittig, 1985). All research methods have distinct advantages and disadvantages, and for this reason, multiple methods should be employed within any program of research—an approach known as "triangulation" (Wallston & Grady, 1985). The chief differences among feminists who pose a radical challenge to psychology lie in the extent to which they endorse the use of nonscientific modes of data gathering, like unstructured interviews or observations, and their willingness to regard nonexperimental or nonscientific ways of gathering information as distinctly "feminist" (Fine & Gordon, 1989).

Despite some important differences among them, feminist psychologists generally are bound by a deep concern with current research practices in psychology. A consensus is building on a number of key issues:

- Science is not, and cannot be, value-free. Values affect all phases of a research project from the choice of what to study to the conclusions drawn from the results. The effects of researchers' values on the works produced are by no means necessarily negative. Indeed, values motivate and enrich all of science. Because scientists' values cannot be obliterated any more than their gender, race, class, and social or educational background, they serve science best when they are acknowledged, examined, and counterbalanced when possible. This position is not an open invitation to indulge biases, wallow in subjectivity, or advocate political causes in the name of science. It simply acknowledges the nature and limits of science and psychological knowledge.

- Although "sex differences" have been studied in psychology since its inception, it is not clear precisely what it is that has been studied. Terms like *sex*, *male*, *female*, *masculine*, and *feminine* have been used too loosely and inclusively to describe everything from the biological sex of participants to social or situational factors considered appropriate to males and females. The term *gender* has been proposed to refer to the complex of biological, social, psychological, and cultural factors braided with the labels "male" and "female" (Unger, 1979). In this formulation, the term *sex* is now largely reserved for biological aspects of males and females. This chapter observes Unger's distinctions.

- Many long-established "sex differences," upon reexamination, do not appear to be main effects that will endure over time (Deaux, 1984; Unger, 1979). Even those few gender differences that have withstood scrutiny tend to be very small and of little social significance (Maccoby & Jacklin, 1974).

- The conventional focus on "sex differences" in sex-role research obscures the many ways in which males and females are similar. A number of biases exist in selecting what findings are reported, published, and cited. Historically, in virtually all cases, this bias has worked in the direction of reporting, publishing, citing, and dramatizing gender differences and overlooking similarities.

- There is a tendency for sex-related differences on many dimensions to be interpreted as originating in innate biological differences, even in the absence of any evidence for biological causation. When gender differences are being explained, all plausible rival explanatory factors must be explored: the biological (e.g., genetic, hormonal, and physiological) and the sociocultural (e.g., familial, peer, economic, and situational), even if all these factors were not explicitly investigated in the study (McHugh et al., 1986).

We believe that psychology, to progress as a science, will continue to rely primarily on quantitative techniques and experimental methods, even as it expands the range of "respectable" techniques and methods to include qualitative and nonexperimental ones. As we hope to demonstrate, quantitative and experimental methods have already made substantial contributions to the psychology of gender and still have much to offer. Like many other feminist psychologists, we believe that the study of gender and psychology generally will benefit by becoming more, and not less, "scientific." But experiments are just one of many scientific methods worth using. As we pose more varied kinds of research questions, we must have available a much wider range of scientific methods.

Before offering a step-by-step guide to the conduct of sex-fair research, we would like to consider three overlapping issues that have concerned feminist critics of mainstream psychology: (1) the role of values in science, (2) a comparison of qualitative and quantitative modes of research, and (3) ethical issues imbedded in the language and conduct of science and research.

The Role of Values in Science

Objectivity is considered a hallmark of science, but it is perhaps most accurately viewed as a retrospective virtue. Science is presented in classrooms and textbooks as the accumulation of dispassionate fact, and teachers and students alike may come to see it that way. But practicing scientists know that it originates with people inspired by ordinary human passions, like ambition, pride, and greed, and constrained by ordinary human limitations imposed by ignorance and prejudice.

At the same time, many scientists possess some extraordinary traits as well. They passionately want to learn the truth about the object of their study. Most are highly committed to the theories they test, the research methods they use, and the conclusions they draw. Without this emotional commitment, it would be difficult to sustain the considerable effort required to receive professional training and launch professional careers in science. Largely because of pervasive beliefs about the objectivity of science and the literary conventions of scientific reporting in fields like psychology, researchers feel compelled to appear completely detached and present their efforts as only the rational exercise of intellect. The fact is, scientists vary considerably in their styles of conceptualizing problems and applying research techniques. There are many different approaches to the pursuit of knowledge using scientific methods. The standardized way of reporting research sanctioned by the American Psychological Association, known as "APA style," which seems to spring from some universally shared approach to problem solving, may obscure some important differences in practice and impose a false unanimity on research reports.

Given what is now known about "experimenter effects" in research and increasing publicity about the incidence of scientific fraud, there are probably very few psychologists today who would argue that perfect objectivity in science is possible. Most would concede that, explicitly or implicitly, every published report unavoidably expresses, to some degree, a point of view or value judgment.

But even those psychologists who reject simplistic notions of value-free science nonetheless seem to embrace more refined versions of the doctrine of objectivity (Schlenker, 1974). If it is impossible to avoid a point of view entirely, most scientific psychologists often do their best to ignore, hide, or downplay its role in research. Researchers who have been forthright about their values, as many feminist psychologists have been, are often dismissed as "advocacy" psychologists (Unger, 1982). There appears to be a widespread, if unspoken, fear among academic psychologists that for a scientist to express values openly or call attention to personal characteristics or values of the scientist in a research report is to compromise the integrity of the research. As Wittig (1985) noted: "One criticism of advocacy in psychology is that when researchers function simultaneously as advocates, their ability to discern facts is compromised and their 'evidence' serves primarily to justify already held beliefs" (p. 804).

It should be recognized that all scientists are, to greater or lesser extents, advocates as well as scholars. The tension between scholarship and advocacy is inevitable and requires constant vigilance on the part of the scientist and surveillance by the scientific community. In this way, the "forced choice" between advocacy and scholarship can be avoided. Campbell's views about the role for advocacy in applied research may well serve as a guide to the basic researcher, particularly those who work in socially relevant or politically sensitive areas like gender (D.T. Campbell, 1969). Campbell saw a role for advocacy in social science research so long as the commitment of the researcher was to explore an issue or help to solve a problem, rather than to advance a particular view of the problem or impose a particular solution. The overarching commitment of all scientists must be to the truth. The distortion of the truth for political or social reasons undermines scientists' trust in the literature and the peer review system. Of course, once revealed, fraud and distortion also undermine the public's trust in science. This trust is essential to the smooth process of science. The personal values of scientists are best expressed by their choices of what is worth studying, the questions worth asking, and the best methods available to probe these questions.

Qualitative versus Quantitative Knowing

Scientists and philosophers have long recognized that there are many critical questions that science cannot address quantitatively, concerning, for example, issues of faith, morality, values, or culture. But even in the cases of questions that are potentially answerable by science, people frequently rely on nonscientific modes of gathering information. People gain a great deal by accepting the conclusions of others rather than by checking or verifying such conclusions by systematic observation. There are many things we could never experience directly, and even for those that we can, our own observations may be less reliable or insightful than those of others. In fact, culture can be viewed as a device for transmitting to people information about events that they have never experienced and may never experience themselves.

Thus, despite the clear advantage of the scientific method of data gathering, there are other ways of knowing besides scientific knowing. According to Buchler (1955), the philosopher Charles Peirce held that there are four ways of obtaining knowledge, or, as he put it, "fixing belief." The first is the method of tenacity, by which people know things to be true because they have always believed them to be true. The second method is the method of authority, whereby information is accepted as true because it has the weight of tradition, expert opinion, or public sanction. The a priori method is the third way of knowing. A priori assumptions are ones that appear to be self-evident or reasonable. The fourth way is the scientific method, whose fundamental hypothesis is that there are "real things whose characters are entirely independent of our opinions about them" (Buchler, 1955, p. 18). According to Peirce, the scientific method has characteristics that no other method of obtaining knowledge possesses: mechanisms of self-correction, objectivity, and appeals to evidence.

Just as there are other ways of knowing besides scientific knowing, there are different ways of scientific knowing. While it can probably be said that there is one scientific approach to problems—one general paradigm of scientific inquiry—there are a number of different research designs and data-gathering techniques that scientists can and do use.

The research design is the overall plan or structure of an investigation. Its purpose is to provide a model of the relationships of the variables of a study and to control variance. Research designs, which will be discussed in detail below, can be classified along a continuum with true or randomized experiments and nonexperimental approaches at the poles. True experiments are characterized by the manipulation of antecedent conditions to create at least two different treatment groups, random assignment of respondents to treatments, constraints upon respondents' behaviors, and the control of extraneous variables. Nonexperimental research designs involve less direct manipulation of antecedent conditions, little control over the assignment of respondents to conditions, fewer constraints on the responses of research participants, and less control over extraneous variables. Case studies, ex post facto studies, and passive- and participant-observational methods exemplify nonexperimental approaches.

Along with choosing a research design, investigators must select strategies for observing respondents or collecting data. It is usually, but not necessarily, the case that experimental research designs are accompanied by quantitative modes of data gathering, and nonexperimental designs by qualitative modes. The distinction between quantitative and qualitative measures is not as clear-cut as those labels imply. The fact is that most observations, from thoughts and feelings to personal and societal products like diaries and documents, can probably be collected systematically and ordered logically on some dimensions and thus quantified. But some kinds of observations are more easily quantified than others. For example, questionnaires with fixed-choice alternatives yield data that lend themselves to categorization and quantification more easily than unstructured interviews. In general, unstructured interviews, sociogram analyses, mappings, many unobtrusive measures, documents, photographs, essays, and casual conversations are examples of what have come to be known as qualitative modes of data gathering.

As many reviewers have noted, both experimental/quantitative and nonexperimental/qualitative approaches to research have advantages and disadvantages, and each has its place in a program of research. Many feminist critics have attempted to increase awareness of lesser-known and little-used research methods, particularly nonexperimental and qualitative ones, and to encourage "triangulation" or "converging operations"—the use of as many different modes of operationalization and measurement of variables as possible within a program of research—as well as replication of studies to establish the reliability and generality of phenomena (Wallston, 1983; Wallston & Grady, 1985).

Like feminist psychologists, European psychologists have taken a broader perspective on the use of research methods than their American counterparts and have been critical of American psychology for its rejection of qualitative modes of knowing. Hall (1990), in his recent description of his impressions of the First European Congress of Psychology, was struck by the common European view that the word *science* has much too narrow a meaning for American psychologists. He paraphrased the keynote address of the eminent Dutch psychologist, Adrian de Groot, who opened the congress this way: "Psychology as a natural science on the model of physics, with an insistence on the sole use of empirical methods as a means of knowing, is an American view. . . . In contrast, the European view of science does not exclude the academic study of the humanities, nor does it consider methods such as anecdotal evidence and reasoning necessarily non- or pre-scientific" (p. 987).

According to Hall, the focus of European criticisms of American psychology involved three fundamental concerns: narrow methodology and topic selection, lack of real concern for theory development and orientation, and an apparent unconcern for the cultural and historical context for understanding human behavior that is characteristic of research in the United States.

Hall also noted that most of the research presented at the congress was data-based, empirical studies, much like research in the United States, with the following subtle differences: wider use of nonexperimental methods, investigation of research topics not often studied in the United States, and more careful consideration given to the theoretical context of studies. He came away from the congress with the view that American psychology, with its many virtues and accomplishments, has much to learn from contemporary European psychology.

In the United States, where experimental and quantitative modes clearly predominate, the issues surrounding choices between nonexperimental/qualitative and experimental/quantitative modes have been hotly debated in some feminist circles. Some feminists have called for the alignment of feminist research with nonexperimental/qualitative methods (Carlson, 1972; Fine & Gordon, 1989).

More typically, feminist critics have argued that no type of method is inherently superior to another and that each makes a unique contribution to the progress of science (Wallston & Grady, 1985). On the whole, though, feminist critics have been highly critical of widely used experimental/quantitative methods on a number of grounds and quite receptive to alternative nonexperimental/qualitative approaches.

Quantitative and experimental methods generally employ a variety of controls to remove or balance extraneous factors, determine which research participants receive which treatments at which times, and limit the possibility of invalid inference. These controls have come under fire from some feminists who regard them as by-products of sexism in science and society and often as unethical, unnatural, stifling, and undermining (Unger, 1983; McHugh et al., 1986). These critics of the quantitative/experimental research paradigm tend to be well-grounded in experimental methodology and able to generate a litany of methodologically sound criticisms. About independent variables, they note that the possible and permissible range of manipulated variables like fear, grief, anger, or guilt is restricted to very low levels in an experiment; the time constraints of an experiment, especially in the laboratory, often impose other serious restrictions on independent variables, so that only acute or reactive forms of some variables, like self-esteem, can be studied. On the dependent variable side, it is by now well established that respondents who know that they are being observed by psychologists are motivated to appear better adjusted and less deviant, more tolerant and rational, more likely to turn the other cheek than retaliate when provoked and to judge others as they themselves would be judged. Psychologists now take it for granted that hypotheses involving antisocial behavior or socially undesirable behavior should be tested outside the laboratory, ideally when respondents do not know that they are being observed (Ellsworth, 1977).

All of these criticisms are true enough, often enough, to encourage feminist psychologists and others to search for alternatives to quantitative and experimental methods. They have warned against the dangers of ignoring relevant qualitative contextual evidence and overrelying on a few quantified abstractions to the neglect of contradictory or supplementary qualitative evidence (Sherif, 1987; Unger, 1983). But qualitative and quantitative methods are not interchangeable; they yield different kinds of information, and the substitution of qualitative techniques for quantitative ones does not seem promising. Quantitative and experimental methods are superior to naturalistic ones for answering causal questions. Of course, not all questions of interest are causal questions, and many important causal questions cannot be probed experimentally due to ethical or practical constraints. Moreover, before relevant variables have been identified and precise causal questions can be formulated in a research area, experimental and quantitative methods may be premature and may even foreclose promising areas of exploration. This said, it remains the case that many of the most important questions that we will ask as scientists or concerned citizens are causal questions. The best way to investigate causal laws is by conducting true or randomized experiments involving manipulated variables in controlled settings. The naturalistic observation of events cannot permit causal inference because of the ubiquitous confounding of selection and treatment. Of necessity, any effort to reduce this inherent equivocality will have the effect of increasing the investigator's control and making conditions more contrived and artificial—that is, more "experimental." Qualitative, quantitative, nonexperimental, and experimental modes of knowing may be best viewed as noninterchangeable but as compatible and complementary.

Despite the chilly climate so many women have encountered in the halls of science generally and the psychological laboratory particularly, many feminist critics recognize that it would be a great mistake for feminists to forsake quantitative and experimental methods or the laboratory for context-rich, confound-laden qualitative and nonexperimental methods. It is undisputed that gender differences are larger and more prevalent in the field than the laboratory (Deaux, 1984). As Unger (1979) noted, far more self-report surveys of sex differences exist than do reports of such differences when actual behavior is observed by others. This finding suggests that many studies of gender differences have not planned well in advance for the sophisticated analysis of those differences and/or their replication. Often, it is only after the painstaking unconfounding of variables that so often covary in naturalistic settings—like gender and status—that we can illuminate how similar the sexes are. It is in the laboratory that much of the work has been done illustrating that many behavioral differences between men and women are the results of conscious self-presentational strategies rather than of different potentials or repertoires (Deaux, 1984), status differences between men and women (Unger, 1979), or differences in how familiar men and women are with experimental stimuli (Eagly, 1978). Time after time, in studies of aggression, influencibility, self-confidence, and helping, to name a few areas, carefully controlled experimental research has been critical in successfully refuting pernicious, long-standing myths about the differences between the genders or about women. The discrete "findings" that have accumulated to form the bodies of literature in psychological studies—the contents of psychology—have often been sexist. But, as Grady (1981) has pointed out, the methods of scientific psychology are valuable to feminists and revolutionaries of all types, as they contain within them the means for challenging the status quo.

Ethical Issues Embedded in the Language and Conduct of Science

It has long been noted that the language of science is itself deeply male-oriented and sexist (Keller, 1974; Sherif, 1987; Unger, 1983) and contributes greatly to the disaffection that some feminists feel from the sciences, including psychology. It is not difficult to generate a list of scientific terms that seem to suggest a preoccupation with power and domination. Thus, we "manipulate" fear and "control" for sex. We "intervene" in field settings and "attack" problems. "Subjects" are "assigned" to treatments and "deceived." Scientists accumulate "hard" facts, and so on. The issues raised by the language of science, like those raised by the literary conventions of the scientific report, are by no means trivial. Language not only reflects but also shapes scientific thought and practice.

At least three different issues are raised by the feminist critique of the language of experimentation. The first issue concerns the perceived adversarial relationship between the experiment and the real world—between the false and contrived and the real and natural, between the distortions of science and the truth of the real world. As noted earlier, it is not clear that anything is gained by conceptualizing science and nature as dichotomies or that feminism should seek to align itself with the "natural" as opposed to the "scientific." The second and related issue concerns the labeling of the objective, rational, and interventionist in science and scientific language as "masculine." Given the apparent human fondness for dualisms and dichotomies, the effect of calling the language of experimentation and quantitative methods "masculine" is to cast the language of subjective, intuitive, and passive observational methods as "feminine." It is not clear that such classifications should be encouraged. Bleier, cited in Lott (1985), has argued, "Science need not be permitted to define objectivity and creativity as that which the male mind does and subjectivity and emotionality as that which the female mind is" (p. 162). Lott goes on to say that the terms *masculinity* and *femininity* are simply cognitive constructs with no independent existence in nature. Statements that tie human characteristics like a "preoccupation with control and dominance" to gender, in Lott's words, "deny the abundance of contradictory evidence and what we know about situational variation in behavior" (p. 162).

The third concern embedded in the feminist response to the language of science is the status differential inherent in the traditional relationship between researchers, especially experimenters, and their research participants and the potential and real abuses of power that flow from this inequity. Perhaps the essence of that differential is captured in the increasingly discredited label "subjects" for research participants. Many feminist researchers seem profoundly uncomfortable with this inequity, which they view as another by-product of sexism in science. Summarizing the point of view of many feminists, McHugh et al. (1986) wrote: "They have suggested that eliciting subjective viewpoints may be one way to 'get behind' the inequality and the limited self-presentation potentially inherent in all researcher-participant interactions. Both the appropriateness and scientific utility of the experimenter's being neutral, disinterested, and nondisclosing have been challenged, especially when the experimenter desires to have participants behave naturally and honestly" (p. 880).

Clearly, the feminist call is for a more respectful, interactive, and "honest" relationship between researchers and research participants. Two implications of this call are that respondents should be consulted about their responses to the experiment and that researchers should disclose to respondents the purposes of the research, or at least refrain from deceiving respondents. There is a growing body of evidence in the psychology of women to suggest that it is essential on scientific as well as moral grounds to elicit the meaning of various aspects of a study from the research participants' point of view. Research situations differ in their salience, familiarity, relevance, and meanings for males and females, as well as for members of different racial and ethnic groups (Richardson & Kaufman, 1983; McHugh et al., 1986). As Richardson and Kaufman stated, gender-by-situation interactions are more the rule than the exception in psychological research, and the failure to explore and specify the meanings that research participants attach to stimuli constitutes a blight on our research literatures.

It is difficult to argue against any of the welcome trends championed by feminist critics that protect the rights and dignity of research participants and make researchers aware of the responsibilities they have to treat participants with respect and caring. Obviously, the gratuitous and uncritical practice of deceiving research participants is completely unwarranted. But there is in fact not good evidence to suggest that research participants feel harmed, violated, or diminished by today's research practices of deception or nondisclosure of the methods and purposes of the research (Abramson, 1977; Mannucci, 1977). As Smith (1983) noted, empirical research on the effects of deception seem to suggest that most respondents regard deception in a scientific context as justifiable and not unethical, especially if respondents have been thoroughly debriefed. According to Smith, respondents view research with deception more favorably than research that is trivial, uninteresting, stressful, or harmful. Mannucci (1977) pointed out that when respondents are presented with a research situation that is not what it seems, they do not always regard themselves as having been "deceived." Of course, the fact that most respondents feel that deception is justifiable does not mean that all respondents feel that way or that respondents would feel that way under all circumstances. Nonetheless, reports of negative attitudes toward research using deception, even where these attitudes were actively solicited, are rare (Smith, 1983).

Aside from respondents' attitudes toward deception, there is the issue of its actual effects on research participants. Again, research on the effects of deception on respondents suggests that there is little, if any, evidence of harm of any kind, including negative effects of inflicted self-knowledge and damage to trust in scientific research or research scientists (West & Gunn, 1978; Reynolds, 1979).

From a scientific standpoint, there is not as yet any evidence to suggest that research participants behave more naturally or honestly when they are aware of the methods and purposes of the research. Smith (1983) reviews a substantial body of evidence that indicates that respondents in fact behave less honestly when they know that they are being observed, when they are asked to take on the roles of those who face moral dilemmas, or when they know the purposes of research. Obviously, even the most vigorous defenders of deception recognize that there are clear limits to its use (Elms, 1982). We need to continue the debate about the extent to which deception-free methods like self-report, role playing, and simulations can be used in place of deception and to continue the development and testing of alternatives to deception.

Feminist critiques of scientific psychology have also been in the forefront of efforts to protect the rights and dignity of research participants, to guard against violations of trust, and to value the totality of respondents' contributions to research. Characteristically, feminist research assigns a high priority to eliciting respondents' viewpoints and explaining fully the meaning and purposes of research at the point of debriefing. These practices have proved to be scientifically, as well as ethically, sound. Feminist research also seeks to avoid or minimize the use of deception and reminds us that there are more important values in society even than the advancement of knowledge. However, it appears that some of the concern about the use of deception and nondisclosure may be exaggerated and that these practices, when carefully monitored and scrupulously implemented, may not be as morally or methodologically problematic as once feared.

A GUIDE TO GENDER-FAIR RESEARCH

We are now prepared to consider each of the stages of the research process, with an eye to noting the pervasive white, middle-class, male bias that has distorted this process. Issues pertaining to formulating research questions, conducting integrative reviews of previous research, choosing research participants and research designs, operationalizing variables, and analyzing and interpreting results will be discussed from a feminist perspective. This orientation owes much to the excellent pioneering work of Kay Deaux, Florence Denmark, Alice Eagly, Irene Hanson Frieze, Kathleen Grady, Randi Daimon Koeske, Maureen Mc-Hugh, Rhoda Unger, and Barbara Strudler Wallston, all of whom have helped to set the standards for the conduct of gender-fair research.

Question Formulation

In recent years, researchers have begun to turn their attention to understudied and undervalued areas—hypothesis generation and question formulation. Traditionally, it has been assumed that research hypotheses are logically derived from theory. Clearly, much of what is described as basic research is derived from theoretical models. But where do these theories come from, and what are, or could be, other sources of our research?

Psychological theories, from the most formal, sweeping, and influential ones like Freud's theory of personality and Piaget's theory of cognitive development, to far less ambitious ones, are often derived from the experiences and observations of the theorists. The overwhelming majority of these theorists in psychology have been men. Some, like Piaget, Kohlberg, and Erikson, have tended to promote standards of healthy behavior based on the experiences of males alone and, like Freud, to depict women more negatively than men. As many feminist psychologists have argued (Sherif, 1987; Unger, 1983; Harding, 1987), up until now, traditional psychology has begun its analysis from men's experience, particularly the experience of white, middle-class males, who have dominated academic psychology. This means that psychology has posed questions about individual and social processes that men find problematic or that men want answered—questions of men, by men, for men. To be sure, many of the traditional topics studied by psychologists have been of great interest to women, and women have been the primary object of study in some lines of research. But asking questions about one sex that could and should be applied to both sexes is sexist. For instance, reports of a relationship between monthly fluctuations in female sex hormones and a woman's ability to perform certain cognitive tasks have recently received widespread attention (Blakeslee, 1988). The daily fluctuations in key male hormones, on the other hand, have not been correlated with male thinking skills. Similarly, the prenatal sexual responsiveness of males but not females has been explored (Brody, 1989). Obviously, the focus on females in the first instance and males in the second lends scientific respectability to stereotypes about female cognitive impairment and male sexual potency that might have been refuted had both genders been studied.

Topics of primary interest to women (e.g., family relationships, female alcoholism, victimization by rape, wife battering) and questions about women that women want answered (e.g., How can corporations change so that women with children can pursue careers at the same time that they raise their families?) have received far less attention than topics of primary interest to men (e.g., work outside the home, male alcoholism, aggression of men toward men, impaired male sexual response) and questions about women that men want answered (e.g., How can women's symptoms of depression and anxiety be treated medically?).

In psychology, we have devoted considerable research attention to the topics of aggression, conflict, achievement, and cognitive processes and less attention to the topics of affiliation, cooperation, and emotional processes. We have studied moral development as it pertains to applying rules and upholding rights in hypothetical situations, not as it pertains to taking care of others and fulfilling responsibilities in actual situations. While no topic or approach is inherently "masculine or "feminine," superior or inferior, the preponderance of topics and approaches studied appears to reflect a masculine bias. More importantly, they reflect a strikingly narrow and distorted view of human behavior.

We are well on our way toward developing a psychology of abstract concepts like "aggression" that lend themselves rather easily to experimental tests in the laboratory. But we have made little progress in developing the psychology of human concerns. It is remarkable that academic psychology has devoted so little attention to the phenomena that occupy people in their daily lives—relating to family and friends, making a living, saving and spending money, educating themselves, enjoying leisure time, to name a few. We have hardly begun to understand the effects on people of being married or committed to a mate, having close friends, believing in God, losing a job, or losing a loved one. We have only recently started studying how climate, geography, crossing time zones, housing and space, and other aspects of the environment affect behavior. The complex relationships between physical health and psychological well-being are only now beginning to receive the attention they deserve from scientific psychologists. Many of the richest, most influential psychological variables we know of—gender, race, ethnicity, age, and educational background—have been given short shrift by psychologists, in part because there may be considerable professional risk involved in studying them.

Some of these areas have been ignored by scientific psychologists because they are regarded as "applied" or "clinical." Applied research is by definition regarded as less generalizable, less important, less prestigious, and more specialized than "basic" or "pure" research. As other investigators have noted, research on topics of particular interest to males is more likely to be regarded as basic, and research of particular interest to females, as applied (McHugh et al., 1986). The psychology of gender and the psychology of women suffer from this classification. Research published in feminist journals like *Psychology of Women Quarterly* and *Sex Roles* is not often cited in mainstream journals in the field as they are seen as specialized and thus of limited interest.

Another reason for avoiding these areas is that they are very difficult to study, particularly with conventional research methods. People cannot be randomly assigned to a belief in God, a Harvard education, or the loss of a loved one. So many variables are confounded with gender and age that interpreting their effects becomes treacherous, especially when one considers the social and political implications of those interpretations.

The "crisis in social psychology" is due in part to the recognition that psychologists have systematically ignored many of the most interesting, important, and pressing questions about nature and social life. Those outside the academic mainstream have not been impressed with the arguments that such questions are only of applied or limited interest or are too difficult to probe with cherished traditional research tools. For one thing, there is increasing evidence that the distinction between basic and applied research is blurring, as applied research becomes more theory-relevant and methodologically rigorous. In fact, scientific psychologists as eminent as Harvard's Howard Gardner see psychology flourishing much more as an applied than a basic field in the future (Blakeslee, 1988). To be sure, new questions do require new assumptions, models, hypotheses, and purposes of inquiry. What we need are new ways of applying scientific techniques of gathering evidence, many of which are seldom used or used mainly in other disciplines. To investigate questions of interest to them, feminist researchers can use any and all of the methods that traditional scientists have used, but use them in different ways to observe behaviors and gain perspectives not previously thought significant.

As an essential corrective to pervasive male bias, the experiences, observations, concerns, and problems of women need to be integrated into psychology. Further, we need to recognize that gender experiences vary across categories of class, race, and culture. As Harding (1987) noted, "Women come only in different classes, races, and cultures; there is no 'woman' and no 'woman's experience' " (p. 7).

Integrative Reviews of Previous Research

Despite the obvious importance of theory, experience, and observation in influencing research questions, most basic researchers probably get their specific ideas from studying other people's research—from the professional literature in a narrow and well-defined area. There are several obvious reasons, including the very obvious practical consideration of fitting one's research into an already existing body of knowledge and having one's contribution recognized as valuable. The problems with this approach from a feminist perspective should be equally obvious. Many bodies of literature in psychology are so tainted by sexist assumptions and research practices that they are unreliable guides for feminist research. How can we review research in such a way that exposes past androcentric biases and enriches future gender-fair research?

All research reports begin with a review of relevant research. Given how influential and ubiquitous they are, it is truly surprising that there are no standards for conducting such reviews. Jackson (1983) explained this by suggesting that, in the past, neither reviewers nor editors attached a great deal of importance to the thoroughness or accuracy of reviews, with the result that most reviews are quite flawed.

Jackson (1983) proposed three components to the process of analyzing previous research in an area: (1) identifying and locating the known universe of relevant studies, (2) noting the systematic methodological strengths and weaknesses of past studies, and (3) judging the implications of these biases and considering how varying characteristics of research participants, treatments, and measures might affect the phenomena of interest. As we consider each component, it should be clear how androcentric biases emerge at each stage of the process.

For most researchers, the universe of relevant studies is strikingly narrow, consisting of the professional literature in a very few scholarly journals. As noted above, to the extent that the professional literature has been dominated by white, middle-class, male theorists and researchers, the literature reflects the values, interests, and concerns of this group. But bias does not exist simply because males have served as the crafters of the research agenda and the gatekeepers of the journals. Bias also exists because sex differences are much more likely to be reported in the mainstream literature than sex similarities, regardless of how unexpected or meaningless they are, because the finding of no differences is not regarded as interpretable. Thus, there is no literature that seeks to integrate the innumerable studies in which no differences are found.

There are only partial correctives for the problem of locating the relevant literature outside the mainstream in areas like the psychology of gender. One remedy lies in expanding the search for studies beyond the small number of mainstream journals with their predictable biases. Relevant journals within the discipline that may have different biases should be sought out, regardless of their circulation or prestige, as should relevant journals from different social science disciplines. Aside from scholarly journals, books, monographs, unpublished doctoral dissertations, and government and other "in-house" publications should also be sought. Papers presented at conventions might be included in the search. Special efforts must be made to incorporate the perspectives of other disciplines, social classes, and cultures representing varying philosophical and political viewpoints. Even this is not enough to redress the imbalance. Aside from deliberately and vigorously expanding the literature search, the reviewer needs to report fully the dimensions of the search strategy so that others may assess its thoroughness, adequacy, and likely sources of bias. Clearly, these prescriptions add significantly to our responsibilities as reviewers, but they are critical if we are ever to strike an essential balance in our efforts to explore complex variables like gender and race.

The second component of the integrative review, according to Jacklin (1983), is the identification of systematic methodological weaknesses and strengths in the bodies of knowledge. A number of feminists have offered cogent criticisms of the research on gender differences and the psychology of women by pointing to pervasive methodological flaws that have systematically distorted results. Jacklin, who has herself conducted some of the most ambitious and well-regarded reviews in these areas, has pointed to some of the most common problems. Although these will be discussed in more detail later, it will suffice here to note briefly the methodological flaws that exist when there are a number of variables confounded with gender, such as status or self-confidence, or when the experimenter's gender produces an effect that interacts with the gender of the respondent, but that interaction is not measured. Another confound exists when the data are obtained by filling out self-reports. There is a well-documented gender difference in the willingness or ability to disclose thoughts and feelings, in the direction of females being more disclosing, and thus there is a concern for researchers in interpreting gender differences obtained with these kinds of measures.

Exploring the implications of methodological biases and speculating about how different research participants, treatments, designs, and measures might affect conclusions are the final component of Jacklin's analyses. Thoughtful critics have already demonstrated what such analyses might yield. For instance, it has been noted that more and larger gender differences have emerged in the field than the laboratory (cf. Unger, 1979) and that the more methodologically controlled the design, the less likely it is that gender differences will emerge (Jacklin, 1983). Unger (1979) has noted that the appearance of gender differences depends upon the age, social class, and cultural background of the respondents. She has also pointed out that males and females ordinarily do not differ in how they respond to stimulus materials used in psychological research, but are especially alike in the stereotypes they have regarding the sexes and how the sexes differ (Unger, 1979). She concluded, then, that gender-of-respondent effects are not nearly as common as gender-of-stimuli effects.

Most feminist psychologists have chosen to regard the psychological literature as a legitimate source of knowledge and have attempted to counteract the many biases of omission and commission from within the discipline (Fine & Gordon, 1989). Feminists need to take a critical stance toward the biases that exist in the psychological literature, biases that necessarily place an extra burden on their integrative reviews. Many feminists have expressed great interest in the alternative to narrative discussions of research studies known as meta-analysis (Glass, 1976; Eagly & Carli, 1981). This approach involves transforming the results of individual studies to some common metric, like significance levels or effect size, and coding various characteristics of the studies. Then, by using conventional statistical procedures, the reviewer can determine whether there are overall effects, subsample effects, and relationships among characteristics of the studies (e.g., use of a correlational design) and the findings of the bodies of literature.

The virtues of this technique from a feminist perspective are significant. Meta-analysis is a systematic and replicable approach. It can accommodate studies with a variety of methodologies and can control for biased findings due to systematic methodological flaws. It can provide estimates of population parameters and permit simultaneous investigation of the relationships among research methods, participants, scope of operationalizations, and the duration of treatment. In probing the extensive, diverse, often contradictory literature on sex-related differences and the psychology of gender, feminists have painstakingly demonstrated how well-established findings on the effects of gender must be qualified by taking into account such variables as task characteristics, response modes, gender of the experimenter, self-presentational strategies, and perceiver's stereotypes about sex-linked behavior, to name a few.

As promising as meta-analytic techniques are and as appealing as they have been to feminist reviewers, we do not mean to suggest that they solve all of the problems of traditional narrative reviews or are themselves without controversy. Some meta-analysts have been criticized for the liberal standards they tend to use in including studies in meta-analysis. The issues of whether and how to exclude studies of poor methodological quality have not been resolved. Of course, not all studies on a given topic can be retrieved for inclusion, and those that cannot are likely to differ systematically on some important characteristics from those that can. For example, retrievable studies are more likely to report differences between treatment conditions and to be published in journals than those that are not retrievable.

Combining effect sizes or significance levels is problematic as a way of estimating treatment effects unless the studies involved used the same or highly similar independent variables. The issue of how broad categories of independent and dependent variables should be has been called the ''apples and oranges'' problem in meta-analysis (Cook & Leviton, 1980). According to these authors, the greater the breadth of the categories used, the more likely the chances that important interaction effects will become impossible to detect and too much confidence will be placed in conclusions about main effects.

Meta-analytic techniques can aid the reviewer in analyzing, categorizing, and weighting past research and promise further clarifications in understanding the effects of gender and related variables. But they do not free the meta-analyst from the responsibility to exercise the same kinds of judgment that has always been expected of traditional reviewers.

Description of Researchers

Because they openly acknowledge the roles of background and values in research, many feminist research methodologists have proposed that researchers make these explicit in their reports (cf. Harding, 1987; Wallston & Grady, 1985). Harding (1987) wrote: "The best feminist analysis insists that the inquirer her/ himself be placed in the same critical plane as the overt subject matter, thereby recovering the entire research process for scrutiny in the results of the research" (p. 9).

There is ample evidence from a wide variety of areas within psychology that the personal attributes, background, and values of researchers distort results. Eagly and Carli (1981) found in their meta-analytic study of conformity and persuasion that the gender of researcher was a determinant of the gender difference in influenceability. Male authors reported larger sex differences than female authors, in the direction of greater persuasibility and conformity among women. Sherwood and Nataupsky (reported in Unger, 1983) found that the conclusions that investigators reached about whether blacks were innately inferior to whites in intelligence could be predicted from biological information about the investigators, including birth order, educational level, birthplace of their parents, and scholastic standing. Psychotherapy outcome studies conducted by researchers who are affiliated with a particular form of psychotherapy and are not blind to treatment condition demonstrate an overwhelming tendency to find that the form of psychotherapy favored by the researcher works best (Kayne & Alloy, 1988). In contrast, when well-controlled comparison experiments are conducted by unbiased assessors, there are usually no differences between the therapies compared.

Many questions arise when we consider the idea of including descriptions of experimenters in research reports. What kinds of information should be included and excluded? How much information is necessary? Where and how should this information be incorporated into the report? Will something be lost when the researcher is no longer portrayed as an invisible, anonymous voice of authority, but as a real, historical, bounded individual?

Obviously, the kind and amount of information that experimenters should include will vary with the research topic and methods. To some extent, the question of what to include is an empirical one. We know, for instance, that gender of the experimenter so often produces an effect that interacts with gender of subject, regardless of the research topic, that gender of experimenter should probably always be noted. If a researcher is comparing forms of treatments, his or her theoretical orientation and affiliation with the treatments under study are of obvious interest to readers. As with descriptions of respondents, the information to be reported reflects the researchers' (or others') "best guess" about which variables other than those directly under study may affect the outcome of the research. Depending upon the research topic, aside from gender, the researchers' ethnic background, subarea, professional socialization, theoretical orientation, and a brief description of research experience are likely candidates for consideration.

To underscore the point that the attributes, background, and beliefs of the researcher are part of the empirical evidence for (or against) the claims advanced in the discussion, the description of the researchers may be inserted in the methods section of the report, alongside the description of respondents. Where this is not possible due to editorial policy, the material should be included in a footnote.

Because of the tendencies within our discipline to minimize the roles of values in science and embrace the "objectivist" stance, we can expect great reluctance among mainstream psychologists to "uncover" the experimenter, as this opens the investigator's perspective to critical scrutiny and may seem to limit or compromise the validity of the research. Given the growing body of evidence that experimenters' beliefs and characteristics affect results, there are solid scientific grounds to argue that this information should be open to scrutiny no less than what has been conventionally defined as relevant information. As Harding (1987) noted: "Introducing the 'subjective element' into the analysis in fact increases the objectivity of the research and decreases the 'objectivism' which hides this kind of evidence from the public" (p. 9).

Sample Selection

Issues and problems related to the selection of research participants have received much attention from psychologists who are interested in gender differences and gender-fair research. Wallston and Grady (1985) point out that, however perfunctory, brief, and inadequate they are, descriptions of respondents in psychological reports almost always include the gender of the respondents. While the routine inclusion of gender is largely due to mere convention, it also reflects pervasive assumptions that gender is a variable that might influence the outcome of research.

Despite widespread beliefs within the discipline that the gender of respondents has the potential to affect the results of a study, psychologists have long recognized the problems with conceptualizing gender as an independent variable. For one thing, gender is a descriptive, rather than a conceptual, variable, with obvious biological (genetic, hormonal, and physiological) and sociocultural (relating to socialization and social, economic, educational, and familial status) components (McHugh et al., 1986). If males and females differ on the dependent variable, it is hardly clear which of the innumerable variables confounded with biological sex actually "caused" the effect.

Psychologists have crafted a number of solutions to the problems associated with the use of gender as an independent variable. Perhaps the most common solution is drawing the same number of males and females from a single setting, specifying the sex composition of the sample, and declaring that one has "controlled for sex." As Wallston and Grady (1985) note, males and females are never randomly assigned to gender and thus are never "equivalent" prior to an intervention. For this reason, studies that compare males and females are in fact quasi-experiments rather than true experiments. As such, any gender comparisons are vulnerable to a variety of threats to internal validity, as we discuss in the section on quasi-experiments below, and inferences based on such comparisons are indeed difficult to support.

It is often overlooked that the sample of males and females available in a given setting are often actually drawn from quite different populations with respect to factors that affect the dependent variables. When the sample is comprised of males and females from different populations, the researcher is essentially "creating" rather than "uncovering" a gender difference. For example, a study of gender differences in marital attitudes using husbands and wives would be quite compromised if the men in the sample were significantly older, better educated, and better paid than the women, even though husbands and wives would presumably be quite similar on a number of other dimensions. Similarly, increasing attention has been paid in recent years to how males and females differ in life span activities (McHugh et al., 1986; Paludi, 1986). Thus, whereas males and females of the same age may be engaged in very different pursuits and express different values and attitudes, males and females engaged in a particular activity or found in the same setting may be at very different ages.

With college students, probably the most common respondent population studied in our discipline, a number of considerations arise. Studies of gender differences may be distorted if the proportions of males and females available are quite different or if one gender is more difficult to recruit or less likely to comply with the requirements of the study. Depending on the research topic, the special characteristics of the males and females who attend a school, choose a major, or enroll in a course should be taken into account. For example, a recent study of the achievement motivation and college enrollment patterns of Italian-American students in the City University of New York (CUNY) suggested that Italian-American women were significantly more achievement-oriented than their male peers and were enrolled in college in greater numbers (Sterzi, 1988). However, subsequent analyses revealed that a strikingly high proportion of the male siblings of female students in the sample were enrolled in or had attended private colleges. Sterzi reasoned that Italian-American parents might be more likely to finance their sons' private college education than their daughters'. Thus, the Italian-American population at a relatively inexpensive public university like CUNY would contain proportionately more achievement-oriented, academically successful Italian-American women than men.

Another historically popular solution to the problems posed by gender-of-respondent effects is the use of single-gender designs. As we noted earlier, traditionally, males have appeared more often as respondents, although there is some evidence that this trend is changing and even reversing itself. There are many reasons given for the choice of studying only one gender. Some are quite practical, as when the investigator points to the need to limit the sample size or avoid costly attempts to recruit the less available gender. Less commonly, the researcher may express a preference for one gender because of beliefs about that gender's reliability in honoring research commitments or ability to endure a treatment. Many researchers use one gender to avoid having to study the vast, murky literature on gender differences, test for gender differences, and interpret any differences that might emerge.

Some investigators offer conceptual reasons for the focus on one gender (Denmark et al., 1988). These reasons are based on the assumption that the research topic is only relevant to one gender. Thus, studies on infant attachment, parental employment effects on children, interpersonal attraction, and the effects of hormonal fluctuations on cognitive ability have tended to use women and girls as respondents, whereas research on aggression, parental absence, homosexuality, antisocial behavior, sexual dysfunction, and sexual responsiveness in infancy have tended to use males.

While often unstated, the assumptions underlying the choice of males in critical theory-building studies appear to be that males are more important, function at higher levels, and behave in ways closer to the "ideal adult" than females. Thus, as we have shown, it is much more common that studies using males are generalized to females than that studies using females are generalized to males (McHugh et al., 1986; Denmark et al., 1988). No major theory of human behavior has gained acceptance within psychology after being tested exclusively on female samples, and yet major theories on achievement motivation and moral development have relied almost exclusively on research with males for their support. Similarly, in animal studies, more theories or evidence for physiological or neurobiological mechanisms have relied almost exclusively on male subjects and are then likely to be generalized to females.

Obviously, as we noted earlier, the use of single-sex designs is sometimes justifiable on theoretical grounds. In a given study, practical considerations may override others in the choice of single-sex designs, so long as the limitations of the design are clearly acknowledged. But overall, the widespread, unexamined practice of studying one sex has been costly to psychology. It has led to the development of theories that were intended to describe both sexes but are relevant only to one, and it has consistently failed to challenge sexist assumptions about the differences in behaviors, interests, and abilities between males and females.

Like the choice of treatment groups, the choice of control groups reflects hypotheses about what variables may affect the dependent variable. As many methodologists recognize, the choice of control groups is not a minor methodological consideration but a major determinant of the interpretability and validity of the study. This choice takes on special significance in the study of gender differences, because males and females are nonequivalent groups and differ on those many variables that are confounded with biological sex. The report by Denmark et al. (1988) on studies of gender differences in job turnover illustrates this point. These studies consistently suggest that women have higher rates of turnover than men. However, it was noted that turnover is correlated with job status, with those in lower-status jobs quitting more often than those in high-status positions. In these studies, gender has been confounded with job status, as women were more likely to hold low-status positions than men. When the appropriate comparison group was selected to control for job status, no gender differences in job turnover emerged.

It should be noted that controlling for variables that are confounded with gender may not be enough (P. B. Campbell, 1983). Some variables are themselves quite biased, such as socioeconomic status, which may use a husband's or father's occupational level or income to determine the woman's status.

A further problem with studying variables like socioeconomic level or occupational level along with gender is that occupations that have a higher proportion of women than men, like elementary school teaching, nursing, and stenography, are frequently less lucrative than occupations that employ more men than women, like plumbing or automobile mechanics, but require higher educational levels. It is important to determine precisely how levels of these variables are determined.

A final, often overlooked issue to be considered in selecting a sample is sample size. Whenever gender is treated as an independent variable, past research suggests that males and females are highly heterogeneous with respect to virtually all dependent variables. Thus, with so many uncontrolled variables present, gender groups might well be comprised of a number of different subgroups that should be considered separately. Under these conditions, only relatively small gender differences can be expected and large samples of males and females may be needed to detect differences. Of course, the larger the sample, the more likely it is that statistically significant differences will be attained. For these reasons, measures of the magnitude of effects should be calculated more regularly in research on gender differences (to be discussed further below), and the practical and social significance of the findings needs to be assessed quite apart from statistical significance.

Research Design

Due to space constraints, the sheer amount of material available on these topics, and the number of excellent treatments elsewhere (Cook & Campbell, 1979; Wallston & Grady, 1985; Wallston, 1983; Richardson & Kaufman, 1983), this treatment of research designs will be relatively brief. It will focus on how feminist concerns affect the choice of research designs and design issues of interest to feminists in the conduct of research rather than on how to implement these designs.

True Experiments

As we have already noted, true or randomized experiments are ones in which respondents are randomly assigned to experimental and control groups. They provide the strongest evidence of all research designs that a treatment causes an effect. When the conditions for experimentation are favorable, true experiments have considerable advantages over other designs in probing causal questions.

Many feminist methodologists who acknowledge the advantages of true experiments have also been quite critical of them in recent years, finding them more "time-consuming, laborious, and costly" than other designs (cf. Wallston, 1983). While this perception is fairly widespread, as Cook and Campbell (1979) note, there is no inherent reason this should be so and little evidence that this is in fact the case. Random assignment to treatment per se usually adds little or nothing to the expenditure of time, labor, or money by the researcher, administrators, or research participants. Even in cases where random assignment is more costly than other modes of selection to treatment, its advantages over other modes of assignment often outweigh any minor inconvenience that its implementation might entail.

Nonetheless, there are many real impediments to conducting true experiments, especially in the field, some disadvantages to them, and many instances in which they are less appropriate than other designs. Obstacles to conducting true experiments may be ethical or practical in nature. Fortunately for humane and ethical reasons, psychologists will never assign people at random to some of life's most powerful and affecting treatments like loss of a loved one, becoming a parent, surviving a catastrophe, or receiving a formal education. In fact, most potent treatments, those that may conceivably cause participants any stress, embarrassment, discomfort, or inconvenience, are no longer permissible under current federal regulations that govern the actions of Institutional Review Boards (IRBs) for the protection of human subjects for research, as well as the guidelines of the American Psychological Association (APA). For these reasons, especially in the laboratory, typical treatments are trivial, short-lived, and unlikely to have large or lasting impacts on participants.

In real world settings, where important, long-term treatments are more feasible, it may be difficult to justify withholding seemingly beneficial or appealing treatments from control groups or administering treatments to groups that vary greatly in perceived attractiveness. Other practical considerations may preclude the conduct of true experiments in the field. Often, these are the result of the investigator's relative lack of control over field settings. Frequently, investigators fail to make the case for random assignment to harried administrators who are mainly concerned about its effects on their constituents and bureaucracy and skeptical about its importance. Even those administrators who appreciate the value of random assignment on scientific grounds may reject it due to the inconvenience, displacement, or resistance that it might cause.

True experiments are ideal when the state of knowledge in an area is advanced enough to permit the experimenter to identify a limited number of important independent variables, specify the relevant levels of those variables, operationalize them adequately, and measure specific effects of those variables with sensitivity and precision. Under the best of conditions, only a small number of independent and dependent variables can be studied in any one experiment, affording true experiments limited opportunity to detect interaction effects, measure the effects of variables at extreme levels, or capture the richness and complexity of a real world setting. Wallston (1981, 1983) has pointed to some of the problems that arise when experiments are performed prematurely: the choice of variables or levels of variables may be arbitrary, operationalizations may be inadequate, and experimental situations may be so unlikely and contrived as to yield misleading findings.

Despite their considerable advantages in establishing the existence of causal relationships (high internal validity and statistical validity), true experiments sometimes compromise the investigator's abilities to generalize to, and across, other operationalizations (construct validity) and other places, people, and times (external validity) due to their artificiality, obtrusiveness, or overreliance on certain kinds of manipulations, measures, research participants, or settings. Thus, while true experiments best equip researchers to probe the question, Does the treatment cause the effect?, they are often less helpful in suggesting what it is that the treatment and effect should be labeled in theory-relevant terms and whether that cause-effect relationship would hold in other settings and times or with other participants.

Problems determining how the treatments and effects should be labeled conceptually—construct validity concerns—are particularly interesting and troubling to psychologists. It is a well-established finding in social science research that when people know that they are being observed, they behave differently than they would otherwise. It is also well documented that when research participants estimate that a particular response is more socially desirable than others, they tend to favor that response over others to present themselves in a more positive light. In this way, demand characteristics—extraneous features of the experimental setting that cue participants about how they should respond—are more likely to operate in true experiments conducted in laboratory settings than in nonexperimental research in the field. Demand characteristics undoubtedly contribute to the finding that gender-of-stimuli effects are more common in the literature than gender-of-respondent effects. Unger (1979) has summarized how demand characteristics may operate when gender-of-stimuli is studied: "Using no stimulus materials other than the label male or female, investigators have found that the sex-of-stimulus person alters people's criteria for mental health, affects their evaluation of the goodness and badness of performance, leads them to make differential attributions about the causes of someone's behavior and induces differential perceptions about the values of others'' (p. 1090).

As problematic as it has been to interpret the meaning of gender-of-stimuli effects in true experiments, attempts to study gender-of-subject effects in true experimental designs have posed even greater difficulties. As Wallston (1983) has pointed out, people cannot be randomly assigned to gender, so that cross-gender comparisons always render a design quasi-experimental and vulnerable to threats to internal validity. This will be discussed below.

Most research psychologists have been far more extensively trained in experimental methods than in alternative designs and have been professionally socialized to revere the true experiment. True experiments have been quite useful to feminist researchers in exploring the effects of gender and exposing sexist myths and will surely continue to serve feminist scientists well. But the limitations of true experiments are increasingly obvious in the study of gender and other variables. Often the choice for researchers is between exploring critical variables like gender, race, age, and central life experiences with nonexperimental methods and avoiding them entirely. Where true experiments are used to study these topics, the information they supply should be supplemented with data gathered using different designs with different assets and shortcomings.

Quasi-Experiments

Quasi-experiments are similar to true experiments in that they are composed of treatment and no-treatment comparison groups. But unlike true experiments, in quasi-experiments assignment to group is not random, and thus groups are nonequivalent at the outset. When experimental groups are different even before the treatment is administered, any differences that emerge among groups at the posttest period cannot be attributed to the treatment in any simple way. Instead, a host of plausible hypotheses that rival the one that the treatment caused the effect must be painstakingly eliminated before a causal relationship can be said to exist between the treatment and the effect. When gender of respondent is studied as an ''independent'' variable, it is incumbent upon the investigator to adduce established scientific laws, research evidence, logic, and common sense to make the case that gender, and not any of the ubiquitous factors to be discussed below, ''caused'' the effect.

Cook and Campbell (1979), guided by their own extensive research experience and substantive readings in social science and philosophy, have compiled the following list of plausible factors, other than the independent variables, that can affect dependent measures. All of the following major threats to the internal validity of an experiment are eliminated when random assignment to conditions is correctly carried out and maintained throughout the experiment; they may, however, operate to reduce the interpretability of many quasi-experiments, including all studies that compare males and females:

- *History*. This is a threat when an effect might be due to an event that takes place between the pretest and posttest other than the treatment. These extraneous events are much more likely to occur in field research than in laboratory settings.
- *Maturation*. This is a threat when an effect might be due to respondents growing older, wiser, more experienced, and so on between the pretest and the posttest periods, when this development is not the variable of interest.
- *Testing*. This is a threat when the effect might be the result of repeated testing. Respondents may become more proficient over time as they become more familiar with the test.
- *Instrumentation*. This is a threat when an effect might be due to a change in the measuring instrument or data-gathering technique between pretest and posttest and not to the treatment.
- *Regression to the mean*. This is a threat due to a particular statistical artifact rather than to the treatment. The statistical artifact is most likely to operate when respondents are selected on the basis of extremely high or low pretest scores. Extreme scores are likely to contain more error than scores closer to the mean and are thus more likely than other scores to "regress" to the mean in a subsequent test. This regression can appear to be a treatment effect.
- *Selection*. This is the most pervasive threat of all to valid inference in quasi-experiments. It operates when an effect may be due to preexisting differences among groups rather than the treatment.
- *Mortality*. This is a threat when an effect may be due to different rates of attrition in treatment and control groups.

"Interactions with selection" threaten validity when any of the foregoing factors interact with selection to produce forces that might spuriously appear as treatment effects.

Males and females are inherently nonequivalent groups that can be expected to differ considerably on life experiences, rates of development, familiarity with stimuli, pretest scores, and so on. Thus, these threats to internal validity commonly operate in studies where males and females are compared and make it difficult to conclude that it was gender alone (leaving aside the issue of identifying what aspect of gender it was) that caused the effect.

Generally, the interpretability of quasi-experimental designs depends upon two factors: how the treatment and control groups are selected and the pattern of the results.

In general, the closer the selection process is to random assignment—the more haphazard the selection process—the stronger the interpretability of the design.

When treatment groups are formed using preexisting, intact groups or, more troublesome still, when respondents are permitted to select themselves into or out of treatment groups, the chances are good that variations among respondents other than the treatment account for posttest differences. The pattern of results, especially when interaction effects are studied, enables the investigator to rule out many of the threats to internal validity that may seem implausible given known features of the sample or well-established scientific laws concerning, for instance, the effects of maturation, statistical regression, and so on.

Two of the most common quasi-experimental designs—and potentially the strongest—are the multiple time-series design and the nonequivalent control group design with pretest and posttest periods. In the nonequivalent control group design the existence of pretests enables the investigator to identify and address the probable preexisting differences between groups. The inclusion of a well-chosen comparison group can help rule out many threats to internal validity. The multiple time-series design is highly similar to the nonequivalent control group design but improves upon it by featuring many pretest and posttest measures for both the treatment and comparison groups. These added observations help investigators assess and rule out threats like history, maturation, statistical regression, and testing with greater confidence than they would have if only a single pretest and posttest measure were available.

If true experiments reign in the laboratory, quasi-experiments are often carried out in real world settings where the investigator does not have full control over the means of assignment to treatment conditions, the implementation of the treatment, or the collection of the data. Clearly, quasi-experiments often represent a compromise between the investigator's desire to exercise control over the independent and dependent variables and the practical constraints of the external environment. Despite their methodological disadvantages relative to true experiments in achieving high internal validity, quasi-experiments are often less contrived, obtrusive, and reactive than true experiments and may possess higher construct and external validity.

However appealing the relative "naturalness" of quasi-experiments is to many feminist researchers, it bears remembering that more evidence in support of sex-role stereotypes and gender differences has been found in field settings than in the laboratory, where confounded variables can be teased apart. Even the strongest quasi-experiments, those that employ similar comparison groups and feature pretests and posttests, require tremendous caution in their interpretation.

Passive Observational Methods

Passive observational methods, sometimes known as correlational designs, are ones in which the investigator neither designs nor controls the "treatment" but merely measures it. Without any control over the independent variable, a potentially limitless number of factors may vary with the variable of interest. As deficient as these designs generally are for probing causal questions, they undeniably have their place in the social sciences for generating research hypotheses and, in their more recent, sophisticated forms, can shed some light on causal relationships.

Passive observational methods are most appropriate when the variables of interest profoundly affect people—for example, unemployment, bereavement, alcoholism, home ownership, inheriting a fortune. Clearly, it is unthinkable on ethical and practical grounds for a researcher to manipulate such events. Further, when exploring a new area of study, passive observation can generate rich hypotheses for future research. Many programs of research are launched with correlational designs that suggest what variables and levels of variables and interactions will be useful to probe in future investigations. These techniques are also indicated when the researcher seeks to establish a relationship among variables and intends to measure the strength of that relationship but is relatively unconcerned with demonstrating a causal connection among variables, as in certain kinds of forecasting.

The measurement techniques used within observational designs are not necessarily different from those that are featured in more controlled designs. There is a tendency for observational studies to rely more heavily than experimental designs on data-gathering techniques like category selection, self-report measures like surveys, interviews, and questionnaires, and the use of historical and archival records.

Feminist methodologists have long recognized and publicized how impressive the range and quality of information gathered through passive observational methods can be (Wallston & Grady, 1985, Sherif, 1987; Fine & Gordon, 1989; Gilligan, 1983). More sophisticated observational designs like cross-lagged panel and path-analytical techniques permit the investigator to probe questions beyond the simple standards in correlational analyses: Is there any kind of relationship between variables? How strong is the relationship? How well can we predict the value of one variable from the value of the other?

Regression approaches enable researchers to ask more complex questions of information gathered using nonexperimental designs: Can a simple rule be formulated for predicting one variable from a combination of others? If so, how good is the rule? Regression analyses are especially useful in applied research, where researchers need to predict future behavior or outcomes based on current available information.

Through the correlational technique of factor analysis, the investigator who is faced with a multitude of items that measure various aspects of a behavior, feeling, attitude, or belief can determine which items are highly intercorrelated and represent a single underlying construct. Factor analyses can be quite helpful to basic researchers who are interested in establishing the discriminant and concomitant validity of their theoretical constructs and to applied researchers working in such areas as survey and questionnaire construction, consumer psychology, and personnel selection who need to isolate the factors that underlie people's perceptions, attitudes, abilities, and so on.

Very recently, methodologists have shown how passive observational methods may be employed for the purpose of causal inference (Cook & Campbell, 1979; Boruch, 1983). The opportunity for exploring the direction of causality between variables exists when there are repeated measures of the same two variables over time. Sophisticated modes of analyses such as path analysis, causal modeling, and cross-lagged panel correlation can be applied to observational data when an adequate number of observations are available, and help the researcher infer which of all possible causal relationships among variables are more or less likely.

Operationalizations

Experimental Stimuli and Tasks

Males and females throughout the life span differ in the ideas, objects, and events to which they are exposed, the behaviors they are able to practice, and the reinforcements they receive in the real world. For these reasons, we can expect them to enter any experimental situation with different orientations, attitudes, perceptions, expectations, and skills. There is a growing body of literature suggesting that males and females in fact do respond to objectively "identical" stimuli differently, at least in part because the stimuli are more familiar, salient, relevant, or meaningful to one gender than the other (Jacklin, 1983). In most cases, the tasks and stimuli employed in psychological studies have tended to favor males and have served to reinforce sexist stereotypes.

One classic example of how differential experience with experimental stimuli can distort findings is provided by Sistrunk and McDavid (1971). They demonstrated that the research indicating that females are more conforming than males was systematically flawed because it was based on experimental tasks that were more relevant and familiar to males than females. Another is the reinterpretation of the literature on short-term persuasion and suggestion by Eagly (1983), who found no evidence for the widely cited finding that females are generally more suggestible than males. Eagly performed an extensive meta-analysis of the experimental literature in these areas and concluded that gender differences are largely due to formal status inequities by which men are more likely than women to have high-status roles.

Perhaps the most dramatic illustration of how differing interpretations of experimental stimuli by males and females can distort results was furnished by Gilligan (1982). She argued that the traditional conceptualizations of moral development offered by Piaget and Kohlberg reflect male experience and thought. Using a variety of research methods, she has shown that females perceive moral dilemmas quite differently from males and respond to different cues in making moral judgments. Her work seriously challenged the assumption underlying the tests of moral reasoning by Piaget and Kohlberg that there is a universal standard of development and a single scale of measurement along which differences can be designated as "higher" or "lower" in the moral sphere.

In this connection, Unger (1979) has written persuasively about the importance of ascertaining the meaning of experimental stimuli and tasks to respondents and the dangers of assuming that all respondents share the investigator's perceptions and assumptions.

As noted above, in the past decade the literature on sex-role research has forced a distinction between gender-of-stimuli effects and gender-of-subject effects. Up until recently, it was not uncommon that "male" versions of a test were offered to men and boys, and "female" versions to women and girls (Jacklin, 1983). Erroneous conclusions about gender differences were commonly deduced from these investigations. When different stimuli are presented to males and females, gender-of-respondents is confounded with gender-of-stimuli. Feminist methodologists have made the point that if the genders are to be compared, identical stimuli must be presented to both genders.

Gender of the Experimenter and Confederates

A common complaint among psychological researchers is that methods sections are typically so sketchily drawn that they rarely contain enough information about the study's materials, procedure, and context to permit replication or even a clear understanding of how extraneous variables may have affected the results. Among the information typically omitted in research reports are the gender of the experimenter and confederates and the gender composition of the sample as a whole or relevant subgroups of the sample. In this manner, researchers themselves refuse or fail to consider that these variables may affect the dependent variables, and they prevent others from making an independent evaluation of the operation of these variables. Such omissions seriously threaten the interpretability and generalizability of the research, as there is strong evidence that the gender of the investigator, confederates, and others in the experimental situation differentially affects the responses of males and females (McHugh et al., 1986). Whenever possible, multiple experimenters and confederates and varied, mixed-gender samples should be employed. In all cases, information on the gender of all participants in the research should be specified.

Single-Gender Designs

In their extensive review of the literature in the areas of aggression and attraction, McKenna and Kessler (1977) found strong evidence for gender bias in the operationalization of variables in single-gender designs. In aggression studies, for example, they found that male respondents were more often exposed to active or direct manipulations than female respondents. Whereas male respondents were frustrated, threatened, or treated in a hostile way in the experimental situation, females more often read vignettes that manipulated aggression less directly.

Dependent Measures

A pervasive gender bias in tests and measures has had a significant impact on entire areas of research. P. B. Campbell (1983) has indicated how sex differences can be created or eliminated through the selection of test items with certain forms and contents. After reviewing the research on gender differences in achievement and aptitude testing, Campbell concluded that girls do better than boys on problems with a stereotypically female orientation, like those dealing with human relationships. Boys, on the other hand, tend to do better than girls on problems with a stereotypically male orientation, like those on the topics of science and economics. Aside from item content, test format also affects the performance of males and females. Females tend to score higher on essay and fill-in-the-blank items than they do on multiple choice items, whereas males do better on multiple choice questions than they do on essay and fill-in-the-blank questions.

When data about feelings, attitudes, beliefs, social or moral judgments, or behaviors are obtained through self-report measures, it must be considered that males and females may differ on their willingness or ability to be candid (P. B. Campbell, 1983). Campbell has found that males are more defensive and less disclosing than females. Richardson and Kaufman (1983) note that males tend to present themselves as confident and self-assured when evaluating or predicting their ability, performance, or self-worth, whereas females tend to be self-effacing in these situations. These differences in response styles, which probably reflect gender-role expectations, strongly suggest that comparisons based on self-report measures should be cautiously interpreted and supplemented with comparisons based on other kinds of measures.

Data Analysis and Interpretation

Traditionally, whenever both genders are studied together, analyses of gender differences tend to be made—whether or not such differences are hypothesized or interpretable. In part because group differences are more interpretable and publishable than findings of no difference and partially because gender differences are more dramatic than similarities, gender differences are more likely to be reported, explained, and integrated into the literature than gender similarities. We have a large and lively literature on ''sex differences'' in psychology, but, as Unger (1979) notes, there is no parallel literature of ''sex similarities'' that seeks to integrate the innumerable studies in which no differences between males and females are found.

In fact, the most thorough, all-inclusive review of the cross-cultural literature on gender differences ever conducted has found strong evidence for very few gender differences (Maccoby & Jacklin, 1974). The work of Maccoby and Jacklin has gone far to dispel many popular myths about gender that have permeated bodies of literatures in psychology and to warn psychologists about the dangers of overgeneralizing gender differences.

Jacklin's (1983) vast experience in evaluating the extensive literature on gender differences has informed her perspective on a number of issues relevant to data interpretation. One concerns the meaning of the word *difference* and how misleading it can be. She notes that one of the largest gender differences to emerge in any body of literature is in the tendency to engage in rough-and-tumble play. Even in this case, 85% of boys are indistinguishable from 85% of girls. This finding speaks to the issue of the size and meaning of gender differences. With a large enough sample, virtually any mean difference between groups will achieve statistical significance. Even the few gender differences that appear to be durable over different peoples, places, and times rarely account for more than 5% of the variance (Deaux, 1984). These findings suggest that there is more variability within gender than between gender, how weak gender of respondent is as a determinant of behavior, and how important it is that researchers report the size of the effect along with comparison tests. Denmark et al. (1988) have cautioned psychologists against exaggerating the size of gender differences or drawing misleading implications from the results of comparison tests in their conclusions. These errors occur when it is suggested, for example, that females should be discouraged from careers in architecture or engineering because they tend to score slightly lower on average than males in tests of spatial ability or that females are less stable or rational than males when subtle performance variations occur with hormonal fluctuations. Other common errors in data interpretation occur when results based on one gender are generalized to both sexes. As noted earlier, this is routine practice with animal research, where, for example, threshold measurements in shock sensitivity for rats have been standardized for males only but are often generalized to both sexes (Denmark et al., 1988). A similar mistake is made when an investigator generalizes from a within-gender difference to a between-gender difference. For instance, if a significant correlation between two variables has been found for one gender but not the other, it cannot be concluded that a gender difference has been found (Jacklin, 1983).

Many feminist methodologists regard the number of variables confounded with gender as the most pervasive problem in interpreting gender differences (Unger, 1979; Deaux, 1984; Wallston & Grady, 1985; Eagly, 1987). As noted above, because males and females are "nonequivalent" at the outset of every experiment, any gender difference that may emerge at the end of the study cannot be attributed to gender per se without tremendous, explicit effort to rule out numerous plausible alternate explanations. In many cases, the males and females sampled in a particular study are drawn from very different populations with respect to the variables under study, especially when volunteers comprise the sample.

Even where gender differences exist, they have frequently been mislabeled in the literature. Many feminist writers have noted the tendency of researchers to assume that gender differences are biologically caused and immutable, although no evidence for either biological origins or inevitability may be presented (Unger, 1979; McHugh et al., 1986; Denmark et al., 1988). They argue that some gender differences may indeed be biologically determined but that the majority of studies offering such interpretations do not specify or measure the presumed causal genetic, hormonal, or physiological mechanisms involved. Frequently such studies rely in their interpretations of differences on "commonsense" notions of gender differences that incorporate popular myths, stereotypes, and prescientific notions of the origins of personality and abilities. Research reports that offer biological explanations for gender differences in the absence of solid evidence also tend to adopt simplistic models of human behavior, based on single factor causation. McHugh et al. (1986) note that most present-day researchers appear to believe that sex-related behaviors originate and are sustained in a context of interactions among biological, social, cultural, and situational factors. Behavior is multiply determined, and it is necessary on scientific as well as moral grounds to consider all possible causal factors—biological, social, cultural, and situational—even though not all variables can be explored in any one study and many are quite difficult to study using currently available research methods.

Among possible causal factors, the special status of biological variables and explanations of gender differences based on them cannot be ignored. Unger (1981) has noted that biological variables are regarded as having unalterable and pervasive effects on behavior, whereas social and cultural variables are seen as having more fleeting and limited effects. Because of the presumed prepotency of biology, those who attribute gender differences to biological factors bear the special burden of seeing their findings overapplied and misapplied over a broad range of social policy issues. Oversimplified conclusions regarding gender differences drawn from such studies can provide "scientific" justification for discriminatory policies that can seriously restrict individual opportunity throughout society. If we can conclude anything from the vast literatures on "sex differences," it is that males and females are more alike on virtually every dimension than they are different. Broad generalizations about gender differences bolstered by the simplistic notion that "biology is destiny" are simply unwarranted.

Finally, when gender differences are reported, value judgments are frequently made about the directions of the differences. Thus, male "rationality" is contrasted with female "emotionality," male "dominance" against female "submissiveness," male "independence" against female "dependence," and male "universal sense of justice" with female "amorality" or "particularity." In most instances, labels with such pejorative connotations are applied to females in the absence of any independent evidence that the behavior or trait being described actually exists or, if it does exist, that it is in any way dysfunctional, pathological, or problematic. The unspoken assumption underlying such evaluations appears to be that if the response is more often associated with females than males, there must be something wrong with it. There is much evidence to suggest that stereotypically male behaviors, attitudes, and values are more highly prized than their presumed female counterparts (Denmark et al., 1988). For example, high mathematical ability, which is regarded as a male strength, is valued more than high verbal proficiency, a traditional area of female superiority. The "male tendency" to control or hide one's emotions is widely seen as more adaptive than the corresponding "female tendency" to express one's feelings, despite the recent work in health psychology suggesting the health dangers of suppressing many emotions and the health benefits of ventilating one's feelings. Instead of permitting sexist or other biased assumptions about the value of behaviors to color their conclusions, researchers would do well to consider the adaptive features of behaviors or traits that have traditionally been viewed with disfavor.

Ironically, females whose responses are closer to the means of males in the sample than females are more often derogated for their nontraditional behavior than lauded for their similarity to the male ideal. Identical performances by males and females will earn males evaluations like "assertive" or "active" and females the more dubious labels of "aggressive" or "deviant" (McHugh et al., 1986). Perhaps one of the most misleading effects of these evaluative labels is that they encourage people to view males and females as poles apart on dimensions along which they hardly differ at all. Value judgments like these also ignore the complexity of human behavior and the context in which behavior takes place and have the effect of diminishing the responses of both men and women.

There continues to be a lively debate among feminist researchers about whether and how to analyze and report gender differences. Some champion routine testing for gender differences and reporting of findings, including failures to detect differences (Eagly, 1987; Rothblum, 1988). On the other hand, some (Baumeister, 1988) favor a gender-neutral psychology that neither studies nor reports gender differences. As Gannon et al. (1992) demonstrate, there is a growing trend within social and developmental subfields not to identify respondents' gender, let alone report on gender differences. Whatever one's position on the issue of the analysis and reporting of gender differences, or gender-neutral psychology, it seems to us that, at the minimum, the gender composition of the sample should always be identified. This will enable future scientists to use that information as they see fit.

IMPLICATIONS OF FEMINIST CONCERNS FOR THE TEACHING OF RESEARCH METHODS

The variable that divides people into males and females is surely one of the most fascinating and important, if enigmatic, that we will ever probe in psychology. As chronicled here and elsewhere, there are so many difficulties in attempting to study gender—and similar factors like race, age, and ethnicity—that most mainstream psychologists have chosen to ignore the study of gender differences and many even disparage efforts to do so (Unger, 1979, 1981). But it is difficult to imagine that an understanding of human behavior will progress when the most central psychological variables are systematically avoided. The kinds of questions raised in probing variables like gender, issues such as the role of values in science, and weighing the advantages of differing research methods will not disappear because they are difficult to address.

Just as many academic psychologists today avoid epistemological issues in their own research and writing, they tend to give short shrift to these topics when they train future scientists. The preponderance of time in courses on research methods and statistical analyses is spent teaching the nuts and bolts of conducting, analyzing, and reporting on simple true experiments in the laboratory. Almost no attention is devoted to the relationship between conceptual frameworks and research methods. When alternatives to true experiments, like passive observational methods, are discussed at all, they are generally compared unfavorably with the more tightly controlled approaches and portrayed as methods of last resort.

Many feminist psychologists have become increasingly concerned about the narrowly focused and distorted training available to students and young psychologists at both the graduate and undergraduate levels (Quina, 1986). Not only have they changed their own modes of considering problems and conducting research, but they have also changed how they instruct their students on the topics of epistemology, research methods, and statistical design. Central to their efforts is the notion that sexism, racism, and other conceptual biases have hobbled psychologists' understanding of the human experience. To that end, they attempt to foster students' awareness of their own everyday assumptions about the nature of reality and help them generate alternative and testable conceptualizations.

Paludi is a feminist psychologist who has successfully restructured graduate and undergraduate statistics and research methods courses along these lines (Bronstein & Paludi, 1988.) She has altered both the form and the content of her courses to convey better the range of perspectives and methodologies available to scientists. We will draw extensively from her work to illustrate what alternative courses might look like.

Even on the most superficial levels, alternative methods courses look quite different in their structure from conventional counterparts. Students may, for example, be seated in discussion rather than lecture formats, and instructors may function more as discussion leaders or facilitators than as lecturers. Because few textbooks in these areas have been written from feminist perspectives, feminist instructors often opt to assemble their own lists of readings to supplement or supplant standard texts in these areas. Reading lists for courses like these often consist of numerous primary sources, representing a much broader range of topics and perspectives than is ordinarily offered to students in more traditional courses. For example, in a research methods course, journal articles on the nature and limits of psychological knowledge, ethics and values in science, and the differences between qualitative and quantitative ways of knowing may appear on reading lists alongside more conventional offerings on how to write the method section of a research report. Such articles can be analyzed in a discussion group where students take on the roles of advocates or critics of the various points of view.

To enhance students' understanding of some knotty methodological issues, a series of classroom or homework exercises or small research projects can be designed. In-class exercises can give students a firsthand sense of how variables like gender of experimenter, gender of stimuli, or others discussed here can operate to affect results. Students can be asked to respond to vignettes like those developed by Bronstein and Paludi (1988), in which the gender (race, age, level of disability, and so on) of the target person is varied, providing students with a clear demonstration of their own stereotypes and encouraging them to acknowledge their own biases. Gender-of-stimuli manipulations can be contrasted with parallel gender-of-respondent manipulations to illustrate the effects of gender role expectations. Similarly, the effects of other demand characteristics as they operate in laboratory (and some field) settings can be demonstrated in classroom exercises.

In statistics courses, an illuminating assignment requires students to vary the ways in which they report a set of data, to see how mode of presentation influences how results are interpreted. Encouraging students to present results in multiple modes—in graphs, tables, and words—and to apply more than one statistical test to the same numbers can help put a data set in perspective. These exercises can fuel the debate on whether statistics do in fact "lie." P. B. Campbell (1988) shows how easy it is to generate data sets where observers are apt to "see" gender differences in a table, but not in a graph, even when the numbers involved are exactly the same. Similarly, one can readily demonstrate how the type of statistical analysis used creates or obscures a difference. For example, applying an analysis of variance to a set of data supplied by males and females, students may find that a statistically significant gender difference emerges. If a regression analysis is applied to the same set of numbers, it will be revealed that respondents' gender accounts for less than 1% of the variance. Another way of helping students explore the meaning of similarities and differences is to induce them to consider the degree or percentage of overlap in the scores of two groups. Assigning students the task of graphing actual gender differences in skill competencies, for example, can demonstrate that the area of overlap—which is at least 90% even in cases of the largest gender differences—is far greater than the area representing group differences (P. B. Campbell, 1988). Most students who complete this assignment readily grasp the point that effect sizes are needed along with exact probability levels for readers to evaluate the real world significance of any difference found.

For the laboratory sections of such courses, instead of focusing exclusively on the design and reporting of a number of true experiments in the laboratory, students might receive a wider range of assignments that introduce them to different research methods. One alternate assignment might be to conduct an unobtrusive observation of a gender, race, or age-relevant interaction. These observations might occur in a real world setting like a restaurant, supermarket, sports arena, or bus. In another assignment, students might be asked to conduct a content analysis of some aspect of popular culture like television commercials, comic books, and magazine ads for gender, race, or age-relevant material (Bronstein & Paludi, 1988).

Instructors who seek to integrate feminist and cross-cultural perspectives into methods courses have also given consideration to modes of evaluating and grading students other than traditional multiple choice tests, which may offer a distorted view of what some students know. In her quest to fit the type of assessment to the material and the student, Paludi, for example, administers what she calls "problem sets" to students in methods courses. After a unit on a particular topic is completed, students are asked a number of long and short essay questions that may, depending upon the topic covered, require them to analyze journal articles as to the biases, ethical violations, and threats to internal, external, construct, and statistical conclusion validity or to comment critically upon justifications of the research hypotheses, research conclusions, and so on contained therein. These problem sets may be quite lengthy and assigned as take-home exercises, or shorter versions can be administered in class. Students may be assigned the reports to be analyzed or may choose research articles on their own, including their own work. In one problem set, Paludi asks students to outline and prepare lectures for their class on topics like the issues involved in follow-up and replication studies or the place of statistics in psychology. These thought-provoking and sophisticated assignments appear to have great educational value and engage the students in ways that more typical assignments clearly do not and may lead to the creative use of statistics as well as the kind of reflective psychology that so many of us seek.

This chapter, along with some others in this volume, may provide some sense of the content that alternative methods courses might offer. One of the major departures from conventional methods courses is the expanded perspective on the research process. Instead of concentrating so heavily on true experimental designs and a few quantitative modes of data gathering, alternative courses attend to all stages of the research process: the role of theory, the review of relevant literature, the formulation of the research question and hypotheses, the selection of a research design that is well suited to the question, the selection of research participants, data analysis, interpretation of the results, publication of the results, and their incorporation into the scientific literature. The sources of bias and error that can enter into the research process at all stages are discussed, guided by Unger's critical point that methodological biases can be traced to conceptual biases such as ideology, political loyalty, values, convention, and personal background.

It is important to stress here that instructors who take a feminist perspective do not disparage or overlook traditional experimental methods or seek to replace them with less methodologically rigorous designs. The unique virtues of the true experiment for probing causal questions guarantee it a central place in any methods course in psychology, regardless of who teaches the course or how it is taught. Nor do such instructors aim to convert methods courses to "psychology of women" courses by focusing only on gender-relevant issues. One of the great contributions of feminist methodologists has been to demonstrate how concerns about gender studies have illuminated many critical and unresolved issues for all social scientists, regardless of their subject areas.

It is also necessary to acknowledge that these approaches to teaching research methods are not always easy to implement. Many feminist instructors who attempt to make alterations in central departmental offerings like statistics or experimental psychology can expect to meet with departmental resistance. Even if they are granted the academic freedom to teach their courses as they wish, they will not readily find the materials, resources, or guidelines that can help them organize their courses. Instructors of alternative courses may spend more time in consultation with students than those in conventional classes because of the "accessible atmosphere" that so many exercises, demonstrations, discussions, and debates can create.

Many questions arise when we consider these and related changes in methods courses. Will students exposed to so many perspectives, techniques, and methods be overwhelmed and confused? If time is spent on such topics as formulating research questions and conducting literature reviews, will students be able to develop the skills to conduct true experiments? If methods other than experiments are taught, will students fail to develop the proper respect for the unique virtues of experiments? Of course, these and similar questions are empirical and should be addressed by research. It may well be the case, for instance, that students need more, as well as different, kinds of methods courses to grasp the kinds of issues raised here.

As difficult as it may be for many of us to contemplate major changes in core courses, there is evidence of increasing concern among educators that the conventional curriculum in psychology is failing our students (Hall & Sandler, 1982). Many of us who have taught traditional research methods courses are well aware of how poorly they prepare most students to conduct or analyze even the simplest experiments and what little enthusiasm most students have for performing experiments or pursuing research careers. We do not mean to suggest that traditional experimental courses are invariably sexist, ineffective, or unappealing to students or that methods courses taught from a feminist perspective have ready solutions to the many problems inherent in training psychologists. Rather, we maintain that if psychologists are determined to eliminate sexism in their research and teaching, acknowledge feminist perspectives, or integrate the new scholarship on women into the appropriate literatures, they must begin by changing the way they conceptualize, use, and teach research methods. Feminist instructors have made some intriguing and worthwhile suggestions along these lines.

We are unaware of any formal evaluations of what or how much students learn about statistical and research methods when they are taught in a nontraditional fashion or how students taught in alternative ways differ in their knowledge, skills, or attitudes from students taught in more conventional ways. We urge that such evaluations take place soon so that they may contribute to the debate on these issues. Meanwhile, our strong, if informal, impression, based on the unsystematic observation of students in nontraditional classes, is that such varied perspectives and pedagogical techniques may be uncommonly effective at engaging students in the research process: getting them to think creatively about research problems, building their confidence to criticize scholarly articles, and exciting them about the prospects of designing their own studies. Perhaps most importantly, these perspectives and techniques offer them far better prospects of conducting research that captures the authenticity and totality of their own experience.

CONCLUSIONS

In our extensive review we have attempted to provide a foundation for designing gender-fair research projects. We began our analysis with a brief review of past feminist critiques of scientific psychology and focused especially on three interdependent areas that have become of concern to feminists: (1) the role of values in science, (2) issues embedded in the language and conduct of science, and (3) a comparison of qualitative and quantitative methods of research. Our general view of research methods has been expressed in various forms throughout this chapter. That is, unbiased consideration of the research questions posed should be the ultimate arbiter of which methods and research strategies should be used.

Throughout this chapter we have referred constantly to the work of Denmark et al. (1988)—*Guidelines for Avoiding Sexism in Psychological Research*. This document encompasses the issues and problems in gender-fair research presented here. It provides specific examples of common avoidable situations and suggestions for minimizing and eliminating such bias. We hope that the guidelines will be seriously considered along with the information provided in this chapter in conjunction with planning research projects.

Finally, the major goal of this chapter was to offer a feminist perspective on the research process, from problem selection to the analysis and interpretation of results. Feminist methodologists will surely continue to challenge the nature of the truths we seek as well as our modes of pursuit. In so doing, they hold forth the promise of a more morally and scientifically sound discipline. We hope that the perspectives we have offered here will sustain this challenge and help to provide a psychology for all people.

REFERENCES

Abramson, P. R. (1977). Ethical requirements for research on human sexual behavior: From the perspective of participating subjects. *Journal of Social Issues, 33*, 184–189.

Adler, T. (1990). Meta-analysis offers precision estimates. *APA Monitor*, September, p. 4.

Baumeister, R. F. (1988). Should we stop studying sex differences altogether? *American Psychologist, 43*, 1092–1095.

Blakeslee, S. (1988). Female sex hormone is tied to ability to perform tasks. *New York Times*, November 18, p. A1.

Bleier, R. (1984). *Science and gender: A critique of biology and its theories on women.* New York: Pergamon Press.

Boruch, R. F. (1983). Causal models: Their import and their triviality. In B. L. Richardson & J. Wirtenberg (Eds.), *Sex role research: Measuring social change* (pp. 215–248). New York: Praeger Press.

Brody, J. E. (1989). Personal health: Childhood sexual expression. *New York Times*, January 26, p. B9.

Bronfenbrenner, U. (1977). Toward an experimental ecology of human development. *American Psychologist, 32*, 513–531.

Bronstein, P., & Paludi, M. A. (1988). The introductory psychology course from a broader human perspective. In P. Bronstein & K. Quina (Eds.), *Teaching the psychology of people: Resources for gender and sociocultural awareness* (pp. 21–36). Washington, DC: American Psychological Association.

Buchler, J. (1955). *Philosophical Writings of Charles Peirce*. New York: Dover.

Campbell, D. T. (1969). Reforms as experiments. *American Psychologist, 24*, 409–429.

Campbell, P. B. (1983). The impact of societal biases on research methods. In J. Wirtenberg and B. L. Richardson (Eds.), *Methodological issues in sex roles and social change* (pp. 197–214). New York: Praeger Press.

Campbell, P. B. (1988). Who's better? Who's worse? Research and the search for differences. Washington, DC: *U.S. Department of Education Publication*.

Carlson, R. (1972). Understanding women: Implications for personality theory and research. *Journal of Social Issues, 28*(2), 17–32.

Carlson, E. R., & Carlson, R. (1960). Male and female subjects in personality research. *Journal of Abnormal and Social Psychology, 61*(3), 482–483.

Cook, T. D., & Campbell, D. T. (1979). *Quasi-experimentation: Design and analysis issues for field settings*. Chicago: Rand-McNally.

Cook, T. D., & Leviton, B. F. (1980). Effects of suspiciousness of deception and perceived legitimacy of deception on task performance in an attitude change experiment. *Journal of Personality, 39*, 204–20.

Deaux, K. (1984). From individual differences to social categories: Analysis of a decade's research on gender. *American Psychologist, 39*, 105–116.

Denmark, F. L. (1988). Personal communication to Rabinowitz.

Denmark, F. L., Russo, N. F., Frieze, I. H., & Sechzer, J. A. (1988). Guidelines for avoiding sexism in psychological research: A report of the APA ad hoc committee on nonsexist research. *American Psychologist, 43*, 582–585.

Eagly, A. H. (1978). Sex differences in influencability. *Psychological Bulletin, 85*, 86–116.

Eagly, A. H. (1983). Gender and social influence: A social psychological analysis. *American Psychologist, 38*, 971–982.

Eagly, A. H. (1987). Reporting sex differences. *American Psychologist, 42*, 876–879.

Eagly, A. H., & Carli, L. L. (1981). Sex researchers and sex-typed communication as determination of sex differences in influencability: A meta-analysis of social influence studies. *Psychological Bulletin, 90*, 1–20.

Ellsworth, P. C. (1977). From abstract ideas to concrete instances. Some guidelines for choosing natural research settings. *American Psychologist, 32*, 604–615.

Elms, A. C. (1982). Keeping deception honest: Justifying conditions for social scientific research strategems. In T. L. Beauchamp, R. R. Faden, R. J. Wallace, Jr., & L. Walters (Eds.), *Ethical issues in social science research* (pp. 232–245). Baltimore: Johns Hopkins University Press.

Fine, M., & Gordon, S. M. (1989). Feminist transformations of / despite psychology. In M. Crawford (Ed.), *Gender and thought* (pp. 146–174). New York: Springer-Verlag.

Gannon, L., Luchetta, T., Rhodes, K., Pardie, L., & Segrist, D. (1992). Sex bias in psychological research: Progress or complacency? *American Psychologist, 47*, 389–396.

Gergen, K. J. (1973). Social psychology as history. *Journal of Personality and Social Psychology, 26*, 309–320.

Gilligan, C. (1982). *In a different voice: Psychological theory and women's development.* Cambridge: Harvard University Press.

Gilligan, C. (1983). New ways of development: New visions of maturity. In J. Wirtenberg & B. L. Richardson (Eds.), *Methodological issues in sex roles and social change* (pp. 17–32). New York: Praeger Press.

Glass, G. V. (1976). Primary, secondary, and meta-analysis research. *Educational Researcher, 5*, 3–8.

Grady, K. E. (1981). Sex bias in research design. *Psychology of Women Quarterly, 5*, 628–636.

Hall, J. P. (1990). Lessons from the First European Congress of Psychology. *American Psychologist, 45*(8), 978–980.

Hall, R. M., & Sandler, B. R. (1982). *The classroom climate: A chilly one for women.* Washington, DC: *Project on the Status of Women and the Association of American Colleges.*

Harding, S. (1987). Is there a feminist method? In S. Harding (Ed.), *Feminism and methodology* (pp. 1–17). Bloomington: Indiana University Press.

Harris, S. (1971). Influence of subject and experimenter sex in psychological research. *Journal of Consulting and Clinical Psychology, 37*, 291–294.

Inquiry urged on sex bias in health studies. (1989, December 18). *New York Times*, p. A20.

Jacklin, C. N. (1983). Methodological issues in the study of sex-related differences. In J. Wirtenberg and B. L. Richardson (Eds.), *Methodological issues in sex roles and social change* (pp. 93–100). New York: Praeger Press.

Jackson, G. B. (1983). Methods for integrative views. In J. Wirtenberg & B. L. Richardson (Eds.), *Methodological issues in sex roles and social change* (pp. 173–196). New York: Praeger Press.

Kayne, N. T., & Alloy, L. B. (1988). Clinician and patient as aberrant actuaries: Expectation-based distortions in assessment of covariation. In L. Y. Abramson (Ed.), *Social cognition and clinical psychology* (pp. 295–365). New York: Guilford Press.

Keller, E. F. (1974). Women in science: An analysis of a social problem. *Harvard Magazine*, Harvard University Press, Boston, p. 14–19.

Keller, E. F. (1982). Feminism and science. *Signs, 7*, 589–602.

Koch, S. (1981). The nature and limits of psychology and knowledge: Lessons of a century qua 'science.' *American Psychologist, 36*, 257–269.

Lott, B. (1985). The potential enrichment of social/personality psychology through feminist research and vice versa. *American Psychologist, 40*, 155–164.

Maccoby, E. E., & Jacklin, C. N. (1974). *The psychology of sex differences.* Stanford, CA: Stanford University Press.

Mannucci, E. (1977). Potential subjects view psychology experiments. (Doctoral dissertation, City University of New York, 1978). *Dissertation Abstracts International, 38*, 3958B–3959B. (University Microfilms, No. DDK 77-32059)

McHugh, M. C., Koeske, R. D., & Frieze, I. H. (1986). Issues in conducting nonsexual psychological research: A guide for researchers. *American Psychologist, 41*, 879–890.

McKenna, W., & Kessler, S. J. (1977). Experimental design as a source of sex bias in social psychology. *Sex Roles, 3*, 117–128.

Paludi, M. A. (1986). Teaching the psychology of gender roles: Some life stage considerations. *Teaching of Psychology, 13*, 133–138.

Paludi, M. A. (1990). Introduction. In M. A. Paludi (Ed.), *Teaching the psychology of women: A manual of resources* (pp. 1–22). Albany, NY: SUNY Press.

Parlee, M. B. (1981). Appropriate control groups in feminist research. *Psychology of Women Quarterly, 5*, 637–644.

Quina, K. (1986). Teaching research methods: A multidimensional feminist curricular transformation plan. *Working paper No. 164*, Wellesley College Center for Research on Women.

Reynolds, P. D. (1979). *Ethical dilemmas and social science research*. San Francisco: Jossey-Bass.

Richardson, B. L., & Kaufman, D. R. (1983). Social science inquiries into female achievement: Recurrent methodological problems. In J. Wirtenberg & B. L. Richardson (Eds.), *Methodological issues in sex roles and social change* (pp. 33–48). New York: Praeger Press.

Rothblum, E. D. (1988). More on reporting sex differences. *American Psychologist, 43*, 1095.

Schlenker, B. R. (1974). Social psychology as a science. *Journal of Personality and Social Psychology, 29*, 1–15.

Sherif, C. W. (1987). Bias in psychology. In S. Harding (Ed.), *Feminism and methodology: Social science issues* (pp. 37–56). Bloomington: Indiana University Press.

Shields, S. A. (1975a). Functionalism, Darwinism, and the psychology of women: A study in social myth. *American Psychologist, 30*, 739–754.

Shields, S. A. (1975b). Ms. Pilgrims Progress: The contributions of Leta Stetter Hollingworth to the psychology of women. *American Psychologist, 30*, 852–857.

Sistrunk, F., & McDavid, J. W. (1971). Sex variable in conforming behavior. *Journal of Personality and Social Psychology, 17*, 200–207.

Smith, C. P. (1983). Ethical issues: Research on deception, informed consent, and debriefing. In *Review of personality and social psychology*, Vol. 4 (pp.297–328). Beverly Hills: Sage.

Sterzi, G. (1988). *Ethnicity, socialization, and academic achievement of Italian-American college students at the City University of New York*. Unpublished doctoral dissertation, CUNY.

Unger, R. (1979). Toward a redefinition of sex and gender. *American Psychologist, 34*, 1085–1094.

Unger, R. K. (1981). Sex as a social reality: Field and laboratory research. *Psychology of Women Quarterly, 5*, 645–653.

Unger, R. (1982). Advocacy versus scholarship revisited: Issues in the psychology of women. *Psychology of Women Quarterly, 7*, 5–17.

Unger, R. (1983). Through the looking glass: No wonderland yet! *Psychology of Women Quarterly, 8*, 9–32.

Wallston, B. S. (1981). What are the questions in the psychology of women: A feminist approach to research. *Psychology of Women Quarterly, 5*, 597–617.

Wallston, B. S. (1983). Overview of research methods in sex roles and social change. In J. Wirtenberg and B. L. Richardson (Eds.), *Methodological issues in sex roles and social change* (pp. 51–76). New York: Praeger Press.

Wallston, B. S., & Grady, K. E. (1985). Integrating the feminist critique and the crisis in social psychology: Another look at research methods. In V. E. O'Leary, R. K. Unger, & B. S. Wallston (Eds.), *Women, gender, and social psychology* (pp. 7–33). Hillsdale, NJ: Erlbaum.

West, S. C., & Gunn, S. P. (1978). Some issues of ethics and social psychology. *American Psychologist*, *33*, 30–38.

Wittig, M. A. (1985). Metatheoretical dilemmas in the psychology of gender. *American Psychologist*, *40*, 800–811.

3

Meta-Analysis in the Psychology of Women

Janet Shibley Hyde and Laurie A. Frost

INTRODUCTION: THE STUDY OF GENDER DIFFERENCES

The tradition of gender differences research has a long history in psychology, much of it predating the modern feminist movement and some of it clearly antifeminist in nature. In the late 1800s, for example, there was great interest in differences in the size of male and female brains and how they might account for the assumed lesser intelligence of women (Hyde, 1990; Shields, 1975). Yet as early as 1910, feminist researchers such as Helen Thompson Woolley wrote well-reasoned critiques of the prevailing research.

In modern psychology, research on gender differences found a home within the field known as differential psychology. Anne Anastasi's *Differential Psychology* first appeared in 1937 and survived to several later editions; it included a chapter on sex differences. Leona Tyler's *The Psychology of Human Differences* had a similar history, first appearing in 1947. The 1958 edition of Anastasi's book, for example, reviewed research on sex differences in abilities (motor skills, perceptual processes, verbal functions, memory, spatial and mechanical aptitudes, numerical aptitudes, and artistic and musical aptitudes), personality (interests and attitudes, sexual behavior, adjustment, aggressiveness and dominance, and masculinity-femininity), and achievement (school achievement and vocational achievement). Anastasi also discussed biological and cultural factors that might contribute to the differences, as well as methodological issues such as the great overlap in distributions for males and females and the effects of selectivity in sampling of male and female populations.

Without doubt, the watershed book on psychological gender differences was Maccoby and Jacklin's *The Psychology of Sex Differences* (1974). Having reviewed more than a thousand studies, they concluded that the following gender differences were fairly well established: (1) girls have greater verbal ability than boys, (2) boys outperform girls in spatial ability, (3) boys perform better than girls on tests of mathematical ability, and (4) males are more aggressive.

Challenging a long-standing tradition of emphasis on gender differences, Maccoby and Jacklin were willing to conclude that some beliefs in gender differences were unfounded, including such beliefs as: (1) girls are more social than boys; (2) girls are more suggestible (imitating and conforming); (3) girls have lower self-esteem; (4) girls are better at low-level cognitive tasks, and boys are better at higher-level cognitive tasks; (5) boys are more analytic; (6) girls are more affected by heredity, boys by environment; (7) girls have less achievement motivation; and (8) girls are more responsive to auditory stimuli, boys to visual stimuli.

Finally, Maccoby and Jacklin concluded that it was still an open question as to whether there were gender differences in the following domains: tactile sensitivity, fear and anxiety, motor activity level, competitiveness, dominance, compliance, and nurturance.

Despite criticisms of Maccoby and Jacklin's methods and conclusions (Block, 1976), the book became an instant classic, and its conclusions continue to be cited as definitive in psychology textbooks to the present day.

In the last decade, feminist psychologists have become increasingly critical of the gender-differences tradition in psychological research. For example, some have argued that the emphasis on gender differences blinds us to gender similarities (Hyde, 1985).

In an important theoretical paper, Hare-Mustin and Marecek (1988) distinguished between alpha bias and beta bias in research and conceptualizations in the psychology of gender. "Alpha bias" refers to the exaggeration of gender differences. "Beta bias," in contrast, refers to the minimizing of gender differences. From a feminist point of view, either bias can be problematic. If differences are exaggerated, for example, the research may serve as a basis for discrimination against women, who are "different." If real differences are minimized or ignored, on the other hand, there are dangers, too; for example, if the large differences in men's and women's wages are ignored, divorce settlements might not provide adequate or equitable support for women and children (Weitzman, 1985).

Meta-analysis is a statistical technique that allows the researcher to synthesize results from numerous studies, and thus it is an especially appropriate tool to apply to questions of gender differences. Moreover, because it yields quantitative results—that is, it provides a measure of the magnitude of the gender difference—it can overcome problems of alpha bias and beta bias. Modern techniques of meta-analysis also can provide a highly nuanced view of gender differences, detecting, for example, those situations in which gender differences in a particular behavior are more likely to occur and those situations in which the gender difference is less likely to be found. This chapter reviews existing meta-analyses of psychological gender differences. Following an introduction to the methods of meta-analysis, we review gender differences in cognitive performance, social behaviors, and motor behaviors.

META-ANALYTIC TECHNIQUES AND METHODOLOGICAL ISSUES

Traditional literature reviews—what might be called narrative reviews—are subject to several criticisms. They are nonquantitative, unsystematic, and subjective, and the task of reviewing 100 or more studies simply exceeds the information-processing capacities of the human reviewer (Hunter, Schmidt & Jackson, 1982).

The review by Maccoby and Jacklin (1974) represented an advance because it made use of systematic vote counting. That is, Maccoby and Jacklin tabled all available studies of gender differences for a particular behavior, permitting the authors and the reader to count the number finding a difference favoring females, the number finding a difference favoring males, and the number finding no difference.

The method of vote counting, unfortunately, also has flaws (Hedges & Olkin, 1985; Hunter et al., 1982). Statisticians have pointed out that vote counting can lead the reviewer to false conclusions (Hunter et al., 1982). For example, if there is a true gender difference in the population, but the studies reviewed have poor statistical power (perhaps because of small sample sizes), the reviewer is likely to conclude that there is no effect because a majority of the studies may find no significant gender difference (for a detailed numerical example of this problem, see Hyde, 1986).

Statistical Methods in Meta-Analysis

Meta-analysis has been defined as the application of "quantitative methods to combining evidence from different studies" (Hedges & Olkin, 1985, p. 13). Essentially, then, it is a quantitative or statistical method for doing a literature review.

A meta-analysis proceeds in several steps. First, the researchers locate as many studies as they can on the particular question of interest. Computerized database searches are very useful in this phase. In the area of psychological gender differences, researchers can often obtain a very large sample of studies. For example, for a meta-analysis of gender differences in verbal ability, we were able to locate 165 studies reporting relevant data (Hyde & Linn, 1988).

Second, the researchers perform a statistical analysis of the statistics reported in each article. For each study, an effect size statistic, d, is computed. For analyses of gender differences, the formula is

$$d = \frac{M_M - M_F}{s}$$

where M_M is the mean of males' scores and M_F is the mean of females' scores; s is the average within-sex standard deviation. Essentially, the d statistic tells us how far apart the male and female means are, in standard deviation units. From a feminist point of view, one of the virtues of the d statistic is that it takes into account not only gender differences (the difference between male and female means), but also female variability and male variability (s, the standard deviation). That is, it recognizes that each sex is not homogeneous.

If means and standard deviations for each sex are not available, d can be computed from other statistics, such as a t test or F test for gender differences. When the dependent variable is dichotomous (e.g., child fights or doesn't) and nonparametric statistics are used, they too can be converted to the effect size d. (For a user-friendly introduction to statistical methods in meta-analysis, see Hedges & Becker, 1986.)

In the third stage of the meta-analysis, the researchers average the d values obtained from all studies. They can then reach conclusions such as the following: Based on 165 studies that reported data on gender differences in verbal ability, the weighted mean effect size (d) was -0.11, indicating a slight female superiority in performance.

Recent developments in meta-analysis make it possible to proceed one step further, to analyzing variations in values of d, that is, in the magnitude of the gender difference, according to various features of the studies (Hedges & Becker, 1986; Hedges & Olkin, 1985). This step is called homogeneity analysis because it analyzes the extent to which the values of d in the set are uniform or homogeneous. If there are large variations in the values of d across studies (and there invariably are), these variations reflect inconsistencies among the studies, and it is the task of the meta-analyst to account for the inconsistencies.

The meta-analysis then proceeds to a model-fitting stage. Either categorical or continuous models can be used. If a categorical model is used, the meta-analyst groups the studies into subsets or categories based on some logical classification system. Statistically, the goal is to find a classification scheme that yields relatively homogeneous values of d within each subset of studies. For example, in an analysis of gender differences in mathematics performance, one could compute an average value of d for studies that measured computation and another value of d for studies that measured mathematical problem solving. Thus investigators can determine whether the gender difference is large for some kinds of mathematics performance and close to zero for others or even if the direction of the gender difference depends on the kinds of mathematics performance assessed; perhaps females perform better on some measures and males on others.

If a continuous model is used in the model-fitting stage, the meta-analyst uses some continuous variable to account for variations among studies in the effect size, d. Essentially, a regression model is fitted in which the effect size is the criterion variable and some relevant continuous variable or variables are the predictors. For example, in studies of aggression, age may be a good predictor of the magnitude of the gender difference (Hyde, 1984).

Methodological Issues

A number of methodological issues in meta-analysis have been raised. Certainly chief among these is an issue of interpretation: When is an effect size large? Because of the way d is computed, it is a statistic much like z, and values can exceed 1. Thus it is impossible to say, in any absolute sense, that a value of .90, or any other value, is large. Cohen (1969) offered the following guidelines: a value of $d = .20$ is small, a value of .50 is moderate, and a value of .80 is large. These guidelines, although useful, are somewhat arbitrary. It is at this stage of interpretation that the problems of alpha bias and beta bias (Hare-Mustin & Marecek, 1988) reappear.

Rosenthal and Rubin (1982c) introduced another scheme for deciding when an effect size is large. They used the Pearson correlation r, rather than d, but the two can easily be translated using the approximation formula $d = 2r$ (or the exact formula $d = 2r\sqrt{(1 - r^2)}$). To assess the magnitude of an effect size, they use the binomial effect size display (BESD). It displays the change in success rate (e.g., recovery from cancer due to treatment with a particular drug compared with an untreated control group) as a function of the effect size. For example, an $r = .30$ ($d = .60$) translates into an improvement in survival from 35% to 65%. Thus, according to Rosenthal and Rubin, effect sizes that appear only small to moderate may represent impressively large effects.

We would argue, however, that impressive effects in curing cancer do not necessarily transfer logically to the study of gender differences. In the latter case, the binomial effect size display can tell us something like the following: An effect size of $d = .40$ means that approximately 40% of one sex falls above the median (40% are above average) and 60% of the other sex falls above the median.

Another approach to interpreting the magnitude of an effect size is to compare it with effect sizes that have been obtained in other meta-analyses, either for related studies in the same field or for studies in other fields. One could compare the effect size for gender differences in mathematics performance with the effect size for gender difference in spatial ability, for example. Or one might compare the effect size for gender differences in mathematics performance with the effect size for social class or ethnic differences in math performance. Table 1 is provided as a guide to making the former kind of comparisons.

Another major methodological issue in meta-analysis concerns the sampling of studies and the potential for sampling bias. Ideally, the sampling procedure should be well defined, systematic, and exhaustive. A poor sampling procedure will produce misleading, if not useless, results. Even with good sampling procedures, however, problems can arise because published results tend to be sta-

Table 1

Average Gender Effect Sizes (*d*) Obtained in Meta-Analyses

Study	Variable	Age	Number of Reports	*d*
COGNITIVE VARIABLES				
Hyde (1981)	Verbal ability	11 and older	12	-.24
	Quantitative ability	11 and older	7	+.43
	Visual-spatial ability	11 and older	8	+.45
	Field articulation	12 and older	14	+.51
Rosenthal & Rubin (1982a)	Verbal ability	11 and older	12	-.30
	Quantitative ability	11 and older	7	+.35
	Visual-spatial ability	11 and older	7	+.50
	Field articulation	12 and older	14	+.51
Meehan (1984)	Propositional logic	All ages	15	+.22
	Combinatorial reasoning	All ages	23	+.10
	Proportional reasoning	All ages	35	+.48
Linn & Petersen (1985)	Spatial perception	All ages	62	+.44
	Mental rotation	All ages	29	+.73
	Spatial visualization	All ages	81	+.13
Whitley et al. (1986)	Attribution of success to ability	Adolescents and adults	29	+.13
	Attribution of success to effort	Adolescents and adults	29	-.04
	Attribution of success to task	Adolescents and adults	29	-.01
	Attribution of success to luck	Adolescents and adults	29	-.07
	Attribution of failure to ability	Adolescents and adults	29	+.16
	Attribution of failure to effort	Adolescents and adults	29	+.15
	Attribution of failure to task	Adolescents and adults	29	-.08
	Attribution of failure to luck	Adolescents and adults	29	-.15
Hyde & Linn (1988)	Vocabulary	All ages	40	-.02
	Analogies	All ages	5	+.16
	Reading comprehension	All ages	18	-.03
	Speech production	All ages	12	-.33
	Essay writing	All ages	5	-.09
	Anagrams	All ages	5	-.22
	General verbal ability	All ages	25	-.20
	SAT-verbal	All ages	4	+.03
Feingold (1988)	DAT verbal reasoning	Adolescents	20	+.05
	DAT spelling	Adolescents	20	-.50
	DAT language	Adolescents	20	-.43
	DAT space relations	Adolescents	20	+.15
	DAT numerical ability	Adolescents	20	+.05
	PSAT-verbal	High school juniors and seniors	6	-.12 - +.01
	PSAT-math	High school juniors and seniors	6	+.12 - +.49
	SAT-verbal	High school juniors and seniors	7	-.06 - +.11
	SAT-math	High school juniors and seniors	7	+.37 - +.51

Table 1 (continued)

Study	Variable	Age	Number of Reports	d
Hyde et al. (1990)	Computation	All ages	45	-.14
	Understanding math concepts	All ages	41	-.03
	Complex problem solving	All ages	48	+.08

SOCIAL VARIABLES

Influenceability and conformity

Cooper (1979)	Group pressure	Adolescents and adults	11	-.28
	Fictitious norm group	Adolescents and adults	3	-.01
	Persuasion	Adolescents and adults	2	-.02
Eagly & Carli (1981)	Group pressure	Adolescents and adults	46	-.32
	Persuasion	Adolescents and adults	33	-.16
	Other conformity	Adolescents and adults	11	-.28
Becker (1986)	Group pressure	Adolescents and adults	35	-.28
	Persuasion	Adolescents and adults	33	-.11
	Other conformity	Adolescents and adults	10	-.13

Aggression

Hyde (1984, 1986)	Aggression (all reports)	All ages	69	+.50
	Mixed aggression	All ages	16	+.43
	Physical aggression	All ages	26	+.60
	Verbal aggression	All ages	6	+.43
	Fantasy	All ages	1	+.84
	Willingness to shock, hurt	All ages	8	+.39
	Imitative	All ages	5	+.49
	Hostility scale	All ages	2	+.02
	Other	All ages	5	+.43
Eagly & Steffen (1986)	Aggression (all reports)	14 and older	50	+.29
	Physical aggression	14 and older	30	+.40
	Psychological aggression	14 and older	20	+.18
	Laboratory studies	14 and older	37	+.35
	Field studies	14 and older	13	+.21

Helping behavior

Eagly & Crowley (1986)	Helping behavior	14 and older	99	+.34

Small group behavior

Carli (cited in Eagly, 1987)	Task behavior	Adults	10	+.59
	Positive socio-emotional behavior	Adults	9	-.59
Wood (1987)	Individual performance	Adults	19	+.38

Table 1 (continued)

Study	Variable	Age	Number of Reports	d
	Group performance	Adults	45	+.39
Leadership behavior				
Dobbins & Platz (1986)	Initiating structure	Adults	8	-.03
	Consideration	Adults	8	-.05
	Subordinate satisfaction	Adults	7	-.08
	Leadership effectiveness	Adults	11	+.18
Eagly & Johnson (1989)	Task style	Adolescents and adults	136	-.04
	Interpersonal style	Adolescents and adults	139	.00
	Democratic vs. autocratic style	Adolescents and adults	23	-.22
Nonverbal behavior				
Hall (1978)	Decoding	All ages	46	-.46
Eisenberg & Lennon (1983)	Empathy (reflexive crying)	Infants	5	-.34
	Empathy to pictures/stories	Children	14	-.11
	Self-report empathy	Children and adults	17	-.91
Stier & Hall (1984)	Initiate touch	All ages	6	-.09
	Receive touch	All ages	5	+.02
Hall (1984)	Decoding skill	All ages	64	-.43
	Face recognition skill	Children and adolescents	5	-.30
		Adults	12	-.35
	Expression skill	All ages	35	-.52
	Facial expressiveness	Adults	5	-1.01
	Social smiling	Children	5	+.04
		Adults	15	-.63
	Gaze	Infants	8	-.41
		Children	10	-.39
		Adults	30	-.68
	Receipt of gaze	Adults	6	-.65
	Distance of approach to others:			
	naturalistic	Adults	17	+.56
	staged	Adults	8	+.12
	projective	Adults	11	+.14
	Distance approached by others:			
	naturalistic	Infants	5	+.98
		Adults	9	+.95
	staged	Adults	5	+.63
	projective	Adults	7	+.85
	Body movement and position:			
	restlessness	Adults	6	+.72
	expansiveness	Adults	6	+1.04
	involvement	Adults	7	-.32
	expressiveness	Adults	7	-.58
	self-consciousness	Adults	5	-.45

Table 1 (continued)

Study	Variable	Age	Number of Reports	d
	Vocal behavior:			
	speech errors	Adolescents and adults	6	+.70
	filled pauses	Adolescents and adults	6	+1.19
	total speech	Adults	12	+.10
Hall & Halberstadt (1986)	Social smiling	Children	5	+.04
	Social smiling	Adults	15	-.42
	Social gazing	Children	11	-.48
	Social gazing	Adults	30	-.69
PSYCHOLOGICAL WELL-BEING				
Hattie (1979)	Self-actualization	Adults	6	-.15
Wood (1987)	Well-being (all reports)	Adults	85	-.01
	Life satisfaction	Adults	17	-.03
	Happiness	Adults	22	-.07
	Positive affect	Adults	6	-.07
	General evaluation	Adults	40	+.06
MOTOR BEHAVIORS				
Thomas & French (1985)	Balance	Children and adolescents	67	+.09
	Catching	Children and adolescents	23	+.43
	Grip strength	Children and adolescents	37	+.66
	Pursuit rotor	Children and adolescents	14	+.11
	Shuttle run	Children and adolescents	28	+.32
	Tapping	Children and adolescents	34	+.13
	Throw velocity	Children and adolescents	12	+2.18
	Vertical jump	Children and adolescents	20	+.18
	Dash	Children and adolescents	66	+.63
	Long jump	Children and adolescents	68	+.54
	Sit-ups	Children and adolescents	29	+.64
	Throw distance	Children and adolescents	47	+1.98
	Agility	Children and adolescents	19	+.21
	Anticipation timing	Children and adolescents	23	+.38
	Arm hang	Children and adolescents	16	+.01
	Fine eye-motor	Children and adolescents	30	-.21
	Flexibility	Children and adolescents	13	-.29
	Reaction time	Children and adolescents	42	+.18
	Throw accuracy	Children and adolescents	14	+.96
	Wall volley	Children and adolescents	32	+.83
Eaton & Enns (1986)	Motor activity level	Prenatal	6	+.33
		Infants	14	+.29
		Preschoolers	58	+.44
		Older children	49	+.64

Note: Positive values of d indicate higher scores by males.

75

tistically significant results. This probably biases published results in the direction of larger effect sizes. In addition, investigators may not publish data that show large and significant effects that run counter to the zeitgeist, a tendency that would serve to maintain the status quo in the literature. One way of guarding against sampling bias is to seek out unpublished studies. Doctoral dissertations are perhaps the best source of unpublished data that may show nonsignificant effects or failures to replicate. One way to assess the threat posed by the ''file drawer'' problem, as it is called, is to determine the number of studies with nonsignificant results that would have to exist in order to invalidate a meta-analytic result. Rosenthal (1979) and Orwin (1983) have worked out file drawer computation procedures for combined probability and effect size data, respectively.

A final issue concerns the validity of meta-analytic research on gender differences. As Eagly (1986) pointed out, both the construct and external validities of the aggregated results of a meta-analysis are probably greater than those of most individual studies. However, threats to that greater validity do exist and cannot be ignored. To the extent that studies in the sample rely on similar measurement instruments or have other features in common, validity may be compromised. Examples are stimulus materials that inadvertently favor one gender over the other, samples that are unrepresentative of the population, and a preponderance of laboratory, as opposed to field, studies. Eagly (1986) recommended using meta-analytic techniques to assess the effects of these study characteristics.

META-ANALYSIS AND GENDER DIFFERENCES IN COGNITIVE PERFORMANCE

Verbal Abilities

In 1974, Maccoby and Jacklin concluded that gender differences in verbal ability were well established in the empirical literature. Hyde (1981) was the first investigator to evaluate that conclusion statistically. Her meta-analysis of the 27 studies of gender differences in verbal ability reviewed by Maccoby and Jacklin yielded a median d of $-.24$ and a median w^2 value of .01. These values indicated a small female advantage and a gender effect that accounted for only 1% of the variance in verbal ability, forcing Hyde to question the practical significance of well-established findings of that magnitude.

Rosenthal and Rubin (1982a) reanalyzed Hyde's data and obtained a statistically significant weighted mean d value of $-.30$, a gender difference they argued was of practical importance. They also showed that there was significant heterogeneity among the d values, some of which was accounted for by recency of publication. The correlation between recency of publication and d was .29, indicating that more recent studies found greater female superiority in verbal ability (although this conclusion does not, in our view, follow logically from their findings). Becker and Hedges (1984) continued with this effort and showed that nearly all of the variability in d across this sample of studies could be accounted for by year of publication and a measure of sample selectivity.

Feingold (1988) added to the evidence that cognitive gender differences are disappearing with his analysis of the four standardizations of the Differential Aptitude Tests (DAT; Bennett, Seashore & Wesman, 1947, 1966, 1974, 1982) and four standardizations of the Preliminary Scholastic Aptitude Test (PSAT; Donlon, 1984) and the Scholastic Aptitude Test (SAT; Donlon, 1984). Three of the DAT scales—Verbal Reasoning, Spelling, and Language—assess verbal abilities, and both the PSAT-Verbal and SAT-Verbal tests contain vocabulary, analogy, and reading comprehension items. The DAT was administered to 8th through 12th graders; the PSAT and SAT, to high school juniors and seniors, respectively. The DAT data were from 1947, 1962, 1972, and 1980; the PSAT data, from 1960, 1966, 1974, and 1983; and the SAT data, from 1960, 1967, 1974, and 1983.

Feingold found that, for each of the three DAT verbal tests, d had grown smaller. In 1947, the effect sizes (averaged across grade) for Verbal Reasoning, Spelling, and Language were .14, $-.54$, and $-.49$, respectively. (Negative values indicate better female performance.) In 1980, these values were $-.02$, $-.45$, and $-.40$. Similar patterns were found for the PSAT and SAT data. Feingold concluded that "gender differences [had] declined precipitously over the years surveyed" (p. 95).

Lastly, Hyde and Linn (1988) added to Hyde's (1981) earlier sample of studies and meta-analyzed 165 reports of gender differences in verbal ability, 120 of which reported data adequate for effect size computations. Three-fourths of the d values were negative, and the mean value was $-.11$, indicating a slight female superiority. Homogeneity analyses revealed that (1) d varied with type of verbal ability (mean $d = -.02$ for vocabulary, .16 for analogies, $-.03$ for reading comprehension, $-.33$ for speech production, $-.09$ for essay writing, $-.22$ for anagrams, and $-.20$ for general verbal ability); (2) d did not vary significantly with type of cognitive process; (3) d did not vary with the mean age of the sample; and (4) studies published before 1974 (the publication date of Maccoby and Jacklin's book) found larger d values (mean $d = -.23$) than did studies published in 1974 or later (mean $d = -.10$). The data from the 1985 administration of the SAT-Verbal test (Ramist & Arbeiter, 1986) were analyzed separately because of the very large number of subjects in the sample. The analysis yielded a d value of .11, indicating slight male superiority. Hyde and Linn concluded that the magnitude of the gender difference in verbal ability is "effectively zero" (p. 64) and recommended that verbal, rather than quantitative, tests be used as selection instruments because they are gender-unbiased.

Spatial, Science, and Quantitative Abilities

Hyde (1981) meta-analyzed the 16 studies of quantitative ability, 10 studies of visual-spatial ability, and 20 studies of field articulation (typically assessed with the Rod-and-Frame Test) cited by Maccoby and Jacklin (1974). She obtained median d values of .43, .45, and .51 (indicating superior male performance) and median w^2 values of .01, .04, and .03, respectively. As in the case of verbal ability, Hyde concluded that the gender effects in these areas of cognitive function are so small in magnitude as to be of dubious practical significance. Rosenthal and Rubin (1982a) and Becker and Hedges (1984) once again used these data to show that gender differences in these three areas have shrunk over time.

Linn and Petersen (1985) focused exclusively on spatial ability in their meta-analysis of studies published since 1974. They culled 172 independent effect sizes from their sample and assigned each of them to one of three categories of spatial ability. For spatial perception (defined as the ability to determine spatial relationships with respect to one's own orientation), they found a mean effect size of .44, indicating better male performance. For mental rotation, the value was .73. For spatial visualization (defined as the ability to perform complex, multistep spatial manipulations), it was .13. These heterogeneous results render as inappropriate all global statements about gender differences in spatial ability.

Linn and Petersen analyzed their data for age trends in the magnitude of the effect sizes. They wanted to assess the evidence for the argument that gender differences in spatial ability are biologically based because they emerge in adolescence. Their results did not support this hypothesis. For example, the mean d for studies of spatial perception in persons under the age of 13 was the same as the mean d for studies of spatial perception in persons between the ages of 13 and 18. (In each case, mean $d = .37$.) Of course, these results do not resolve the issue of the origin of gender differences in spatial ability because not all biological explanations posit a pubertal onset.

Feingold's (1988) report on trends over time in female and male performance on the DAT revealed similar patterns in the data for quantitative and spatial tests as described above for verbal ones. For example, from 1947 to 1980, the effect size for gender differences in performance on the spatial relations test went from .37 to .15, and the effect size for the numerical ability test went from .21 to $-.10$. These values indicate that the gender gap is narrowing, and in some cases female performance is surpassing male performance. The data for the PSAT and SAT contain the same trend; however, especially for the SAT, the magnitude of the effect size—which favors males—is still moderately large ($d = .42$).

Hyde, Fennema, and Lamon (1990) meta-analyzed 100 studies of mathematics performance, assessing the evidence for the effects of gender, task, and age. Across studies of samples of the general population, they obtained an average value of $-.05$, indicating a negligible female advantage. When they looked at computation, understanding of mathematical concepts, and complex problem solving separately, they obtained mean d values of $-.14$, $-.03$, and .08, respectively. An analysis of age trends revealed that females outperform males in computation in both elementary (mean $d = -.20$) and middle school (mean $d = -.22$) and that males outperform females in problem solving in high school (mean $d = .29$) and college (mean $d = .32$). Hyde et al. also found an effect for sample selectivity, in that studies of highly selective or precocious subjects produced the largest gender differences. Finally, they provided still more evidence that cognitive gender differences are getting smaller: the mean effect size for studies published before 1974 was .31, whereas the mean d value for later studies was .14. Hyde et al. argued that Maccoby and Jacklin's (1974) conclusion that "boys excel in mathematical ability" (p. 352) is oversimplified and is by now outdated. The meta-analyses reported here used mathematics performance on standardized tests as the measure. If one looks instead at math grades in school, girls perform better than boys (Kimball, 1989).

Formal Operational Thought

Meehan (1984) conducted a meta-analysis of 53 studies of formal operational thought in children, adolescents, and adults. For the most part, gender differences were not the primary focus of these studies. Meehan grouped the studies by type of task, with task being defined according to Inhelder and Piaget's (1958) work on formal operations. Separate meta-analyses were carried out on each group of studies. Meehan obtained mean d values of .22, .10, and .48 for studies of propositional logic, combinatorial reasoning, and proportional reasoning, respectively. In each case, males outperformed females. The pattern of results was the same for younger (mean age less than or equal to 17 years) and older samples. Meehan suggested that task format (e.g., manipulative versus written), experimenter's gender, and the confounding of formal and spatial reasoning skills may underlie observed gender differences in formal thought.

Gender-Role Identity and Cognitive Performance

Signorella and Jamison (1986) used meta-analytic techniques to assess the evidence for Nash's (1979) hypothesis that individuals perform well on a task to the extent that its gender stereotype is consistent with their self-concept. Nash has argued that her hypothesis can account for observed gender differences in cognitive performance as the result of socialization processes. Signorella and Jamison examined the correlations between gender role identity (as measured by bipolar measures, like the Gough Femininity Inventory, or androgyny measures, like the Bem Sex Role Inventory) and performance on spatial, mathematical, and verbal tasks for females and males separately. The spatial tasks were further subdivided into spatial perception, mental rotation, and spatial visualization categories, according to Linn and Petersen's (1985) typology. The authors found support for Nash's hypothesis on both spatial and mathematical tasks, but not on verbal tasks.

For females, the average correlations between M-F (amount of masculinity, as measured by a bipolar instrument) and spatial perception, mental rotation, and spatial visualization were .29, .10, and .10, respectively. The average correlations between performance on these three types of tasks and F (femininity, as measured by an androgyny scale) were $-.13$, $-.04$, and $-.08$; and the average correlations between performance and M (masculinity, as measured by an androgyny scale) were .05, .19, and .13. For mathematical tasks, the average correlations between performance and M-F, F, and M were .15, $-.07$, and .07, respectively. The analogous values for verbal tasks were .01, .04, and $-.05$. Some of these relationships varied with the mean age of the sample and the year of publication.

For males, Signorella and Jamison obtained the following mean effect sizes (r): M-F and spatial perception, .05; F and spatial perception, .06; M and spatial perception, .01; M-F and mental rotation, .16; F and mental rotation, $-.07$; M and mental rotation, .15; M-F and spatial visualization, .10; F and spatial visualization, .01; M and spatial visualization, .06; M-F and math, .11; F and math, $-.03$; M and math, .03; M-F and verbal performance, .04; F and verbal performance, .05; and M and verbal performance, .00. Again, the mean age of the sample and publication date modified some of these relationships, but all of them are small.

Achievement Attributions

Sohn (1982) performed an effect size analysis on 28 reports of gender differences in achievement attributions, using w^2 as his effect size measure. For ability attributions, he obtained a nonsignificant average effect size of .004. For luck, effort, and task difficulty performance attributions, the values were .01, .00, and .00, respectively. When Sohn computed the average effect sizes for ability, luck, effort, and task difficulty attributions under success and failure conditions separately, he obtained values of .01 or less in each case. Clearly, he could only conclude that females and males do not differ in their attributional styles for success and failure.

Frieze and her colleagues (Frieze et al., 1982; Whitley et al., 1986) conducted two meta-analyses of gender differences in achievement attributions. Their goal was to evaluate the empirical evidence for each of three theoretical models of gender effects in this arena—general externality, self-derogation, and low expectancy. The models have in common the prediction that women tend not to attribute their successes to ability, but differ in their other predictions. Because the more recent study includes the data from, and reaches the same conclusions as, the earlier one, we will present only the more recent one.

Whitley et al.'s (1986) sample comprised 21 studies that used causally worded questions (e.g., "To what extent do you think your performance on this task was caused by luck?") and 7 studies that used informationally worded ones (e.g., "How much ability to perform this task do you think you have?"). Using Hedges's (1981, 1982b) unbiased effect size as their dependent measure, they found that—for success—men made slightly more attributions to ability than do women (mean $g = .13$) and women made slightly more attributions to luck (mean $g = -.07$). For failure, the mean effect sizes were $-.08$ for task difficulty, $-.15$ for luck, $.16$ for ability, and $.15$ for effort. An analysis of the effect of question wording on g allowed for some refinement of these results. Specifically, for success attributions, although women made more luck attributions in response to causal questions, men made more luck attributions to informational ones. For failure, men made more effort attributions to informational questions, but not to causal ones, and women made more luck attributions to causal questions, but not to informational ones. Within gender, meta-analyses of success-versus-failure attributions to each of the four sources indicated that women's and men's overall patterns of achievement attributions are quite similar. In view of the small effect sizes, Whitley et al. concluded that not only are each of the three models lacking in empirical validity but that their common premise is unfounded.

Mathematics Attitudes and Affect

Hyde and her colleagues (Hyde, Fennema, Ryan, Frost & Hopp, 1990) examined 70 reports of gender differences in mathematics attitudes and affect, as measured by such instruments as the Fennema-Sherman Scales (1976) and the Mathematics Anxiety Ratings Scales (Richardson & Suinn, 1972). The dependent variables included, for example, mathematics anxiety, mathematics self-concept, parental attitudes toward the subject's participation in mathematics, and mathematics success and failure attributions. The effects on d of the age of the subjects, the year of publication, and the selectivity of the sample were evaluated. For the Fennema-Sherman Scales, Hyde et al. found mostly small effect sizes (more than half were one-tenth of a standard deviation or less) for all age groups combined. The one exception to this pattern was the stereotyping of math as a male domain. It yielded a large effect size (mean $d = -.90$), indicating that males stereotype mathematics as a masculine activity more than females do. Homogeneity analyses revealed that this gender difference in stereotyping—as well as gender differences (that favored boys) in parents' and teachers' attitudes toward the subject's participation in mathematics—peaks in the high school years. The pattern of generally small effect sizes, a few of which increase with the age of the subjects, was repeated for measures of mathematics attitudes and affect other than the Fennema-Sherman Scales. Not surprisingly, the size of the gender difference in mathematics anxiety was associated with the selectivity of the sample: it was lowest in highly selected, precocious samples (mean $d = +.09$) and highest in remedial and math anxiety classes (mean $d = +.30$). Regression analyses of the Fennema-Sherman effect size data showed that male students reported more positive parental and teacher attitudes in the 1970s but that female students reported more positive attitudes in the 1980s and that the gender difference in the stereotyping of mathematics as a male domain has decreased somewhat over time. The authors urged caution in interpreting the former result, however, because one cannot tell from the data whether the attitudes of significant adults have become more positive toward girls or more negative toward boys. Overall, Hyde et al. concluded that gender differences in mathematics attitudes and affect are small—too small to account for females' underrepresentation in mathematics-related occupations (thus urging us to look elsewhere for an explanation), but not so small that they can be ignored (the cumulative effect of many small disadvantages for females may still be a powerful one).

META-ANALYSIS OF GENDER DIFFERENCES IN SOCIAL BEHAVIOR

Influenceability and Conformity Behavior

In their narrative review of the extant literature on gender differences in compliance with peer pressure (which they examined separately from compliance with adult demands and expectations), Maccoby and Jacklin (1974) concluded that no gender differences occur in relatively impersonal situations, as epitomized by the persuasive communication paradigm. However, they concluded that in face-to-face encounters like the Asch situation, women are somewhat more influenceable than are men. After highlighting the tremendous inconsistency of findings across studies, Maccoby and Jacklin speculated that the "femininity" or "masculinity" of the items used in an Asch-type study might account for some of that variability (Sistrunk & McDavid, 1971).

In one of the earliest meta-analyses of gender differences, Cooper (1979) evaluated the 47 studies of influenceability and conformity behavior reviewed by Maccoby and Jacklin. The analysis was part of a demonstration of the then new meta-analytic procedures and their advantages over narrative review. After excluding Sistrunk and McDavid's (1971) study because of "its special place in the literature" (p. 137) and 8 others for a variety of methodological reasons (e.g., they were correlational studies or were performed on non-American subject populations), Cooper statistically evaluated the conclusions drawn by Maccoby and Jacklin. When he considered all 38 studies taken together, he concluded that females do, indeed, conform more than do males. When he separated the 38 studies according to experimental paradigm—that is, Asch-type group pressure, fictitious group norm, or persuasive communication—he found gender differences only for the face-to-face Asch-type studies. These results were in basic agreement with Maccoby and Jacklin's conclusions. However, whereas Maccoby and Jacklin had been struck by the inconsistency of findings across the group pressure studies, Cooper argued that there was, in fact, impressive consistency. Overall, Cooper claimed that the cumulated evidence available to Maccoby and Jacklin in 1974 suggested a small but consistent tendency for females to show more conformity behavior, at least in face-to-face, group pressure situations. He drew the same conclusion when he meta-analyzed the 145 studies of gender differences in conformity behavior reviewed by Eagly (1978).

Cooper's work has been criticized (Sohn, 1980) for containing a statistical error (he used the standard error of the mean for d, rather than the standard deviation of the sample d values, in computing the confidence interval for d) and for not making proper use of effect size data to support its conclusions. Furthermore, it should be noted that Cooper had adequate quantitative information on only 18 of the 38 studies he included in his analysis.

Eagly and Carli (1981) performed a more thorough meta-analysis of 148 studies of gender differences in adolescent and adult conformity behavior published between 1949 and 1977. The 148 studies—most of which had been reviewed narratively by Eagly in 1978—comprised 61 persuasion studies, 64 conformity studies involving group pressure, and 23 conformity studies not involving group pressure. d values could be calculated for 90 of the studies. Eagly and Carli obtained mean d values of $-.16$, $-.32$, and $-.28$ for the persuasion studies, group pressure conformity studies, and other conformity studies, respectively. (Negative values of d indicate greater female conformity.) Across all three types of studies, the mean effect size was .26. Eagly and Carli also evaluated the relationships between content of stimulus materials and effect size and between author's gender and effect size. Surprisingly, they did not find an overrepresentation of masculine content in the persuasion studies. (Similar analyses were not done for the conformity studies because of the impossibility of rating the stimulus material.) They did, however, find a strong and consistent relationship between author's gender (scored dichotomously: $1 = 50\%$ or more female authors, $2 = 50\%$ or more male authors) and obtained effect size. The point-biserial correlation between author's gender and d was .43 ($p < .05$) for the persuasion studies, .27 ($p = .07$) for the group pressure conformity studies, .78 ($p < .01$) for the other conformity studies, and .41 ($p < .001$) for all types of studies combined. Looked at another way, the mean effect size obtained in studies (all types combined) authored primarily by women was $-.02$, whereas the mean effect size obtained in studies authored primarily by men was $-.34$. In other words, male authors found greater female influenceability while female authors did not. In their effort to make sense of this striking result, Eagly and Carli did a similar analysis of Hall's (1978) sample of 75 studies of gender differences in decoding nonverbal cues. Here, they found male authorship to be associated with less inaccurate decoding by males and female authorship to be associated with more inaccurate decoding by males. Eagly and Carli concluded that both female and male researchers may unintentionally present their own gender more favorably than do researchers of the other gender. They also speculated that researcher gender differences may influence aspects of experimental design, choice of stimuli, and willingness to publish findings of no gender differences that challenge gender-based stereotypes.

Becker (1986) reanalyzed the set of studies reviewed by Eagly and Carli (1981), using the more rigorous statistical techniques developed by Hedges (1981, 1982a, 1982b) in the intervening years (see above). She also examined the effects of several study characteristics on d, including type of subjects studied, type of outcome measure used, number of items in the outcome measure (more items yield higher reliability), number and gender of confederates, and gender of experimenter. Only 78 independent effect sizes could be gleaned from the studies using the new methods. Becker obtained mean effect sizes of $-.11$, $-.28$, and $-.13$ for the persuasion, group pressure, and other conformity studies, respectively. Planned linear contrasts indicated that the mean effect size for the group pressure studies was significantly higher than the other two, suggesting—at first glance—that greater female influenceability is particularly apparent in group pressure situations. However, further analyses indicated that paradigm type was confounded with type of outcome measure (e.g., change score versus posttest) and that type of outcome measure was significantly related to d in both the group pressure and persuasion studies. For the other conformity studies, percentage of male authors, number of items in the outcome measure, and number of confederates all related to effect size. Becker concluded:

An oversimplification of these results is that women conform more. But this conclusion is based on just less than half of the available studies. Most often, results were unreported, and hence effect sizes were not computed, because there was no finding of a significant gender difference. Since significance depends on effect size, we would suppose that large effects are not "hidden" in the other studies. It is unlikely that the true (population) gender difference [in influenceability] is much larger than that reported here. (p. 205)

Aggression

Maccoby and Jacklin's (1974) conclusion regarding gender differences in aggression was one of their least qualified. They found males to be more aggressive than females wherever they looked, across cultures, across ages, and across types of aggression. All that remained to be discovered, it seemed, was the source of this well-established gender difference.

Using the primitive meta-analytic technique of probability combining—which can give only a yes-no answer to the question of whether there is a significant gender difference across a group of studies—Tieger (1980) and Maccoby and Jacklin (1980) debated just this issue. Tieger argued against biological causation, buttressing his argument with his failure to find a gender difference in studies of young children (age 6 years or less). Maccoby and Jacklin were critical of his analysis, in part because he had treated dependent measures as if they were independent. When they corrected his error, they found a highly significant gender difference in aggression for this age range. Unfortunately, this whole approach to the issue of biological versus environmental causation is somewhat misguided because many biologically determined gender differences make delayed appearances. Consider, for example, the growth of facial hair.

Hyde (1984, 1986) applied the newer and more sophisticated meta-analytic procedures to a set of 143 studies of gender differences in aggression. Seventy-five of the studies were those cited by Maccoby and Jacklin (1974). An additional 68 studies were gleaned from the 1979 through 1981 issues of *Psychological*

Abstracts. Only studies of American and Canadian subjects were included, and there were no restrictions on subjects' age. Eighty-three independent effect sizes could be calculated from the studies.

When Hyde eliminated the 14 clinical and other selective samples from the set, she obtained a mean d value of .50 for the remaining 69 general samples. (The selective samples had a mean d value of .82.) Using Rosenthal and Rubin's (1982b) Z statistic for a linear contrast, Hyde found a significant age trend in the data, indicating that the gender difference in aggression varied inversely with the average age of subjects in the study. That is, gender differences in aggression were larger among preschoolers (median $d = .58$) and smaller among college students (median $d = .27$).

Using Hedges's (1982a, 1982b) homogeneity statistics, Hyde found that type of research design (i.e., experimental versus naturalistic), method of measurement (e.g., direct observation, self-report, parent or teacher report, and so on), and type of aggression sampled (e.g., physical, verbal, and so on) all produced significant between-category differences. (None of the three categorization strategies reduced within-category heterogeneity to a nonsignificant level, but that would be difficult to achieve with so many effect sizes.) When Hyde evaluated her data for between-category differences in d, she found that the naturalistic/correlational studies yielded significantly larger gender differences in aggression than did the experimental studies (mean $d = .56$ versus mean $d = .29$). However, she did not find significant differences between studies that used direct observation and studies that used other methods of measurement or between studies of physical aggression and studies of verbal aggression. In a regression-type model-fitting analysis, however, Hyde did find both method of measurement and type of aggression to be significant predictors of d when age was used as a covariate.

In summing up the results of her analyses, Hyde (1986) stated that there appears to be a moderate and fairly consistent gender difference in aggression. However, she also cautioned that her statistical results cannot and do not inform us about either the origin of that difference or the value interpretation we should give to it.

At about the same time that Hyde's work appeared, Eagly and Steffen (1986) published a meta-analysis of gender differences in aggression that had been reported in the experimental social psychological literature. They restricted their sample to studies of subjects 14 years of age and older (most were college-age samples) and to studies in which the dependent variable was a behavioral measure of aggression toward another person. These restrictions resulted in a fairly homogeneous group of laboratory and field studies wherein relatively brief encounters with strangers were assessed. Eagly and Steffen used social role theory to select their predictors of gender differences.

The sample of 63 studies yielded 81 reports of gender differences and 50 independent effect sizes for the analysis. Across all 50 values, the mean weighted effect size was .29, indicating greater male aggressiveness. However, as might be expected, there was significant heterogeneity among the 50 values. When they tested several categorical models on the effect size data, Eagly and Steffen found that the mean d was greater for the laboratory (.35) than for the field (.21) studies and greater for studies of physical (.40) than psychological (.18) aggression. They also found that the gender difference was larger for semiprivate than for public experimental settings (.38 versus .17) and larger when aggression was required rather than freely chosen (.37 versus .24). As with the Hyde data reviewed above, no model successfully reduced the within-class heterogeneity to a nonsignificant level. Also of note is the fact that every mean effect size calculated was positive in sign, indicating great consistency in the direction of the gender difference (even though there is clearly great inconsistency in its size).

As part of their effort to fit continuous models to their effect size data, Eagly and Steffen had 200 undergraduates rate brief descriptions of the aggressive behaviors described in the studies in their sample for (1) harmfulness to the target, (2) anxiety/guilt for the subject, and (3) dangerousness for the subject. The subjects were also asked how likely they thought it to be that (1) they, (2) the average woman, and (3) the average man would enact the aggressive behavior. The group's responses to these six questions, scored for gender differences, were included in the set of predictor variables used in the regression-type analysis. A series of univariate and multivariate tests revealed several significant predictors of d, in particular, the gender difference in the undergraduate respondents' assessment of how much anxiety/guilt and danger they would feel had they perpetrated such an act of aggression. That is, to the extent that the women respondents reported that they would feel more anxiety/guilt and danger in that situation than the men reported they would feel, d was large. The results of this set of analyses were, by and large, interpretable within the framework of Eagly's (1987) social role theory.

Eagly and Steffen also looked at gender effects for the target person, or victim. The mean weighted d for the 20 values was .13, indicating more aggression toward men. The pattern of relationships they found between various study features (e.g., laboratory versus field setting, physical versus psychological aggression, and so on) and the effect size for the subject's gender also held for the effect size for the target's gender. For 13 studies, Eagly and Steffen were able to calculate both effect sizes. They found them to be negatively but nonsignificantly correlated, $r(11) = -.25$. Were this value to reach significance as more studies are added to the small sample, it would indicate that smaller effect sizes for target/victim gender are associated with larger effect sizes for subject/perpetrator gender. That is, under conditions in which men show more aggression than women, the gender of the victim is less salient.

Helping Behavior

A meta-analysis of gender differences in helping behavior was performed by Eagly and Crowley (1986) and is as deeply rooted in social role theory as is

Eagly and Steffen's (1986) work on gender differences in aggression. There are also many structural similarities between the two reports, for example, the criteria used to select studies for the analysis, the use of a questionnaire study with undergraduates to obtain gender-based ratings for each of the helping behaviors described in the studies, and the evaluation of target gender differences.

Eagly and Crowley were able to cull 99 effect sizes from the 172 studies they found. The mean weighted effect size, across all 99 of them, was .34. The positive sign indicates greater helping behavior among men. This result seems, at first, counterintuitive, because helping is central to the female role. However, it is exactly what social role theory predicts. The key to understanding this result is an appreciation of the dynamics of the typical social psychological study of helping behavior (which was the only type of study Eagly and Crowley included in their sample). As was the case in the social psychological studies of aggression, these studies examined relatively brief encounters with strangers, encounters that call for "chivalrous acts and nonroutine acts of rescuing" (p. 300). As Eagly and Crowley argued quite convincingly, these are exactly the types of helping behaviors that the male gender role fosters. The female gender role, in contrast, fosters caretaking and helping behaviors primarily in the context of ongoing close relationships, which are not assessed in psychologists' typical research.

The results of Eagly and Crowley's categorical model-fitting analyses indicated that the gender difference in helping behavior was larger (in the male direction) in off-campus settings than in the laboratory, when there were other people around to witness the act than when there were not, when other helpers were available than when there were not, and when the appeal for help was a presentation of a need rather than a direct request. The results of their continuous model-fitting analyses indicated that larger effect sizes (again, in the male direction) were associated with earlier publication date; gender differences in the undergraduate raters' reports of how competent, comfortable, and endangered they would feel performing the helping behavior; gender differences in the undergraduates' reports of how likely they would be to perform the helping behavior; and the undergraduate raters' judgment that the average man would be more likely to perform the helping behavior than would the average woman. In other words, to the extent that the male undergraduate raters said that they would be more likely to perform the helping behavior and feel more competent, more comfortable, and less endangered doing it than did the female raters and to the extent that all of the undergraduate raters thought that the average man would be more likely to perform the behavior than would the average woman, the behavior was associated with a larger gender difference. Eagly and Crowley's multivariate analyses of the effect size data allowed for some refinement of these results, all of which are easily accounted for by social role theory.

As mentioned earlier, Eagly and Crowley also analyzed the target—or requester—gender effects. Across 36 values, the mean weighted effect size was −.46, indicating that women receive more help than do men. The correlation between the effect size for the target's gender and the effect size for the subject's gender was negative and significant, r (34) $= -.40$, $p < .01$. Thus, not surprisingly, the study characteristics that related significantly to subject gender effect size (i.e., setting, surveillance, availability of helpers, type of request) were also related to target gender effect size, though in the opposite direction. Further analysis of these data revealed that men were more likely to help women than men, but received help from men and women about the same; whereas women were equally likely to help men and women, but more often received help from men than from women.

Small Group Behavior

Anderson and Blanchard (1982) performed a meta-analysis of gender differences in small group behavior. Their sample size was small (two to eight gender difference reports, depending on the analysis), and they used only Rosenthal's (1978) Z statistic for estimating an overall significance level across studies, so their results must be viewed as tentative.

Anderson and Blanchard reviewed five observational studies that had used Bales's (1950) Interaction Process Analysis protocol for assessing small group behavior and two others that had measured only total participation rate. The Bales system codes two important dimensions of group interaction, task behavior and socioemotional behavior. Socioemotional behavior can be coded as either positive or negative; task behavior is coded as either active or passive. The results of the analyses revealed (1) no gender difference in total participation (in either same or mixed-sex groups), (2) significantly more positive socioemotional behavior by women than men (in both mixed-sex and all groups combined), and (3) significantly more active task behavior by men than women (in same-sex, mixed-sex, and all groups combined). The authors concluded that "general cultural sex roles are manifest in task group interaction" (p. 119); however, they also pointed out that "in none of the studies were women found to engage 'predominantly' in social-emotional behavior; both men and women devote the majority of their interaction to the group's task activity" (p. 119).

Carli (cited in Eagly, 1987) drew similar conclusions from her more sophisticated effect size analysis. She obtained average effect sizes of .59 (across 10 values) for task behavior and $-.59$ (across 9 values) for positive socioemotional behavior, indicating more task behavior among men and more positive socioemotional behavior among women. Like Anderson and Blanchard, Carli did not find evidence of a gender difference in total participation. She did, however, find statistical evidence that group discussion topics that favor the interests or knowledge of one gender over the other elicit more task and more socioemotional behavior from the favored gender. Her interpretation of this finding was that the subjects' experiences in their social roles outside of the group influenced their behavior in the group.

In her analysis of studies of gender differences in other types of small group behavior, Carli found that women allocate smaller rewards to themselves than do men (mean effect size of − .29 across 11 values) and that men divide rewards among group members more equitably (i.e., according to the members' input) than do women (mean effect size of .20 across 10 values), but that men and women do not differ in their tendency to reward group members equally. She also found no gender difference in level of cooperation in the Prisoner's Dilemma game in same-sex groups, but a tendency for greater male cooperation in mixed-sex groups (mean effect size of .28 across 6 values).

Wood (1987) focused her meta-analysis on gender differences in group productivity. She restricted her review to laboratory studies in which an objective measure of performance on the assigned task was used. The 52 studies she found were coded for a variety of attributes, the most important of which had to do with the nature of the dependent measure. For example, the studies were coded for whether group members worked on the task individually or together, how it was scored (for creativity, number of solutions, time to completion, number of errors, and so on), and whether it required task-oriented or social activity for better performance. Wood found that men outperformed women when working individually in same-sex groups (mean effect size of .38 across 19 values) and when working together in same-sex groups (mean effect size of .39 across 45 values). She found no evidence of a gender difference in individual performance while working in mixed-sex groups (5 studies only) and only a nonsignificant tendency for mixed groups to outperform single-sex groups of either gender (8 studies only).

Wood's categorical model-fitting analyses (done only on the same-sex data) yielded only two significant effects. First, when the dependent measure was number of solutions, there was better male performance when group members worked alone (mean $d = .78$), but not when they worked together (mean $d = − .05$). That is, men generated more solutions than did women when they worked alone in same-sex groups, but the two sexes generated equal numbers of solutions when they worked in groups together with other members of their own gender. Second, on tasks that require task-oriented behavior for good performance, men outperform women whether they are working individually (mean $d = .25$) or together (mean $d = .34$); whereas on tasks that require social behavior for good performance, women perform slightly better (mean $d = − .11$). Study variables that accounted for small, but significant, portions of the variance in gender effect size were male authorship and more recent year of publication: a greater percentage of male authors and more recent year of publication were associated with larger effects. Wood called for greater appreciation, in the workplace, of the specific facilitative effects of women's interaction style on group productivity.

Leadership Behavior

In the same paper in which they reviewed the literature on gender differences in small group behavior, Anderson and Blanchard (1982) assessed a small set of findings on gender differences in leadership behavior, leadership effectiveness, and attitudes toward male and female leaders. Again, using only Rosenthal's (1978) Z statistic, they found no significant systematic gender effects.

Four years later, Dobbins and Platz (1986) conducted a somewhat larger review and analysis of the literature. They found 17 studies that reported on gender differences in leadership behaviors (specifically, initiating structure and consideration, which are analogous to task-oriented and socioemotional behavior, respectively), leadership effectiveness, or subordinate satisfaction. Six were field studies, 6 were laboratory experiments, and 5 were laboratory simulations. They found no gender differences in initiating structure, consideration, or subordinate satisfaction (mean $d = -.03$, $-.05$, and $-.08$, respectively), and the gender difference they found for leadership effectiveness (mean $d = .18$) proved to be restricted to laboratory settings. Their negative findings prompted Dobbins and Platz to call for "a moratorium on research that simply compares male and female leaders" (p. 125) and an increase in research that identifies the factors by which gender stereotypes are maintained.

Eagly and Johnson (1989) recently completed a thorough quantitative review of the leadership literature. They evaluated gender differences in autocratic versus democratic (also known as directive versus participative) leadership style, as well as in task versus interpersonal orientation. The 144 studies in their analysis included laboratory experiments, assessment studies, and field studies in organizational settings. Because of their belief that, in real life settings, male and female leaders are selected according to the same criteria, Eagly and Johnson predicted that they would find smaller gender differences in the field studies than in the other two types of reports. Their prediction was supported by their results.

Across all 329 effect sizes they computed, Eagly and Johnson obtained a mean value of .03, indicating virtually no gender difference. They found similarly near-zero mean effect sizes across all gender comparisons on interpersonal style measures, task style measures, and bipolar measures that assessed the two styles simultaneously. In stark contrast was the comparatively large gender difference they found for democratic versus autocratic style (mean $d = -.22$), a finding that suggests women are more democratic than men in their leadership style.

When they looked at the three types of studies (organizational, assessment, laboratory) in their sample separately, Eagly and Johnson found strong support for their major prediction regarding field studies, as well as consistent evidence for a gender difference in democratic versus autocratic style. More specifically, across the effect sizes gleaned from the 269 organizational studies, they obtained mean values of .01, $-.02$, .03, and $-.21$ for interpersonal style, task style, interpersonal versus task style, and democratic versus autocratic style, respectively. The analogous values for the 43 assessment studies were $-.25$, .08, .04, and $-.29$; and the values for the 17 laboratory studies were $-.37$, .19, $-.12$, and $-.20$. Thus, with the exception of democratic versus autocratic style, larger gender differences were obtained in studies of subjects who do not actually occupy leadership positions and who are evaluated in artificial and contrived settings. In these studies, men behave in a more task-oriented fashion and women, in a more interpersonally oriented one. The tendency for women to lead in a more democratic way and men to do so in a more autocratic way, in contrast, is found across all types of studies. Indeed, the authors found that 92% of the gender comparisons on this dimension were in the stereotypic direction. Eagly and Johnson suggested that female and male leaders bring to their leadership positions a wealth of gender-based experience. Consequently, though they may be selected according to the same criteria, they are not equivalent persons. Eagly and Johnson also suggested that female leaders may attempt to placate their coworkers by asking for their input, in order to cope with continued institutional hostility toward women leaders. Lastly, although Eagly and Johnson did not argue for the greater effectiveness of a participative leadership style, they did note the current trend away from rigid, hierarchical management practices, a trend presumably guided by that belief.

Nonverbal Communication

Hall (1978) reviewed 75 studies of gender differences in the ability to decode nonverbal communication and found that 68% of the studies reported superior female performance. Approximately half of those results were statistically significant. Hall obtained a significant mean effect size of .40 across the 46 values that could be computed, another indicator of a female advantage. When she categorized the studies according to type of stimulus material, Hall found that audiovisual stimuli (mean $d = 1.02$) produced larger gender differences than did either auditory (mean $d = .18$) or visual (mean $d = .32$) stimuli. This pattern is consistent with Rosenthal and DePaulo's (1979) finding of a greater female nonverbal sensitivity advantage for facial cues (.33) than for body (.22) or vocal tone cues (.12).

Hall found nonsignificant relationships between effect size and age of subject, age of sender, and sex of sender, suggesting that the gender effect is a robust one. She also found a tendency for recent studies to obtain larger gender effects, a finding that she accounted for by their greater use of audiovisual stimulus materials and the greater precision and reliability of their measurement instruments. Hall viewed her finding that women more accurately interpret nonverbal communication as consistent with gender role theory, approached from either an early learning or evolutionary stance. She encouraged researchers to study other primates in order to resolve the issue. Hall also argued that nonverbal sensitivity is an asset, not a liability, and suggested that boys and men be given special training.

Eisenberg and Lennon (1983) reviewed the literature on gender differences in affective empathy, which they defined as "emotional matching and/or sympathetic responding" (p. 101). They evaluated studies that used one of the following seven types of empathy measures: infants' reflexive crying (i.e., crying in response to another infant's cry), self-report in response to viewing emotional pictures or hearing emotional stories, self-report in simulated distress situations, observer ratings of subjects' responses to another's emotional state, physiological responsiveness to another's emotional state, self-report empathy measures, and other-report empathy measures. Although limitations in the individual reports prevented Eisenberg and Lennon from doing meta-analyses on every group of studies, they found that (1) female infants do more reflexive crying than male infants (mean $d = -.34$); (2) girls show more empathy in response to pictures and stories than boys (mean $d = -.11$); and (3) females of all ages report more empathy on paper-and-pencil inventories than males (mean $d = -.91$).

Stier and Hall (1984) reviewed 43 observational studies of gender differences in touch and obtained a complex and somewhat ambiguous pattern of results. Looking first at the direction of the findings, they found that 63% of the studies reported more female-to-male than male-to-female touching, 71% reported more female-to-female than male-to-male touching, 64% reported more touch initiated by females, and 61% reported more touch received by females. However, the average effect sizes associated with each of these four variables were all near zero (.02, .00, $-.09$, and .02, respectively). Stier and Hall also reported that the majority of studies found that females react more favorably to touch than do males, although they did not include an average effect size. Their failure to find clear-cut evidence for an asymmetry in touching behavior in opposite-gender dyads forced Stier and Hall to conclude that Henley's (1977) power hypothesis did not have a strong empirical base. They did, however, suggest a modification. Drawing on Goldstein and Jeffords's (1981) finding that lower-status legislators touched higher-status legislators more often than the other way around, Stier and Hall speculated that touching may be more consistent with lower, rather than higher, status and reflect the individual's "strong desire either to redress the status imbalance or to establish a bond of solidarity" (p. 456).

In her review of the literature on gender differences in nonverbal communicative behaviors, Hall (1984) devoted a chapter to each of the following topics, quantifying the evidence wherever possible: interpersonal sensitivity and judgment accuracy, expression accuracy, facial behavior, gaze, interpersonal distance and orientation, touch, body movement and position, and voice. In her concluding chapter, she provided a table (Table 11.1, p. 142) in which the average point-biserial correlations between gender and performance for 21 nonverbal behaviors are displayed. (These values have been included in Table 1. Again, to obtain a rough comparability of statistics, $d = 2r$.) Each average effect size is based on at least five independent studies, and, where they exist, separate results are reported for infants, children, and adolescents. The data indicate that women are better at decoding nonverbal communication ($r = -.21$), recognizing faces ($r = -.17$), and expressing emotions nonverbally ($r = -.25$); that they have more expressive faces ($r = -.45$), smile ($r = -.30$) and gaze ($r = -.32$) more, receive more gaze ($r = -.31$), approach ($r = -.27$) and are approached by others ($r = -.43$) more closely, and make fewer speech errors ($r = .33$) and filled pauses ($r = .51$); and that their body movements are less restless ($r = .34$), less expansive ($r = .46$), more involved ($r = -.16$), more expressive ($r = -.28$), and more self-conscious ($r = -.22$). Surely it was this set of results that led Hall and Halberstadt (1986) to comment, two years later, "In sum, based on a literature of hundreds of studies, it appears that women occupy a more nonverbally conscious, positive, and interpersonally engaged world than men do" (p. 137).

Hall and Halberstadt (1986) meta-analyzed the literature on gender differences in social smiling and gazing, in part to evaluate the warmth-affiliation, dominance-status, and social tension-nervousness accounts of women's tendency to smile and gaze more. As construed by Hall and Halberstadt, the warmth-affiliation hypothesis suggests that it is because of women's greater socioemotional orientation; the dominance-status hypothesis, that it is because of women's weaker position in the social hierarchy; and the social tension-nervousness hypothesis, that it is because of women's greater attempts to increase interpersonal comfort.

For social smiling, Hall and Halberstadt found no gender difference for children (ages 2 through 12, mean $d = .04$, 5 studies), but a significant gender effect for adults, in favor of women (mean $d = -.42$, 15 studies). In comparison, they found that girls do significantly more social gazing than do boys (mean $d = -.48$, 11 studies) and that women do more social gazing than do men (mean $d = -.69$, 30 studies). The results of their model-fitting analyses did not provide unequivocal support for any one of the three hypotheses.

META-ANALYSIS AND GENDER DIFFERENCES IN PSYCHOLOGICAL WELL-BEING

Hattie (1979) reported a quantitative summary of six studies of gender differences in performance on the Personal Orientation Inventory (Shostrom, 1966), a self-report measure of self-actualization. He found an average effect size of $-.15$, indicating a slight female superiority, and concluded that there was no need for separate test norms for each gender.

Bassoff and Glass (1982) conducted a meta-analysis of 26 studies of sex roles and mental health, in an effort to determine statistically whether the cumulated evidence pointed to a stronger association between mental health and sex-typed or androgynous identity. They computed 227 correlation coefficients on the data reported in the 26 studies, grouped them according to type of gender role identity being compared (e.g., masculine female versus androgynous female), and calculated the mean correlation for each group of correlations. Bassoff and Glass found the largest correlations between gender role identity and mental health (i.e., the largest differences) for the following pairs of sex roles: masculine versus feminine males (mean $r = .49$), androgynous versus feminine males (mean $r = .44$), androgynous versus feminine females (mean $r = .39$), and masculine versus feminine females (mean $r = .34$). (Note: In each pair, the positively coded gender role identity is listed first.) They found much smaller differences between masculine and androgynous females (mean $r = -.11$) and between masculine and androgynous males (mean $r = .07$). Bassoff and Glass concluded that, although the notion that psychological androgyny promotes mental health has much appeal, the data do not support it. Rather, the data point to a strong, positive relationship between masculinity and mental health that holds across gender, sample selectivity, and type of sex role measure. Further, they argued from their results, any relationship between androgyny and mental health appears to be the result of the masculinity component of androgyny, not the integration of masculinity and femininity.

Taylor and Hall (1982) drew similar conclusions from their meta-analytic review of 107 reports of the effects of masculinity and femininity on self-esteem, adjustment, ego development, or other measures of mental health. They conducted their analysis in the context of a theoretical reconceptualization of androgyny within the framework of a two-way analysis of variance. According to this approach, Bem's (1974) model of androgyny predicts a significant interaction, whereas Spence, Helmreich, and Stapp's (1975) model predicts significant main effects for both masculinity and femininity.

Across all 107 reports, Taylor and Hall found that 91% of the associations between masculinity and psychological health were positive, whereas only 79% of the associations between femininity and psychological health were positive. Furthermore, the strength of the association between masculinity and mental health was stronger than that between femininity and mental health, both for each gender and for each type of dependent measure. For example, the average correlation between masculinity and adjustment was .53 for men and .31 for women, whereas the average correlation between femininity and adjustment was .05 for men and .04 for women. Lastly, Taylor and Hall found that, of the results that addressed the issue, about half favored psychologically balanced individuals and half favored sex-typed individuals.

Taylor and Hall concluded that the traditional notion that feminine women and masculine men embody psychological health clearly must be rejected and that the balance model of androgyny has minimal and inconsistent empirical support. Rather, they argued, for each gender, "it is primarily masculinity that pays off" (p. 362).

Whitley (1983, 1984) performed parallel meta-analyses of 35 studies of sex-role orientation and self-esteem and 32 studies of sex-role orientation and psychological well-being. In each report, he used the proportion of variance accounted for as his effect size (ES) and also computed combined probability levels (Zma).

Whitley found both masculinity ($ES = .27$) and femininity ($ES = .03$) to be significantly related to self-esteem, with no gender differences in this pattern. He also found significant effects for masculinity, femininity, and their interaction ($ES = .12, .01,$ and $.01$, respectively) in a subset of eight studies in which the additive and interactive effects of masculinity and femininity could be assessed separately. Whitley himself questioned the real world significance of the small statistical effects for femininity and the masculinity-femininity interaction and concluded that the strongest support was for the link between masculinity and self-esteem. Additional analyses indicated that the Personal Attributes Questionnaire (Spence, Helmreich & Stapp, 1974, 1975) yielded stronger associations between masculinity and self-esteem than did the Bem Sex Role Inventory (Bem, 1974) and that masculinity was more strongly associated with social, rather than global, measures of self-esteem.

In his review of studies of well-being, Whitley (1984) included reports of gender differences in depression and reports of gender differences in general adjustment. He found a negative relationship ($ES = -.07$) between masculinity and depression, essentially no relationship ($ES = -.01$) between femininity and depression, and positive relationships between masculinity and general adjustment ($ES = .11$) and femininity and general adjustment ($ES = .03$). There were no differences in ES as a function of the subject's gender or the gender by sex-role interaction. Again, Whitley concluded that the evidence strongly supports the masculinity model of mental health, rather than the congruence model or the androgyny model.

Haring-Hidore and her colleagues (Haring, Stock, & Okun, 1984; Haring-Hidore, Stock, Okun, & Witter, 1985; Stock, Okun, Haring, & Witter, 1983) did a series of three meta-analytic reviews of several correlates of subjective well-being. Of relevance here, they found that well-being is positively related to age and that this association is significantly stronger for men than for women (Stock et al., 1983). (The first-order correlation between percent of sample male and effect size was .12.) They also found a positive correlation between subjective well-being and being married, again, a relationship that proved to be significantly stronger for men ($r = .17$) than for women ($r = .12$) (Haring et al., 1984; Haring-Hidore et al., 1985).

Wood, Rhodes, and Whelan (1989) conducted a meta-analytic review of 93 studies of gender differences in life satisfaction and well-being. They were particularly interested in the effects associated with marriage, which they predicted would be especially salutory for women. Because studies of life satisfaction tend to be done disproportionately on elderly and disabled subjects, Wood et al. ran validation analyses on a subset of 18 studies with samples that were representative of the U.S. population.

Across the 85 effect sizes that could be computed, Wood et al. obtained a nonsignificant mean value of $-.01$. The mean effect size for the 18 representative samples was $-.05$, indicating that women's reports were significantly more positive than men's. Effect size varied with type of measure, in that measures of life satisfaction (mean $d = -.03$) and happiness (mean $d = -.07$) yielded more favorable outcomes for women, measures of positive affect (mean $d = -.07$) yielded a trend that favored women, and measures of general evaluation (mean $d = .09$) yielded results that favored men. Studies published before 1978 yielded an effect that favored women (mean $d = -.05$), whereas later studies reported an effect that favored men (mean $d = .06$); however, this effect did not hold for the representative subset, and all effect sizes are small. Studies with a higher percentage of employed subjects obtained more favorable outcomes for women, but not enough data were available to do a complete analysis of this variable. Age was not significantly related to effect size.

To assess the effect of marital status, Wood et al. used the percent of the subjects in the sample who were married as a predictor variable in a regression-type analysis. The effect was significant (standardized $b = -.44$) and indicated that studies with a higher percent of married subjects obtained larger effect sizes favoring women. The validation analysis yielded the same result, and the general finding held for each type of dependent measure. Additional analyses revealed that marriage is associated with enhanced well-being for both men and women but that this difference tends to be greater for women. Wood et al. accounted for this result within the framework of social role theory. They argued that women's social role is associated with greater emotional sensitivity, expressiveness, and skillfulness and that marriage and family life provide women with greater opportunities to fulfill their gender role of "emotional specialist."

META-ANALYSIS AND GENDER DIFFERENCES IN MOTOR ACTIVITY LEVEL AND MOTOR PERFORMANCE

Motor activity level has been defined as an "individual's customary level of energy expenditure through movement" (Eaton & Enns, 1986, p. 19). It is conceived of as an important component of temperament and can even be measured prenatally (e.g., Robertson, Dierker, Sorokin & Rosen, 1982). After reviewing the literature available at the time, Maccoby and Jacklin (1974) concluded that there are no gender differences in activity level during the first year of life and that the data are inconsistent for older children. They found that under some conditions, boys are more active, whereas under others, boys and girls are no different from one another. This led Maccoby and Jacklin to conclude that although males may be biologically predisposed to respond more actively under some conditions, "it is not accurate to describe [them] as generally more active" (p. 177).

The single meta-analysis performed to date on gender differences in motor activity level was done by Eaton and Enns (1986). They evaluated 127 independent effect sizes taken from 90 different research reports and examined the effects of developmental factors, situational factors, measurement factors, and investigator factors on the size of d. It is important to note that in 90% of the studies included in the analysis, the mean age of the sample was 15 years or less. Consequently, the results of the Eaton and Enns work are not necessarily applicable to older subjects. Across all studies, Eaton and Enns obtained an average effect size of $+.49$ ($SD = .44$), indicating a higher activity level for males. Expressed in other terms, they obtained a point-biserial correlation between gender and activity level of .24 (that is, gender accounted for about 5% of the variance in activity level). Eaton and Enns found small and significant correlations between d and subjects' age ($r = .26$), the restrictiveness of the setting where the measurements were taken (e.g., playground versus classroom; $r = -.22$), and the inclusiveness of the measurement instrument used (e.g., a low-inclusive instrument would be one that measured arm movements, whereas a high-inclusive instrument would be one that measured whole body movements and general activity level; $r = -.28$). A multiple regression analysis, performed because of the nonorthogonality within the sets of study characteristics, indicated that larger effect sizes were found in studies of older (i.e., preadolescent and adolescent) subjects whose behavior was assessed in nonstressful, unrestrictive settings and in the presence of peers.

Thomas and French (1985) performed a meta-analysis on 64 studies of gender differences in motor performance, from which they gleaned 702 effect sizes. More than half of the studies they used yielded two or more effect sizes, and 16 of the studies yielded more than three values of d. They defended their decision to treat the multiple effect sizes obtained from a single study as if they were independent by arguing that the correlations between performances on these motor tasks are typically low. Thomas and French were especially interested in identifying age-related trends in the accumulated data on motor performance. Of the 20 motor tasks included in the analysis (because they met the criterion of having been included in at least three individual studies), 12 were found to yield age-related effect size curves. For 8 of these tasks (balancing, catching, grip strength, pursuit rotor, shuttle run, tapping, throw velocity, and vertical jump), the relationship between age and d was a positive linear one; for the remaining 4 (dash, long jump, sit-ups, and throw distance), the relationship was a quadratic one (U-shaped). The 8 tasks that did not yield age-related gender differences were agility, anticipation timing, arm hang, fine eye-motor, flexibility, reaction time, throw accuracy, and wall volley. For 18 of the 20 tasks, the mean effect size across studies was positive, indicating better performance by males. Most of these values ranged between .01 and .66, with the mean effect sizes for throw velocity and throw distance being much larger (2.18 and 1.98, respectively). Only the fine eye-motor and flexibility tasks yielded negative mean effect sizes ($-.21$ and $-.29$, respectively), indicating better female performance.

Thomas and French concluded that the data "do not support the notion of uniform development of gender differences in motor performance across childhood and adolescence" (p. 273). They argued that before puberty, the performance differences between girls and boys are typically small to moderate (d's of .20 to .50), meaning that many girls are outperforming many boys. They further argued that these prepubertal differences are most likely the result of environmental factors (e.g., parent and teacher expectations and encouragement, practice opportunities, and so on), and not biological ones. Then, at puberty, the greater increase in boys' size and muscle development—combined with the continued and perhaps intensified environmental influences—results in a greater gender gap in motor performance that continues through adolescence. Evidence (Linn & Hyde, 1989) that female Olympic athletes have continued to close the gender-related performance gap on both the 100-meter dash and 100-meter free-style events suggests that gender differences in motor performance are highly responsive to environmental forces such as training and need not persist into adulthood.

CONCLUSION

We believe that meta-analysis is a useful tool that can advance the study of gender differences, for several reasons:

1. Meta-analysis indicates not only whether there is a significant gender difference, but also how large the gender difference is. Therefore, it can be used to determine which psychological gender differences are large and which are not.

2. Meta-analysis represents an advance over years of psychological doctrine stating that one could never accept the null hypothesis. We believe that some effect sizes obtained through meta-analysis are so small that the null hypothesis of no gender difference can be accepted (Hyde & Linn, 1988). We recommend that any effect size < .10 be interpreted as no difference. This in turn will allow researchers to lay to rest some persisting rumors of psychological gender differences that are simply unfounded.

3. One of the most important trends in gender research today is the investigation of gender x situation interactions; meta-analysis permits some powerful analyses of this sort. Eagly's report of the situations that promote different patterns of gender differences in helping behaviors is an excellent example (Eagly & Crowley, 1986).

4. Meta-analysis can be a powerful tool to analyze issues other than gender differences. Examples are the analyses of the role of androgyny and masculinity in psychological well-being (e.g., Bassoff & Glass, 1982; Taylor & Hall, 1982). As a further example, feminist psychologists are increasingly interested in investigating the joint effects of gender and ethnicity; meta-analysis can be used here as well. For example, Hyde, Fennema, and Lamon (1990) examined gender differences in math performance as a function of ethnicity and found mean d values of $-.02$, $.00$, $-.09$, $.13$, $.11$, and $.09$ for blacks, Hispanics, Asian-Americans, whites, Australians, and Canadians, respectively.

5. Meta-analyses can be theory-grounded and can be used to test theories of gender. Good examples are Eagly's application of social role theory in predicting patterns of gender differences in aggression and in helping behaviors (Eagly & Crowley, 1986; Eagly & Steffen, 1986).

REFERENCES

Anastasi, A. (1958). *Differential psychology: Individual and group differences in behavior* (3rd ed.). New York: Macmillan.

Anderson, L. R., & Blanchard, P. N. (1982). Sex differences in task and social-emotional behavior. *Basic and Applied Social Psychology, 3*, 109–139.

Bales, R. F. (1950). *Interaction process analysis*. Reading, MA: Addison-Wesley.

Bassoff, E. S., & Glass, G. V. (1982). The relationship between sex roles and mental health: A meta-analysis of 26 studies. *Counseling Psychologist, 10*, 105–112.

Becker, B. J. (1986). Influence again: An examination of reviews and studies of gender differences in social influence. In J. S. Hyde & M. C. Linn (Eds.), *The psychology of gender: Advances through meta-analysis* (pp. 178–209). Baltimore: Johns Hopkins University Press.

Becker, B. J., & Hedges, L. V. (1984). Meta-analysis of cognitive gender differences: A comment on an analysis by Rosenthal and Rubin. *Journal of Educational Psychology, 76*, 583–587.

Bem, S. L. (1974). The measurement of psychological androgyny. *Journal of Consulting and Clinical Psychology, 42*, 155–162.

Bennett, G. K., Seashore, H. G., & Wesman, A. G. (1947). *Manual for the Differential Aptitude Tests*. New York: Psychological Corporation.

Bennet, G. K., Seashore, H. G., & Wesman, A. G. (1966). *Fourth edition manual for the Differential Aptitude Tests*. New York: Psychological Corporation.

Bennett, G. K., Seashore, H. G., & Wesman, A. G. (1974). *Fifth edition manual for the Differential Aptitude Tests*. New York: Psychological Corporation.

Bennett, G. K., Seashore, H. G., & Wesman, A. G. (1982). *Differential Aptitude Tests Form V and W: Administrator's handbook*. New York: Psychological Corporation.

Block, J. (1976). Issues, problems, and pitfalls in assessing sex differences: A critical review of *The psychology of sex differences*. *Merrill-Palmer Quarterly, 22*, 283–308.

Cohen, J. (1969). *Statistical power analysis for the behavioral sciences*. New York: Academic Press.

Cooper, H. M. (1979). Statistically combining independent studies: A meta-analysis of sex differences in conformity research. *Journal of Personality and Social Psychology, 37*, 131–146.

Dobbins, G. H., & Platz, S. J. (1986). Sex differences in leadership: How real are they? *Academy of Management Review, 11*, 118–127.

Donlon, T. F. (1984). *The College Board technical handbook for the Scholastic Aptitude Test and Achievement Tests*. New York: College Entrance Examination Board.

Eagly, A. H. (1978). Sex differences in influenceability. *Journal of Personality and Social Psychology, 85*, 86–116.

Eagly, A. H. (1986). Some meta-analytic approaches to examining the validity of gender-difference research. In J. S. Hyde & M. C. Linn (Eds.), *The psychology of gender: Advances through meta-analysis* (pp. 159–177). Baltimore: Johns Hopkins University Press.

Eagly, A. H. (1987). *Sex differences in social behavior: A social-role interpretation*. Hillsdale, NJ: Erlbaum.

Eagly, A. H., & Carli, L. L. (1981). Sex of researcher and sex-typed communications as determinants of sex differences in influenceability: A meta-analysis of social influence studies. *Psychological Bulletin, 90*, 1–20.

Eagly, A. H., & Crowley, M. (1986). Gender and helping behavior: A meta-analytic review of the social psychological literature. *Psychological Bulletin, 100*, 283–308.

Eagly, A. H., & Johnson, B. T. (1989). Gender and leadership style: A meta-analysis. Manuscript submitted for publication.

Eagly, A. H., & Steffen, V. J. (1986). Gender and aggressive behavior: A meta-analytic review of the social psychological literature. *Psychological Bulletin, 100*, 309–330.

Eaton, W. O., & Enns, L. R. (1986). Sex differences in human motor activity level. *Psychological Bulletin, 100*, 19–28.

Eisenberg, N., & Lennon, R. (1983). Sex differences in empathy and related capacities. *Psychological Bulletin, 94*, 100–131.

Feingold, A. (1988). Cognitive differences are disappearing. *American Psychologist, 43*, 95–103.

Fennema, E., & Sherman, J. A. (1976). Fennema-Sherman Mathematics Attitudes Scales: Instruments designed to measure attitudes toward the learning of mathematics by females and males. *JSAS Catalog of Selected Documents in Psychology, 6*, 31. (Ms. No. 1225.) (Reprinted by Wisconsin Center for Education Research, University of Wisconsin-Madison.)

Frieze, I. H., Whitley, B. E., Jr., Hanusa, B., & McHugh, M. C. (1982). Assessing the theoretical models for sex differences in causal attributions for success and failure. *Sex Roles, 8*, 333–343.

Goldstein, A. G., & Jeffords, J. (1981). Status and touching behavior. *Bulletin of the Psychonomic Society, 17*, 79–81.

Hall, J. A. (1978). Gender effects in decoding nonverbal cues. *Psychological Bulletin, 85*, 845–875.

Hall, J. A. (1984). *Nonverbal sex differences: Communication accuracy and expressive style*. Baltimore: Johns Hopkins.

Hall, J. A., & Halberstadt, A. G. (1986). Smiling and gazing. In J. S. Hyde & M. C. Linn (Eds.), *The psychology of gender: Advances through meta-analysis* (pp. 136–158). Baltimore: Johns Hopkins.

Hare-Mustin, R. T., & Marecek, J. (1988). The meaning of difference: Gender theory, postmodernism, and psychology. *American Psychologist, 43*, 455–464.

Haring, M. J., Stock, W. A., & Okun, M. A. (1984). A research synthesis of gender and social class as correlates of subjective well-being. *Human Relations, 37*, 645–657.

Haring-Hidore, M. J., Stock, W. A., Okun, M. A., & Witter, R. A. (1985). Marital status and subjective well-being: A research synthesis. *Journal of Marriage and the Family, 47*, 947–953.

Hattie, J. (1979). Stability of results across many studies: Sex differences on the Personal Orientation Inventory. *Journal of Personality Assessment, 43*, 627–628.

Hedges, L. V. (1981). Distribution theory for Glass' estimator of effect size and related estimators. *Journal of Educational Statistics, 6*, 107–128.

Hedges, L. V. (1982a). Fitting categorical models to effect sizes from a series of experiments. *Journal of Educational Statistics, 7*, 119–137.

Hedges, L. V. (1982b). Fitting continuous models to effect size data. *Journal of Educational Statistics, 7*, 245–270.

Hedges, L. V., & Becker, B. J. (1986). Statistical methods in the meta-analysis of research on gender differences. In J. S. Hyde & M. C. Linn (Eds.), *The psychology of gender: Advances through meta-analysis* (pp. 14–50). Baltimore: Johns Hopkins University Press.

Hedges, L. V., & Olkin, I. (1985). *Statistical methods for meta-analysis*. New York: Academic Press.

Henley N. M. (1977). *Body politics: Power, sex, and nonverbal communication*. Englewood Cliffs, NJ: Prentice-Hall.

Hunter, J. E., Schmidt, F. L., & Jackson, G. B. (1982). *Meta-analysis: Cumulating research findings across studies.* Beverly Hills: Sage.

Hyde, J. S. (1981). How large are cognitive gender differences? A meta-analysis using w^2 and *d. American Psychologist, 36,* 892–901.

Hyde, J. S. (1984). How large are gender differences in aggression? A developmental meta-analysis. *Developmental Psychology, 20,* 722–736.

Hyde, J. S. (1985). *Half the human experience: The psychology of women* (3rd ed.). Lexington, MA: D. C. Heath.

Hyde, J. S. (1986). Introduction: Meta-analysis and the psychology of gender. In J. S. Hyde & M. C. Linn (Eds.), *The psychology of gender: Advances through meta-analysis* (pp. 1–13). Baltimore: Johns Hopkins.

Hyde, J. S. (1990). Review essay: Meta-analysis and the psychology of gender differences. *Signs, 16,* 55–73.

Hyde, J. S., Fennema, E., & Lamon, S. J. (1990). Gender differences in mathematics performance: A meta-analysis. *Psychological Bulletin, 107,* 139–155.

Hyde, J. S., Fennema, E., Ryan, M., Frost, L. A., & Hopp, C. (1990). Gender differences in mathematics attitudes and affect: A meta-analysis. *Psychology of Women Quarterly, 14,* 299–324.

Hyde, J. S., & Linn, M. C. (1988). Gender differences in verbal ability: A meta-analysis. *Psychological Bulletin, 104,* 53–69.

Inhelder, B., & Piaget, J. (1958). *The growth of logical thinking from childhood to adolescence.* New York: Basic Books.

Kimball, M. M. (1989). A new perspective on women's math achievement. *Psychological Bulletin, 105,* 198–214.

Linn, M. C., & Hyde, J. S. (1989). Gender, mathematics, and science. *Educational Researcher, 18* (8), 17–27.

Linn, M. C., & Petersen, A. C. (1985). Emergence and characterization of sex differences in spatial ability: A meta-analysis. *Child Development, 56,* 1479–1498.

Maccoby E. E., & Jacklin, C. N. (1974). *The psychology of sex differences.* Stanford, CA: Stanford University Press.

Maccoby, E. E., & Jacklin, C. N. (1980). Sex differences in aggression: A rejoinder and reprise. *Child Development, 51,* 964–980.

Meehan, A. M. (1984). A meta-analysis of sex differences in formal operational thought. *Child Development, 55,* 1110–1124.

Nash, S. C. (1979). Sex role as a mediator of intellectual functioning. In M. A. Wittig & A. C. Petersen (Eds.), *Sex-related differences in cognitive functioning* (pp. 263–302). New York: Academic Press.

Orwin, R. G. (1983). A fail-safe *N* for effect size. *Journal of Educational Statistics, 8,* 157–159.

Ramist, L., & Arbeiter, S. (1986). *Profiles, college-bound seniors, 1985.* New York: College Entrance Examination Board.

Richardson, F. C., & Suinn, R. M. (1972). The Mathematics Anxiety Ratings Scales: Psychometric data. *Journal of Counseling Psychology, 19,* 551–554.

Robertson, S. S., Dierker, L. J., Sorokin, Y., & Rosen, M. G. (1982). Human fetal movement: Spontaneous oscillations near one cycle per minute. *Science, 218,* 1327–1330.

Rosenthal, R. (1978). Combining results of independent studies. *Psychological Bulletin, 85,* 185–193.

Rosenthal, R. (1979). The "file drawer problem" and tolerance for null results. *Psychological Bulletin, 86,* 638–641.

Rosenthal, R., & DePaulo, B. M. (1979). Sex differences in accommodation in nonverbal communication. In R. Rosenthal (Ed.), *Skill in nonverbal communication* (pp. 68–103). Cambridge, MA: Oelgeschlager, Gunn, & Hain.

Rosenthal, R., & Rubin, D. B. (1982a). Further meta-analytic procedures for assessing cognitive gender differences. *Journal of Educational Psychology, 74,* 708–712.

Rosenthal, R., & Rubin, D. B. (1982b). Comparing effect sizes of independent studies. *Psychological Bulletin, 92,* 500–504.

Rosenthal, R., & Rubin, D. B. (1982c). A simple, general purpose display of the magnitude of experimental effect. *Journal of Educational Psychology, 74,* 166–169.

Shields, S. (1975). Functionalism, Darwinism, and the psychology of women: A study in social myth. *American Psychologist, 30,* 739–754.

Shostrom, E. L. (1966). *Manual, Personal Orientation Inventory.* San Diego, CA: Educational and Industrial Testing Service.

Signorella, M. G., & Jamison, W. (1986). Masculinity, femininity, androgyny, and cognitive performance: A meta-analysis. *Psychological Bulletin, 100,* 207–228.

Sistrunk, F., & McDavid, J. (1971). Sex variable in conformity behavior. *Journal of Personality and Social Psychology, 17,* 200–207.

Sohn, D. (1980). Critique of Cooper's meta-analytic assessment of the findings on sex differences in conformity behavior. *Journal of Personality and Social Psychology, 39,* 1215–1221.

Sohn, D. (1982). Sex differences in achievement self-attributions: An effect size analysis. *Sex Roles, 8,* 345–357.

Spence, J. T., Helmreich, R., & Stapp, J. (1974). The Personal Attributes Questionnaire: A measure of sex-role stereotypes and masculinity-femininity. *JSAS Catalog of Selected Documents in Psychology, 4,* 43. (Ms. No. 617)

Spence, J. T., Helmreich, R., & Stapp, J. (1975). Ratings of self and peers on sex role attributes and their relation to self-esteem and conceptions of masculinity and femininity. *Journal of Personality and Social Psychology, 32,* 29–39.

Stier, D. S., & Hall, J. A. (1984). Gender differences in touch: An empirical and theoretical review. *Journal of Personality and Social Psychology, 47,* 440–459.

Stock, M. A., Okun, M. A., Haring, M. J., & Witter, R. A. (1983). Age differences in subjective well-being: A meta-analysis. In R. J. Light (Ed.), *Evaluation studies: Review annual* (Vol. 8, pp. 279–302). Beverly Hills: Sage.

Taylor, M. C., & Hall, J. A. (1982). Psychological androgyny: Theories, methods, and conclusions. *Psychological Bulletin, 92,* 347–366.

Thomas, J. R., & French, K. E. (1985). Gender differences across age in motor performance: A meta-analysis. *Psychological Bulletin, 98,* 260–282.

Tieger, T. (1980). On the biological basis of sex differences in aggression. *Child Development, 51,* 943–963.

Tyler, L. (1947). *The psychology of human differences.* New York: Appleton-Century-Crofts.

Weitzman, L. J. (1985). *The divorce revolution: The unexpected social and economic consequences for women and children in America.* New York: Free Press.

Whitley, B. E., Jr. (1983). Sex-role orientation and self-esteem: A critical meta-analytic review. *Journal of Personality and Social Psychology, 44,* 765–778.

Whitley, B. E., Jr. (1984). Sex-role orientation and psychological well-being: Two meta-analyses. *Sex Roles*, *12*, 207–225.

Whitley, B. E., Jr., McHugh, M. C., & Frieze, I. H. (1986). Assessing the theoretical models for sex differences in causal attributions of success and failure. In J. S. Hyde & M. C. Linn (Eds.), *The psychology of gender: Advances through meta-analysis* (pp. 102–135). Baltimore: Johns Hopkins.

Wood, W. (1987). Meta-analytic review of sex differences in group performance. *Psychological Bulletin*, *102*, 53–71.

Wood, W., Rhodes, N., & Whelan, M. (1989). Sex differences in positive well-being: A consideration of emotional style and marital status. *Psychological Bulletin*, *106*, 249–264.

Woolley, H. T. (1910). A review of the recent literature on the psychology of sex. *Psychological Bulletin*, *7*, 335–342.

Part II

Society's View of Women

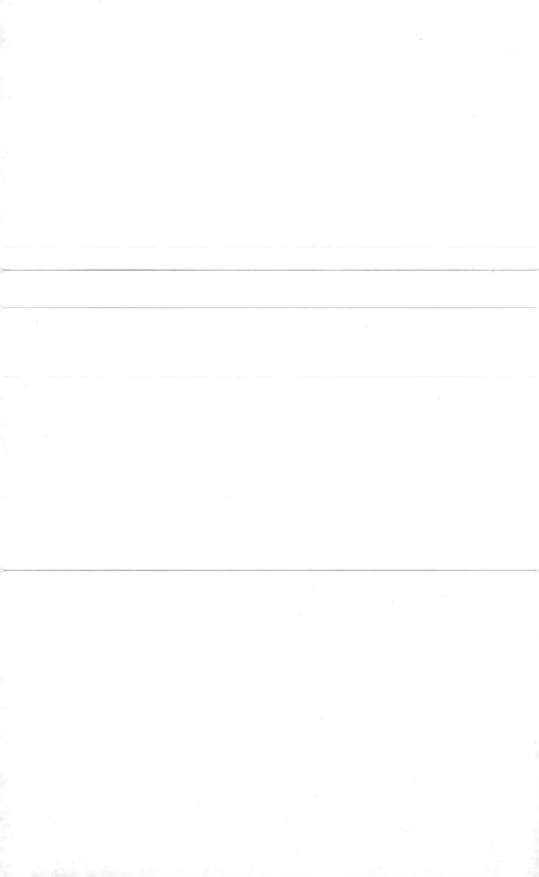

4

Gender Stereotypes

Kay Deaux and Mary Kite

The subtle influence of sex upon a person's perceptions may vary with each observer and play both an unconscious and conscious role in influencing actions taken.

—Gesell, 1990, p. 9

Judge Gerhard Gesell of the U.S. Court of Appeals wrote these words in his precedent-setting decision awarding a partnership to a woman who had been discriminated against on the basis of gender. In 1982, Ann Hopkins was denied promotion to partnership at the accounting firm of Price Waterhouse, despite a strong record of performance. She was the only woman considered for partnership that year; at the time the company had only seven women among their 662 partners. Hopkins was not told to work harder. Rather, she was given advice that focused on her makeup, her jewelry, and her style of walk and talk. Hopkins sued the firm and won, and she continued to win as the case was appealed, heard by the Supreme Court, and returned to the court of appeals (on a legal issue of burden of proof), where Judge Gesell made his decision awarding her a partnership.

The case of *Price-Waterhouse v. Hopkins* marked a rite of passage for research on gender stereotypes. The empirical and theoretical literature of social scientists was an integral part of the process, first represented at the lower court in expert witness testimony (Fiske, 1989) and later in an *amicus brief* filed with the Supreme Court (Fiske, Bersoff, Borgida, Deaux, & Heilman, 1990). At each level of decision, the courts recognized the role that gender stereotypes had played in the evaluation of Hopkins. Yet the prevalence of gender stereotyping and the consequences of such stereotypes for other women and men will surely not be altered by the decision in this single case.

"We has met the enemy, and it is us," Walt Kelly had Pogo say (Bartlett, 1980). And so it is with stereotyping, a ubiquitous process to which we all succumb. In this chapter, we will consider why that is the case, what conditions support stereotypes, and what functions they serve. We will review both theoretical analyses and empirical findings as they relate to the content of gender stereotypes and subtypes, the development of stereotypes, and individual differences in their use. Finally, we will consider possibilities for change, both in cultural endorsement and individual usage.

THEORETICAL ORIENTATIONS TO STEREOTYPING

Stereotypes about gender are multidetermined. As is true of other hypothetical constructs such as attitudes (Eagly & Chaiken, 1993) and schemas (Fiske & Taylor, 1991) that we use to help us explain people's beliefs and behaviors, stereotypes are subject to multiple interpretations. Over the years, a number of different theoretical perspectives have been offered, each presenting a somewhat different window on the causes and consequences of stereotypes. Borrowing from the analyses of Ashmore and Del Boca (1976, 1981) with slight modifications, we consider three general theoretical orientations to the study of stereotyping and prejudice: sociocultural, motivational, and cognitive. Depending on which framework is adopted, one makes different assumptions, asks somewhat different questions, and often uses different methodologies to examine the issues. Together, however, these frameworks capture the richness and complexity of stereotyping and prejudice.

Sociocultural Perspective

In observing that many stereotypes are provided by one's culture, Lippmann (1922) laid the foundation for the sociocultural perspective. According to this view, stereotypes are shared belief systems, and an individual's personal beliefs reflect the larger societal view. The classic approaches to assessing stereotypes reflected these assumptions. In the method developed by Katz and Braly (1933), for example, respondents used an adjective checklist to indicate which characteristics they thought were associated with which groups. Majority agreement then defined the stereotype. Initially developed to measure ethnic stereotypes, the method was used to assess gender stereotypes as well (Broverman, Vogel, Broverman, Clarkson, & Rosenkrantz, 1972; Rosenkrantz, Vogel, Bee, Broverman, & Broverman, 1968; Sheriffs & McKee, 1957; Williams & Best, 1982).

Within the general sociocultural perspective, two variants can be distinguished: (1) a cultural and (2) a structural approach. Both agree that society is the source of shared stereotypes, but they differ in their interpretations of when and how information is acquired.

Cultural Approach

The general premise of the cultural approach is that children are socialized to act in accordance with the cultural dictates, presumably through the social rewards and punishments that accompany adoption of society's values and norms. This acceptance of culture and its continuation into adulthood lead to the reinforcement and perpetuation of stereotyping. Ashmore and Del Boca (1981) argue that much of gender stereotyping research is, at least implicitly, committed to this perspective.

Research on media stereotypes reflects the cultural approach. Two steps are involved in this research. The first step is to demonstrate that men and women are presented in consistently stereotypical ways in the media. The second step is to test the assumption that by continually viewing these presentations, people develop stereotypes of women and men that are consistent with these depictions and that, in many respects, provide the normative information we use to characterize the sexes. The pervasiveness of gender stereotypes in the media is well documented. The forum for these stereotypes includes women's magazines (Friedan, 1963; Ruggiero & Weston, 1985; Sullivan & O'Connor, 1988), television programs (Mayes & Valentine, 1979; Sternglanz & Serbin, 1974), television commercials (Manstead & McColloch, 1981; McArthur & Resko, 1975), comic strips (Brabant & Mooney, 1986; Chavez, 1985; Potkay & Potkay, 1984), and rock music videos (Brown, 1985). Although the direct effect of these presentations on the endorsement of stereotypes is more difficult to establish, some longitudinal work has linked amount of media exposure to children's acceptance of gender stereotypes (Eron, Huesmann, Brice, Fischer & Mermelstein, 1983; Morgan, 1982). In an experimental study of media effects, women who viewed stereotyped commercials conveyed fewer achievement themes when asked to describe their lives 10 years in the future (Geis, Brown, Jennings [Walstedt] & Porter, 1984).

Structural Approach

This version of the sociocultural perspective emphasizes the common positions that certain groups occupy within the social structure. Rather than emphasizing early socialization experiences, adherents of this approach focus on the ongoing structural constraints that channel our experience, from the family to the societal level.

Eagly's (1987) social-role theory is the best example of this approach. According to her theory, stereotypes of men and women (or any subgroup) are derived, at least in part, from observing individuals in their societal roles. Men and women, for example, occupy different social positions: men are more likely to assume the occupational role, and women are more likely to assume the domestic role. From observing the sexes in these varied roles, people derive gender-role expectations for others as well as their own sex-typed behaviors. To the extent that people adopt a role congruent with what they have observed to be appropriate to their sex, sex differences and accompanying stereotypes become self-perpetuating. If, according to this analysis, roles change, then beliefs about women and men will change accordingly.

In support of this theory, Eagly and Steffen (1984, 1986) found that occupational roles are a strong determinant of the traits ascribed to women and men, outweighing gender information. Employed people are regarded as more agentic than people in the domestic role, regardless of their gender. Moreover, part-time employees are seen as less agentic than full-time employees, suggesting that type of employment also has a considerable impact on how women and men are perceived. Individuals with higher-status jobs are perceived to have more agentic qualities than individuals in lower-status occupations. Age stereotypes can be similarly modified by providing employment information. Older men and women are viewed as less agentic than younger men and women, but only when they are described as "average." When the individuals are known to be employed, older women and men are not thought to be less agentic than younger women and men (Kite, 1990).

Motivational Perspective

Research in the motivational framework has its roots in psychodynamic models. Early theorists believed that stereotyping and prejudice fulfilled goals of personality integration. Accordingly, stereotypes were thought to be motivationally based and served to strengthen one's personal identity. The question of interest at that time was whether overarching personality differences could predict how people would respond to stereotyped groups. More recently, the questions have been expanded to include how motives and goals relate to stereotyping and prejudice.

The benchmark work in this perspective is that of Adorno and his colleagues (Adorno, Frenkel-Brunswik, Levinson & Sanford, 1950), who examined the relationship between authoritarianism and prejudice. They found, for example, that when people high in authoritarianism discussed sexual relations, they revealed negative feelings about sexuality and the other sex in general. Related research on tolerance for ambiguity also takes a motivational perspective (Frenkel-Brunswik, 1949; Larsen, 1984), as does recent work on self-esteem and prejudice. In each case, there is an attempt to show that certain stable personality dispositions predict a person's willingness to evaluate negatively members of some outgroup.

The relationship between self-esteem and prejudice is not as simple as once believed, however. People who have low self-esteem are more prejudiced, in general, than people with high self-esteem (see Ashmore & Del Boca, 1976, for a review), a tendency that appears to be quite global. However, people with low self-esteem are biased even toward members of the same social group

(Crocker & Schwartz, 1985), suggesting that an ethnocentric bias does not account for this phenomenon. Moreover, when the self-concept is threatened, it is those persons high in self-esteem, not those low in self-esteem, who respond by derogating the outgroup (Crocker, Thompson, McGraw & Ingerman, 1987).

Functional theories of attitude also emphasize motivational factors, stressing that people can hold similar attitudes for very different reasons (D. Katz, 1960; Smith, Bruner & White, 1956). For example, two people may agree that women should not have the same rights and responsibilities as men, yet the psychological mechanisms underlying their beliefs may be quite dissimilar. For one, strong religious beliefs may be the basis for this perspective, while the other's beliefs may be expressed to gain favor with colleagues. In redirecting attention to functional causes, Herek (1986a, 1986b, 1987) suggests that people can benefit either from holding an attitude about the attitude object itself or from expressing the attitude. In the first case, attitudes have an experiential function that helps people make sense of the world in terms of past experience. In the second case, attitudes serve an expressive function that is tied to the person's identity and self-esteem, either serving basic values, seeking social acceptance, or protecting defensive needs. As applied to the case of gender, this approach would suggest that the endorsement of stereotypes can be understood only through a more individual analysis of function.

Cognitive Orientation

The dominant contemporary orientation to stereotyping stresses not individual needs for holding a stereotype, but rather the inherent information-processing capacity of human beings. From this perspective, stereotyping is one example of a more general categorization process, necessary for people to deal with the complexities of human existence. To cope with a potentially unmanageable amount of information, people learn to streamline information processing by grouping people, objects, and events into manageable categories based on some similarity among members. Efficient as this system can be, it is also fraught with biases. People may see things that are not there while ignoring things that are (Hamilton, 1979; Taylor & Crocker, 1981). These misperceptions, in turn, can serve to confirm the expectancies that a person has about members of stereotyped groups and ultimately perpetuate those stereotypes.

These ideas are not new; their roots are in the writings of Lippman (1922), Allport (1954), and other early theorists. Yet it was not until Tajfel's (1969) landmark paper that the principle of categorization received widespread attention. Tajfel believed that categorization is an essential component of the stereotyping process, but unlike Allport and Lippman, who viewed stereotypes as oversimplified, rigid, and incorrect, Tajfel pointed out that categorization is a normal and not necessarily inaccurate part of cognitive functioning.

The strength of the cognitive approach lies in its attention to the ways in which these categories are used—how they influence the encoding of information, memory, and subsequent inferences and judgments (Fiske & Taylor, 1991; Hamilton, 1979). Rather than an end in themselves, stereotypes and other categorical representations are considered in terms of their consequences. Of most interest to cognitive theorists is not what is stored in a particular schematic representation, but rather how the information is used and the consequences of this utilization.

The cognitive approach to stereotyping dominates contemporary thinking on the issues (see Messick & Mackie, 1989; Sherman, Judd & Park, 1989, for recent reviews). Some attempts to integrate cognitive and motivation perspectives are developing as well (Fiske & Neuberg, 1990; Fiske & Pavelchak, 1986; Srull & Wyer, 1986). Although these analyses have only infrequently been concerned with gender, the implications for gender stereotypes are quite clear (see Fiske, 1989). Accordingly, our subsequent analysis of gender stereotypes will be strongly influenced by this perspective, particularly when dealing with issues of structure and change.

Are Stereotypes True or False?

Concern with the accuracy of stereotypes is to some degree contingent on one's theoretical stance. Early motivational approaches, for example, emphasized the inevitable distortions in stereotypes, regarding stereotypes as less a reflection of reality than a manifestation of individual needs. Alternatively, it is argued that all stereotypes contain a "kernel of truth," however surrounded by exaggeration and oversimplification. With the more recent cognitive models of stereotypes, the question of truthfulness tends to be finessed. These models emphasize the representations of the perceiver rather than the intrinsic characteristics of the target (though they do alert us to the ways in which distortions can occur). Thus, to begin to frame an answer to the question posed above, one must first declare one's theoretical stance. Yet despite the elusiveness of the answer, some general comments can be made.

There is little question that some aspects of the gender belief system correspond (albeit imperfectly) to objective differences in the behaviors, activities, and/or distribution of women and men in the social system. Occupational patterns, for example, show marked sex differences, as does task division of labor within the household. By observing these differences in the distribution of men and women to social roles, Eagly (1987) argues, people derive their stereotypic beliefs about the sexes. Yet the causal sequence is not unidirectional. Stereotypes acquire a prescriptive character as well, thereby channeling the activities and choices that individuals make and, in some instances, reinforcing the distinctions between women and men.

Whereas some proponents of the kernel of truth point to social roles as the origin of stereotypes, others claim biological determinism, arguing that certain sex differences are "hard-wired" and thus basic to distinguishing men from women. Even if one agrees that there are some biological differences between the sexes, the debate is not resolved. One needs to question further how subject any biological factors are to environmental alteration.[1] Although fascinating, the discussion of the origin of observed sex differences is tangential to our concerns here.

The issue of stereotype accuracy really has two parts: first, the accuracy of the hypothetical average as a description of the total population, and second, the fit of the general category to the individual case. The first of these issues is sometimes less controversial and more easily answered (depending on the concrete or abstract nature of the behavior or trait in question). If one believes that women are more likely to be secretaries than are men and that men are more likely to be marines, there are informational sources that can confirm those beliefs. Such sources are less readily available, however, if the attribute is a more abstract emotion or personality trait. Assessing probabilities of "emotional" women or "aggressive" men, for example, requires a level of agreement as to what constitutes emotionality or aggression that is difficult to attain.[2] It is just these kinds of abstractions that most often define the turf of gender stereotypes.

The more pernicious aspect of stereotypes lies in the application of the general category, however imperfectly defined, to the case of the individual. Given the wide within-sex variation in virtually every trait or behavior associated with gender stereotypes, overgeneralization is axiomatic. At minimum, stereotypes should be considered probabilistic estimates rather than absolute ascriptions. Yet unless they have a good reason to demand more individuating information, people will often be content to use the average as a "best fit estimate" and judge members of the category accordingly (Fiske, 1989; Fiske & Neuberg, 1990). Thus even the stereotype that is accurate at the group level may be quite inappropriately applied at the individual level. The consequences of this process are covered more directly in Chapter 7.

THE CONTENT AND STRUCTURE OF GENDER STEREOTYPES

Gender stereotypes have a familiar quality. Nearly any person stopped on the street could probably reel off a list of characteristics associated with one sex or the other. Indeed, early research on gender stereotypes focused on just this type of descriptive listing. Current analyses have become more complex, recognizing that both the dimensions of description and the targets of that description are best represented in multiple, rather than singular, terms.

The Content of Gender Stereotypes

The traits associated with women and men are well documented (Broverman et al., 1972; Rosenkrantz et al., 1968; Spence, Helmreich, & Stapp, 1974) and concentrate in two dimensions: beliefs that women are concerned for the welfare of other people (labeled expressive or communal) and beliefs that men are assertive and controlling (labeled instrumental or agentic). People are equally willing to apply these traits to themselves as to others, indicating that self-description is linked to the stereotypic assessment of others. Moreover, these stereotypic beliefs are not limited to U.S. populations. In research covering 30 different nations, Williams and Best (1982) observed considerable consensus in the perceived attributes of women and men. Men were typically seen as stronger and more active, characterized by high needs for achievement, dominance, autonomy, and aggression. Women, in contrast, were believed to be more concerned with affiliation, nurturance, and deference.

In terms of the relative desirability of these two trait dimensions, there has been some confusion over the years. Rosenkrantz and his colleagues (1968) originally reported that there were a larger number of masculine traits than feminine traits that were evaluated positively. Yet in terms of mean ratings, there was no difference in the average "goodness" of these two stereotypical clusters. Recent work by Eagly and her colleagues (Eagly & Mladinic, 1989; Eagly, Mladinic & Otto, 1990) suggests that traits assigned to women are actually more favorable than those assigned to men, at least among the college student samples they have tested.

Is it possible that gender stereotypes are changing? For the most part, stereotypes have shown remarkable durability across time and place. Bergen and Williams (1989, cited in Bergen, 1989) for example, compared stereotype ratings of men and women in 1972 and 1988 and found no important differences. Yet one Norwegian study did show a shift toward greater favorability of the female stereotype (Bjerke, Williams & Wathne, 1989, reported in Bergen, 1989). Werner and LaRussa (1985), comparing U.S. data collected in 1978 with data collected 20 years earlier, also found evidence of some shifts. Although many aspects of gender stereotypes remained unchanged over the 20-year interval, there was also evidence that the male stereotype was becoming less favorable and the female stereotype more favorable. Perhaps Eagly's recent data reflect these changes. It will be important to continue doing longitudinal studies of gender stereotypes to determine how permanent these changes are and what form they take.

Most of the early research on the content of gender stereotypes concentrated on personality traits associated with women and men. Yet it is obvious that many other domains are also linked to gender in most people's minds. Indeed, the aforementioned person in the street would very likely invoke sports, hobbies, occupations, and a range of other domains in which the sexes were believed to differ. Deaux and Lewis (1983, 1984) reported that stereotypes of gender can be differentiated on the basis of role behaviors, physical characteristics, and occupational status. Other investigators have confirmed this multidimensional approach (Ashmore & Del Boca, 1979; Freeman, 1987; see also Huston, 1983, for a discussion of the independence of various gender components). These dimensions (as well as others that might be identified) are not perfectly correlated, a finding that is consistent with the notion of stereotypes as a kind of "fuzzy set.'' However, the dimensions are interrelated to the extent that information about one dimension can influence inferences about other dimensions, suggesting that the network of beliefs is interwoven (Deaux & Lewis, 1984; Jackson & Cash, 1985).

Stereotypes and Subtypes

Stereotypes of women and men are very general categories. In theory, each gender stereotype refers to approximately half of the world's population. Almost by definition, such general categories lack discriminatory power; as a consequence, people develop beliefs about particular kinds of women and men that may or may not share features with the more general categories.

Before considering some of these specific subtypes, however, we should note limitations on the assumptions about 50% of the world's population. Investigators of gender stereotypes typically assume that the terms *women* and *men* are not limited to any particular ethnic group or social class. Yet there is evidence that the well-established stereotypes of men and women are limited in both respects. Landrine (1985) varied race (black and white) and class (middle and lower) information in asking people to evaluate the category of woman. Her results suggest that both factors make a difference. For example, black women were believed to be dirtier, more hostile, and more superstitious than white women; white women were thought to be more dependent, more emotional, and more passive than black women. Dimensions on which the social classes differed included impulsivity, superstition, consideration, and responsibility. More importantly, the ratings of white women were much more similar to the standard findings for the stereotype of ''woman'' than were the ratings of black women, suggesting that race is an implicit, but unrecognized, variable in much stereotype research.[3] Studies of black women are few; studies of other women of color are virtually nonexistent. Hence the 50% assumption is quite unjustified.

Subtypes are formed because the more global, superordinate category proves unsatisfactory (Rothbart & John, 1985). In its generality, the general stereotype of woman or man fails to speak to specific features that people believe are characteristic of particular groups (e.g., ''These modern career types aren't like the women I used to know''). Thus people develop categories that they think are more accurate descriptions of a subgroup (e.g., ''Businesswoman are pushy, lack charm'').

The particular subtypes that are formed depend on both context and experience. In one of the first explorations of subtypes, Clifton, McGrath & Wick (1976) identified ''housewife'' and ''bunny'' as two distinct female stereotypes. Noseworthy and Lott (1984) pointed to four clear subtypes: sex object, career woman, housewife, and athlete. The same four categories of women were reported by Deaux, Winton, Crowley, and Lewis (1985); in addition, they identified common male categories of businessman, athletic man, blue-collar workingman, and macho man. Suggesting how specific context can create specific subtypes, Holland and Davidson (1983) report a male category of "fratty-bagger" used by undergraduates at the University of North Carolina.

In the studies just discussed, investigators relied on respondents to identify categories of common usage. Using a different approach, some investigators decide on categories of interest in advance and then ask respondents to make inferences about characteristics of a person who fits that category label. With this strategy, the investigator typically defines the domain of attributes as well, asking respondents to evaluate a specific set of traits and behaviors associated with the general male-female stereotype.

Gender stereotypes associated with sexual orientation is one such example. Beliefs about homosexual women and men show how easily male and female are conceptualized in oppositional terms. Lesbians are believed to have characteristics typically associated with men, while gay men are believed to have predominantly feminine characteristics (Kite & Deaux, 1987). Apparently, people hold an implicit belief in Freud's inversion theory, even though there is scant evidence to support this belief in the actual characteristics of homosexual men and women (Storms, 1978a, 1978b).

Age also modifies gender stereotypes, although far less dramatically. People generally believe that 65-year-olds—both men and women—are less likely to have masculine traits, to engage in traditionally masculine role behaviors, and to have physical characteristics such as strong muscles or a deep voice. Older men and women are also believed to be less likely to engage in feminine role behaviors than are 35-year-olds. Yet the perceived distinctions between women and men remain constant across the two age groups, even though the baseline is lowered for some characteristics (Kite, Deaux & Miele, 1991). Further, open-ended responses by subjects in this study showed that age distinctions were much stronger than gender distinctions, again emphasizing the importance of considering groups defined more specifically than by gender alone.

Beliefs about the agentic and communal traits of women and men also vary with information about employment status. Specifically, agency is associated with full-time employment, and communion is associated with the homemaker role for both women and men (Eagly & Steffen, 1984, 1986). Similarly, when the leadership roles of a marital couple are specifically described, the powerful person is assumed to be agentic and the nonpowerful person assumed to be communal, regardless of sex of the marital partner (Gerber, 1988). Even a title of address can evoke stereotypic images: women using "Ms." are perceived to be more achievement-oriented and assertive, but less interpersonally warm than women with a more traditional "Miss" or "Mrs." (Dion, 1987).

There is some evidence that subtypes of women are more clearly articulated than those of men. Ashmore, Del Boca, and Titus (1984), for example, found that multidimensional scaling solutions for women identified three clear types (wife/mother, sexual woman, and independent career woman), while the solution for men was less definite. Deaux and Sinnett (1989) consulted dictionaries for terms used to describe women and men and asked people to categorize the terms into meaningful categories or types of women and of men. In a parallel study, subjects sorted photographs of men and women collected from magazines and newspapers. In both cases, people had more consistently defined categories of women than of men. The reasons for these differences are not clear. To check the nature of the bias, Deaux and Sinnett (1989) conducted a third study using an identical set of verbal descriptors with instructions to consider them in reference to either women or men. In this case, there were no differences, suggesting that the categorization reflects the observed distribution of women and men in the society (or in our vocabulary and our magazines) rather than a biased perspective by the respondents. Women are more different among each other than are men, this analysis would suggest. Research that simultaneously considers race and gender also suggests that differences between stereotypes of black and white men are less pronounced than the differences between black and white women (Deaux & Kite, 1985).

Many stereotypes of women and men are triggered by visual cues. Allport recognized the importance of physical appearance to prejudicial judgments. "Visibility and identifiability aid categorization," he remarked in a statement that is as applicable to gender as to the racial case he originally considered (1954, p. 127). The primacy of visual information is a key: people are often characterized on the basis of their appearance before other kinds of descriptive information become available (McArthur, 1982; Fiske & Taylor, 1991). Often a particular physical feature or article of clothing (e.g, briefcase or bikini) can cue subordinate categories of belief. A number of investigations have shown that information about physical appearance is more potent than other types of information in eliciting stereotypic inferences (Deaux & Lewis, 1984; Freeman, 1987).

Some researchers have suggested that information about physical appearance, and in particular physical attractiveness, might be more crucial to impressions of women than of men. However, a recent meta-analysis of research on the physical attractiveness stereotype by Eagly, Ashmore, et al. (1991) finds no support for this supposed difference. Specifically, the belief that "beauty is good" is equally true when judging women or men. Further, in considering aspects of appearance more broadly than facial attractiveness, we believe that physical cues are equally important to the male and female stereotypes.

In summary, current research on gender stereotypes has revealed a picture much more complex than the two general dimensions of male-female difference isolated by Broverman, Rosenkrantz, and their colleagues. There is little doubt that beliefs about these general dimensions persist. At the same time, some evidence is beginning to suggest there may be a few dents in the stereotypic armor, at least along evaluative lines. Beyond these general dimensions, people have a variety of gender subtypes that they find useful. It seems likely that these subtypes are formed because the more superordinate category proves unsatisfactory (Rothbart & John, 1985). In the course of interaction, the person presumably selects that stereotypic subtype that seems to fit most closely the case at hand. In part, this choice is influenced by the available information. In addition, however, context probably exerts considerable influence, affecting not only what information is available but what categories are salient as well. The implications of this multiplicity for maintenance and change will be considered further in a later section.

INDIVIDUAL DIFFERENCES IN GENDER STEREOTYPING

Individual differences in the tendency to endorse and use gender stereotypes are still not well understood. Traditional assumptions about the consensual basis of stereotypes certainly delayed an investigation of individual differences. If one assumes that stereotypes are shared by the culture as a whole, then the question of individual differences in beliefs about gender is effectively finessed (Ashmore & Del Boca, 1981). A second conceptual retardant was the assumption that stereotyping is a global tendency, that is, that a person will be more or less prone to stereotype members of stigmatized groups in general, with no important distinctions between particular target groups. Research on the authoritarian personality, which set out to define what personality characteristics lead to prejudicial attitudes, exemplified this second assumption. The evidence to support this assumption is weak, however. In fact, generality cannot be assumed even within a domain (see Gardner, Lalonde, Nero & Young, 1988, on measures of ethnic stereotypes). Both conceptual issues and methodological strategies have challenged the early global assumptions.

The increased interest in gender as a target of stereotyping has resulted in an outpouring of measures to assess beliefs and attitudes related to gender roles. Beere's (1990) recent handbook of tests lists 18 scales measuring stereotypes, 24 scales assessing attitudes toward men's and women's employee roles, 26 scales measuring beliefs about marital and parental roles, 30 scales assessing multiple roles in general, and 56 additional scales measuring various issues associated with women and men. These tests represent a real potpourri. Some of the measures are very specific, such as those directed at beliefs about feminism or attitudes toward policewomen. Others are designed to be more general assessments, covering a variety of issues within a single measure. Some were created specifically for research with children. Not all of these measures are used to assess individual differences in beliefs and attitudes; some have been used only to assess average group response to a particular target or set of information. It is also worth noting that although cross-cultural extensions are available in some cases (e.g., Britain, Ireland, India), none of the scales is directed at uncovering within-culture ethnic differences in stereotyping.

Much of the work on individual differences in gender stereotyping reflects empirical concerns. Thus, the developer's main goal is to create an instrument that will assess beliefs about the specified target group—women, men, some subset of women and men, or some gender-related attitudinal domain. In addition, however, some theoretical debates have emerged. Not surprisingly, given the current theoretical climate, these debates typically invoke models from social cognition. The most prominent of these concerns is the concept of gender schema. We will review that debate in some detail and then consider other theoretical and empirical approaches to assessing gender stereotyping. We will also discuss some of the issues that continue to face investigators in this area.

Categorizing Gender: Who's Got the Schema?

Bem (1981, 1985) proposed gender schema theory to account for individual differences in the processing of gender-linked information. By her account, sex typing derives, at least in part, from the tendency to use such schematic processing. Some persons, termed gender schematic, are believed to have a generalized readiness to process information on the basis of sex-linked categories and will use this dimension in preference to all other possible bases of categorization. People who do not use this basis of categorization are termed gender aschematic. For those who are schematic, Bem assumes that this way of viewing the world is pervasive, influencing information processing and evaluation across a broad range of experience.

To assess individual differences in gender schematicity, Bem relies on people's scores on the Bem Sex Role Inventory (BSRI; Bem, 1974).[4] Sex-typed persons (males above the median in masculinity and below the median in femininity and females with the reverse scoring pattern) are proposed to be gender schematic, while androgynous and undifferentiated persons (above or below the median, respectively, on both scales) are not. Predictions for cross-sex typed persons (those who endorse sex-discrepant characteristics and deny sex-congruent characteristics) are unclear (Bem, 1985), and results of studies examining their actual responses are inconsistent (Bem, 1981; Frable & Bem, 1985).

Bem and her colleagues have used gender schema theory to predict a variety of behaviors, including categorization effects in recall (Bem, 1981; Frable & Bem, 1985), response latency in judging the self-relevance of traits (Bem, 1981), the influence of a partner's appearance on social interaction (Andersen & Bem, 1981), judgments of the appropriateness of sports behavior (Matteo, 1988), perceptions of gender in movement (Frable, 1987), and acceptance of gender ideology (Frable, 1989). Accompanying these supportive findings, however, are a number of studies that fail to replicate previously reported findings or do not support hypotheses derived from the theory. Evidence for use of gender as an organizing principle in free recall is particularly problematic (Deaux, Kite & Lewis, 1985; Kite & Deaux, 1986; Edwards & Spence, 1987; Payne, Connor & Colletti, 1987). Payne et al. (1987) also failed to replicate Bem's (1981) response latency data. Similarly, Stangor (1988) found no relationship between the BSRI and recognition sensitivity, another form of memory measure.

Effects of gender schematicity have been difficult to obtain in other domains as well, including expectancy confirmation paradigms (Lewis, 1985) and the "who said what" studies in which observers are asked to recall the comments of particular speakers (Beauvais & Spence, 1987; Branscombe, Deaux, & Lerner, 1985). In contrast, Frable (1989) recently reported that sex-typed, that is, gender schematic, individuals are more likely to accept culturally appropriate gender rules, pay attention to the sex of job applicants, devalue women, and (for men only) endorse sexist language.

Not only are the outcome measures inconsistent, but questions have been raised about the criteria used to define gender schematicity as well. Markus (1977; Markus et al., 1982), in extending her self-schema theory to gender-related domains, proposed that masculinity and femininity are represented as separate self-schemas and that a person may be masculine schematic, feminine schematic, or both (or neither).[5] Predictions from this model and that of Bem diverge most sharply for the person who is high in both masculinity and femininity: Markus and her colleagues predict that this group would be most likely to be gender schematic while Bem argues they are the least schematic. Attempts to pit these two models against each other have yielded mixed results (Hungerford & Sobolew-Shubin, 1987; Payne et al., 1987; Edwards & Spence, 1987).

In assessing this diverse set of results, it seems clear that the domains in which gender schematicity operates need to be more clearly defined. Studies of information processing present the weakest case for gender schema theory, often failing to distinguish between those who are supposedly gender schematic and those who are not. In some cases, other dimensions are simply more salient than gender for everyone (Kite & Deaux, 1986). Another reason for the mixed pattern of results, Skitka and Maslach (1990) suggest, is that investigators have failed to make a distinction between the simple use of sex as a category and more subtle inferences about psychological gender. In fact, there is considerable evidence that sex is a generally available social category used by all (Devine, 1989; Hamilton, 1979). Thus gender schematics and gender aschematics alike should respond to this dimension. The differences between gender schematics and aschematics should be most likely to appear, according to Skitka and Maslach (1990), when cues related to gender are more subtle, requiring more inferential work on the part of the perceiver. It is in these cases that gender schematics should tap into their schemas. The hypothesis is an intriguing one and merits further consideration. It may help to explain, for example, why studies that deal directly with social interaction or move beyond the simple stereotypic trait associations (Andersen & Bem, 1981; Frable, 1989) appear to demonstrate gender schematicity more clearly.

Evidence that gender schematics use their schema selectively is also provided by McKenzie-Mohr and Zanna (1990). They suggest that the use of such schemas depends both on their availability and on the degree to which they are primed by the situation. To demonstrate this, they exposed both schematic and aschematic men to either a pornographic film or a neutral discussion in the Canadian House of Commons. When subsequently interacting with a female interviewer, only those men who were schematic and who had watched the film showed sexist behavior, illustrating the situational dependence of gender schemas.

Cognitive Accessibility and Expertise

In another analysis of individual differences using models from social cognition, Stangor (1988) derived a measure of stereotyping based on the assumption that people differ in the degree to which gender is readily accessible, that is, able to be retrieved from memory. Chronic accessibility was assessed by asking subjects to list characteristics of different types of people (e.g., someone you frequently encounter); these terms were then rated for their gender linkage. Thus, in contrast to the self-descriptive traits that are used by Bem and Markus to define gender schematicity, Stangor relies on the characteristics people use to describe others. Using this measure, Stangor showed that people high in gender accessibility were more likely to process subsequent behavioral descriptions in gender-related terms.

Stangor's analysis of accessibility bears some relationship to cognitive conceptions of expertise (Chase & Simon, 1973; Reitman, 1976). From this perspective, one makes the assumption that experts are better able to organize and retrieve information relevant to their particular area of expertise than are nonexperts; they also can vary the strategies they use when processing information related to that area. Markus, Smith, and Moreland (1985) relied on these analyses of expertise to link their self-referent concept of schematicity to perceptions of others. They found that masculine schematics who viewed the videotaped actions of another person behaving in masculine ways consistently chunked information into larger units and could vary their information-processing strategy when the situation required it.

Additional work on expertise (Taylor et al., 1978) considered its potential relation to stereotyping by examining the number of within-sex (or race) errors made by members of the stereotyped group, compared to nonmembers. Taylor et al. (1978) reasoned that expertise ought to be greatest for those persons who were members of a stereotyped group; thus, these individuals should make the fewest recall errors. However, their results showed no differences between women and men in the number of times they confused members of either the same or opposite sex, nor were stereotype ratings affected by group membership. (Similarly, racial group membership did not influence the within-race error rate.) These authors concluded that, although familiarity may be advantageous to a point, there is no added advantage once a basic level of expertise has been obtained. One problem in extending expertise to social domains is that it is difficult to find objective criteria to assess "expert status." Certainly the idea that group membership alone implies expertise, when the groups are as large and heterogeneous as women and men, is too simple. Furthermore, Catrambone and Markus (1987) have argued that expertise should influence judgments of others only when perceivers are encouraged or required to go beyond the information given and reach their own conclusions about a target person. In contrast, experts should be no better or worse at recalling information presented about a target person, a conclusion that echoes the analysis of gender schema findings.

Empirically Derived Measures

Numerous other measures of gender stereotypes are available, for the most part less theoretical in their origin and more diverse in their content. In some cases, a single measure has been offered to assess both self-evaluations and gender stereotypes (Spence et al., 1974). A variety of other measures are domain-specific, and the relationships between these more narrowly targeted instruments and the more general stereotypes have yet to be untangled. We can discuss only a few of the available measures here; for more information, readers are advised to consult Beere (1990).

Ratio Measure of Sex Stereotyping

C. L. Martin (1987) developed a measure of individual differences in sex stereotyping by applying the ratio approach suggested by McCauley and Stitt (1978) to a set of instrumental, expressive, and neutral attributes. Respondents are asked to estimate the percentage of women and the percentage of men who possess each attribute; these estimates yield a ratio score that indicates the extent to which the person believes men and women differ from one another. In comparing stereotype scores obtained on this measure to group norms, C. L. Martin (1987) found that the stereotyped beliefs about differences between women and men were more extreme than the distributions of self-reported differences, suggesting that stereotypes are exaggerations of reality.[6] We know of no further work testing the predictive utility of this measure of stereotyping, but the approach seems promising and could easily be extended to other attribute domains.

Free Response Measures

Berninger and DeSoto (1985) find clear individual differences in the type of information people produce about stereotyped groups. When asked to respond to the descriptor "warm female," for example, some people focus on traits and psychological dimensions to define that person while others use status variables, exemplars, or descriptions of what the person is not like as a means of characterizing the target person. Still others use a mixture of various types of information. Unfortunately, the authors provide no insight as to how these individual differences might be used to examine the stereotyping process or make predictions about behavior. Eagly and Mladinic (1989) assessed individual differences by asking people to list five characteristics of a target person, then to rate the percentage of people in each group who have that characteristic, and finally to rate each characteristic on an evaluative scale. A score for each person is created following Fishbein and Ajzen's (1975; Ajzen & Fishbein, 1980) Expectancy X Value method of aggregating evaluative beliefs. Like Berninger and DeSoto's measure, this score represents the individual's beliefs about the target group rather than their ratings on items selected by the researcher. Yet Eagly and Mladinic extend these ideas by providing an easily quantified measure of these beliefs.

Attitudes Toward Rights and Roles

Many instruments have been developed to assess attitudes toward equal rights, traditional roles, and the appropriate responsibilities for women and men (Beere, 1990). The most widely used of these measures is the Attitude Toward Women Scale (AWS), developed by Spence and Helmreich (1972). It is not totally clear how these measures of attitudes toward specific domains of male and female involvement relate to trait-based stereotypes. On the one hand, Spence and her colleagues report substantial correlations between trait stereotype ratings and AWS scores (Spence, Helmreich & Stapp, 1975). In contrast, Eagly and Mladinic (1989) find no association between scores on the AWS and attitudes toward women as assessed on an evaluative semantic differential measure. These latter authors suggest that there is an important distinction between beliefs about the rights and responsibilities of women and attitudes toward the general category of women. In fact, attitudes toward rights and responsibilities can probably not be considered a single dimension, either. A. Martin (1990), for example, has isolated two distinct and unrelated factors in men's attitudes toward women, one assessing traditional and primarily interpersonal roles and the other focusing on more public issues of equal opportunity and fair employment. Clearly there is room for a great deal of psychometric work in this area.

Prospects for Assessing Individual Differences

The profusion of measures of gender-related beliefs testifies to the vitality of the field, but it also presents its own set of problems. The terrain needs to be more clearly mapped, both conceptually and psychometrically. Just as investigators of self-reported "masculinity" and "femininity" had to contend with the multiplicity of gender-related characteristics (Spence, 1984, 1985), so too will those concerned with stereotypes and attitudes have to do some of the more systematic spadework.

As exploration of individual differences continues, researchers would be wise to consider those issues that have plagued attitude-behavior research for decades. Given the substantial number of beliefs that are relevant to gender, the specificity-generality issue (Ajzen & Fishbein, 1977) has clear relevance to predicting gender-linked responding. That is, beliefs measured at a global level should best predict reactions toward women and men when those behaviors are also measured in broad terms, such as by using appropriately designed multiple-act criteria. The strategies for adequately assessing behavior must also be considered, such as the value of aggregating across a variety of conceptually related behaviors and occasions (Ajzen, 1988; Fishbein & Ajzen, 1975; Epstein, 1980, 1983).

Understanding the links between stereotyped beliefs and actions is not only a methodological issue. Already it is clear that the possession of stereotypic beliefs does not guarantee discriminatory action. Indeed, research by Devine (1989) and others shows that virtually everybody has encoded stereotypic beliefs about gender, ethnicity, age, and other prominent social categories. Both traditionalists and egalitarians, despite differences in their avowed beliefs, show commonality in some basic associations about women and men. Thus it may be more important for researchers to understand when stereotypes are used than who has them, as the research of McKenzie-Mohr and Zanna (1990) suggests. Analyses of attitude accessibility as a key to the attitude-behavior relationship is relevant here (Fazio, 1986). So too is the interactive model of Deaux and Major (1987), which suggests conditions under which gender stereotypes are more or less likely to be invoked. In adopting these frameworks, concern will shift from the more taxonomic question of who holds gender stereotypes to the more process-oriented question of when gender stereotypes have consequences.

THE DEVELOPMENT OF STEREOTYPES

How boys and girls acquire their own gender identity is the focus of Chapter 9. Here we address a more specific aspect of the socialization process by asking how children acquire gender stereotypes.

The Acquisition Process

Children's knowledge of gender begins at a very early age, as children learn both to recognize their own gender assignment and to understand the ways in which certain behaviors and activities are associated with gender categories. By the age of 3, children can categorize people on the basis of gender, and in fact they begin to learn about stereotypes and sex-typed behaviors even before the notion of gender constancy (the understanding that sex remains constant over time) is understood (Huston, 1983; Stangor & Ruble, 1987). Possession of this simple gender schema—girls and boys—allows children to encode and organize a wide range of information into one of two basic categories (Bem, 1983; Martin & Halverson, 1981).

The acquisition of gender stereotypes is a continuing process, representing a gradual increase in amount and complexity of information as the child grows older (Huston, 1983; Williams, Bennett & Best, 1975). In earlier years, perceived differences between the sexes focus on activities and toys. With increasing age, children add abstract traits to their gender stereotypes and develop increasingly complex understandings of what masculinity and femininity mean (Huston, 1983; Martin, 1989). On the one hand, these increments mean there are more ways of differentiating males and females. At the same time, however, children become more flexible in their use of stereotyping, recognizing the diversity that exists within each sex group (Huston, 1983). The coexistence of these trends reminds us again that the availability of particular knowledge about gender needs to be distinguished from the tendency to use that knowledge to process information or guide behavior (Stangor & Ruble, 1987).

Children learn information and elaborate schemas about their own sex earlier than they do for the other sex (Martin & Halverson, 1981; Martin, Wood & Little, 1989; Stangor & Ruble, 1987). For example, a 4-year-old girl will associate liking dolls with liking kitchen sets before she makes a connection between liking trucks and liking airplanes (Martin, et al., 1989). Evaluative differences are evident as well, particularly among younger children. More positive attributes are associated with one's own sex and more negative attributes with the other sex (Albert & Porter, 1983; Etaugh, Levine & Mennella, 1984). Boys seem to be more stereotypical in their thinking than girls, and within the United States, at least, black children appear to be less stereotyped than white children. Social class, in contrast, seems to make no difference (Huston, 1983).

With development, the child's process of inference becomes increasingly sophisticated. Very young children are able to infer properties of boys and girls when presented those categories, but cannot reliably infer the category given the property (Gelman, Collman & Maccoby, 1986). Somewhat later, children are able to make predictions about a target person's behavior based on provided labels, but they tend not to use component information if it contradicts the label (Berndt & Heller, 1986; Martin, 1989). If told that a boy liked to play with dolls, for example, children of 4 to 5 would predict that he would like football more than tea sets. With increasing age, children use more of the available information to make more differentiated judgments. This increasing complexity allows children to see that not all girls and not all boys are alike. Yet the perceived linkages among stereotypical components persist in conjunction with this differentiation (Berndt & Heller, 1986; Deaux & Lewis, 1984).

Socialization Sources

Society is generous in providing information about gender. Few institutions or socializing agents can be ignored when we try to determine just how children learn about gender. Recognizing the multiplicity of these influences is important; parceling out the relative contribution of the various agents may well be impossible.

Traditionally, people have looked to the family as a source of stereotype acquisition. Both by example and by instruction, parents are believed to communicate their beliefs about gender-appropriate behaviors. Yet even the family unit does not define a single set of influences, as P. A. Katz (1987) has shown. The family constellation includes not only parents but also siblings, and often extended family members as well, each of whom can convey separate and distinct beliefs about gender. Families also differ in terms of ethnicity, socioeconomic class, and maternal employment, and each of these factors may be associated with different patterns of gender beliefs. Further, as P. A. Katz (1987) points out, the effect of parental influence may vary substantially with age of the child, both in its immediate and its long-term influence.

Schools are also a potent source of information about gender, both with regard to category salience as well as the content of gender schemas. Particularly in early school years, the salience of gender as a category can be emphasized through the segregation of boys and girls, even on tasks where gender is irrelevant (Stanworth, 1983). In addition, specific gender-related knowledge is learned from teachers, from classmates, and from the instructional materials used (Meece, 1987). Peers, in fact, appear to be a particularly strong force for conservatism in the preschool years (Huston, 1983). Much knowledge of gender has typically been acquired before the child enters school, of course, and thus the schools may do little to instill new beliefs. Further, children themselves show a strong preference for same-sex play groups, even when the tasks involved are neutral rather than sex-typed (Maccoby, 1990). However, an assessment of the literature suggests that the schools play a significant role in reinforcing preestablished distinctions and are less successful in introducing ideas of variability and flexibility (Meece, 1987).

The media, television, in particular, have long been recognized as important sources of gender-related information. Indeed, given statistics on the extensive exposure of children to TV, averaging two to four hours a day from early preschool years on, it is difficult to ignore this medium's potential (Calvert & Huston, 1987). As in the case of school, children bring their already-established schemas to the experience; yet in the case of television, the exposure is so early and often so extensive that it seems likely to have more impact. Because so many studies have documented the stereotypy of television programming, content, and theme, it is assumed that heavy television viewing should be associated with greater gender stereotypy. The evidence for this link is inconsistent, however (Huston, 1983), in part because the methodological issues are so complex. The one-shot exposure of experimental studies does not capture the phenomena, and naturalistic studies require attention to so many factors, such as amount of exposure, program content, and parental guidance, that causal certainty is elusive.

In analyzing the impact of any of these socialization agents, it is clear that the messages are multifaceted and the impact uneven. Most agents probably display a full range of stereotypic and not-so-stereotypic behaviors, varying either by domain, immediate context, or in more random fashion. For this reason, it is especially important to recognize the active role that children themselves play in learning about stereotypes. Individual differences in the child's gender schema will, to some degree, affect what new material is encoded and stored and thus shape the contents of gender stereotypes (Calvert & Huston, 1987; Signorella, 1987). Thus idiosyncratic beliefs about gender can coexist with the more consensual views.

USING AND CHANGING STEREOTYPES

If the learning of stereotypes is inevitable, must their persistence be assumed as well? There are at least two ways to approach this question. The first is to ask whether, at a consensual or group level, the general stereotypes of women and men endure. Are there any changes in the patterns of gender beliefs, and, if so, what factors might lead to change? A second approach is to focus on the use of stereotypes, rather than their existence. Even if people have stereotypes, can they learn to circumvent them? What conditions make stereotype usage more or less likely?

Stability and Change in Gender Beliefs

Gender stereotypes have shown remarkable staying power. Several studies have been conducted in the United States, comparing the views of 10-20 years ago with current views (Bergen, 1989; Liben & Bigler, 1987; Ruble, 1983; Snodgrass, 1990; Werner & LaRussa, 1985). In each case, the investigators report little change in people's perceptions of the characteristics possessed by the typical woman and man. As noted earlier, there is some suggestion that the positive-negative evaluation of the sexes has shifted slightly, with views of women becoming more favorable and those of men less favorable. Yet the core beliefs in the instrumental and agentic qualities of men and the emotional and communal attributes of women persist.

The stability of gender stereotypes stands in interesting contrast to measured changes in people's attitudes about the appropriate rights and roles for women and men. In numerous longitudinal comparisons, contemporary respondents report themselves much more favorable to women's employment, equal payment in the workplace, and, to a lesser extent, division of labor in the household than did those surveyed decades ago (Helmreich, Spence & Gibson, 1982; Mason, Czajka & Arber, 1976; Simon & Landis, 1989). In part, we suspect this difference between gender stereotypes and attitudes toward specific role domains is explained by the force of legislation and court decisions, a case of beliefs being reshaped to fit the legal realities. Whereas law may speak to the allowable domains of women and men, however, it cannot mandate the "nature" of women and men, thus allowing beliefs about these "essences" to persist.

Analysis of stereotype maintenance and change often reflects the theoretical stance one takes with regard to why stereotypes form in the first place. A psychodynamic model, for example, suggests that individuals will maintain stereotypic beliefs as long as their psychic needs and defense mechanisms remain unchanged. Eagly's (1987) social-role model points to the relative stability in the division of labor between the sexes as the basis for persisting stereotypes. According to this model, stereotypes will persist as long as women and men engage in different behaviors in the household and participate differentially in the labor market. Sharp social rearrangements must occur before stereotypes will change. Other macrolevel explanations could point to continuing economic discrimination or to the stability of the dominant power structure as factors contributing to the maintenance of stereotypes.

From the perspective of the currently prominent cognitive models, changes in stereotypes are considered at the level of individual. Like larger social systems, individual cognitive structures resist change. Established schemas operate in a highly conservative mode, hospitable to compatible information and resistant to information and events that do not fit the existent pattern. This tendency to "cognitive efficiency" can be understood as a rational solution to the demands of processing excessive information. At the same time, it makes attempts to change stereotypes quite difficult.

Evidence for the biasing properties of schemas is substantial, tested over a broad range of categories including gender. Hepburn (1985), for example, showed that individuals who observe male and female actors engaging in an equal number of sex-typed and neutral activities recalled a greater number of schema-consistent activities. Even imagined, rather than actual, events can serve to perpetuate stereotypic beliefs (Slusher & Anderson, 1987). Further, as Stangor and Ruble (1989) have shown, when people have a large amount of prior information available, they are more likely to form impressions congruent with their prior expectancies than when their information is more limited. Certainly in the case of gender, where schemas are established early and used often, this experience factor is important in explaining stereotype persistence.

In considering how stereotypes might change, cognitive theorists have raised a number of questions. Are stereotypes more likely to change gradually through the accumulation of inconsistent information? Are changes more sudden, responsive to dramatic instances of nonstereotypic behavior? The latter case appears to be rare, in that such dramatic instances are typically discounted, attributed to an unrepresentative individual rather than to group properties (Rothbart & John, 1985; Weber & Crocker, 1983). (If that individual previously has been shown to be a particularly good example of the category, however, even a single person's behavior may have some impact on the general stereotype.) Unexpected behavior shared by only a few members of the group will often lead to the formation of subtypes, allowing categorization of the "deviants" and preservation of the more general category (Rothbart & John, 1985; Weber & Crocker, 1983). In contrast, if the inconsistent behavior is associated with numerous members of the category, then change in the categorical beliefs is more likely (Weber & Crocker, 1983). Further, some preliminary evidence reported by Rothbart (1989) suggests that stereotypes change more readily at the subtype level than at the superordinate level.

More longitudinal work is needed to answer some of these questions about cognitive structures and change. For the most part, however, this research suggests that stereotypes are quite resistant to change. Indeed, the work of Devine (1989) and others within the cognitive tradition points to the intractability of gender stereotypes. Even for those who claim to endorse equal rights, liberalization of roles, and the like, stereotypic associations to gender are virtually automatic, emerging without any obvious conscious processing when a person is confronted with a member of the category. Without massive social change, it is unlikely that these associations will disappear or even weaken very much.

The Use of Gender Stereotypes

If the prospect for change in the overall endorsement of gender stereotypes is somewhat dismal, the possibilities for alterations in their usage are considerably more promising. People may not be able to prevent themselves from learning gender stereotypes, but they can learn to override them.

When do people ignore categorical beliefs and attend instead to the individuating characteristics of a particular person? This question has elicited considerable debate (Krueger & Rothbart, 1988; Locksley, Borgida, Brekke & Hepburn, 1980; Rasinski, Crocker & Hastie, 1985). The best answer is a conditional one. Single instances of individuating information are rarely sufficient to overcome a strong categorical belief. Thus, learning that a father changed his daughter's diapers on one occasion probably does little to alter stereotypes about that man's fathering role. Evidence of continuous deviation from the stereotype, however, may override the categorical bias. Thus, the father described as changing diapers daily and tending to feeding schedules as well will most likely be judged on his own terms.

The willingness of people to ignore the category and concentrate on specific information about the target person depends both on the category and on the case. Some categories, such as woman or man, are so general that we may readily abandon them in the face of more specific information. In contrast, categories such as football players or career women may be constructed more tightly, with associated attributes rated more extremely than in the general man-woman case and endorsed with greater certainty. In these cases, the categories are more persistent influences on judgment (Krueger & Rothbart, 1988). The nature of the individuating information is also important. Information that is vivid and not easily refutable, for example, would be much more influential than information acquired thirdhand from an unreliable source.

The willingness of people to abandon categorical beliefs also depends on the kind of judgment that is required. In trying to predict which rest room a person will use, for example, individuating information is probably not very useful. Unfortunately, it is not only rest rooms that are divided so sharply between his and hers. Occupations may also be based on strict categorical assumptions (Glick, Zion & Nelson, 1988). In the Glick et al. study, people given stereotype-inconsistent information about a male or female applicant altered their inferences about the applicant's personality and about his or her suitability for the job, showing a reliance on specific case information rather than on the gender stereotype. Nonetheless, these subjects still indicated that they would be significantly more likely to interview a man than a woman for a traditionally male job and more likely to interview a woman than a man for a traditionally female job. Thus people can alter their judgments of a particular individual, based on specific case information—but the criterion for the decision or outcome has to be ungendered as well.

There are a number of ways in which one can weaken the grip of stereotypes. Simpler judgments are less likely to depend on stereotypes than are more complex judgments (Bodenhausen & Lichtenstein, 1987), and so one might want to split complex decisions (e.g., should a person be promoted) into smaller pieces where performance could be assessed more clearly. Ambiguous criteria also foster the use of stereotypes. If people are motivated to be accurate when they make judgments about another person, then they are less likely to rely on stereotypes (Neuberg & Fiske, 1987). Similarly, if people are held accountable for their decisions, they are less likely to use broad generalizations (Tetlock, 1983; Tetlock & Kim, 1987). More generally, as Fiske (1989) has argued, getting people to pay attention to each other is a key to reducing the use of stereotypes. With attention directed clearly to the individual, a person is less likely to make categorical judgments and more likely to incorporate individuating characteristics in any subsequent judgment. People do not forget about the category in these circumstances—but they do see individual attributes as more informative than the general categorical information.

A FINAL NOTE

Like Pogo, we find that the enemy is us. The ubiquity of stereotypes is evidence that they are not limited to the belief system of a few prejudiced individuals, but rather that they are part of the fabric of general societal beliefs and norms. Further, like an act of the quick-change artist, gender stereotypes can alter their form, shifting from general beliefs about women and men to more specific, but still categorical, assumptions about black women, pregnant women, career women, and the like.

Yet the existence of stereotypes does not mandate their use. People can learn to apply alternative interpretations to events, bringing attention and intention to bear. Stereotypes will not quickly fade away—but with effort and constant vigilance, their utility can be questioned and their use appropriately constrained.

NOTES

We thank Yael Bat-Chava, Alice Eagly, Carol Martin, Janet Spence, and Bernie Whitley for their very helpful comments on an earlier version of this manuscript. Preparation of this article was facilitated by a National Science Foundation grant (BNS-8746412) to the first author and a New Faculty Grant from Ball State University to the second author.

1. Gould (1980) has written superbly on these issues, pointing out that heritability cannot be equated with biological determinism.

2. The whole research tradition of assessing sex differences, of course, attempts to do just that, using operational definitions to tie down the abstractions. Yet this literature provides strikingly few examples of clear sex differences. Main effects when obtained are typically modified by task and situational features, making the picture far more complex than simple stereotypes would have it (Hyde & Linn, 1986).

3. This use of white as the standard is reminiscent of Eagly and Kite's (1987) findings regarding nationality stereotypes. In that case, males were the standard used in forming stereotypes of nations, and the female stereotypes were typically quite divergent.

4. Although the psychometrically similar Personal Attributes Questionnaire (Spence et al., 1975) is sometimes used to categorize gender schematics as well, this use is not consistent with the rationale of its development. Spence acknowledges the appeal of gender schematicity on a conceptual level, but she and her colleagues argue that constructs such as roles, masculinity-femininity, and gender schema are complex, multifaceted, and not adequately tapped by measures that essentially assess expressiveness and instrumentality.

5. Markus, like Bem, uses the terms *masculinity* and *femininity* in a very general sense, while relying on measures that primarily assess expressiveness and instrumentality. Although we agree with Spence and her colleagues (Spence, 1984; Spence & Helmreich, 1981) that masculinity and femininity are multidimensional concepts connoting more than the trait dimensions, we use the terms here as Bem and Markus have used them.

6. This comparison is an imperfect test in that we do not know the degree to which men and women actually possess a trait, as compared to their self-reports. If self-reports tend to minimize sex differences, then the difference may be less than C. L. Martin (1987) suggests. In contrast, if people tend to exaggerate self-reported sex differences, at least partially buying the stereotypes themselves, then the difference between stereotypes and reality may be even sharper than Martin observed.

REFERENCES

Adorno, T. W., Frenkel-Brunswik, E., Levinson, D. J., & Sanford, R. N. (1950). *The authoritarian personality*. New York: Harper & Row.

Ajzen, I. (1988). *Attitudes, personality, and behavior*. Chicago: Dorsey Press.

Ajzen, I., & Fishbein, M. (1977). Attitude-behavior relations: A theoretical analysis and review of empirical research. *Psychological Bulletin, 84*, 888–918.

Ajzen, I., & Fishbein, M. (1980). *Understanding attitudes and predicting social behavior*. Englewood Cliffs, NJ: Prentice-Hall.

Albert, A. A., & Porter, J. R. (1983). Age patterns in the development of children's gender-role stereotypes. *Sex Roles, 9*, 59–67.

Allport, G. W. (1954). *The nature of prejudice*. New York: Addison-Wesley.

Andersen, S. M., & Bem, S. L. (1981). Sex typing and androgyny in dyadic interaction: Individual differences in responsiveness to physical attractiveness. *Journal of Personality and Social Psychology, 41*, 74–86.

Ashmore, R. D., & Del Boca, F. K. (1976). Psychological approaches to understanding intergroup conflict. In P. Katz (Ed.), *Towards the elimination of racism* (pp. 73-123). New York: Pergamon Press.

Ashmore, R. D., & Del Boca, F. K. (1979). Sex stereotypes and implicit personality theory: Toward a cognitive-social psychological conceptualization. *Sex Roles, 5*, 219–248.

Ashmore, R. D., & Del Boca, F. K. (1981). Conceptual approaches to stereotypes and stereotyping. In D. L. Hamilton (Ed.), *Cognitive processes in stereotyping and intergroup behavior* (pp. 1–35). Hillsdale, NJ: Erlbaum.

Ashmore, R. D., Del Boca, F. K., & Titus, D. (1984). *Types of women and men: Yours, mine, and ours.* Paper presented at the meeting of the American Psychological Association, Toronto.

Bartlett, J. (1980). *Familiar quotations.* Boston: Little, Brown.

Beauvais, C., & Spence, J. T. (1987). Gender, prejudice, and categorization. *Sex Roles, 16,* 89–100.

Beere, C. A. (1990). *Gender roles: A handbook of tests and measures.* New York: Greenwood Press.

Bem, S. L. (1974). The measurement of psychological androgyny. *Journal of Consulting and Clinical Psychology, 42,* 155–162.

Bem, S. L. (1981). Gender schema theory: A cognitive account of sex typing. *Psychological Review, 88,* 354–364.

Bem, S. L. (1983). Gender schema theory and its implications for child development: Raising gender-aschematic children in a gender-schematic society. *Signs, 8,* 598–616.

Bem, S. L. (1985). Androgyny and gender schema theory: A conceptual and empirical integration. In T. B. Sonderegger (Ed.), *Nebraska symposium on motivation: Psychology and gender* (pp. 179–226). Lincoln: University of Nebraska Press.

Bergen, D. J. (1989). *Sex stereotypes in the United States of America revisited.* Thesis submitted to Department of Psychology, Wake Forest University, Winston-Salem, NC.

Berndt, T. J., & Heller, K. A. (1986). Gender stereotypes and social inferences: A developmental study. *Journal of Personality and ,ocial Psychology, 50,* 889–898.

Berninger, V. W., & DeSoto, C. (1985). Cognitive representation of personal stereotypes. *European Journal of Social Psychology, 15,* 189–211.

Bodenhausen, G. V., & Lichtenstein, M. (1987). Social stereotypes and information-processing strategies: The impact of task complexity. *Journal of Personality and Social Psychology, 52,* 871–880.

Brabant, S., & Mooney, L. (1986). Sex role stereotyping in the Sunday comics: Ten years later. *Sex Roles, 14,* 141–148.

Branscombe, N. R., Deaux, K., & Lerner, M. S. (1985). Individual differences and the influence of context on categorization and prejudice. *Representative Research in Social Psychology, 15,* 25–35.

Broverman, I. K., Vogel, S. R., Broverman, D. M., Clarkson, F. E., & Rosenkrantz, P. S. (1972). Sex-role stereotypes: A current appraisal. *Journal of Social Issues, 28* (2), 59–78.

Brown, J. D. (1985). Race and gender in rock video. *Social Science Newsletter, 70,* 82–86.

Calvert, S. L., & Huston, A. C. (1987). Television and children's gender schemata. In L. S. Liben & M. L. Signorella (Eds.), *Children's gender schemata* (pp. 75–88). San Francisco: Jossey-Bass.

Catrambone, R., & Markus, H. (1987). The role of self-schemas in going beyond the information given. *Social Cognition, 5,* 349–368.

Chase, W. G., & Simon, H. A. (1973). Perception and chess. *Cognitive Psychology, 4,* 55–81.

Chavez, D. (1985). Perpetuation of gender inequality: A content analysis of comic strips. *Sex Roles, 13,* 93–102.

Clifton, A. K., McGrath, D., & Wick, B. (1976). Stereotypes of women: A single category? *Sex Roles, 2*, 135–148.

Crocker, J., & Schwartz, I. (1985). Prejudice and ingroup favoritism in a minimal intergroup situation: Effects of self-esteem. *Personality and Social Psychology Bulletin, 11*, 379–386.

Crocker, J., Thompson, L. L., McGraw, K. M., & Ingerman, C. (1987). Downward comparison, prejudice, and evaluations of others: Effects of self-esteem and threat. *Journal of Personality and Social Psychology, 52*, 907–916.

Deaux, K., & Kite, M. (1985). Gender stereotypes: Some thoughts on the cognitive organization of gender-related information. *Academic Psychology Bulletin, 7*, 123–144.

Deaux, K., Kite, M. E., & Lewis, L. L. (1985). Clustering and gender schemata: An uncertain link. *Personality and Social Psychology Bulletin, 11*, 387–397.

Deaux, K., & Lewis, L. L. (1983). Components of gender stereotypes. *Psychological Documents, 13*, 25. (Cat. #2583)

Deaux, K., & Lewis, L. L. (1984). Structure of gender stereotypes: Interrelationships among components and gender label. *Journal of Personality and Social Psychology, 46*, 991–1004.

Deaux, K., & Major, B. (1987). Putting gender into context: An interactive model of gender-related behavior. *Psychological Review, 94*, 369–389.

Deaux, K., & Sinnett, L. (1989). *Categories of women and men*. Manuscript in preparation.

Deaux, K., Winton, W., Crowley, M., & Lewis, L. L. (1985). Level of categorization and content of gender stereotypes. *Social Cognition, 3*, 145–167.

Devine, P. G. (1989). Stereotypes and prejudice: Their automatic and controlled components. *Journal of Personality and Social Psychology, 56*, 5–18.

Dion, K. L. (1987). What's in a title? The Ms. stereotype and images of women's titles of address. *Psychology of Women Quarterly, 11*, 21–36.

Eagly, A. H. (1987). *Sex differences in social behavior: A social-role interpretation.* Hillsdale, NJ: Erlbaum.

Eagly, A. H., Ashmore, R. D., Makhijani, M. G., & Longo L. C. (1991). What is beautiful is good, but . . . : A meta-analytic review of research on the physical attractiveness stereotype. *Psychological Bulletin, 110* (1), 109–128.

Eagly, A. H., & Chaiken, S. (1993). *The psychology of attitudes.* San Diego, CA: Harcourt Brace Jovanovich.

Eagly, A. H., & Kite, M. E. (1987). Are stereotypes of nationalities applied to both women and men? *Journal of Personality and Social Psychology, 53*, 451–462.

Eagly, A. H., & Mladinic, A. (1989). Gender stereotypes and attitudes toward women and men. *Personality and Social Psychology Bulletin, 15*, 543–558.

Eagly, A. H., Mladinic, A., & Otto, S. (1990). *Are women evaluated more favorably than men? An analysis of attitudes, beliefs, and emotions.* Unpublished manuscript, Purdue University, West Lafayette, IN.

Eagly, A. H., & Steffen, V. J. (1984). Gender stereotypes stem from the distribution of women and men into social roles. *Journal of Personality and Social Psychology, 46*, 735–754.

Eagly, A. H., & Steffen, V. J. (1986). Gender stereotypes, occupational roles, and beliefs about part-time employees. *Psychology of Women Quarterly, 10*, 252–262.

Edwards, V. J., & Spence, J. T. (1987). Gender-related traits, stereotypes, and schemata. *Journal of Personality and Social Psychology, 53*, 146–154.

Epstein, S. (1980). The stability of behavior: II. Implications for psychological research. *American Psychologist, 35*, 790–806.

Epstein, S. (1983). Aggregation and beyond: Some basic issues on the prediction of behavior. *Journal of Personality, 51*, 360–392.

Eron, L. D., Huesmann, L. R., Brice, P., Fischer, P., & Mermelstein, R. (1983). Age trends in the development of aggression, sex typing, and related television habits. *Developmental Psychology, 19*, 71–77.

Etaugh, C., Levine, D., & Mennella, A. (1984). Development of sex biases in children: 40 years later. *Sex Roles, 10*, 913–924.

Fazio, R. H. (1986). How do attitudes guide behavior? In R. M. Sorrentino and E. T. Higgins (Eds.), *The handbook of motivation and cognition: Foundations of social behavior* (pp. 204–243). New York: Guilford Press.

Fishbein, M., & Ajzen, I. (1975). *Belief, attitude, intention, and behavior: An introduction to theory and research*. Reading, MA: Addison-Wesley.

Fiske, S. T. (1989, August). *Interdependence and stereotyping: From the laboratory to the Supreme Court (and back)*. Paper presented at the meeting of the American Psychological Association, New Orleans.

Fiske, S. T., Bersoff, D. N., Borgida, E., Deaux, K., & Heilman, M. E. (1990). *Stereotyping research on trial: APA's Amicus Curiae brief in Price Waterhouse v. Hopkins*. Unpublished manuscript.

Fiske, S. T., & Neuberg, S. L. (1990). A continuum of impression formation, from category-based to individuating processes: Influences of information and motivation on attention and interpretation. *Advances in Experimental Social Psychology, 23*, 1–74.

Fiske, S. T., & Pavelchak, M. A. (1986). Category-based versus piecemeal-based affective responses: Developments in schema-triggered affect. In R. M. Sorrentino & E. T. Higgins (Eds.), *Handbook of motivation and cognition: Foundations of social behavior* (pp. 167–203). New York: Guilford.

Fiske, S. T., & Taylor, S. (1991). *Social Cognition* (2nd ed.). New York: Random House.

Frable, D. E. S. (1987). Sex-typed execution and perception of expressive movement. *Journal of Personality and Social Psychology, 53*, 391–396.

Frable, D. E. S. (1989). Sex typing and gender ideology: Two facets of the individual's gender psychology that go together. *Journal of Personality and Social Psychology, 56*, 95–108.

Frable, D. E. S., & Bem, S. L. (1985). If you're gender-schematic, all members of the opposite sex look alike. *Journal of Personality and Social Psychology, 49*, 459–468.

Freeman, H. R. (1987). Structure and content of gender stereotypes: Effects of somatic appearance and trait information. *Psychology of Women Quarterly, 11*, 59–68.

Frenkel-Brunswik, E. (1949). Intolerance of ambiguity as an emotional and perceptual personality variable. *Journal of Personality, 18*, 108–143.

Friedan, B. (1963). *The feminine mystique*. New York: W. W. Norton.

Gardner, R. C., Lalonde, R. N., Nero, A. M., & Young, M. Y. (1988). Ethnic stereotypes: Implications of measurement strategy. *Social Cognition, 6*, 40–60.

Geis, F. L., Brown, V., Walstedt, J. J., & Porter, N. (1984). TV commercials as achievement scripts for women. *Sex Roles, 10*, 513–525.

Gelman, S. A., Collman, P., & Maccoby, E. E. (1986). Inferring properties from categories versus inferring categories from properties: The case of gender. *Child Development, 57*, 396–404.

Gerber, G. L. (1988). Leadership roles and the gender stereotype traits. *Sex Roles, 18*, 649–668.

Gesell, G. (1990). *Findings of fact and conclusions on law of remand.* Court Action 84-3040, Ann B. Hopkins v. Price Waterhouse.

Glick, P., Zion, C., & Nelson, C. (1988). What mediates sex discrimination in hiring decisions? *Journal of Personality and Social Psychology, 55*, 178–186.

Gould, S. J. (1980). *The panda's thumb: More reflections in natural history.* New York: W. W. Norton.

Hamilton, D. L. (1979). A cognitive-attributional analysis of stereotyping. *Advances in Experimental Social Psychology, 12*, 53–84.

Helmreich, R. L., Spence, J. T., & Gibson, R. H. (1982). Sex-role attitudes: 1972-1980. *Personality and Social Psychology Bulletin, 8*, 656–663.

Hepburn, C. (1985). Memory for the frequency of sex-typed versus neutral behaviors: Implications for the maintenance of sex stereotypes. *Sex Roles, 12*, 771–776.

Herek, G. M. (1986a). The instrumentality of attitudes: Toward a neofunctional theory. *Journal of Social Issues, 42*, 99–114.

Herek, G. M. (1986b). The social psychology of homophobia: Toward a practical theory. *Review of Law and Social Change, 14*, 923–934.

Herek, G. M. (1987). Can functions be measured? A new perspective on the functional approach to attitudes. *Social Psychology Quarterly, 50*, 285–303.

Holland, D., & Davidson, D. (1983, May). *Labeling the opposite sex: Metaphors and themes in American folk models of gender.* Paper presented at conference on folk models, Institute for Advanced Study, Princeton University.

Hungerford, J. K., & Sobolew-Shubin, A. P. (1987). Sex-role identity, gender identity, and self-schemata. *Psychology of Women Quarterly, 11*, 1–9.

Huston, A. C. (1983). Sex-typing. In P. H. Mussen (Ed.), *Handbook of child psychology* (Vol. 4, pp. 387–467). New York: John Wiley.

Hyde, J. S., & Linn, M. C. (Eds.). (1986). *The psychology of gender: Advances through meta-analysis.* Baltimore: Johns Hopkins University Press.

Jackson, L. A., & Cash, T. F. (1985). Components of gender stereotypes: Their implications for inferences on stereotypic and nonstereotypic dimensions. *Personality and Social Psychology Bulletin, 11*, 326–344.

Katz, D. (1960). The functional approach to the study of attitudes. *Public Opinion Quarterly, 24*, 163–204.

Katz, D., & Braly, K. (1933). Racial prejudice and racial stereotypes. *Journal of Abnormal and Social Psychology, 28*, 280–290.

Katz, P. A. (1987). Variations in family constellation: Effects on gender schemata. In L. S. Liben & M. L. Signorella (Eds.), *Children's gender schemata* (pp. 39–56). San Francisco: Jossey-Bass.

Kite, M. E. (1990). *Age, gender, and employment: A test of social role theory.* Paper presented at the meeting of the American Psychological Association, Boston, MA.

Kite, M. E., & Deaux, K. (1986). Gender versus category clustering in free recall: A test of gender schema theory. *Representative Research in Social Psychology, 16*, 38–43.

Kite, M. E., & Deaux, K. (1987). Gender belief systems: Homosexuality and implicit inversion theory. *Psychology of Women Quarterly, 11*, 83–96.

Kite, M. E., Deaux, K., & Miele, M. (1991). Stereotypes of the elderly: Does age outweigh gender? *Psychology and Aging, 6*, 19–27.

Krueger, J., & Rothbart, M. (1988). The use of categorical and individuating information in making inferences about personality. *Journal of Personality and Social Psychology, 55*, 187–195.

Landrine, H. (1985). Race x class stereotypes of women. *Sex Roles, 13*, 65–75.

Larsen, R. J. (1984). *Tolerance for ambiguity in the personality attributes of others.* Unpublished manuscript, University of Illinois, Urbana.

Lewis, L. L. (1985). *The influence of individual differences in gender stereotyping on the interpersonal expectancy process.* Unpublished doctoral dissertation, Purdue University, West Lafayette, IN.

Liben, L. S., & Bigler, R. S. (1987). Reformulating children's gender schemata. In L. S. Liben & M. L. Signorella (Eds.), *Children's gender schemata* (pp. 89–105). San Francisco: Jossey-Bass.

Lippmann, W. (1922). *Public opinion.* New York: Harcourt, Brace.

Locksley, A., Borgida, E., Brekke, N., & Hepburn, C. (1980). Sex stereotypes and social judgment. *Journal of Personality and Social Psychology, 39*, 821–831.

Maccoby, E. E. (1990). Gender and relationships: A developmental account. *American Psychologist, 45*, 513–520.

Manstead, A. S. R., & McCulloch, C. (1981). Sex-role stereotyping in British television advertisements. *British Journal of Social Psychology, 20*, 171–180.

Markus, H. (1977). Self-schemata and processing information about the self. *Journal of Personality and Social Psychology, 35*, 63–78.

Markus, H., Crane, M., Bernstein, S., & Siladi, M. (1982). Self-schemas and gender. *Journal of Personality and Social Psychology, 42*, 38–50.

Markus, H., Smith, J., & Moreland, R. L. (1985). Role of the self-concept in the perception of others. *Journal of Personality and Social Psychology, 49*, 1494–1512.

Martin, A. J. (1990). *Men's ambivalence toward women: Implications for evaluations of rape victims.* Unpublished doctoral dissertation, City University of New York.

Martin, C. L. (1987). A ratio measure of sex stereotyping. *Journal of Personality and Social Psychology, 52*, 489–499.

Martin, C. L. (1989). Children's use of gender-related information in making social judgments. *Developmental Psychology, 25*, 80–88.

Martin, C. L., & Halverson, C. F. (1981). A schematic processing model of sex typing and stereotyping in children. *Child Development, 52*, 1119–1134.

Martin, C. L., Wood, C. H., & Little, J. K. (1989). The development of gender stereotypes. Unpublished manuscript, Arizona State University, Tempe.

Mason, K. O., Czajka, J. L., & Arber, S. (1976). Change in U.S. women's sex-role attitudes, 1964-1974. *American Sociological Review, 41*, 573–596.

Matteo, S. (1988). The effect of gender-schematic processing on decisions about sex-inappropriate sport behavior. *Sex Roles, 18*, 41–58.

Mayes, S., & Valentine, K. (1979). Sex-role stereotyping in Saturday morning cartoon shows. *Journal of Broadcasting, 23*, 41–50.

McArthur, L. Z. (1982). Judging a book by its cover: A cognitive analysis of the relationship between physical appearance and stereotyping. In A. H. Hastorf & A. M. Isen (Eds.), *Cognitive social psychology* (pp. 149–211). New York: Elsevier.

McArthur, L. Z., & Resko, B. G. (1975). The portrayal of men and women in American television commercials. *Journal of Social Psychology, 97,* 209–220.

McCauley, C., & Stitt, C. L. (1978). An individual and quantitative measure of stereotypes. *Journal of Personality and Social Psychology, 36,* 929–940.

McKenzie-Mohr, D., & Zanna, M. P. (1990). Treating women as sexual objects: Look to the (gender schematic) male who has viewed pornography. *Personality and Social Psychology Bulletin, 16,* 296–308.

Meece, J. L. (1987). The influence of school experiences on the development of gender schemata. In L. S. Liben & M. L. Signorella (Eds.), *Children's gender schemata* (pp. 57–73). San Francisco: Jossey-Bass.

Messick, D. M., & Mackie, D. M. (1989). Intergroup relations. *Annual Review of Psychology, 40,* 45–81.

Morgan, M. (1982). Television and adolescents' sex role stereotypes: A longitudinal study. *Journal of Personality and Social Psychology, 43,* 947–955.

Neuberg, S. L., & Fiske, S. T. (1987). Motivational influences on impression formation: Outcome dependency, accuracy-driven attention, and individuating processes. *Journal of Personality and Social Psychology, 53,* 431–444.

Noseworthy, C. M., & Lott, A. J. (1984). The cognitive organization of gender-stereotypic categories. *Personality and Social Psychology Bulletin, 10,* 474–481.

Payne, T. J., Connor, J. M., & Colletti, G. (1987). Gender-based schematic processing: An empirical investigation and reevaluation. *Journal of Personality and Social Psychology, 52,* 937–945.

Potkay, C. R., & Potkay, C. E. (1984). Perceptions of female and male comic strip characters: Favorability and identification are different dimensions. *Sex Roles, 10,* 119–128.

Rasinski, K. A., Crocker, J., & Hastie, R. (1985). Another look at sex stereotypes and social judgments: An analysis of the social perceiver's use of subjective probabilities. *Journal of Personality and Social Psychology, 49,* 317–326.

Reitman, J. (1976). Skilled perception in GO: Deducing memory structures from inter-response times. *Cognitive Psychology, 8,* 336–356.

Rosenkrantz, P., Vogel, S., Bee, H., Broverman, I., & Broverman, D. M. (1968). Sex-role stereotypes and self-concepts in college students. *Journal of Consulting and Clinical Psychology, 32,* 286–295.

Rothbart, M. (1989, October). Paper presented at meeting of Society of Experimental Social Psychology, Santa Monica, CA.

Rothbart, M., & John, O. P. (1985). Social categorization and behavioral episodes: A cognitive analysis of the effects of intergroup contact. *Journal of Social Issues, 41* (3), 81–104.

Ruble, T. L. (1983). Sex stereotypes: Issues of change in the 1970s. *Sex Roles, 9,* 397–402.

Ruggiero, J. A., & Weston, L. C. (1985). Work options for women in women's magazines: The medium and the message. *Sex Roles, 12,* 535–547.

Sheriffs, A. C., & McKee, J. P. (1957). Qualitative aspects of beliefs about men and women. *Journal of Personality, 25*, 451–464.

Sherman, S. J., Judd, C. M., & Park, B. (1989). Social cognition. *Annual Review of Psychology, 40*, 281–326.

Signorella, M. L. (1987). Gender schemata: Individual differences and context effects. In L. S. Liben & M. L. Signorella (Eds.), *Children's gender schemata* (pp. 23–37). San Francisco: Jossey-Bass.

Simon, R. J., & Landis, J. M. (1989). Women's and men's attitudes about a woman's place and role. *Public Opinion Quarterly, 53*, 265–276.

Skitka, L. J., & Maslach, C. (1990). Gender roles and the categorization of gender-relevant behavior. *Sex Roles, 22*, 133–150.

Slusher, M. P., & Anderson, C. A. (1987). When reality monitoring fails: The role of imagination in stereotype maintenance. *Journal of Personality and Social Psychology, 52*, 653–662.

Smith, M. B., Bruner, J. S., & White, R. W. (1956). *Opinions and personality*. New York: Wiley.

Snodgrass, S. E. (1990, August). *Sex role stereotypes are alive and well*. Paper presented at meeting of American Psychological Association, Boston.

Spence, J. T. (1984). Masculinity, femininity, and gender-related traits: A conceptual analysis and critique of current research. *Progress in Experimental Personality Research, 13*, 1–97.

Spence, J. T. (1985). Gender identity and its implications for concepts of masculinity and femininity. In T. Sonderegger (Ed.), *Nebraska Symposium on Motivation: Psychology and gender* (pp. 59–95). Lincoln: University of Nebraska Press.

Spence, J. T., & Helmreich, R. L. (1972). The Attitudes toward Women Scale: An objective instrument to measure attitudes toward the rights and roles of women in contemporary society. *JSAS Catalog of Selected Documents in Psychology, 2*, 667–668.

Spence, J. T., & Helmreich, R. L. (1981). Androgyny versus gender schema: A comment on Bem's gender schema theory. *Psychological Review, 88*, 365–368.

Spence, J. T., Helmreich, R. L., & Stapp, J. (1974). The personal attributes questionnaire: A measure of sex-role stereotypes and masculinity/femininity. *JSAS Catalog of Selected Documents in Psychology, 4*, 43.

Spence, J. T., Helmreich, R., & Stapp, J. (1975). Ratings of self and peers on sex role attributes and their relation to self-esteem and conceptions of masculinity and femininity. *Journal of Personality and Social Psychology, 32*, 29–39.

Srull, T. K., & Wyer, R. S., Jr. (1986). The role of chronic and temporary goals in social information processing. In R. M. Sorrentino & E. T. Higgins (Eds.), *The handbook of motivation and cognition: Foundations of social behavior* (pp. 503–549). New York: Guilford Press.

Stangor, C. (1988). Stereotype accessibility and information processing. *Personality and Social Psychology Bulletin, 14*, 694–708.

Stangor, C., & Ruble, D. N. (1987). Development of gender role knowledge and gender constancy. In L. S. Liben & M. L. Signorella (Eds.), *Children's gender schemata* (pp. 5–22). San Francisco: Jossey-Bass.

Stangor, C., & Ruble, D. N. (1989). Strength of expectancies and memory for social information: What we remember depends on how much we know. *Journal of Experimental Social Psychology, 25*, 18–35.

Stanworth, M. (1983). *Gender and schooling: A study of sexual divisions in the classroom.* London: Hutchinson.

Sternglanz, S. H., & Serbin, L. A. (1974). Sex role stereotyping in children's television programs. *Developmental Psychology, 10,* 710–715.

Storms, M. D. (1978a). Attitudes toward homosexuality and femininity in men. *Journal of Homosexuality, 3,* 257–263.

Storms, M. D. (1978b). Sexual orientation and self-perception. In P. Pliner, K. R. Blankstein, I. M. Spigel, T. Alloway, & L. Krames (Eds.), *Advances in the study of communication and affect (Vol. 5): Perception of emotion in self and others.* New York: Plenum.

Sullivan, G. L., & O'Connor, P. J. (1988). Women's role portrayals in magazine advertising: 1958-1983. *Sex Roles, 18,* 181–188.

Tajfel, H. (1969). Cognitive aspects of prejudice. *Journal of Social Issues, 25,* 79–97.

Taylor, S. E., & Crocker, J. (1981). Schematic bases of social information processing. In E. T. Higgins, C. P. Herman, & M. P. Zanna (Eds.), *Social cognition: The Ontario Symposium* (Vol. 1, pp. 89–134). Hillsdale, NJ: Erlbaum.

Taylor, S. E., Fiske, S. T., Etcoff, N. L., & Ruderman, A. J. (1978). Categorical and contextual bases of personal memory and stereotyping. *Journal of Personality and Social Psychology, 36,* 778–793.

Tetlock, P. E. (1983). Accountability and complexity of thought. *Journal of Personality and Social Psychology, 45,* 74–83.

Tetlock, P. E., & Kim, J. I. (1987). Accountability and judgment processes in a personality prediction task. *Journal of Personality and Social Psychology, 52,* 700–709.

Weber, R., & Crocker, J. (1983). Cognitive processes in the revision of stereotypic beliefs. *Journal of Personality and Social Psychology, 45,* 961–977.

Werner, P. D., & LaRussa, G. W. (1985). Persistence and change in sex-role stereotypes. *Sex Roles, 12,* 1089–1100.

Williams, J. E., & Best, D. L. (1982). *Measuring sex stereotypes: A thirty-nation study.* Beverly Hills: Sage.

Williams, J. E., Bennett, S. M., & Best, D. L. (1975). Awareness and expression of sex stereotypes in young children. *Developmental Psychology, 11,* 635–642.

5

Sexism: An Integrated Perspective

Rhoda Unger and Saundra

DEFINITIONAL ISSUES

Even though a number of different definitions of prejudice, discrimination, and sexism exist, there is general agreement about the essential meaning of these concepts. Allport (1954) defined prejudice as "an antipathy based on a faulty and inflexible generalization. It may be directed toward a group as a whole, or toward an individual because he [sic] is a member of that group" (p. 9). Jones (1972) extended this definition: "Prejudice is a negative attitude toward a person or group based upon a social comparison process in which the individual's own group is taken as the point of reference" (p. 3). This negative bias is maintained in disregard of facts that contradict it. These definitions emphasize the cognitive aspects of prejudice. However, prejudice is generally characterized as having an affective and behavioral component as well as a cognitive one (Harding, Proshansky, Kutner, & Chein, 1969).

While prejudice is an attitude, discrimination is defined as selectively unjustified negative behavior toward members of the target group. According to Allport (1954), discrimination involves denying "individuals or groups of people equality of treatment which they may wish" (p. 51). Jones (1972) defines it "as those actions designed to maintain own-group characteristics and favored position at the expense of the comparison group" (p. 4).

Sexism is a newer term than prejudice or discrimination. It refers to prejudice and discrimination against women as members of a social category. Many researchers distinguish between individual sexism, which involves the attitudes and behaviors of particular people, and institutional sexism, which refers to intentional or unintentional manipulation or toleration of institutional policies that unfairly restrict the opportunities of women as compared with men. The gender gap in salaries is one example of the effect of institutional sexism, although, as we shall see, individual attitudes may also contribute to the existence of such a gap.

It is impossible to provide inclusive documentation of discrimination against women in a single book chapter. We have chosen, therefore, to provide a theoretical structure in which to place specific examples of discrimination and their effect. We have several purposes in constructing this framework. First, by providing examples of sexism at various levels of analysis, we hope to demonstrate that sexism is a sociocultural phenomenon as much as it is an individual problem. Second, by focusing upon elements common to various levels of analysis, we hope to provide clues to the underlying processes that maintain sexism in our society. Third, by examining and comparing findings at various levels, we hope to explore the limitations of theories that are generated through consideration of data from only one level.

Forms of sexism may be classified as occurring at four levels, defined by the way they are measured. Moving from the particular to the general, these levels are individual, social/structural, institutional, and cultural. Individual sexism may be the most familiar to those involved in the discipline of psychology. It is examined by means of methodologies that look at negative biases against women that exist "inside the heads of individuals." Such biases include stereotypes, categorization involving in-group and out-group distinctions, and evaluation and attributional biases. Application of these biases in the "real world" of employment in terms of recruitment, screening, and promotional practices that favor men over women may also be included. The basis for considering all of these processes as exemplars of individual sexism is that they all occur whether or not the target individual is present. Although the conditions in which evaluation takes place may play an important role in judgment, measurement of these forms of discrimination is not changed by the presence of other persons within the evaluatory situation.

Social/structural sexism involves interaction between individuals—either as dyads or within groups. Forms of sexism that may be included in this category include nonverbal behaviors connoting status and power (especially those involving the use of space and the regulation of interpersonal communication) and the differential effect of target sex on helping and aggression. On a group level, the selection and identification of leaders and the isolation of tokens or deviants on the basis of sex may be included. All of these measures involve behavior with reference to another person or persons who are actually present in the situation. Although it is possible to look at the perceptions of others as a function of the group context or the sex ratio of its membership, sociostructural sexism differs from individual sexism because it involves behavior with respect to people from a particular sexual category.

Institutional sexism is most frequently studied by sociologists. It involves the effects of various institutional structures in terms of their differential impact upon men and women in our society. The focus of these studies is people as collectivities rather than as individuals who interact with others. Institutional sexism includes the effect of educational level and years of work experience, the impact of sex ratios within organizations and occupations, and the effects of occupational status on women and men.

Finally, cultural sexism looks at the cultural meaning of sex. Analyses of cultural sexism are more diffuse and generalized than the other levels discussed above. They seek to explain the value of sex and gender categories for the culture as a whole. Obviously, the meaning of sex distinction depends upon whether one is a member of the dominant or subordinate group. Cultural sexism, therefore, includes the phenomenology of being a victim of prejudice as well as analyses of the general social practices that maintain sexism within a society. Such practices include gender as a system of categorization and cultural practices that create and maintain social deviance. In sum, cultural analyses of sexism focus upon the latent assumptions and beliefs about gender and their effect upon individuals within a particular culture.

At the end of this chapter, we will review important themes that appear in analyses of sexism at all levels. By means of such themes we hope to link findings at various levels and avoid some of the limitations of theoretical formulations that utilize only some of the available information.

SOME CAVEATS: THE INTERSECTION OF RACISM AND SEXISM

Sexism is obviously not the only way in which people discriminate against others. All of the definitions used earlier in this chapter were, in fact, drawn with modifications from definitions of racism. Throughout this chapter we will be drawing analogies between sexism and racism. The similarities and differences between the two phenomena should help to further our understanding of both. We shall try, however, to avoid ranking forms of oppression. Prejudice and discrimination are destructive to members of all subordinate social categories.

We are particularly interested in one group of individuals who are missing from most analyses of both racism and sexism—minority women. To paraphrase the title of a book on black women's studies (Hull, Scott & Smith, 1982), all the blacks are men and all the women are white in most empirical studies of prejudice and discrimination. We have included as many studies of minority women as we could find. These studies, however, are frequently more ethnomethodological and personal in tone than those done in the laboratory. Some readers may find the mixture of "data" and viewpoint jarring. We would argue that personal stories are an important source of information about oppression and constitute a valid form of evidence. To understand the issues raised by the possession of two stigmatized social identities, social scientists must listen to all kinds of voices.

The exclusion of minority women from research is itself a form of discrimination. In a recent review of 28 psychology of women textbooks, Brown and her associates (Brown, Goodwin, Hall & Jackson-Lowman, 1985) found that 18 offered token or no reference to black women. In a further analysis of the material on minority women that did appear in these texts, they found that only 6 discussed studies that used an experimental design to obtain information while 13 used case histories or anecdotal data. The lack of comparability between studies of white women and nonwhite "others" obviously limits the conclusions that can be drawn by this review.

Some scholars (Zinn, Cannon, Higginbotham & Dill, 1986) have argued that there are institutional structures that limit the contributions of women of color and women from working-class backgrounds to the field of women's studies. For example, during 1983–1984 there were no women of color (except one Japanese-American woman) among the editors of the leading interdisciplinary journals in women's studies, and there was only token representation in positions below the editorial level. There are relatively few black faculty members at prestigious institutions where research and scholarship are encouraged (Exum, 1983). Consequently, women of color and working-class women are not in decision-making positions with regard to the conduct and publication of relevant research. Zinn and her associates note that work from such women may be rejected because it does not conform to the established research paradigm.

The exclusion/omission of the contributions of those women who are least likely to be part of the academy has significant consequences for the understanding of commonalities and differences between sexism and racism, in particular, black women's experience of sexism and racism. In a pioneering issue of the *Journal of Social Issues* that explored these issues for black women, Smith and Stewart (1983) suggested that contextual interactive designs and comparison of multiple gender/race groups as alternative research approaches would provide more comprehensive information on the effects of sexism and racism on the lives of black women. This information would inform us about aspects of white women's experience that have been hitherto ignored as well.

INDIVIDUAL SEXISM

Current Cognitive and Informational Approaches

Within psychology, the study of sexism is now typically embedded in the larger theoretical context of the role of cognitive processes in intergroup behavior. The cognitive perspective emphasizes the role of categorization and biases in information processing in the production and maintenance of gender stereotypes (see chapter 4). The focus is on the role of mental representations in encoding, storing, and retrieving information about persons and social events.

One of the fundamental processes underlying stereotypes is the categorization of people as in-group and out-group members. Members of out-groups are evaluated less favorably, receive fewer rewards, and are seen as having fewer desirable characteristics than members of the in-group (Hamilton & Trolier, 1986). People tend to see members of the out-group as similar to each other and different from themselves. Women have been found to be subject to out-group categorization (Taylor, Fiske, Etcoff & Ruderman, 1978). Both sexes, moreover, appear to agree that males have significantly more advantages and significantly fewer disadvantages than females (Fabes & Laner, 1986). Further evidence of the consequences of out-group categorization is evident from a large number of studies demonstrating evaluation and attributional biases against women.

Evaluation and Attributional Biases

Early Work in the Area

Evaluation bias refers to the tendency of people to evaluate the work or performance of women and men differently. The classic work in this area was done by Goldberg in 1968. In this study, he provided female college students with identical essays that had purportedly been written by a male or a female. The essays were on topics that were either stereotypically "masculine" (law and city planning), stereotypically "feminine" (elementary school teaching and dietetics), or gender-neutral (linguistics and art history). The results showed that the work of women tended to be devalued. Essays with a female name were rated as less valuable and their authors less competent than were essays with a male name attached. The effect of the author's sex was significant for masculine and neutral fields, but not for feminine ones.

The finding that women may discriminate against other women had a great deal of impact, especially at the beginning of the women's movement. A number of studies followed up the original finding, varying the sex of the subject population, the nature of the tasks performed, and the kind of evaluations made. These studies extended the range of the original pro-male finding. Thus, Pheterson, Kiesler, and Goldberg (1971) found that college students of both sexes rated abstract paintings by women as less good than the same paintings attributed to a male artist. Deaux and Emswiller (1974) found that male performance on a perceptual discrimination task was seen as more skillful than the equivalent female performance, whether the task was sex-typed as male (discrimination of mechanical objects) or female (discrimination of household objects). When women and men were portrayed as responding the same way in an emergency situation, the man was judged as behaving in a more logical way than the woman (Taynor & Deaux, 1975). Adolescents (Etaugh & Rose, 1975) and children (Etaugh & Brown, 1975) were found to have evaluation biases against women similar to those found for adult subjects.

Other studies demonstrated attributional biases in the evaluation of the performance or behavior of women and men. Attributional bias may be defined as the tendency to explain identical behavior in men and women as due to different causes. A number of different attributional biases related to sex have been identified. For example, when women were portrayed as performing equally as well as men in an objective situation (e.g., attaining a medical degree), the cause of their success was attributed more to effort than to ability (Feldman-Summers & Kiesler, 1974). Similarly, female success in school courses has been attributed to easy courses whereas the identical success of males has been attributed to ability (Feather & Simon, 1975). Women's competent performance may also be attributed more to luck and men's more to skill (Deaux & Emswiller, 1974).

Attributions about females and males have a similar pattern. Female success is attributed to external and/or unstable causes—factors that are not under the control of the person—whereas male success is attributed to internal and/or stable factors. In general, both sexes tend to share the tendency to make different attributions about the performance of women and men (Wallston & O'Leary, 1981). Such differential attributions about identical performance undermine the objective competence of women. The attribution of good performance to factors that do not suggest future predictability makes any single positive evaluation virtually meaningless (Nieva & Gutek, 1980).

Biases against women have not always been found. For example, the work of women artists was not perceived to be inferior to that of men when subjects were informed that the work they were evaluating was by the winner of an art show rather than an entrant (Pheterson et al., 1971). Women were not evaluated more poorly than men if they were portrayed to have professional stature (Kaschak, 1978). In fact, some researchers (Abramson, Goldberg, Greenberg & Abramson, 1978) have found that female attorneys and paralegal workers were rated as having more vocational competence than identical males. They termed these results "the talking platypus phenomenon." The label refers to the idea that when a woman engages in extremely out-of-role behavior, it is evaluated more positively than the same behavior in men because it is so unexpected that she can perform well at all.

Current Work on Evaluation and Attributional Bias: The Interaction of Sex and Gender

Findings on evaluation bias have continued to be inconsistent (see review of this area by Ruble, Cohen, & Ruble, 1984). Although men appeared to be favored more than women, a substantial number of studies found either a pro-female bias or no main effect for the sex of the target individual. This kind of pattern suggests that other variables besides stimulus sex are operating. Recent studies have, therefore, focused upon the interaction of other gender-related variables with target sex. One such variable is the gender typing or presumed masculinity or femininity of the task to be evaluated. For example, Paludi and Strayer (1985) asked 300 college students to evaluate an academic article in the field of politics (stereotypically masculine), psychology of women (stereotypically feminine), or education (neutral) that had been signed with a male name, a female name, a sexually ambiguous name, with initials, or with no name attached. They found that, in general, an article written by a male was valued more positively than if the author was not male.

Perhaps more interesting than findings of pro-male evaluation bias, however, were findings on the assumptions made by subjects when they saw an article with no name given or with initials or a sexually ambiguous name attached. Eighty-seven % of the subjects attributed an article on politics to a male and 96% attributed an article on the psychology of women to a female. Explanations given by the subjects for decisions were based upon traditional stereotypes: for example, ''Men are associated with business, economics, and politics''; ''The author seems to have insight into women's feelings''; or ''The author is male— because the style is abrupt.''

This study illustrates the impact that the implicit assumptions about sex and gender that subjects carry with them to the experimental situation may have upon evaluation. These assumptions are not easily manipulated. They may help to account for some of the inconsistency in results of various studies.

Another important interacting variable is the sex composition of the group in which the ratings are made. An early study by Starer and Denmark (1974) demonstrated that males showed more pro-male evaluation bias when they made judgments in the presence of all-male groups than when they were alone, whereas the opposite effect occurred for females. Similarly, Toder (1980) found that male-authored articles were rated more highly than female-authored articles in groups with equal numbers of women and men, but not in all-female groups. Women in all-female groups also endorsed more profeminist ideas after reading articles by females than did women in mixed-sex groups. Both these articles suggest that males in groups tend to trigger negative biases against women.

A more recent study that looked at the effect of the presence of males on evaluation bias included male or female experimenters as well as all-female, all-male, or mixed-sex groups (Etaugh, Houtler & Ptasnik, 1988). They found that subjects in mixed-sex groups generally evaluated the female more favorably in the presence of a female, as compared with a male, experimenter. Male subjects were more influenced than females by the experimenter's sex, tending to give higher ratings to the stimulus person of the same sex as the experimenter. As we shall see later, the sex of individuals who are apparently irrelevant to an evaluation may increase the salience of gender. These studies also suggest that men's discrimination against women may be heightened in group situations or with a male authority figure present.

Assumptions about Attractiveness and Gender

Recent studies on gender stereotypes using cognitive methodology have shown that besides traits, beliefs about occupational roles and physical characteristics are closely associated in images of women and men (Deaux, Winton, Crowley & Lewis, 1985; see also chapter 4). It is, therefore, not surprising that evaluational bias effects are found using these correlated variables. For example, physical attractiveness enhanced the evaluations of both male and female essayists (Cash & Trimer, 1984). For females, however, attractiveness was less beneficial for masculine than for feminine topics. Sexism appeared as an interactive effect of attractiveness. As usual, the women subjects in this study did not evaluate the sexes differently than did men subjects.

Attractiveness also had different consequences for men and women when people were asked to explain their rapid rise as corporate executives (Heilman & Stopeck, 1985). Luck was viewed as more responsible for the success of attractive women as compared to unattractive women and for the success of unattractive men as compared to attractive men. Attractiveness was viewed as associated more with political know-how and less with effort for both sexes.

The differential effects of attractiveness for women and men seems to be linked to its association with appropriate gender (Unger, 1985). Attractive men are seen as masculine whereas attractive women are seen as feminine. Masculine characteristics appear to be preferred in decision-making positions. In one study that looked at the effect of female applicants' dress on the hiring recommendations of personnel administrators, there was a positive correlation between the masculinity of the costume and the favorability of the recommendations received (Forsythe, Drake & Cox, 1985). In another study in which male and female undergraduates interviewed a female confederate who was supposedly applying for an entry-level managerial position, women who engaged in "too many" feminine strategies (combining smiling, eye contact, an informal posture, and the use of perfume) were rated as less desirable than confederates who used only one such strategy (Baron, 1986).

These studies have some sexist assumptions because they examine the effect of the manipulation of perceived gender only for female stimulus persons. There is reason to believe that assumptions about gender and attractiveness also influence perceptions about the employability of men. Thus, Unger, Hilderbrand, and Madar (1982) found that unattractive men were perceived as more likely to aspire to stereotypically traditional female occupations such as librarian and nurse than were their more attractive counterparts.

The Effect of Minority Status

Discrimination in the form of evaluation bias has also been found when the target persons were members of an ethnic minority group. It is difficult to do such studies because of the reactive nature of stimulus materials in which minority group membership is denoted. However, it has been demonstrated that individuals of both sexes attribute significantly greater ability, less effort, and less luck to a white man with a successful banking career as compared with either a black man, a white woman, or a black woman (Yarkin, Town & Wallston, 1982). Their attributions for the latter three groups did not differ from each other.

Interestingly, even an apparent lack of awareness of ethnic identity can produce prejudicial biases. A study that clearly demonstrates this effect asked Chicana and Anglo women to respond to verbal descriptions in which an Anglo, black, or Chicana woman experienced either success or failure in her first year as an assistant professor (Romero & Garza, 1986). In comparison with Anglo subjects, Chicana subjects were more likely to attribute both occupational success and failure to luck, ethnicity, and sex. Under failure conditions, Anglo women credited all the target individuals with significantly less competence than did Chicana women. The attributions of Chicana women indicated that ethnic origin played a greater role in success and a significantly lesser role in failure for Anglo actors than for black or Chicana actors. Anglo women, in contrast, made strikingly similar attributions for the success or failure of all actors regardless of ethnicity. This color blindness appears to have blinded them to the impact of structural factors on the success and failure of minority individuals.

Blaming the Victim (and Those Associated with Her)

The most extreme form of attributional bias involves attributing responsibility for victimization to those who have been victimized. Such bias punishes the victim a second time. Most attention has been paid to victim blaming in cases of rape. At least one recent study has found, however, that more blame was attributed to female than to male victims across several types of assault and in different situations (Howard, 1984). Undergraduates who read transcripts—ostensibly of interviews by a police detective of a man or woman who had been assaulted while jogging—blamed women more than men, but did not blame those who had been raped more than those who had been robbed.

The specific sources of blame were different for the two sexes. The highest level of characterological blame (due to undesirable personality traits) was attributed to a female victim of a robbery whereas the highest level of behavioral blame (being in the wrong place or doing the wrong thing) was attributed to a male victim of a robbery. These differences were most marked in individuals who were most traditional in their attitudes about the sexes. They were willing to make attributions about very specific characteristics and behaviors of the victims despite having been offered no data about them. A similar difference in characterological attributions has been found for female versus male victims of negligence. Women were seen as more emotional and meriting more assistance than men who had experienced the same misfortune (Barnett & King, 1985).

Women are victimized twice by such attributions. First, they are blamed more than men. Second, since characterological attributions are more stable than behavioral ones, women may find it more difficult to defend themselves against accusations that they were either responsible for their own undoing or more unhinged by it.

The effects of evaluation and attributional bias appear to extend beyond judgments about the target individuals themselves. In one study that demonstrated such effects, subjects were presented with a 50-minute audiotape of a rape trial and saw photographs of both the victim and the defendant (Villemur & Hyde, 1983). The variables examined included the sex of the defense attorney, the age of the victim, the attractiveness of the victim, and the sex of the jurors. The most striking finding was the higher acquittal rate under a female attorney (71%)

than under a male attorney (49%). Jurors also attributed more fault to the victim and less to the defendant when the defense attorney was female. There were no other significant main effects. This study appears to indicate that putative rapists are blamed less and their victims blamed more if they can find a woman to defend them.

Another effect involving the transference of attributions to the victim has been demonstrated using a situation in which a defense attorney (who is always defending a white male) was portrayed as either black or white (Kirkland, Greenberg & Pyszczynski, 1987). When a confederate, posing as a subject, made an ethnic slur in the presence of genuine subjects, both the attorney and defendant received negative evaluations. Especially harsh verdicts were made against defendants who were associated with a black attorney who had been the target of a derogatory ethnic label as compared to either black or white attorneys who had been the target of a nonethnic label.

The Application of Attributional and Evaluation Bias to Issues Involving Employment

Attributional and evaluation bias directed against women has mainly been examined in terms of achievement. It is, therefore, not surprising that techniques designed to study individual sexism have been applied outside the laboratory to the "real world of work." Such studies have examined sex biases in recruitment, screening, and promotional practices. Overwhelmingly, they demonstrate that women job applicants are treated less well than men applicants at every level of the selection process.

Recruitment Practices

One of the earliest studies in this area was conducted by Levinson (1975) as part of a course in sociological methodology. Male and female students in this class made job inquiries in response to 256 different classified advertisements. For each job, a person deemed sex-"inappropriate" for the position phoned first, followed by an "appropriate"-sex inquirer a half hour later. Clear-cut sex discrimination was found in over one-third of the telephoned inquiries (defined by an inquirer's being informed that the job was restricted by sex or being told that the position was filled when a subsequent inquirer was told it was still open). Although clear-cut discrimination was more common against male than female callers (44% versus 28%), indirect discrimination was more commonly directed against female nonconventional applicants. For example, men who applied for a "female" job (83% of these were secretary, receptionist, waitress, or maid) were sometimes told about a better-paying job that was available. They were also told that the jobs were too simple, dull, or low-paying. Nonconventional women applicants, on the other hand, were told the jobs were too difficult, had long or night hours, or required too much physical strength.

A recent study using the same methodology (Winston, 1988) found that instances of outright discrimination had been reduced by 50% (the good news is that no discrimination was found in 61.8% of the positions!). She also found no sex difference in the treatment of nonconventional job applicants. Female applicants, however, still experienced more indirect discrimination than male applicants. While men were more likely to be discriminated against monetarily, women were more frequently told that their qualifications were inadequate, more frequently experienced put-downs, and were more often denied the opportunity to talk with the employer over the telephone. These studies document the degree of sex bias in recruitment practices, but they do not tell us how the sex typing of a job influences the sex ratio of the applicant pool for each position. An older study by Bem and Bem (1973), however, demonstrated that the language by which a position is advertised influences the applicant pool. For example, changing the job title of a telephone "lineman" to a more sex-neutral term increased the number of women who applied for the position. In a study of high school students, Heilman (1979) told them that two occupations currently dominated by men would achieve an even balance in sex ratios in 15 years. The anticipated balance increased the occupational interest of girls, but reduced the interest of boys.

All of the studies in this area suggest that sex biases are present at the very beginning of the application process and, indeed, help to determine the probable sex of applicants. As we shall see, the sex composition of occupations is an important determinant of their relative status and financial rewards. These data show how both internal and external psychological barriers operate at the entry level to maintain a sex-segregated status quo.

Screening Practices

The issue of sex bias in evaluation and decision-making processes is probably one of the most investigated areas in applied psychology. Although the weight of the evidence supports the idea that women applicants receive lower evaluations than men with the same objective qualifications, sex biases are not always found and may even be reversed at times (see reviews by Powell, 1987; Ruble et al., 1984). Rather than attempt to include all the relevant studies in the area we will review some of the theories put forth to explain when sex bias is present and discuss the implications of findings in terms of the general issue of individual sexism.

The Presence of Relevant and/or Individuating Information

A number of researchers have suggested that relevant information significantly reduces or even eliminates sex biases in judgments about occupational suitability (see reviews by Kalin & Hodgins, 1984; Nieva & Gutek, 1980; Tosi & Einbender, 1985). These argue that personal information takes precedence over, and obviates the need for, category information. For example, Tosi and Einbender did a meta-analysis of 21 studies that had been designed to test for sex discrimination in some stage of personnel selection. They found that of the 11 studies that showed sex discrimination, 10 fell into the category in which less information about applicants had been provided. Studies that found no sex discrimination provided more varied forms of information about each applicant.

Quantity of information, however, may be less important than the kind of information provided. The same meta-analysis showed that more gender-salient information was provided in studies that showed discrimination than in those that did not. In this context, gender-salient information was defined as the use of sex-segregated occupational categories.

It is impossible to avoid gender salience according to this definition since most occupations are, in reality, sex-segregated. Heilman (1980) conducted one of the few experimental studies that directly examined the relationship between the sex ratios within occupations and hiring decisions. She asked interviewers to evaluate an application from a woman along with those of seven additional candidates. The applicant pool was manipulated so that it included between 12.5% and 100% women candidates. When women represented 25% or less of the total pool, the same application from a woman was rated more unfavorably than if the pool reflected a higher percentage of women.

Individuating information about competence may have little impact if evaluators have different attributions about the causes of good work performance in men and women. In a laboratory study of the relationship between attributional processes and reward allocation, Heilman and Guzzo (1978) found attributing performance to ability led to higher ratings of promotability than if the equivalent performance was seen as being due to effort, task difficulty, or luck. This pattern occurred regardless of the sex of the employee. If this attributional pattern is applied to women more than men, it helps to explain why they receive lower rewards for equal performance. There is some evidence of a general tendency to explain achievements by males by more internal, stable causes and to explain the same behaviors in females by more external causes (see review by Hansen & O'Leary, 1985).

Sex-Congruence Between the Applicant and the Job

A major source of sex discrimination may be perceptions of a lack of fit between the candidate and the job (Heilman, 1983). This model suggests that gatekeepers will be equally negative about women who apply for a job seen as requiring masculine attributes and men who apply for a job seen as requiring feminine attributes. Although the evidence in this area is somewhat inconsistent (Powell, 1987), a considerable body of evidence suggests that perceived sex and gender fit do play a role in selection decisions.

Perceived fit appears to be affected by a number of gender-related variables. These include sex typing of the occupation (Gardner & Discenza, 1988); the degree to which credentials fit the job demands (Plake et al., 1987); and inferences about personality traits assumed to be consistent with the position (Dipboye & Wiley, 1977, 1978; Gerdes & Garber, 1983). When, however, individuals were given individuating information that eliminated sex-typed personality attributions about male and female applicants and their perceived job suitability, sex discrimination was not eliminated (Glick, Zion & Nelson, 1988). The responses of 212 business professionals indicated a strong preference for male applicants for a stereotypically masculine job even when similar information on the résumés of women and men had led to perceptions of similar personality traits. In this study, perceived gender played a role independent of other aspects of personality. Masculine traits were positively related to the likelihood that either sex applicant would be interviewed for stereotypically masculine, feminine, or sex-neutral jobs.

It is difficult to determine in advance what information will be defined by evaluators as gender-relevant. For example, when one of four identical résumés (which varied the sex of the applicant and whether his or her scholastic ability was high or average) was sent at random to 100 personnel directors for an accounting position, both the number of replies and the number of positive responses were greater for an applicant with initials as compared with one with a female name (Zikmund, Hitt & Pickens, 1978). This difference was greatest for applicants with a high grade point average.

Equal Employment, Affirmative Action, and Feminism: Variables That Add to Sex Bias

Some clues appear to increase the probability of biases in the selection process. Clues about feminist ideology or about possible advancement through affirmative action policies appear to be particularly potent stimuli that evoke discrimination. For example, Hitt and Zikmund (1985) found that female applicants with an M.B.A. were preferred over applicants who used only initials, but only if their résumé showed no evidence of feminist ideology. Applications from women with no thesis received more favorable replies than those from women whose identical résumés included a thesis on sex discrimination. Similarly, minority candidates to graduate school were rated as less qualified when their undergraduate institution had an affirmative action policy (Garcia, Erskine, Hawn & Casmay, 1981).

It is not always easy to predict how biases will emerge. For example, provision of both a strong and a weak affirmative action policy eliminated sex discrimination in the selection of a manager by municipal administrators, but lower starting salaries were recommended for women in the strong fair employment policy statement condition (Rosen & Mericle, 1979). The researchers suggested that low salary recommendations may have reflected a reaction against perceived hiring constraints and a subtle attempt to undermine the career prospects of newly hired females.

The Incremental Effects of Evaluation Bias

Favorable evaluation of task-specific performance does not necessarily lead to a favorable evaluation of long-term potential or general ability. For example, subjects showed only a small difference in terms of sex in their ratings of 12 applicants for a management trainee position. When, however, they were told that only one opening could be filled, male candidates were far more likely to be selected (Dipboye, Arvey & Terpstra, 1977). In a study using actual evaluations of subordinate performance by supervisors (most of whom were male), Gupta and her associates (Gupta, Jenkins & Beehr, 1983) found that women received more positive evaluations than did men and that opposite-sex evaluators were more positive than evaluators of the same sex. Nevertheless, male subordinates received more promotions and same-sex subordinates received more pay increases. Forced choice studies of this kind are more reflective of reality since in most cases a manager has to choose one person for advancement and not just rate many.

To sum up the findings so far, individual sexism does not appear to occur only under conditions of ambiguity or uncertainty. While task-relevant and/or individuating information may sometimes play a role in making decisions, more egalitarian, gender-relevant information from a variety of sources may be used as a basis for sex bias. An important point that emerges from these studies is that evaluation and actual rewards are not necessarily closely related (and may, in fact, have a differential relationship for men and women).

It is also important to note that the criteria for evaluation may change as a function of the characteristics of the candidates. One intriguing study in this regard found, for example, that interview scores were counted more heavily for women than for men in arriving at a final ranking for admission to medical school (Clayton, Baird & Levinson, 1984). Women were, in addition, generally rated more poorly than men in such interviews. This finding is intriguingly similar to reports in the popular press that some highly competitive colleges have begun to count admission essays more heavily in response to the high number of Asian students with high SATs who are "flooding" their applicant pool.

The effects of individual sexism in employment practices can best be viewed in terms of a sequence of more and more narrowly gauged filters. Biases enter into the sequence at every level: recruitment of applicants in terms of the perceived sex-appropriateness of the occupation; responses to applicants; screening of candidates; rating of applicants who reach the interview stage; hiring and salary decisions; and, finally, promotional decisions once someone has been in the organization for a while. The consequences of these practices is a highly sex-segregated work force. This, in turn, influences the perception of what is an appropriate occupation for a woman or a man—altering the sex ratio of the applicant pool without any need for sexism in advertising.

Why Are Women Rewarded Less Well Than Men?

Current studies of individual sexism in the work world have concentrated on cognitive explanations of why women are rewarded less well than men. These studies indicate that inferences involving sex-related differences in factors other than achievement may influence reward allocations. For example, Rusbult and her associates (Rusbult, Lowery, Hubbard, Maravankin & Neises, 1988) found that, consistent with their predictions, undergraduates asked to act as managers of a baseball team allocated higher salaries to more deserving employees and those with high competence and dedication. Their allocations, however, were also influenced by employee mobility. Highly competent employees with greater mobility were given a greater share of the available rewards than were competent but entrapped employees. This tendency was particularly pronounced under conditions of low resources and low employee availability. The researchers characterized this pattern as "rational selective exploitation." Similarly, undergraduate business students engaged in a corporate simulation differed in their response to labor shortages in male versus female sex-typed jobs (Buttner & Rosen, 1987). They favored raising salaries for male sex-typed jobs, but favored alternatives to salary increases for female sex-typed jobs at the entry and middle (but not the professional) level.

In moderate-status occupations, lower pay was perceived as fairer for female employees than for gender-neutral employees in the same occupations (Jackson & Grabski, 1988). Jobs enacted by men were rated as higher in responsibility, in persuasive ability requirements, and in monetary worth than the same jobs enacted by women (McArthur & Obrant, 1986). All of these studies indicate that perceptions about appropriate rewards may be more sex-biased than are perceptions about competence. They also indicate that reward allocations are influenced by institutional factors that are different in nature from the individual's perception of males and females. These factors are produced by the current structure of the world of employment; for example, men have more employment mobility, men's occupations have higher status, men's occupations are viewed as more socially desirable, and so on. They are also influenced by culture, which values men and what men do more than women and what women do. These individual perceptions are not, therefore, the product of informational biases— they are a veridical picture of current reality. They point out some of the limitations of a model of sexism based only upon what is inside the head of our subjects. Contemporary, real world instances of sexism cannot be explained solely by biases in cognitive functioning. Individual sexism is too pervasive and too consistent to be simply a product of each individual's effort to deal with a complex social world. We must ask, for example, why some social categories are much more likely to induce biased responses than are others, for example, female rather than male, black rather than white, and so on.

Little attention has been paid to motivational and social learning processes. Social categories do more than segment and systematize the social world. They provide an important basis for the individual's self-identity and self-esteem (Tajfel, 1982). They provide a model for the way individuals are supposed to function within the social system of which they are a part. In other words, social categories provide a model for actions as well as thoughts. We need to look to other levels of sexism besides the individual one to understand the functional value of sexism for both the individual and society.

SOCIOSTRUCTURAL SEXISM

The kinds of sexism discussed above range on a continuum from prejudice to discrimination. Negative biases against women discriminate against them whether or not the women happen to be present when the judgment occurs. Evidence of discrimination makes more of an impact, however, when it is behavioral, but such discrimination is more difficult to demonstrate under laboratory conditions when the norms mandate that people are "subjects" without a personal or cultural history (Unger, 1981). Most of the studies of negative behaviors directed against people of different social categories are, therefore, indirect. They include three major categories, which we will discuss separately: unobtrusive measures of nonverbal behaviors; examination of behaviors directed toward or against another individual (helping and aggression); and some of the dynamics of behaviors within groups, particularly those involving participation and the identification or selection of leaders. Since each of these areas deserves a chapter or a book of its own, our coverage will not attempt to be inclusive. Instead, we shall try to survey some of the current research in each area and to note processes that seem to be similar across levels of sexism and that may help to explain the interrelationship between these levels.

Unobtrusive Measures of Nonverbal Behavior

The classic work in this area remains that of Henley (1977). Citing Goffman's early (1956) observation that relations between persons of unequal status are asymmetrical, she documented many studies showing that norms governing posture, gesture, movement, use of space, touching, and facial expressions reflect and support the low power position of women. The male-female differences found follow the same pattern generally found in interactions between any persons of unequal status (see also reviews by Frieze & Ramsey, 1976; Unger, 1976, 1978).

Current studies have found nothing to contradict the idea that status and sex are highly confounded in our society. For example, Lott (1987) observed previously unacquainted pairs of men, women, and mixed-sex pairs during a 10-minute task in which each pair constructed a domino structure for a contest. As predicted, women's behavior did not change as a function of the sex of their partner, but men distanced themselves more from a female than from a male partner. They turned their faces or bodies away, they made more negative comments, they followed their partner's advice less often, and they placed the dominoes closer to themselves. Women smiled more than men no matter with whom they were interacting. Paper-and-pencil measures had not revealed evidence of any gender stereotypes or sexist biases.

Of course, one could argue that such studies reflect gender norms rather than status norms. Several recent studies, however, have addressed this question directly. Leffler, Gillespie, and Conaty (1982) assigned status-differentiated positions (teacher and student) to students randomly. They found that high-status subjects, whatever their sex, claimed more direct space with their bodies, talked more, and attempted more interruptions than low-status subjects. Males, whatever their status assignment, used more horizontal space, touched more frequently, and laughed less than females. Their study suggests that the greater use of space is a mark of higher status, but the way this space is organized may depend upon the particular kind of status—specific or diffuse or achieved rather than ascribed. This kind of use of space by white subjects to distance themselves from blacks has also been found in a number of studies (see review by Crosby, Bromley & Saxe, 1980).

Dovidio and his colleagues (Dovidio, Ellyson, Keating, Heltman & Brown, 1988) manipulated the extent to which male and female subjects in their experiment possessed expert or reward power relative to their partners. In these mixed-sex pairs, both women and men high in expertise or reward power displayed high visual dominance as defined by looking more while speaking than looking while listening. In conditions where men and women did not have differential power, visual behavior was related to sex. Men displayed visual behavior similar to the patterns found under conditions of high expertise and high reward whereas the women exhibited visual behavior similar to those found under conditions of low expertise and reward.

The two studies above suggest that sex as a status cue may be overridden by specific information about other relevant forms of status. It is not as clear that this can easily occur outside of a laboratory situation. For example, Brooks (1982) has found that male students interrupt significantly more in female professors' than in male professors' classrooms. They also showed more assertiveness as measured by the frequency and duration of speech. No significant differences in speech between male and female students were found in male professors' classes. Data on group processes (to be discussed below) suggest that power relationships between the sexes are sensitive to the group context and may be easier to manipulate when only one person of each sex category is present.

The Intersection of Sex and Power

These studies demonstrate how social expectations are reflected in nonverbal power displays. Messages concerning dominance and relative power may be communicated without the awareness of either the sender or the receiver. Dominance and power, however, are associated with males even when no nonverbal messages are exchanged. For example, an early study by Johnson (1976) found that subjects of both sexes believed that messages from an unseen partner communicating referent, helpless, and indirect power were more likely to have been sent by women than men. In contrast, messages communicating expert, legitimate, and informational power were seen as more likely to have been sent by men than women.

More recent studies suggest that the sexes are also evaluated differently on the basis of dominance and submissiveness. Keating (1985) has found that both men and women gave significantly higher dominance ratings to male faces with mature, rather than immature, features. There was no effect of facial features on ratings of the dominance of female faces. Male faces with mature features were also rated as more attractive, especially by women. Female faces were perceived as attractive when they displayed characteristics that made male faces look submissive and unattractive. This study demonstrates that gender and at-tractiveness are related in terms of perceived dominance. Males are seen to be more attractive when they are dominant whereas females are seen as more attractive when they are subordinate.

Women are not expected to possess power and authority in our society. There are a number of studies documenting negative evaluations of women who do. For example, women directing men received less positive evaluations and were seen as acting out of role when compared with men directing either men or women, or women directing only women (Jacobson, Antonelli, Winning & Opeil, 1977). Experienced managers asked to evaluate a dialogue between two individuals in a corporate setting, in which one person successfully persuaded the other to adopt a specific plan of action, perceived influential men as significantly more powerful, as higher in corporate position, and warmer than women in identical situations (Wiley & Eskilson, 1982). Men were seen as more effective and active when they used expert power whereas women were seen as more effective when they used reward power. Men and women who were believed to be equal in position were assumed to have the same power, but different personalities. The evaluations of the women were far colder than those of the men.

Power is also seen as a more relevant dimension in judgments about people in jobs that are sex-typed as male rather than female (Hartman, Griffeth, Miller, & Kinicki, 1988). Undergraduates rated people of both sexes who performed well as computer programmers as more masculine and more active and powerful than those who performed poorly. There were no differences in the perceptions of power between individuals who performed well or poorly as nurses. Pro-gramming was also seen as more socially desirable than nursing.

Negative evaluations of women who possess power and authority appear to be related to the issue of whom they are perceived to have power over. For example, when students viewed videotapes of women who were in positions of authority over men, the men were seen as weaker than men who were subordinate to other men (Denmark & McKenna in Denmark, 1980). White men appear to have equal difficulty accepting either a white woman or a black man as more competent than themselves even when relative competence had been explicitly manipulated by the experimenters (Dovidio & Gaertner, 1981, 1983).

Helping as an Unobtrusive Measure of Sexism

Helping studies provide researchers with another opportunity to examine status versus gender norms as explanations for relations between the sexes. For example, norms mandate that we help the helpless, but a body of evidence suggests that people are less likely to help people who are physically stigmatized or are members of social categories different from their own (see review by Piliavin & Unger, 1985). The only exception to this phenomenon appears to be in terms of sexual categories where women appear to be helped more than men and men help more than women. These differences, however, appear to be limited to highly specific conditions in which women need help in travel away from their homes (Piliavin & Unger, 1985). They may be related to cross-cultural norms that mandate that women remain apart from the public sphere.

Eagly (1987) also notes that apparently greater male helpfulness may be due to definitions of help in terms of heroic and chivalrous acts. What these explanations have in common is that the woman is in a culturally defined dependent relationship vis-à-vis the man.

What happens to helping when the woman needing assistance has higher status than the man? An extremely interesting study by Dovidio and Gaertner (1983) has examined this relationship. They conducted an experiment in which male and female subjects interacted with a man or woman who was introduced as either their supervisor or their subordinate and who was purportedly either higher or lower in ability than themselves. Before the subjects interacted with the confederate on the task that was supposed to be the subject of the study, he or she "accidently" knocked a container of pencils to the ground. Helping was unobtrusively measured by the extent to which the subjects assisted in picking them up.

They found that status, but not ability, influenced the frequency with which women were helped, whereas ability, not status, primarily influenced the degree to which men were helped. Men and women helped high- and low-ability female partners equally as often, but they helped high-ability male partners much more than low-ability males. In contrast, both sexes helped female supervisors less than female subordinates, but did not discriminate between male supervisors and subordinates. Dovidio and Gaertner (1981) had previously found a similar reluctance by white males to help black males who were supposedly supervising them. Relative ability also had no effect on helpfulness toward black males although the high-ability white confederate was helped significantly more than his low-ability counterpart.

We have discussed these studies in great detail because they illustrate a number of common processes that appear to underlie discrimination against individuals in subordinate social categories. First, people of a higher-status group appear to be reluctant to recognize ability differences in individuals with a lower status than their own. Second, discriminatory biases may be aroused when traditional role relationships are threatened and helping behavior may be motivated by a desire to restore the traditional status hierarchy. Third, the potential for discrimination may be greater than social scientists believe because it is frequently masked by the individual's desire to behave in a socially desirable manner. Studies such as these, which use indirect and unobtrusive measures, indicate a level of sexism and racism (Crosby et al., 1980) of which the subjects themselves may not be aware.

Of course, it is possible to find some studies that show more direct discrimination against women. For example, college students of both sexes worked less hard in a card-sorting task when they were informed that the quota had been set by a female as compared to a male engineering student (Sanders & Schmidt, 1980). Several studies (Stead & Zinkhan, 1986; Zinkhan & Stoiadin, 1984) have found that men receive service priority in department stores even when they arrive at the same time as a woman customer. The men were assisted first twice as often as were the women. Women are helped more than men in such situations only when norms of dependency are evoked (Unger, Raymond & Levine, 1974; Weimann, 1985).

Indirect Aggression Against Women

Since there are several chapters in this volume on violence against women, we will limit ourselves only to a brief survey of those laboratory studies that have examined variables that are consistent with the helping studies discussed above. Since strong norms about public violence against women exist, most such studies utilize indirect or covert measures of aggression. White (1983), in her survey of sex and gender issues in aggression research, concludes that male violence against women increases when sex role expectations have been violated—that is, if the female becomes aggressive. For example, male Japanese students retaliated more against a woman who gave them severe rather than mild electric shocks (Ohbuchi & Izutsu, 1984). When the attack was severe, however, they retaliated less against an attractive than an unattractive woman. As we have said before, attractiveness carries with it connotations of femininity and dependency, which may have ameliorated the perception that traditional sex roles had been violated.

There is increasing evidence that men who accept traditional sex roles may be more willing to aggress against women. Thus, Nirenberg and Gaebelein (1979) found that males with traditional attitudes about the sexes were more willing to instigate aggression against females than against males while those with liberal attitudes instigated less aggression and directed it equally against women and men. A recent study by Malamuth (1988) found that traditional attitudes toward women were significantly correlated with the amount of aversive noise given women, but not men. Stereotyping was not, unlike the other measures used, correlated with punishment levels, but was correlated with the level of rewards withheld from women, but not from men. Malamuth suggests that highly stereotypic males may resent a woman who does not know her place but also believe it is inappropriate to aggress against the weaker sex. Hence, they may make greater use of covert aggression. It is important to stress that his study indicates that specific factors contribute to aggression against women and that these factors must be examined within the larger context of sexist relations.

The studies on helping and aggression summarized above indicate that women are particularly likely to be the target of sexist behaviors when they violate norms about women's inferior status. There are a large number of ways in which women can violate such norms. Direct violations include having a position within an organization that confers power over men, behaving aggressively, or telling men what to do. All of these violations involve women's being in positions of authority. As we shall see below, there is reason to believe that it is the subordinate's claim to authority, rather than competence, that may be more potent in evoking discriminatory behavior.

Indirect violations of traditional norms about sex and power may also provoke sexist responses. For example, less attractive women are extended less help and subjected to more aggression. Women are also helped more than men when they evoke norms of dependency. Greater belief in stereotypic sex roles appears to be strongly related to negative responses to women who are out of place.

Intragroup Processes

The Confounding of Maleness and Competence

If social/structural sexism is tied to societal norms, sexist effects should appear most clearly in group contexts. The impact of sex-related variables in groups is extremely complex (see review by Dion, 1985). In addition to all of the variables discussed in terms of individual and dyadic relationships, one must also take into account such factors as the percentage of each sex present in the group, the task in which the group is engaged, whether leaders are elected or emerge, and the position of the group within the more general institutional framework. In this section of the chapter, we will review some of the recent work on groups that seems to relate to some of the issues discussed earlier.

As noted above, experimental manipulations of the relative competence of women and men can change the nonverbal behaviors customarily emitted by the two sexes. Similar manipulations in a mixed-group context also appear to change sex-related patterns of task-related behavior. Wood and Karten (1986) observed students interacting in four-person, mixed-sex groups. When subjects were given only information about each other's name and sex, men were perceived by themselves and by other group members to be higher in competence than women. The men also engaged in a greater amount of active task behavior (giving information and opinions) whereas women exhibited a greater amount of positive social behaviors (agreeing and acting friendly). In groups where status was manipulated by providing false feedback about high intellectual and moral aptitude, high-status members were perceived to be more competent and engaged in more active task and less positive social behaviors than low-status members. In this condition, no sex differences were obtained. These data suggest that when status is not specified, traditional gender differences occur because of the belief that men are more competent than women.

A number of other studies have also shown that men are believed to be more competent in groups than are women (Craig & Sherif, 1986; Izraeli, 1983; Pugh & Wahrman, 1983). The study by Izraeli is particularly compelling because she examined real groups of men and women—those who had been elected to work-ers' committees in their organizations. She examined the effects of the sex composition of the group of which they were a part on men's and women's perceptions about their own effectiveness and that of others in the group. Men held more sex stereotypic and pro-male attitudes than did women regardless of the sex composition of the committee. However, the sex composition of the group did have an effect on women's attitudes. In groups in which they were a small minority, women perceived themselves as less influential than men. They also viewed themselves as having been elected to look after women and to represent them. The proportion of women on sex-skewed committees who had this belief was actually greater than the proportion of men who did.

Pugh and Wahrman (1983) attempted to manipulate perceptions about the relative superiority of men and women in order to reduce men's influence in group decisions involving spatial judgment. When no experimental intervention took place, women deferred to men significantly more often than men deferred to women. Both sexes seemed to agree that men were more competent than women. The only manipulation that changed this traditional pattern was rigging a task so that women would perform better than men. Under these circumstances, women became more influential and men became less, but these purportedly more competent women still did not gain a significant advantage over their male partners. In a study that they were still conducting when they reported on the present one, the researchers noted that when no information was provided, blacks deferred to whites in a manner similar to the way women deferred to men. This finding indicates differences in social influence are mediated by perceptions of relative status rather than beliefs about sex-related competencies.

Sources of Sex-Related Differences in Intragroup Behavior

Manipulation of norms involving sex and status appears to influence traditional sex-related differences quite easily in mixed-sex groups. For example, Snodgrass (1985) found that subordinates were more sensitive than leaders to feelings of other group members. She found no main effect of sex independent of role on interpersonal sensitivity. Porter and her associates (Porter, Geis, Cooper & New-man, 1985) examined the leadership behavior of mixed-sex dyads where both individuals were either sex-typed or androgynous. When dyads were reminded of their gender-role beliefs before discussion, androgynous men and women shared leadership more and sex-typed partners less. In comparable dyads without such reminders, men dominated regardless of androgyny.

Social constraints from outside of the group context can also be important. Sexism in the media may have a particularly strong impact. For example, Swarz and his associates (Swarz, Wagner, Bannert & Mathes, 1987) found that women who were exposed to advertisements that portrayed women in their traditional role as homemakers reported less favorable attitudes toward political participation than did women who were not exposed to such advertisements. Similarly, women who were exposed to traditional commercials de-emphasized achievement in favor of homemaking in images of their future lives in comparison with women who had been exposed to role-reversed commercials (Geis, Brown, Jennings & Porter, 1984).

Group Processes: Sex and the Selection of Leaders

It is clear from the studies cited above that both women and men perceive women as less competent in groups than are men. This difference, in turn, may cause women to engage in fewer task-oriented activities and attempts to influence the group process. These behaviors make women less likely to be perceived as influential members of the groups of which they are a part. It is important to note, however, that even when women and men engage in identical behavior, it is difficult to change traditional sex-related perceptions of relative competence. The most effective manipulations in this regard are changes in ''official'' status within the group so that women are labeled as leaders and men are labeled as subordinates. Demonstrations of actual performance superiority by women are also effective. Even these manipulations, however, may not be acknowledged, and it appears that women must be objectively better in order to be seen as just as good (Pugh & Wahrman, 1983).

Under these conditions, it is not surprising that women are chosen as leaders of groups less often than are men (Dion, 1985). The reluctance to select a woman as leader is particularly strong in the political arena. For example, in a simulated mayoral election in which individuals of different race, sex, and age with equivalent qualifications were each pitted in two-candidate races against a control candidate (a white, middle-aged male), he was able to win four of the five contests (Sigelman & Sigelman, 1982). A younger white male was the only candidate able to beat him.

In another study by the same researchers (Sigelman, Thomas, Sigelman & Ribich, 1986), undergraduates evaluated six challengers to an incumbent in either a mayoral or a county clerk's race. They found that men, but not women, consistently discriminated against women candidates. They also found that physical attractiveness was less consistently an asset for female than for male candidates.

Social surveys about the electability of black and/or female candidates indicate that a marginal political view or social identity does not necessarily predict voting for a member of a socially subordinate group. For example, liberals were more likely than conservatives to vote for a black candidate but not for a woman (Hedlund, Freeman, Hamm & Stein, 1979). Black men were also significantly less likely to vote for a woman candidate than were black women or whites of both sexes (Sigelman & Welch, 1984).

A recent national NORC (National Opinion Research Council) sample indicated that black males are more sex-role traditional than white males (Ransford & Miller, 1983). Forty-nine % of the black men sampled agreed that women's place was in the home compared to 33% of white men. Sixty % versus 44% agreed that women are emotionally unsuited for politics. It is noteworthy that black men were not more traditional than white men on questions about women's working outside the home. In fact, one recent study using the Attitudes toward Women Scale found that white men were the most conservative group and black women were the most liberal in their attitudes about equality of the sexes (Brenner & Tomkiewicz, 1986). However, black men appear to be particularly negative about women's taking political positions in the community.

The Impact of the Group Context: Tokenism

Much of the research on sex differences in groups is derived from expectation states theory (Berger, Cohen & Zelditch, 1972). This theory argues that in the absence of some kind of intervention, group members will develop expectations about the potential value of each other's contributions by generalizing from the value placed on certain external characteristics of individuals. If those characteristics are disvalued in a society, group members will be likely to assume that the task contributions of a person possessing them will not be valuable either. These expectations, in turn, lead the group's members both to offer opportunities to participate and to appreciate the contributions of those who have valued characteristics and to withhold both opportunities for participation and appreciation from those with socially devalued characteristics. Diffuse status characteristics such as sex and race theoretically have properties that make them especially likely to be used in organizing task behavior.

The effect of diffuse status characteristics is particularly strong when individuals who are socially devalued are in a numerical minority within their group. The limiting condition of this phenomenon is, of course, when only one member of the devalued group is present. This is the phenomenon that has been christened "tokenism."

Kanter (1977) has argued that when the proportion of women within a group is small, they are more visible and isolated from the men who, because of their numerical dominance, determine the culture of the group. Laboratory studies have demonstrated that lone females have less ability to influence group decision making than do males who have identical credentials and behaviors (Wahrman & Pugh, 1974). Women members of otherwise all-male groups may be ignored or socially isolated. In one study (Wolman & Frank, 1975), the behavior of men toward solo women in formerly all-male peer groups was so hostile and negative that it drove most of them from the groups.

Tokens are either evaluated unfairly or evaluated on the basis of their normative reactions to differential treatment by majority group members. An interesting experiment by Lord and Saenz (1985) indicates that tokenism can be induced in anyone, regardless of social status. College students were led to believe they were sharing their views on everyday topics with three other students (actually videotaped confederates) who were all either the student's own sex or all of the opposite sex. In a later memory task, token participants remembered fewer of the opinions expressed in the group than did nontokens. This study suggests that the phenomenon of tokenism induces cognitive deficits in people even when they are not treated differently as a result of being a token. Preoccupation with distinctiveness may distract attention from the substance of the ongoing group interaction even if the other members of the group do nothing but merely be present. These effects may be due to implicit status labels since the use of videotapes ruled out differential treatment of the token.

The consequences of tokenism are not simply due to the numerical dominance of one group. Token status appears to intensify stereotypic beliefs so that male tokens are seen as more masculine and/or powerful than when they are present in larger numbers (Kanter, 1977). Male tokens in primarily female groups are not socially isolated. For example, male nurses (41 of 322 nursing students) were not disadvantaged in terms of acquiring information about how to get around formal rules, strategies for impressing superiors, and personal information that could affect their performance (Fairhurst & Snavely, 1983). Crocker and McGraw (1984) conducted an experiment that varied the sex composition of task-oriented groups and found that the consequences of having solo status were markedly different for solo males and females. Solo females were unlikely to be selected as group leaders; overall group satisfaction was lowest when a solo female was present; and gender-related issues were most likely to be raised in groups that included a solo female. Solo males, on the other hand, tended to be integrated into their groups as leaders, resulting in smoother group functioning.

Men were seen by others in the group as more masculine when they had solo status whereas women were perceived to be least feminine when they had solo status. Such sex stereotypical expectancies could account for why solo males were likely to be chosen as group leaders. There was no room in these groups, however, for a solo with low status. For example, there were no subservient roles, such as that of secretary, available.

These studies demonstrate that tokenism is not simply a result of numerical dominance. Numerical dominance is situationally dependent (based, e.g., on who might form a committee). Tokenism, however, exerts its effects through cultural dominance, which is a constant. Those who dominate a field of action over time come to determine the rules of interaction for strangers who chance to penetrate the boundaries. Neither their culture nor their power is neutralized by numerical reshuffling (Izraeli, 1983).

INSTITUTIONALIZED SEXISM

The studies reviewed above involve processes that are the product of individual behavior. Although they reflect and, in turn, influence the formal structures that regulate our lives, examination of attitudes and behaviors alone does not make clear the extent to which sexism permeates our society. To understand sexism, we must also look at occupational segregation and the forces that maintain it. A number of recent analyses indicate that occupational segregation is a key factor in the differential relationship among education, experience, and income for men and women. Gender inequality in paid employment cannot be explained simply in terms of the relationships between individual women and men.

Some Data on Gender Inequality in Paid Employment

According to U.S. Department of Labor figures, between 1950 and 1985, the proportion of American women in the labor force rose dramatically from 34% to 55% (England & McCreary, 1987). By 1985, 53% of married women with children under 6 years of age were in the labor force. Nevertheless, women in the labor force outside the home are employed primarily in traditional women's occupations. The segregation of job categories by sex represents an institution-alized pattern of discrimination. Sex segregation exists both across occupations (most occupations are sex-typed) and within organizations. The work force within most companies is structured so that the managers are almost entirely male, the clerical staff is almost entirely female, the technical staff is mixed (although better-paying jobs are dominated by men), and the janitorial staff is comprised of minorities, many of them minority women (see Benokraitis & Feagin, 1986, for a more extensive discussion of occupational segregation).

Benokraitis and Feagin argue that sex segregation is not part of the "natural order of things." Job categories have been intentionally segregated. For example, as late as 1920 the majority of clerical work was done by men; as recently as 1950 about 40% of clerical employees were male (Glenn & Feldberg, 1984). One result of this trend was a decline in wages paid to (women) clerical employees. Today men work in far more types of occupations than women, who are heavily concentrated in just 30 of the 400 to 500 major job categories in the United States.

An Examination of Explanations for Gender Inequality in Paid Employment

In addition to documenting sex segregation in occupations, a number of researchers have explored various explanations that have been put forth to explain this gender gap. The kinds of explanations examined include psychological, sociological, and economic factors. We shall review briefly some of these theories and their critiques.

At the psychological level, sex differences in occupations have been explained as a result of the differential socialization of girls and boys and its effect upon occupational choice. However, knowledge about sex discrimination may also affect occupational preferences since there is little point in preparing for a job if one does not expect to be hired for it (England & McCreary, 1987). Studies demonstrating changes in girls' and boys' occupational interests when information about the sex ratios of people in particular occupations was manipulated have been discussed earlier (Heilman, 1979). Other studies showed that fewer girls expected to work in male jobs than those who aspired to such nontraditional jobs (Marini & Brinton, 1984) and that 34% of girls in a large-scale survey thought sex would be a barrier to getting jobs (Bachman, Johnson & O'Malley, 1980). The correlation between the sex composition of young women's occupational preferences and their later jobs has been found to be quite low—about .25 (Jacobs, 1987). If early socialization explained most job segregation, one would expect a higher correlation than this.

Sex differences in years of work experience have also been used to explain occupational segregation. However, women with continuous work experience are not more likely than other women to be employed in predominantly male jobs (England & McCreary, 1987). Neither women's ages nor their number of children (which might correlate with work experience) is related to the percentage of women within particular occupations. Extensive sex segregation exists in entry-level positions, where neither men nor women have any experience.

Occupations in which women predominate offer considerably lower salaries than those in which men predominate (Benokraitis & Feagin, 1986). Differential work experience, on-the-job training, and the number of years an employee remains at a particular job can explain the gap only if these factors have substantial effects on earnings (Corcoran & Duncan, 1979). If, for example, workers who lost time from work to take care of family members are paid the same as workers who miss no work, then the fact that women, on average, tend to miss somewhat more work for this reason does not explain why they earn less than men. This is the case—job continuity has little effect on wages.

In another test of explanations for the earnings gap, Treiman and Roos (1983) looked at nine different industrial nations to see if evidence supported one of the following explanations: a human capital hypothesis—women earn less because they have less education and experience; a dual career hypothesis—women earn less because they adjust their work behavior to meet the demands of family obligations; and an occupational segregation hypothesis—women earn less because of their concentration in low-level jobs. None of these hypotheses received much support in any country, leaving open the possibility that the earnings differences are due to deeply entrenched institutional arrangements that limit women's opportunities and achievements.

In every country investigated, the researchers found a characteristic pattern of men's and women's work. They also found that, on the average, women working full-time earned less than two-thirds of what their male coworkers earned. For the men in all countries, education had a positive effect on income. For women, this relationship was less consistent. In five countries the correlation was not significantly different from zero. Although not marrying had significant costs for men in most of the countries investigated (on the average, married men earned 20% more than single men), married women who worked full-time did not earn less than single women. These data argue that having a dual career has no effect on the earnings of married women who work full-time. Finally, differences in the distribution of women and men over major occupational groups had virtually no effect on income. Sex differences in income were, on average, just as large within each of the major occupational groups as they were for the labor force as a whole.

Using still a different method of analysis, Bielby and Baron (1986) looked at occupational roles in a diverse sample of California companies. They found only 8% of the workers in their sample shared job titles, and in those few instances in which men and women performed similar work roles, the jobs were typically done in distinct organizational settings. When a company employed both sexes in the same occupation, the women and men were typically assigned different job titles. Their findings are consistent with a theory of statistical discrimination; for example, employers reserve some jobs for men and some for women. There is little evidence that this reflects efficient and rational responses to sex-related differences in skills or in turnover costs.

It has been argued that women choose female sex-typed occupations because they offer maximal lifetime earnings for those who are intermittently employed. When education and experience are controlled, however, women have higher lifetime earnings if they work in predominantly male occupations (England, 1984). In fact, both men and women who work in predominantly female occupations are discriminated against in terms of salary (England, Farkas, Kilbourne & Dou, 1988; Izraeli & Gaier, 1979). One intriguing study (Pfeffer & Davis-Blake, 1987) looked at the effect of the proportion of women administrators on the salaries of both men and women in administrative positions in colleges and universities. They found an inverse relationship between the proportion of women and the salaries of both sexes. These findings are particularly impressive because they looked at variation in the proportion of women in a similar set of positions across similar institutions. The negative effects were found not only for positions customarily held by women, but also for other positions held by men and women in the administrative hierarchy.

Segregation of occupations by race appears to follow a pattern similar to that found in sex segregation. Years of formal education explain only about one-third of the wage gap between white and black men and only 11% of the wage gap between black and white women (England & McCreary, 1987). At present, minority women appear to be more affected by sex discrimination than by race discrimination. In fact, Almquist (1987) has noted that labor market gender inequality is greatest among smaller, more affluent minorities, many of whom are recent immigrants. Her findings point out that achievement relative to the majority group is quite different than gender inequality within a group. Black women contribute more income and share more family power with their spouses than do white women from families with a comparable income (Richardson, 1982). The level of gender inequality within any group reflects both the amount of resources available and the way in which these resources are distributed between men and women within the group.

There is evidence that minority women with the same education and vocational training are tracked into less well-paying, racially homogeneous jobs (Hillsman & Levenson, 1975; Treas, 1978). For example, Deaux (1984) found that white women were far less likely to be janitors compared with their proportion among steelworkers (although women were overrepresented as compared with men) and Hispanic women were far more likely to be employed in this job category. Janitorial and nonjanitorial groups did not differ in education and seniority.

Salary appears to be a function of the percentage of women in a job category. One study found that each 1% of women in an occupation had a net depressing effect on the annual earnings of workers in that occupation of $30 for men and $17 for women (England, Chassie & McCormack, 1982). This means that the difference between the median annual earnings in two occupations comparable on their skill demands, but differing in that one is 100% male and one is 100% female, is $1,682 for women and $3,005 for men. This is the sort of wage discrimination that is at issue in "comparable worth." It is a form of wage discrimination different from lack of equal pay for equal work.

Do Nonmonetary Job Rewards Compensate for the Gender Gap in Salaries?

It has been argued that women select female sex-typed occupations because they offer nonmonetary rewards that compensate for lower wages. Some of the suggested forms of compensation are less effort and commitment required, convenient work hours, and congenial work conditions and coworkers. There is no evidence, however, that women allocate less effort to work because of their family and household responsibilities. On average, women reported allocating more effort to work than did men, even though they also reported spending twice as much time as men on household chores (Bielby & Bielby, 1988). As women added work roles to their family roles, they generated the energy necessary to fulfill their commitments to both sets of activities. The effort expended was only slightly related to compensation.

Contrary to a theory of alternative compensations, women in blue- and white-collar jobs attributed more importance to pay and work conditions than to congenial coworkers (O'Farrell & Harlan, 1982). However, a sizable minority of women in blue-collar jobs reported less satisfaction with work because of harassment from male coworkers. Gutek and Cohen (1987) have coined the phrase "sex-role spillover" for the carryover of gender-based roles into the work setting. Behavior associated with gender become incorporated into work roles. In male-dominated jobs, activity, rationality, and aggressiveness are emphasized, whereas nurturance and passivity are associated with "women's work." This process is exacerbated by having a highly skewed ratio of the sexes in the work environment. Some studies have indicated more reports of harassment from women employed in nontraditional occupations where there are few other women present than from women employed in more sex-segregated settings.

These findings suggest that occupational segregation has important psychological as well as economic consequences. Women who work in integrated or nontraditional jobs face the problem of being visible role deviants. As we shall see in our discussion of cultural sexism, one response to role deviance is to call attention to the social category of the "deviant." For women, one aspect of such categorization is to be seen as sex objects (Yoder & Adams, 1984). Because of their visibility, tokens also experience performance pressures and serious problems with self-esteem (Yoder, 1985). However, token women in nontraditional occupations also earn more than women in traditional occupations. Thus, being a token is not completely negative since women may derive self-esteem from their higher salary and identification with male power and status. The mixed effects of tokenism may account for some of the discrepancies in studies in this area.

Although tokenism may be explored in terms of social sexism, it is also a consequence of institutional sexism—the normative sex-segregated structure of the occupational world. Tokenism can affect anyone, but not everyone is equally likely to become a token. It is this aspect of sex-related reality that cultural sexism explores.

CULTURAL SEXISM

The previous sections of this chapter document the existence of sexism at individual, social, and institutional levels of analysis. The studies discussed above also indicate that a complete analysis of sexism cannot be obtained from consideration of data from only one of these levels. For example, it has been argued that individual biases against women are a form of faulty information processing. However, it may be impossible to eliminate information about gender from our cognitive processes. Gender "sneaks into" evaluations by way of assumptions about attractiveness, personality traits, social roles, and job appropriateness. Information that is inconsistent with gender norms is readily ignored or rationalized as exceptional. Moreover, gender biases may be validated by women's own behaviors within group contexts or by their relative absence from certain jobs or positions of authority within the world of employment. Such confirmation is the consequence of gender-biased social and institutional practices in addition to individual biases.

In turn, it is the absence of women from most task-oriented groups and influential positions that makes them vulnerable to social processes that justify their continued exclusion. As noted earlier, although the psychological processes that create tokens may affect anyone, everyone does not have an equal probability of becoming a token. A focus upon an individual level of analysis ignores the impact that cultural constructions have on the way individuals from different social categories behave.

Cultural sexism may be examined as both a system for the regulation of society and the processes that regulate the behaviors of individual members of a society. In the interest of symmetry, we shall begin this section with a brief consideration of sexism as a form of social control and end it with some descriptions of specific mechanisms by which control is exerted. Such an organization will, in a sense, get us back to where we have begun—inside the heads of some people. This time, however, the people will be the victims of sexism instead of its perpetrators.

Labeling Women Deviant

Most of the studies discussed above indicate that women are a social category. They are not simply different from men, but are socially subordinate to them. It is women's lower social status and power that are key features in any cultural analysis of sexism.

Becker wrote the classic book on cultural mechanisms of social control in 1963. He argued that "social groups create deviance by making the rules whose infraction constitutes deviance, and by applying these rules to particular people and labeling them as outsiders" (p. 9). He also argued that labeling is largely a matter of some persons' or groups' imposing their rules on others. Ultimately, who is defined as deviant and for what is a question of political and economic power. Power and intergroup conflict are key determinants of deviance outcomes. Definitions of deviance operate to impose control. Those who define deviance benefit through the labeling of others as deviant.

More recently, Schur (1983) has argued that gender is a norm system in which women are labeled deviant. Individual women and their acts acquire their "deviantness" through a characteristic pattern of meaning-attachment. How people perceive and react to a given behavior or condition is what counts most socially. This is because the very same behavior or condition may be defined and responded to differently by different persons. For example, an unmarried woman who has an active and varied sex life may be labeled either "promiscuous" or "liberated" depending upon the value system of the person doing the labeling.

What is important about Schur's analysis is that he provides a framework for examining the entire social category of "woman" as a status which, in itself, carries with it a certain degree of stigma. Women's vulnerability to stigmatization rests on their general social subordination and their relatively poor power position vis-à-vis men. At the same time, when women are effectively stigmatized, their relative subordination is reinforced. Schur describes four grounds for accepting womanhood as a devalued status. Examples of each have been described extensively both in this chapter and in this book as a whole. They are:

1. The well-documented existence of sex inequality within our social and economic system. Devalued persons, i.e., women, are systemically relegated to the lower echelons of the socioeconomic and economic prestige ladder. Occupancy of such positions, in turn, tends to be a basis for evaluating people unfavorably.

2. Widespread evidence of categorization and objectification tendencies.

3. Pervasive devaluation of women in cultural symbolism, for example, the mass media, language, and pornography.

4. Both the multitude of specific "deviances" imputed to women and the failure strongly to condemn male offenses against them illustrate the low cultural value placed on femaleness.

It is the perception of threat, regardless of whether or not the perception is well founded, that triggers efforts at systematic devaluation. The evidence discussed above indicates that women are most likely to be devalued when they are in economic competition with men or when men fear that they may lose control of economic and political institutions.

Deviance and the Construction of Double Binds

Women typically face a myriad of double binds or no-win situations with respect to gender norms. Double binds represent a form of contradiction for individuals. They are situations that are so structured that a woman within them must incur some social penalty regardless of her behavior. This kind of social paradox is not the result of accidental circumstances, but is due to the way social roles for women in our society are constructed and behaviorally maintained (Unger, 1988).

Double binds exist because so many contradictory definitions about women exist that one can be evoked to match almost any possible behavior. For example, it is difficult to find a behavior that does not fit some feature of "mother," "sex object," "pet," or "iron maiden," which have been described by some theorists as the four archetypal roles for women in Western society (Kanter, 1977; Wood & Conrad, 1983). Behavior conforming to any of these prototypes may be rewarded, while at the same time, behavior inconsistent with another prototype may be ignored or punished. These roles are particularly problematic for the target individual because she has not constructed them herself, nor can she be sure what definition is being used by other participants in the situation.

Double binds are most apt to occur within social contexts in which sexism is also most easily documented (Unger, 1988). For example, double binds occur when the woman is "out of place," when she is perceived as a threat either because of her position or behavior, and when she is one of the few members of her social category present (a token). Double binds are created through the power of dominant members of a culture to define its reality and because subordinate members tend to accept dominant definitions.

One of the subtlest forms of definitional binds for women is the use of "exceptionalist" labels. For example, a focus upon "superwomen" is not only just an assertion that most women cannot do such things, but is also an assertion that "typical," "normal," and "natural" women do not, cannot, and should not do them (Schur, 1983). The success of a few exceptional women supports the status quo by providing examples that encourage others to look inward for the sources of their own "failure" (Yoder, 1985).

Tokenism as a Form of Double Bind

Tokenism is a subtle form of the double bind. As we have seen above, the situation is devised, whether intentionally or inadvertently, to assure the failure of the token. However, her lack of success is seen as personal or as a function of her social category and can be used to jeopardize whatever standards of affirmative action currently exist. The social isolation of the token—a situation in which deviance definitions are most potent—encourages her to seek personal, rather than structural, change.

Tokenism produces a variety of negative effects. Several reports indicate widespread feelings of loneliness and isolation among employed women and women in leadership positions (Apfelbaum, 1986; Bhatnagar, 1988). Tokenism may also result in a loss of self-esteem (Yoder, 1985). This may be partly a consequence of perceptions by others (discussed above) that those who received their position because of affirmative action are less deserving. But it may also be due to performance pressures due to visibility within a group of socially dominant individuals. For example, Alexander and Thoits (1985) examined achievement as measured by grade point average of men and women in departments that were either heavily skewed or only slightly tilted toward one sex or the other. They found that tokenism decreased the achievement of women, but had no effect on the achievement of men.

While tokenism has disadvantages for the token, it provides a number of institutional and cultural advantages for members of the dominant group. For example, as long ago as 1975, Laws argued that "tokenism is the means by which the dominant group advertises a promise of mobility so long as tokens do not change the system they enter" (pp. 51–52). Tokenism may also inhibit female bonding because a token woman may not wish to emphasize her own gender deviance by associating with others in a devalued category.

The Definition of Deviance as a Cultural Construction

If sexism is culturally as well as individually based, few differences between individuals in prejudice and discrimination against women should be found. Cultural sexism would help to explain the puzzling finding that gender stereotypes are not well correlated to other measures of personality and attitudes (Goldberg, 1974; Spence & Helmreich, 1978). It would also help explain consistent findings that women and men do not differ significantly in their evaluations of target individuals who differ in sex (Wallston & O'Leary, 1981). There should be few individual differences in normative beliefs about gender.

Individual difference studies may show, in fact, that those who are more in tune with social norms are more prejudiced. One recent study has found, for example, that high self-monitors were more likely to use information about personal appearance in evaluating job applicants than were low self-monitors (Snyder, Berscheid & Matwychuk, 1988). High-authoritarian personnel managers of both sexes have also been found to favor males more than females (Simas & McCarrey, 1979).

The Cultural Value of Sexism

Social distinctions provide justification for a nonegalitarian status quo. Such distinctions have bidirectional causality (Konrad & Gutek, 1987). By altering the contingencies for the reward and punishment of members of social groups, they increase group differences in social behavior. Once such behavioral distinctions are created, observers can look to them for reasons they treat members of different social groups differently. Thus, we justify paying men more than women because men are performing different jobs, men are in more important jobs, or men are more competitive and aggressive. The extensive literature on gender differences can be used as a justification for maintaining gender as an important social distinction. The role of individual, social, and institutional practices in creating these distinctions are ignored or defined as transitory whereas the differences themselves are defined as universal and permanent.

THE PHENOMENOLOGICAL CONSEQUENCES OF SEXISM

One of the paradoxes in the study of sexism is the extent to which women deny its relevance to themselves. For example, in a large-scale survey of 400 adults in a Boston suburb, Crosby (1982) found no significant differences between employed women and men in measures of job-related grievances, satisfaction, or deservedness. This subjective equality existed despite the fact that employed women made significantly less money than employed men at equivalent job levels. The women felt no sense of personal discrimination, even though they were keenly aware of sex discrimination in general.

Lack of awareness of personal discrimination is partly due to lack of information with which to make group comparisons (Crosby, 1984). It is also partly due to a tendency for people to make judgments about themselves differently than they make about others (Unger & Sussman, 1986). Such cognitive biases are likely to be found in both sexes.

Other important responses, however, are more a function of the isolated social position and lower status of women. For example, academic women in departments that were male-dominated were less likely to perceive sex discrimination and more accepting of the concept of meritocracy than were women in departments that were not male-dominated (Reid, 1987). Very powerful women leaders indicated a lack of a sense of entitlement as distinct from a lack of competence, which was never in question in their minds (Apfelbaum, 1986). They reported a sense of being a token because someone of their sex was needed by those in power. They questioned the legitimacy of their own authority.

This sense of undeservedness may reflect women's awareness of their categorical membership. In an intriguing study in which Heilman and her associates (Heilman, Simon & Repper, 1987) distributed rewards based either on performance or on gender, men and women serving as task leaders differed in their response to the method of selection. Only women's self-perceptions and self-evaluations were negatively affected by selection based on sex in comparison with selection based on merit. When selected on the basis of sex, women devalued their leadership performance, took less credit for successful outcomes, and reported less interest in persisting as leader of their group. They also characterized themselves as more deficient in general leadership skills. Categorical reward had no effect on men's view of themselves or their worth (perhaps because it is a meaningless distinction for them since they are the normative category). This study has obvious implications in terms of affirmative action programs in which members of subordinate groups are "told" that they have received their positions because of their sexual or racial category.

Other studies also suggest that women's devaluation of their own worth is a response to sexual categorization. Thus, Chacko (1982) found that women who attributed their selection as managers mainly to being women were dissatisfied with their work in general and experienced a great deal of work-related role conflict. She coined the phrase *procedural stigma* to describe how being selected by way of procedures perceived as unfair leaves the person selected feeling stigmatized. These women's perceptions appear to reflect similar perceptions in others. Female undergraduates who read a story in which a protagonist received a research award expected poorer subsequent evaluations when they believed that selection criteria had included preferential treatment because of sex (Nacoste & Lehman, 1987).

Feelings of lack of entitlement extend to monetary rewards as well as acceptance of personal power. Studies have consistently found that women pay themselves less than men do when allocating rewards between themselves and others (see review by Major & Deaux, 1982). This difference appears to be due to women's feelings of lesser personal entitlement with respect to monetary payment for work performed. In the absence of social comparison information and in a private work environment, women perceived less money as fair pay for their work and paid themselves less money than men did, despite similar perceived work inputs (Major, McFarlin & Gagnon, 1984). They worked longer, did more work, did more correct work, and were more efficient than men for the same amount of pay.

This study suggests why employers may have a stake in a sex-segregated work force. It is only when external bases of social comparison are unavailable that individuals rely on internal, same-sex norms (Berger, Rosenholtz & Zelditch, 1980). As long as women lack information about the reward structure for men, they will be willing to work for less pay.

A recent study by Moore (1987) suggests that the nature of women's and men's comparison groups has an effect upon the extent of relative deprivation that they perceive. She found no significant differences between women and men nor between occupational groups in the amount of individual relative deprivation perceived. However, women in masculine occupations reported lower levels of deprivation despite the fact that they actually earned less than men in these occupations. This seeming paradox may be due to the use of other women (primarily in lower-paid feminine occupations) as a comparison group. Nontraditional women appear to feel they have no reason to complain because, on the average, they earn more than those with whom they compare their state. Like all other women, these non-traditional women also undervalue their inputs and see themselves as meriting less than comparable men.

Women's willingness to give themselves lower pay for identical work done by men is consistent with a model of cultural sexism. Women appear to be responding to cultural norms about the relative worth of women and men. Gender differences in personal entitlement do not appear to be related to differences in personal history. For example, Major et al. (1984) found no relationship between past pay history and either self-pay or time worked. In another recent study in which 87 male and female certified management accountants were matched, women had lower salaries, fewer career experiences, and lower expectations than men, but still rated themselves as successful as men (Keys, 1985) In addition, Crosby (1982) found no support for the hypothesis that men value money more than women do.

SEXISM AND RACISM COMBINED

Ironically, the experience of being a token does not necessarily have an undermining effect for some black professional women, but, rather, served as a motivating factor for them (Epstein, 1973). "Being a black woman. . . . It's made me fight harder. . . . If I had been white with the same abilities, I'm not sure the drive would have been the same" (p. 169). The preceding quotation was a typical comment among black women interviewed. Furthermore, these black professional women indicated that they deserved whatever benefits they gained as a result of being used on the basis of sex and race. Epstein encountered less self-hatred among the black professional women she interviewed than among comparable white professional women. In addition, black professional women had a higher regard for each other than did white professional women.

Research on the combined effects of sexism and racism has, however, yielded inconsistent results. For example, in a study of college graduates, 74% of the black women versus only 49% of the white women interviewed thought that they had personalities conducive to careers as business executives (Fichter, 1964). These black women were, however, graduates of predominantly black colleges and so may have benefited from an absence of tokenism during their formative years. In contrast, Leggon's (1980) interviews of black professional women revealed that the combined status of race and sex worked to their disadvantage. The black women in this study attributed their lack of advancement in their careers to racial discrimination rather than sexual discrimination.

Awareness of the sexist and racist biases of others appears to ameliorate their negative effects. Dion (1975) performed an experiment in which female subjects believed they were competing against several unseen opponents (who were either male or female) and that they had failed either mildly or severely in this competition. His hypothesis that women's self-esteem may be more vulnerable to interpersonal rejection and discrimination by males than by females was confirmed, especially when severe failure was experienced. However, women who attributed their severe failure at the hands of their putative male opponents to prejudice had stronger self-esteem and more positive feminine identification than women who did not attribute their failure to men's sexist bias. Dion has reported similar effects with Oriental and French-Canadian minorities (Dion, Earn & Yee, 1978).

In sum, the studies reported above suggest that women share cultural assumptions about the lesser worth of women to an astonishing extent. These assumptions are conveyed to women by negative attitudes and behaviors directed toward them in everyday life situations. However, overtly negative responses may not be necessary to communicate social stigma. In daily interaction, women are often perceived and responded to in terms of their categorical membership— as females, first and foremost. Such responses may themselves carry a certain degree of stigma, since, relatively speaking, femaleness is a devalued status. "Other things being equal, the greater the consistency, duration, and intensity with which a definition is promoted by others about an actor, the greater the likelihood the actor will embrace that definition as truly applicable to himself" (Lofland, 1969, p. 122). Systematic devaluation implies a strong likelihood of impaired self-esteem.

SUMMING UP

Sexism exists at a variety of levels, which interact with each other. All are worth examining, but some factors may be more important than others and more resistant to change. The following areas appear to be particularly important in terms of the relationship between various levels of analysis.

At the individual level, a key issue appears to be the confounding of dominance, masculinity, competence, and attractiveness for men. A woman is unlikely to be rewarded for the former three qualities, and their possession may penalize her by stigmatizing her as unfeminine and/or unattractive. Recent studies seem to suggest that dominance may be a more potent predictor of negative views about women than competence.

On a social level, a key issue appears to be women in authority. Women have particular difficulty in influencing groups and in being elected to leadership positions. Women in authority are helped less than those in a clearly subordinate position. The critical issue is not so much that a woman appears to be competent in a masculine domain, but that she outperforms a man. When a woman has authority over men of the same age and social class, she is seen to reduce their status rather than enhancing her own.

At an institutional level, a key issue continues to be the sex segregation of occupations. Occupational distinctions extend beyond simple work roles. Occupational segregation limits interpersonal contact between the sexes and reduces the opportunity for men to receive disconfirming information about the characteristics of women. At the same time, occupational segregation makes it less likely that women will receive social comparison information that will lead them to demand equal compensation for equal work.

Tokenism appears to be the extreme example of occupational segregation in which any women at all may be found. Thus, it is an important phenomenon to examine in terms of the impact of unbalanced sex ratios. Tokenism has a number of effects at various levels of analysis. It affects the performance of tokens as well as perceptions of that performance. It leads to enhancement of the peer values of majority group members, but only if that majority consists of members of the dominant group. Although the psychological processes underlying tokenism appear to be universal, the sociological variables—especially status differentials—are not. Therefore, tokenism is an asymmetrical phenomenon that illustrates the limits of looking at sexism at only one level of analysis.

At a cultural level, a key issue is the way assumptions shared by members of the same culture function to create differences between women and men. Psychologists, in particular, appear to be reluctant to accept the idea that gender is a system for creating social distinctions. In one of his last papers, Tajfel (1984) pointed out that it is not the difference that matters in our status-dominated societies, but the distinction. Distinction is the active social process that creates, expresses, and maintains differences. The power and status of dominant groups confer upon them the power to originate and diffuse powerful social myths. These myths affect the extent to which individuals as members of social groups are able to achieve recognition of their individuality.

The power to define is exemplified by the creation of double binds for women in our society. Double binds require acceptance both of conflicting definitions and of the belief that no conflict exists. They illustrate the power of social myths to protect the individual (dominant and dominated) from cognitive conflict. People are even protected from the need to admit that their beliefs are not as rationally coherent as they should be. Social myths may explain why individuals appear to be unaware of their own personal victimization.

The fact that some forms of discrimination can be manipulated within the laboratory to produce effects on anyone who is a target does not change the fact that, in reality, women are the normative targets of sexism. The fact that forms of sexism exist within our heads does not change the fact that sexism reflects real world distinctions. The fact that individuating information can sometimes reduce the effects of sexism does not change the fact that any information can be defined as gender-related under some conditions. The fact that demonstration of behavioral equality can sometimes alter biased perceptions does not change the fact that opportunities for such disconfirmation are limited by segregation of the sexes within the occupational world.

In other words, psychological analysis of prejudice and discrimination is not sufficient to explain sexism. We must look at social, institutional, and cultural factors as well as individual processes. Ironically, by way of cultural processes, sexism comes full circle and must be analyzed within all of our heads—male and female, white and black, members of dominant and subordinate groups. However, sexism cannot be changed merely within our heads because it is an accurate reflection of a nonegalitarian reality.

REFERENCES

Abramson, P. R., Goldberg, P. A., Greenberg, J. H., & Abramson, L. M. (1978). The talking platypus phenomenon: Competency ratings as a function of sex and professional status. *Psychology of Women Quarterly, 2,* 114–124.

Alexander, V. D., & Thoits, P. A. (1985). Token achievement: An examination of proportional representation and performance outcomes. *Social Forces, 64,* 332–340.

Allport, G. W. (1954). *The nature of prejudice.* Reading, MA: Addison-Wesley.

Almquist, E. M. (1987). Labor market gender inequality in minority groups. *Gender & Society, 1* 400–414.

Apfelbaum, E. (1986). *Women in leadership positions.* The Henri Tajfel Memorial Lecture presented at the meeting of the British Psychological Association, University of Sussex.

Bachman, J. G., Johnson, L. D., & O'Malley, P. M. (1980). *Monitoring the future: Questionnaire responses from the nation's high school seniors.* Ann Arbor: Institute for Social Research, University of Michigan.

Barnett, M. A., & King, L. M. (1985). Undergraduates' punish-help judgments: The effect of transgressor's and victim's sex. *Sex Roles, 12,* 579–586.

Baron, R. A. (1986). Self-presentation in job interviews: When there can be "too much of a good thing." *Journal of Applied Social Psychology, 16,* 16–28.

Becker, H. S. (1963). *Outsiders.* New York: Free Press.

Bem, S. L., & Bem, D. J. (1973). Does sex-biased job advertising "aid and abet" sex discrimination? *Journal of Applied Social Psychology, 3,* 6–18.

Benokraitis, N. V., & Feagin, J. R. (1986). *Modern sexism: Blatant, subtle, and covert discrimination.* Englewood Cliffs, NJ: Prentice-Hall.

Berger, J., Cohen, B. P., & Zelditch, M. (1972). Status conceptions and social interactions. *American Sociological Review, 37,* 241–255.

Berger, J., Rosenholtz, S. J., & Zelditch, M. (1980). Status organizing processes. *Annual Review of Sociology, 6,* 479–508.

Bhatnagar, D. (1988). Professional women in organizations: New paradigms for research and action. *Sex Roles, 18,* 343–355.

Bielby, D. D., & Bielby, W. T. (1988). She works hard for the money: Household responsibility and the allocation of work effort. *American Journal of Sociology, 93,* 1031–1059.

Bielby, W. T., & Baron, J. N. (1986). Men and women at work: Sex segregation and statistical discrimination. *American Journal of Sociology, 91*, 759–799.

Brenner, O. C., & Tomkiewicz, J. (1986). Race differences in attitudes of American business school graduates toward the role of women. *Journal of Social Psychology, 126*, 251–253.

Brooks, V. R. (1982). Sex differences in student dominance in female and male professors' classrooms. *Sex Roles, 8*, 683–690.

Brown, A., Goodwin, B. J., Hall, B. A., & Jackson-Lowman, H. (1985). A review of psychology of women textbooks: Focus on the Afro-American woman. *Psychology of Women Quarterly, 9*, 29–38.

Buttner, E. H., & Rosen, B. (1987). The effects of labor shortages on starting salaries for sex-typed jobs. *Sex Roles, 17*, 59–71.

Cash, T. F., & Trimer, C. A. (1984). Sexism and beautyism in women's evaluation of peer performance. *Sex Roles, 10*, 87–98.

Chacko, T. I. (1982). Women and equal employment opportunity: Some unintended effects. *Journal of Applied Psychology, 67*, 119–123.

Clayton, O., Jr., Baird, A. C., & Levinson, R. M. (1984). Subjective decision making in medical school admissions: Potentials for discrimination. *Sex Roles, 10*, 527–532.

Corcoran, M., & Duncan, G. J. (1979). Work history, labor force attachment, and earnings differences between the races and the sexes. *Journal of Human Resources, 14*, 3–20.

Craig, J. M., & Sherif, C. W. (1986). The effectiveness of men and women in problem-solving groups as a function of group gender composition. *Sex Roles, 14*, 453–466.

Crocker, J., & McGraw, K. M. (1984). What's good for the goose is not good for the gander: Solo status as an obstacle to occupational achievement for males and females. *American Behavioral Scientist, 27*, 357–369.

Crosby, F. (1982). *Relative deprivation and working women.* New York: Oxford University Press.

Crosby, F. (1984). The denial of personal discrimination. *American Behavioral Scientist, 27*, 371–386.

Crosby, F., Bromley, S., & Saxe, L. (1980). Recent unobtrusive studies of black and white discrimination and prejudice: A literature review. *Psychological Bulletin, 87*, 546–563.

Deaux, K. (1984). Blue-collar barriers. *American Behavioral Scientist, 27*, 287–300.

Deaux, K., & Emswiller, T. (1974). Explanations of successful performance on sex-linked tasks: What's skill for the male is luck for the female. *Journal of Personality and Social Psychology, 29*, 80–85.

Deaux, K., Winton, W., Crowley, M., & Lewis, L. L. (1985). Level of categorization and content of gender stereotypes. *Social Cognition, 3*, 145–167.

Denmark, F. L. (1980). Psyche: From rocking the cradle to rocking the boat. *American Psychologist, 35*, 1057–1065.

Dion, K. L. (1975). Women's reaction to discrimination from members of the same or opposite sex. *Journal of Research in Personality, 9*, 294–306.

Dion, K. L. (1985). Sex, gender, and groups. In V. E. O'Leary, R. K. Unger, & B. S. Wallston (Eds.), *Women, gender, and social psychology* (pp. 293–347). Hillsdale, NJ: Erlbaum.

Dion, K. L., Earn, B. M., & Yee, P. H. N. (1978). The experience of being a victim of prejudice: An experimental approach. *International Journal of Psychology*, *13*, 197–214.

Dipboye, R. L., Arvey, R. D., & Terpstra, D. E. (1977). Sex and physical attractiveness of raters and applicants as determinants of resume evaluations. *Journal of Applied Psychology*, *62*, 288–294.

Dipboye, R. L., & Wiley, J. W. (1977). Reactions of college recruiters to interviewee sex and self-presentation style. *Journal of Vocational Behavior*, *10*, 1–12.

Dipboye, R. L., & Wiley, J. W. (1978). Reactions of male raters to interviewee self-presentation style and sex: Extensions of previous research. *Journal of Vocational Behavior*, *13*, 192–203.

Dovidio, J. F., Ellyson, S. L., Keating, C. F., Heltman, K., & Brown, C. E. (1988). The relationship of social power to visual displays of dominance between men and women. *Journal of Personality and Social Psychology*, *54*, 233–242.

Dovidio, J. F., & Gaertner, S. L. (1981). The effects of race, status, and ability on helping behavior. *Social Psychology Quarterly*, *44*, 192–203.

Dovidio, J. F., & Gaertner, S. L. (1983). The effects of sex, status, and ability on helping behavior. *Journal of Applied Social Psychology*, *13*, 191–205.

Eagly, A. H. (1987). *Sex differences in social behavior: A social-role interpretation.* Hillsdale, NJ: Erlbaum.

England, P. (1984). Wage appreciation and depreciation: A test of neoclassical economic explanations of occupational sex segregation. *Social Forces*, *62*, 726–749.

England, P., Chassie, H., & McCormack, L. (1982). Skill demands and earnings in female and male occupations. *Sociology and Social Research*, *66*, 147–168.

England, P., Farkas, G., Kilbourne, B. S., & Dou, T. (1988). Explaining occupational sex segregation and wages: Findings from a model with fixed effects. *American Sociological Review*, *53*, 544–558.

England, P., & McCreary, L. (1987). Gender inequality in paid employment. In B. B. Hess & M. M. Ferree (Eds.), *Analyzing gender*. Newbury Park, CA: Sage.

Epstein, C. (1973). The positive effects of the multiple negative: Explaining the success of black professional women. In J. Huber (Ed.), *Changing women in a changing society* (pp. 150–173). Chicago: University of Chicago Press.

Etaugh, C., & Brown, B. (1975). Perceiving the causes of success and failure of male and female performers. *Developmental Psychology*, *11*, 103.

Etaugh, C., Houtler, B. D., & Ptasnik, P. (1988). Evaluating competence of women and men: Effects of experimenter gender and group gender composition. *Psychology of Women Quarterly*, *12*, 191–200.

Etaugh, C., & Rose, S. (1975, April). Adolescents' sex bias in evaluation of performance. Paper presented at the meeting of the Eastern Psychological Association, New York City.

Exum, W. (1983). Climbing the crystal stair: Values, affirmative action and minority faculty. *Social Problems*, *30*, 383–397.

Fabes, R. A., & Laner, M. R. (1986). How the sexes perceive each other: Advantages and disadvantages. *Sex Roles*, *15*, 129–143.

Fairhurst, G. T., & Snavely, B. K. (1983). A test of the social isolation of male tokens. *Academy of Management Journal*, *26*, 353–361.

Feather, N. T., & Simon, J. G. (1975). Reactions to male and female success and failure in sex-linked occupations: Impressions of personality, causal attributions, and perceived likelihood of different consequences. *Journal of Personality and Social Psychology*, *31*, 20–31.

Feldman-Summers, S., & Kiesler, J. (1974). Those who are number two try harder: The effects of sex on attributions of causality. *Journal of Personality and Social Psychology*, *30*, 846–855.

Fichter, J. H. (1964). Graduates of predominantly negro colleges—class of 1964. Public Health Services Publication, no. 1571. Washington DC: Government Printing Office.

Forsythe, S., Drake, M. F., & Cox, C. E. (1985). Influence of applicant's dress on interviewer's selection decisions. *Journal of Applied Psychology*, *70*, 374–378.

Frieze, I. H., & Ramsey, S. J. (1976). Nonverbal maintenance of sex roles. *Journal of Social Issues*, *32*, 133–142.

Garcia, L. T., Erskine, N., Hawn, K., & Casmay, S. R. (1981). The effect of affirmative action on attributions about minority group members. *Journal of Personality*, *49*, 427–437.

Gardner, D. G., & Discenza, R. (1988). Sex effects in evaluating applicant qualifications: A reexamination. *Sex Roles*, *18*, 297–308.

Geis, F. L., Brown, V., Jennings, J., & Porter, N. (1984). TV commercials as achievement scripts for women. *Sex Roles*, *10*, 513–525.

Gerdes, E. P., & Garber, D. M. (1983). Sex bias in hiring: Effects of job demands and applicant competence. *Sex Roles*, *9*, 307–319.

Glenn, E., & Feldberg, R. (1984). Clerical work: The female occupation. In J. Freeman (Ed.), *Women: A feminist perspective*. Palo Alto, CA: Mayfield.

Glick, P., Zion, C., & Nelson, C. (1988). What mediates sex discrimination in hiring decisions? *Journal of Personality and Social Psychology*, *55*, 178–186.

Goffman, E. (1956). The nature of deference and demeanor. *American Anthropologist*, *58*, 473–502.

Goldberg, P. A. (1968). Are women prejudiced against women? *Transaction*, *5*, 28–30.

Goldberg, P. A. (1974). Prejudice toward women: Some personality correlates. *International Journal of Group Tensions*, *4*, 53–63.

Gupta, N., Jenkins, C. D., Jr., & Beehr, T. A. (1983). Employee gender, gender similarity, and supervisor-subordinate cross-evaluations. *Psychology of Women Quarterly*, *8*, 174–184.

Gutek, B. A., & Cohen, A. G. (1987). Sex ratios, sex role spillover, and sex at work: A comparison of men's and women's experiences. *Human Relations*, *40*, 97–115.

Hamilton, D. L., & Trolier, T. K. (1986). Stereotypes and stereotyping: An overview of the cognitive approach. In J. F. Dovidio & S. L. Gaertner (Eds.), *Prejudice, discrimination, and racism*. New York: Academic Press.

Hansen, R. D., & O'Leary, V. E. (1985). Sex-determined attributions. In V. E. O'Leary, R. K. Unger, & B. S. Wallston (Eds.), *Women, gender, and social psychology*. Hillsdale, NJ: Erlbaum.

Harding, J., Proshansky, H., Kutner, B., & Chein, I. (1969). Prejudice and ethnic relations. In G. Lindzey & A. Aronson (Eds.), *The handbook of social psychology* (2nd ed.). Reading, MA: Addison-Wesley.

Hartman, S. J., Griffeth, R. W., Miller, L., & Kinicki, A. J. (1988). The impact of occupation, performance, and sex on sex role stereotyping. *Journal of Social Psychology*, *128*, 451–463.

Hedlund, R. D., Freeman, P. K., Hamm, K. E., & Stein, R. M. (1979). The electability of women candidates: The effects of sex role stereotypes. *Journal of Politics, 41*, 513–524.

Heilman, M. E. (1979). High school students' occupational interest as a function of projected sex ratios in male-dominated professions. *Journal of Applied Psychology, 64*, 275–279.

Heilman, M. E. (1980). The impact of situational factors on personnel decisions concerning women: Varying the sex composition of the applicant pool. *Organizational Behavior and Human Performance, 26*, 386–396.

Heilman, M. E. (1983). Sex bias in work settings: The lack of fit model. *Research in Organizational Behavior, 5*, 269–298.

Heilman, M. E., & Guzzo, R. A. (1978). The perceived cause of work success as a mediator of sex discrimination in organizations. *Organizational Behavior and Human Performance, 21*, 346–357.

Heilman, M. E., Simon, M. C., & Repper, D. P. (1987). Intentionally favored, unintentionally harmed? Impact of sex-based preferential selection on self-perceptions and self-evaluations. *Journal of Applied Psychology, 72*, 62–68.

Heilman, M. E., & Stopeck, M. H. (1985). Attractiveness and corporate success: Differential causal attributions for males and females. *Journal of Applied Psychology, 70*, 379–388.

Henley, N. M. (1977). *Body politics*. Englewood Cliffs, NJ: Prentice-Hall.

Hillsman, S. T., & Levenson, B. (1975). Job opportunities of black and white working-class women. *Social Problems, 22*, 510–532.

Hitt, M. A., & Zikmund, W. G. (1985). Forewarned is fore-armed: Potential between and within sex discrimination. *Sex Roles, 12*, 807–812.

Howard, J. A. (1984). Societal influences on attribution: Blaming some victims more than others. *Journal of Personality and Social Psychology, 47*, 494–505.

Hull, A., Scott, P., & Smith, B. (1982). *All the women are white, all the blacks are men, but some of us are brave: Black women's studies*. Westbury, NY: Feminist Press.

Izraeli, D. N. (1983). Sex effects or structural effects? An empirical test of Kanter's theory of proportions. *Social Forces, 62*, 153–165.

Izraeli, D. N., & Gaier, K. (1979). Sex and interoccupational wage differences in Israel. *Industrial Relations, 18*, 227–232.

Jackson, L. A., & Grabski, S. V. (1988). Perceptions of fair pay and the gender wage gap. *Journal of Applied Social Psychology, 18*, 606–625.

Jacobs, J. (1987). The sex typing of aspirations and occupations: Instability during the careers of young women. *Social Science Quarterly, 68*, 722–737.

Jacobson, M. B., Antonelli, J., Winning, P. U., & Opeil, D. (1977). Women as authority figures: The use and misuse of authority. *Sex Roles, 3*, 365–375.

Johnson, P. (1976). Women and power: Toward a theory of effectiveness. *Journal of Social Issues, 32*, 99–110.

Jones, J. M. (1972). *Prejudice and racism*. Reading, MA: Addison-Wesley.

Kalin, R., & Hodgins, D. C. (1984). Sex bias in judgments of occupational suitability. *Canadian Journal of Behavioral Science, 16*, 311–325.

Kanter, R. M. (1977). *Men and women of the corporation*. New York: Basic Books.

Kaschak, E. (1978). Sex bias in student evaluations of college professors. *Psychology of Women Quarterly, 3*, 235–243.

Keating, C. F. (1985). Gender and the physiognomy of dominance and attractiveness. *Social Psychology Quarterly*, *48*, 61–70.

Keys, D. E. (1985). Gender, sex role, and career decision making of certified management accountants. *Sex Roles*, *13*, 33–46.

Kirkland, S. L., Greenberg, J., & Pyszczynski, T. (1987). Further evidence of the deleterious effects of overhead derogatory ethnic labels: Derogation beyond the target. *Personality and Social Psychology Bulletin*, *13*, 216–227.

Konrad, A. M., & Gutek, B. A. (1987). Theory and research on group composition: Applications to the status of women and ethnic minorities. In S. Oscamp and S. Spacapan (Eds.), *Interpersonal processes: The Claremont Symposium on applied social psychology* (pp. 85–121). Newbury Park, CA: Sage.

Laws, J. L. (1975). The psychology of tokenism: An analysis. *Sex Roles*, *1*, 51–67.

Leffler, A., Gillespie, D. L., & Conaty, J. C. (1982). The effects of status differentiation on nonverbal behavior. *Social Psychology Quarterly*, *45*, 153–161.

Leggon, C. (1980). Black female professionals: Dilemmas and contradictions of status. In L. Rodgers-Rose (Ed.), *The black woman* (pp. 189–201). Beverly Hills: Sage.

Levinson, R. M. (1975). Sex discrimination and employment practices: An experiment with unconventional job inquiries. *Social Problems*, *22*, 533–543.

Lofland, J. (1969). *Deviance and identity*. Englewood Cliffs, NJ: Prentice-Hall.

Lord, C. G., & Saenz, D. S. (1985). Memory deficits and memory surfeits: Differential cognitive consequences of tokenism for tokens and observers. *Journal of Personality and Social Psychology*, *49*, 918–926.

Lott, B. (1985). The devaluation of women's competence. *Journal of Social Issues*, *41*, 43–60.

Lott, B. (1987). Sexist discrimination as distancing behavior: I. A laboratory demonstration. *Psychology of Women Quarterly*, *11*, 47–58.

Major, B., & Deaux, K. (1982). Individual differences in justice behavior. In J. Greenberg & R. L. Cohen (Eds.), *Equity and justice in social behavior*. New York: Academic Press.

Major, B., McFarlin, D. B., & Gagnon, D. (1984). Overworked and underpaid: On the nature of gender differences in personal entitlement. *Journal of Personality and Social Psychology*, *47*, 1399–1412.

Malamuth, N. M. (1988). Predicting laboratory aggression against female and male targets: Implications for sexual aggression. *Journal of Research in Personality*, *22*, 474–495.

Marini, M., & Brinton, M. (1984). Sex typing in occupational socialization. In B. Reskin (Ed.), *Sex segregation in the workplace*. Washington DC: National Academy Press.

McArthur, L. Z., & Obrant, S. W. (1986). Sex biases in comparable worth analysis. *Journal of Applied Social Psychology*, *16*, 757–770.

Moore, D. (1987). Relative deprivation in the labor market. *Israel Social Science Research*, *5*, 121–137.

Nacoste, R. W., & Lehman, D. (1987). Procedural stigma. *Representative Research in Social Psychology*, *17*, 25–38.

Nieva, V. F., & Gutek, B. A. (1980). Sex effects on evaluation. *Academy of Management Review*, *5*, 267–276.

Nirenberg, T. D., & Gaebelein, J. W. (White). (1979). Third party instigated aggression:

Traditional versus liberal sex role attitudes. *Personality and Social Psychology Bulletin*, 5, 348–351.

O'Farrell, B., & Harlan, S. L. (1982). Craftworkers and clerks: The effect of male co-worker hostility on women's satisfaction with non-traditional jobs. *Social Problems*, 29, 252–265.

Ohbuchi, K., & Izutsu, T. (1984). Retaliation by male victims: Effects of physical attractiveness and intensity of attack by female attackers. *Personality and Social Psychology Bulletin*, 10, 216–224.

Paludi, M. A., & Strayer, L. A. (1985). What's in an author's name? Differential evaluations of performance as a function of author's name. *Sex Roles*, 12, 353–361.

Pfeffer, J., & Davis-Blake, A. (1987). The effect of the proportion of women on salaries: The case of college administrators. *Administrative Science Quarterly*, 32, 1–24.

Pheterson, G. I., Kiesler, S. B., & Goldberg, P. A. (1971). Evaluation of the performance of women as a function of their sex, achievement, and personal history. *Journal of Personality and Social Psychology*, 19, 114–118.

Piliavin, J. A., & Unger, R. K. (1985). The helpful but helpless female: Myth or reality? In V. E. O'Leary, R. K. Unger, & B. S. Wallston (Eds.), *Women, gender, and social psychology* (pp. 149–190). Hillsdale, NJ: Erlbaum.

Plake, B. S., Murphy-Berman, V., Derscheid, L. E., Gerber, R. W., Miller, S. K., Speth, C. A., & Tomas, R. E. (1987). Access decisions by personnel directors: Subtle forms of sex bias in hiring. *Psychology of Women Quarterly*, 11, 255–263.

Porter, N., Geis, F. L., Cooper, E., & Newman, E. (1985). Androgyny and leadership in mixed-sex groups. *Journal of Personality and Social Psychology*, 49, 808–823.

Powell, G. N. (1987). The effects of sex and gender on recruitment. *Academy of Management Review*, 12, 731–743.

Pugh, M. D., & Wahrman, R. (1983). Neutralizing sexism in mixed-sex groups: Do women have to be better than men? *American Journal of Sociology*, 88, 746–762.

Ransford, H. E., & Miller, J. (1983). Race, sex, and feminist outlooks. *American Sociological Review*, 48, 46–59.

Reid, P. T. (1987). Perceptions of sex discrimination among female university faculty and staff. *Psychology of Women Quarterly*, 11, 123–127.

Richardson, M. S. (1982). Sources of tension in the psychology of women. *Psychology of Women Quarterly*, 7, 45–54.

Romero, G. J., & Garza, R. T. (1986). Attributions for the occupational success/failure of ethnic minority and nonminority women. *Sex Roles*, 14, 445–452.

Rosen, B., & Mericle, M. F. (1979). Influence of strong versus weak fair employment policies and applicant's sex on selection decisions and salary recommendations in a management simulation. *Journal of Applied Psychology*, 64, 435–439.

Ruble, T. L., Cohen, R., & Ruble, D. N. (1984). Sex stereotypes: Occupational barriers for women. *American Behavioral Scientist*, 27, 339–356.

Rusbult, C. E., Lowery, D., Hubbard, M. L., Maravankin, O. J., & Neises, M. (1988). Impact of employee mobility and employee performance on allocation of rewards under conditions of constraint. *Journal of Personality and Social Psychology*, 54, 605–615.

Sanders, G. S., & Schmidt, T. (1980). Behavioral discrimination against women. *Personality and Social Psychology Bulletin, 6*, 484–488.

Schur, E. M. (1983). *Labeling women deviant: Gender, stigma, and social control*. New York: Random House.

Sigelman, C. K., Thomas, D. B., Sigelman, L., & Ribich, F. D. (1986). Gender, physical attractiveness, and electability: An experimental investigation of voter biases. *Journal of Applied Social Psychology, 16*, 229–248.

Sigelman, L., & Sigelman, C. K. (1982). Sexism, racism, and ageism in voting behavior: An experimental analysis. *Social Psychology Quarterly, 45*, 263–269.

Sigelman, L., & Welch, S. (1984). Race, gender, and opinion toward black and female presidential candidates. *Public Opinion Quarterly, 48*, 467–475.

Simas, K., & McCarrey, M. (1979). Impact of recruiter authoritarianism and applicant sex on evaluation and selection decisions in a recruitment interview analogue study. *Journal of Applied Psychology, 64*, 483–491.

Smith, A., & Stewart, A. (1983). Approaches to studying racism and sexism in black women's lives. *Journal of Social Issues, 39*, 1–15.

Snodgrass, S. E. (1985). Women's intuition: The effect of subordinate role on interpersonal sensitivity. *Journal of Personality and Social Psychology, 49*, 146–155.

Snyder, M., Berscheid, E., & Matwychuk, A. (1988). Orientations toward personnel selection: Differential reliance on appearance and personality. *Journal of Personality and Social Psychology, 54*, 972–979.

Spence, J. T., & Helmreich, R. H. (1978). *Masculinity and femininity*. Austin: University of Texas Press.

Starer, R., & Denmark, F. L. (1974). Discrimination against aspiring women. *International Journal of Group Tensions, 4*, 65–71.

Stead, B. A., & Zinkhan, G. M. (1986). Service priority in department stores: The effect of customer gender and sex. *Sex Roles, 15*, 601–611.

Swarz, N., Wagner, D., Bannert, M., & Mathes, L. (1987). Cognitive accessibility of sex role concepts and attitudes toward political participation: The impact of sexist advertisements. *Sex Roles, 17*, 593–601.

Tajfel, H. (1982). Social psychology of intergroup relations. *Annual Review of Psychology, 33*, 1–39.

Tajfel, H. (1984). Intergroup relations, social myths, and social justice in social psychology. In H. Tajfel (Ed.), *The social dimension* (Vol. 2). Cambridge: Cambridge University Press.

Taylor, S. E., Fiske, S. T., Etcoff, N. L., & Ruderman, A. J. (1978). Categorical and contextual basis of person memory and stereotyping. *Journal of Personality and Social Psychology, 36*, 778–793.

Taynor, J., & Deaux, K. (1975). Equity and perceived sex differences: Role behavior as defined by the task, the mode, and the actor. *Journal of Personality and Social Psychology, 32*, 381–390.

Toder, N. L. (1980). The effect of the sexual composition of a group on discrimination against women and sex-role attitudes. *Psychology of Women Quarterly, 5*, 292–310.

Tosi, H. L., & Einbender, S. W. (1985). The effects of the type and amount of information in sex discrimination research: A meta-analysis. *Academy of Management Journal, 28*, 712–723.

Treas, J. (1978). Differential achievement: Race, sex, and jobs. *Sociology and Social Research, 62,* 387–400.

Treiman, D. J., & Roos, P. A. (1983). Sex and earnings in industrial society: A nine-nation comparison. *American Journal of Sociology, 89,* 612–650.

Unger, R. K. (1976). Male is greater than female: The socialization of status inequality. *Counseling Psychologist, 6,* 2–9.

Unger, R. K. (1978). The politics of gender. In J. Sherman & F. Denmark (Eds.), *Psychology of women: Future directions of research.* New York: Psychological Dimensions.

Unger, R. K. (1981). Sex as a social reality: Field and laboratory research. *Psychology of Women Quarterly, 5,* 645–653.

Unger, R. K. (1985). Personal appearance and social control. In M. Safir, M. Mednick, D. Izraeli, & J. Bernard (Eds.), *Women's worlds: The new scholarship.* New York: Praeger.

Unger, R. K. (1988). Psychological, feminist, and personal epistemology: Transcending contradiction. In M. Gergen (Ed.), *Feminist thought and the structure of knowledge.* New York: New York University Press.

Unger, R. K., Hilderbrand, M., & Madar, T. (1982). Physical attractiveness and assumptions about social deviance: Some sex by sex comparisons. *Personality and Social Psychology Bulletin, 8,* 293–301.

Unger, R. K., Raymond, B. J., & Levine, S. (1974). Are women discriminated against? Sometimes! *International Journal of Group Tensions, 4,* 71–81.

Unger, R. K., & Sussman, L. E. (1986). "I and thou": Another barrier to societal change? *Sex Roles, 14,* 629–636.

Villemur, N. K., & Hyde, J. S. (1983). Effects of sex of defense attorney, sex of juror, and age and attractiveness of the victim on mock jury decision making in a rape case. *Sex Roles, 9,* 879–889.

Wahrman, R., & Pugh, M. D. (1974). Sex, nonconformity, and influence. *Sociometry, 37,* 137–147.

Wallston, B. S., & O'Leary, V. E. (1981). Sex makes a difference: Differential perceptions of women and men. In L. Wheeler (Ed.), *Review of personality and social psychology* (Vol. 2). Beverly Hills: Sage.

Weimann, G. (1985). Sex differences in dealing with bureaucracy. *Sex Roles, 12,* 777–790.

White, J. W. (1983). Sex and gender issues in aggression research. In R. G. Geen & E. I. Donnerstein (Eds.), *Aggression: Theoretical and empirical reviews* (Vol. 2). New York: Academic Press.

Wiley, M. G., & Eskilson, A. (1982). Coping in the corporation: Sex role constraints. *Journal of Applied Social Psychology, 12,* 1–11.

Winston, N. A. (1988). Sex-bias responses to telephoned job inquiries, Tampa, 1987. *Society and Social Research, 72,* 121–124.

Wolman, C., & Frank, H. (1975). The solo woman in a professional peer group. *American Journal of Orthopsychiatry, 45,* 164–171.

Wood, J. T., & Conrad, C. (1983). Paradox in the experience of professional women. *Western Journal of Speech Communication, 47,* 305–322.

Wood, W., & Karten, S. J. (1986). Sex differences in interactive style as a product of perceived sex differences in competence. *Journal of Personality and Social Psychology, 50,* 341–347.

Yarkin, K. L., Town, J. P., & Wallston, B. S. (1982). Blacks and women must try harder: Stimulus persons' race and sex attributions of causality. *Personality and Social Psychology Bulletin*, *8*, 21–30.

Yoder, J. D. (1985). An academic woman as a token: A case study. *Journal of Social Issues*, *41*, 61–72.

Yoder, J. D., & Adams, J. (1984). Women entering nontraditional roles: When work demands and sex-roles conflict. *International Journal of Women's Studies*, *7*, 260–272.

Zikmund, W. G., Hitt, M. A., & Pickens, B. A. (1978). Influence of sex and scholastic performance on reactions to job applicant resumes. *Journal of Applied Psychology*, *63*, 252–254.

Zinkhan, G. M., & Stoiadin, L. F. (1984). Impact of sex role stereotypes on service priority in department stores. *Journal of Applied Psychology*, *69*, 691–693.

Zinn, M., Cannon, L., Higginbotham, E., & Dill, B. (1986). The costs of exclusionary practices in women's studies. *Signs*, *11*, 290–303.

Part III

Social, Personality, and Cognitive Development Across the Life Span

6

Developmental Psychology of Women: Conception to Adolescence

Pamela T. Reid and Michele A. Paludi

The development of girls into women is a process that includes a variety of interacting, complex factors, involving physical, social, and psychological domains. In this chapter we will attempt to examine a number of these factors and to explain how they interact with one another. We will also present a relatively comprehensive perspective of the conditions and circumstances that influence the gender-role specific development of girls from conception through adolescence. During this examination of relevant questions and issues of development, we will take care to consider the ethnic, cultural, and social class diversity of girls and women in order to provide some understanding of the range of behavior possibilities that exist in our society.

THE DEVELOPMENTAL APPROACH

We define "development" as a combination of quantitative and qualitative growth that occurs over time. We see growth as a young girl becomes not only larger, but more dexterous and more coordinated. Development is evidenced during pubescence, as a girl's body grows into that of a woman's. We see the results of development in her increasing grasp of language and social skills and in greater intellectual achievements. Development is also obvious in the young woman's developing recognition of societal expectations and her possible acceptance of limits on her future behavior and aspirations.

The developmental approach to studying behavior is an attempt to establish the rules for the changes that may be observed over time (Newman & Newman, 1987). Although everyone can observe the same child and note identical changes, different theoretical perspectives have evolved to explain these changes. The differences in theoretical perspective are due to the initial assumptions made about human behavior. In fact, much of developmental theory may be found to revolve about a core set of issues. Over the years the focus of developmental psychology has been on men's development (Rabinowitz & Sechzer, this volume; Unger, 1981). Men, especially white men, represented the standard of "human behavior." In recent decades, however, researchers have increasingly recognized the importance of defining standards for women's behavior as different from that for men (Samelson, 1978; Wallston & Grady, 1985). Although white people remain the most frequently studied participants in research investigations, there is a growing realization among psychologists that differences among ethnic, racial, and cultural populations should be considered important in determining patterns of behavior and development (Bronstein & Quina, 1988). For the study of women's development, these issues remain essential as we address questions of why and how women's development occurs.

Major Developmental Issues

Nature versus Nurture

The question of whether development occurs due to the forces of nature (genetic, biological, and inherited factors) or nurture (learned, experiential, and environmental factors) lies at the root of almost all developmental research. While early investigators posed the issue as an "either-or" question, many researchers today see it as a question of degree. It may seem reasonable and logical to recognize the contributions of both nature and nurture; still, the debate remains heated concerning which factor contributes more significantly. On one hand, the search for the biological underpinnings of girls' and women's behavior is frequently interpreted as an attempt to set unchangeable limits on their opportunities. On the other hand, attempts to explain all of women's traits in terms of environmental factors is seen as a denial of the genetic realities of human behavior. Obviously, an understanding of both the biological concomitants of behavior and the external influences on that behavior is necessary for a psychology of women that is accurate and complete.

Critical Periods versus Plasticity

Another major issue for developmental research is the question of whether there exist optimal or critical times during which a particular behavior must develop. At the present time there has been no great effort to determine whether characteristics of girls' and women's behavior must be developed along a critical time period. Although some biologically based questions may be seen as related to critical periods, for example, concern about the development of maternal behavior or whether there is an optimal age for onset of menstruation, there has been little speculation about the more clearly social characteristics in girls and women, for example, questioning the possibility of changes from a very stereotypical feminine behavior pattern to a less stereotypical one. As more research focuses on women's development, issues of critical periods may receive more attention (Doyle & Paludi, 1990).

Additional Theoretical Issues

There are two remaining issues that have been included as essential areas of differences among developmental research, activity versus passivity and continuity versus discontinuity. "Activity versus passivity" refers to the role that people play in their own development. The cognitive-developmental theorists, such as Piaget (1947) and Kohlberg (1976), believe that children actively engage the environment. This theoretical perspective views people as biologically prepared to interpret and organize their world. Other theoretical views, social-learning, for example, see individuals as more passive recipients and reactors to stimuli (Bandura & Walters, 1963). The issue of activity versus passivity has been related only indirectly to girls' and women's development. Empirical findings have often been interpreted in ways that imply that women's behavior is more passive than that of men's. For example, in the area of moral development, researchers frequently conclude that girls are less rational and less mature in their ability to make judgments of good and bad (Kohlberg, 1976).

The issue of "continuity versus discontinuity" refers to the question of whether development progresses at a steady rate, with quantitative changes building upon past experiences; or at an uneven pace, taking qualitative leaps from one stage to another. This final issue is one for which no specific attention has been paid to women's development. Yet, the question may have to be posed eventually if the understanding of the developmental patterns is to be complete. In all areas of development, physical, personality, and social, the major issues of development will need to be reconsidered in order to include questions that address girls' and women's developmental patterns.

SOCIETAL EXPECTATIONS AND GENDER-ROLE PRESCRIPTIONS

Every society has clear and distinct behavioral expectations for girls and women. These expectations and the demands that accompany them constitute the roles that the society prescribes for girls and women (Bem, 1981). The behavior our society accepts as appropriate for either a 2-year-old girl or a 16-year-old has been defined and carefully socialized into our consciousness through a variety of sources. While we may expect some differences in behavior based on culture and ethnicity, there is a surprisingly strong consensus across groups as to what constitutes appropriate behavior for girls and women (Lott, 1987). For example, girls are expected to be gentle and quiet, docile and obedient, caring and nurturant and eventually to become mothers (Russo, 1976). Girls as young as 4 years of age have demonstrated that the mother role is distinguishable for them. For example, Reid, Tate, and Berman (1989) found that when presenting themselves in the "mother role," girls stood closer to infants, touched them more, and smiled more. However, increasingly, young women are adopting nonstereotypic behavior and accepting other responsibilities for themselves; for example, girls are preparing to be workers, adventurers, supervisors, and athletes.

Researchers are examining the ways in which girls prepare themselves to fill these new roles and how their new images may affect their lives. While current psychological theory promotes the notion that "feminine" and "masculine" characteristics are both necessary and complementary components of a well-adjusted adult (Bem, 1983), in practice psychologists and the general public have been somewhat resistant to relinquishing the notion that gender-role related characteristics are bipolar, that is, opposite and contradictory. It is still somewhat surprising to most of us for a girl or young woman to be both competent and feminine. Our ingrained expectation is that she can be one or the other, not both (Sedney, 1989).

Influences of Parents and Culture

To understand the impact of the societal expectations on girls, we should recognize that gender-role related information emanates from many sources. Obviously, the primary source during the early years of childhood is in the home. Family members, especially parents, contribute much to the shaping of a girl's development of gender-role appropriate behaviors and ideas (Reid, 1981). Surveys and discussions with parents of young children demonstrate a general consensus that girls are expected to be verbal, compliant, passive, physically weak, quiet, and clean (Basow, 1992). Even before birth parents project fetal activity as representative of assumed gender-role related differences; that is, very active fetal movement is assumed to characterize a boy rather than a girl. For newborns, both parents, but fathers especially, perceive their daughters as smaller, more delicate, less active, and weaker than they perceive sons (Rubin, Provenzano & Luria, 1974). In more recent studies of adults, it was again demonstrated that adults perceived an infant's behavior as "feminine" if the child was labeled "girl" (Delk, Madden, Livingston, & Ryan, 1986; Paludi & Gullo, 1986).

In addition to holding stereotypic expectations, parents encourage gender-role appropriate activities by providing children with sex-typed toys and clothing (Doyle & Paludi, 1990). Girls are given dolls, dollhouses, and miniature household appliances. Boys are provided with building blocks, sports equipment, models of vehicles and animals. Parents also behave differently toward their daughters and sons. They have been found to engage in more "rescuing" behavior with girls, that is, assisting and accompanying girls more often than necessary (Matlin, 1993; Newson & Newson, 1968). Their consistent willingness to help girls suggests both expectation for, and support of, high levels of dependency in girls. It has been suggested that in many nonverbal ways parents convey anxiety to their daughters when attempts at independence are made.

While there has been some consistency of findings, we should note that most investigators have focused on white, middle-class families. There is some evidence that parental responses may vary considerably based on both ethnicity and social class (Paludi, 1988). While Romer and Cherry (1980) found few differences in gender-role related expectations of middle-class black parents compared with white parents of the middle class, Price-Bonham and Skeen (1982) did find racial differences. Racial differences were also found in a study of preschool girls and boys. Reid et al. (1989) found both sex and race influenced children's responses to babies. Little empirical data exist on gender-role expectations for other ethnic groups; however, anecdotal information suggests that Asian American and Hispanic American parents may expect their daughters to be even more submissive and dependent than those of white American families. With respect to social class, Carr and Mednick (1988) suggested that socialization of feminine gender-role behavior does vary with social class and that this socialization would impact directly the achievement behavior exhibited by girls. Their study of black preschool children supported this contention. They found that girls with greater nontraditional gender-role training were higher in achievement. Other researchers have found class differences among black families that suggest that working-class girls will have fewer gender-role constraints (Casenave, 1979; Romer & Cherry, 1980). Studies of social class differences on other ethnic groups have been conducted infrequently.

Hill (1988) noted that lesbian mothers perceived their daughters and their sons to be more similar in characteristics than did heterosexual mothers. Lesbian mothers held less stereotypic ideas relating to the feminine role and encouraged more traditionally masculine role expectations of their daughters. Daughters of employed mothers also perceived women's role as involving freedom of choice and satisfaction (Baruch & Barnett, 1986).

According to Jacklin and Maccoby (1983), parents appear to modify their treatment of their children as they become older. Thus, the individual personality of a girl may eventually exert more influence than her sex. Parents cannot be considered the sole agent of gender-role typing through the childhood and adolescent years, and some research suggests that parental influence on children's attitudes is weak (Baruch & Barnett, 1986). We must, therefore, consider other socialization agents to understand fully the influences on gender-role development.

Influences of School

Although parents and the family lay the foundation for early gender-role expectations, in our society children are also exposed to societal expectations through the school. In school situations both teachers and peers have been found to serve as strong agents for appropriate gender-role–related behaviors. For example, teachers support the dependency needs of young girls by attending to them primarily when they remain in close proximity (Halliday, McNaughton & Glynn, 1985; Serbin, O'Leary, Kent & Tonick, 1973). Girls received more disapproval for lack of knowledge from teachers than boys and they were less likely to be mentioned by teachers as being creative. Teachers reported having higher expectations and "favoring" girls more in languages; boys were favored in science.

Social class differences also seem to affect teachers' responses to children. Quay and Jarrett (1986) found that preschool teachers of lower-class children had fewer verbal interactions with them; however, their interactions did not vary by sex, as did the interactions of teachers of middle-class children.

Peers also encourage passivity and gender-role stereotyped choices for both girls and boys (Connor, Serbin & Ender, 1978). Even young girls are seen behaving in deferent ways to boys who have not yet developed "superior strength or size." In observations of preschool children, W. S. Mathews (1975) reported that one 3-year-old girl in a playhouse situation asked a boy of the same height to help her reach a toy iron placed out of her reach. The girl acted as though the boy were more competent at this physical task than she could be. In a number of situations girls accept the subordinate position, even when they may possess superior knowledge and expertise (Lockheed & Hall, 1976).

Girls appear to learn the appropriate gender-role–related behavior through a number of mechanisms. In addition to the overt instructions from parents and teachers, the subtle cues presented by women and men models have been found to exert a strong influence on children. In our society many of the women models to which girls are exposed seem to behave in stereotypically feminine ways. Thus, while societal sanctions are often not particularly severe for girls who fail to maintain feminine standards of behavior, the models for any nonfeminine behavior are so rare that there may be little incentive for girls to act in nontraditional ways. For example, while women dominate the teaching field at the preschool and elementary levels, more than 80% of elementary school principals are men (Parelius & Parelius, 1978). These men represent both authority and masculinity. Girls grow to expect that these characteristics belong together. As children progress through school, it becomes increasingly clear that women are also not expected to develop interests in math, science, or computers. The lack of women models in these areas acts to convince girls that their attention to these subjects are inappropriate and ill-advised (see Betz, this volume).

Media Images and Influences

Although parents and adults in children's communities are obvious models of appropriate and expected behavior, the behavior of characters from a variety of media sources also plays a role in the development of gender-role expectations. Casual observation, as well as serious investigation, reveals that print, film, and television images influence the behavior of girls in demonstrable ways. For the most part, reviews of research indicate that the overwhelming majority of media images of girls and women conform to both racial and gender stereotypes (Mayes & Valentine, 1979; Ruble, Balaban & Cooper, 1981). Both popular literature and children's schoolbooks portray females as dull, neat, and passive (McArthur & Eisen, 1976). Although black girls and women were rare, they are also presented in very stereotypic ways (Dickerson, 1982). Characters represented in stories read for school and for pleasure are often intended to expose children to new vistas and allow them to share vicariously experiences of other people. For girls, however, they may also receive through stereotyped characters confirmation of societal expectations that girls do not take risks, accomplish exciting feats, or leave the security of their homes and the protection of men.

While books are impactful, no one will argue with the more powerful influence of television. Virtually every household in America has a television set, and children of all ages have been shown to watch upward of 20 hours per week. Television models, too, present stereotyped images of girls and women. Stern-glanz and Serbin (1974), in an early study of children's television programs, found that girls and women were depicted as nurturant, succorant, relatively inactive, and ineffective. Black female characters on television were even more stereotyped relative to black males (Reid, 1979).

Preschool girls have been shown to make sex-typed choices based on the television characters they observe (Ruble et al., 1981), and even identification with characters depends on their traditional gender-role–related portrayal (McGhee & Frueh, 1980). Interestingly, girls are found to model verbal labeling rather than the active behaviors modeled by boys after observing televised characters. Of course, even the absence of girls and women models conveys a message that the group is not important enough to be represented. This must be the impression given to girls who are Chicanas, Puerto Rican, Native American, and Asian. For it is rare indeed when characters from these groups are depicted in a significant way in any national media (Reid, 1979).

Stereotypes about women's and men's behavior are also clearly observable in rock music videos (Freudinger & Almquist, 1978). Girls and women are depicted as emotional, deceitful, illogical, frivolous, dependent, and passive. Boys and men are portrayed as sexually aggressive, rational, demanding, and adventuresome. Rock music videos frequently depict gratuitous violence against women and women as sex objects. The interface of racism and sexism is also apparent in the videos. For example, in "All She Wants to Do Is Dance," a Third World woman is depicted as hedonistic and sexual while a revolution is going on. Men step on her image in a mirror (Basow, 1986). Frequent exposure to rock music videos increases the probability that subsequent women's and men's behavior will be appraised in the context of the gender-role stereotypic schemas, even for preschool and young children (Waite & Paludi, 1987).

Influences of Culture, Race, and Social Class

As we have suggested throughout this chapter, the development of girls and young women is a process influenced by numerous interacting factors. Within the United States the role expectations for girls have many commonalities, but they also vary somewhat depending upon social class and the ethnicity of the family and the surrounding community. It has been found that greater flexibility and permissiveness exist in middle-class homes regardless of ethnicity. This flexibility leads to the availability of masculine activity choices for girls. In working-class homes, on the other hand, parents are more concerned that their children adhere strictly to gender-role appropriate behavior, as it is stereotypically defined (Hall & Keith, 1964; Mussen, Conger & Kagen, 1963). Surveys conducted with black and white families indicated that lower-class blacks subscribed even more strongly than whites to the belief that boys should hold dominant positions in the family (Ten Houten, 1970). However, Ten Houten also found that black mothers tended to dominate in specific areas (e.g., working toward educational goals) more than did white mothers. A review of several studies by Smith and Midlarsky (1985) suggests that black women and men actually demonstrate overall less stereotyping than white women and men. Although little empirical research exists on gender norms and expectations accepted as appropriate among ethnic groups in this country, Williams (1982) studied stereotypes held by women and men in 25 different countries. Results indicated both similarities and differences across cultural groups. Apparently, stereotypic notions about feminine and masculine characteristics do not vary widely.

It is not surprising that children adopt gender-role–related patterns of behavior early in their lives. Although social pressures to conform to gender-role expectations have typically been less stringent for girls than for boys (Hall & Keith, 1964), girls are well aware of the stereotypic feminine preferences that they are expected to hold. Expressions of girls' awareness of gender-role stereotypes will be discussed in the next sections of this chapter, girls' physical and cognitive development in childhood and adolescence.

PHYSICAL DEVELOPMENT

Although Freud's notion that "biology is destiny" is no longer uncritically accepted, the fact remains that physical development and biological events are important to women throughout the life span. Beginning with the prenatal growth period, girls are found to follow a faster biological timetable than boys. Girls continue to mature at a differential rate and with different behavioral results (Jacklin, 1989; Shaffer, 1989). In reviewing the stages of physical development, it is important to address how the biological "clock" influences girls' physical abilities and to examine the relationship between inherited and experiential factors in development. Recognition must also be given to a key biological event in girls' lives, menarche. As part of our discussion of the concept of physical femininity, we must consider current social trends that encourage girls' participation in sports and athletic activities. Finally, an examination of physical and biological issues as discrete aspects of development leads us to consider the interrelationship of physical competency with personal autonomy and self-esteem. For example, body image among girls has been found to influence self-esteem and other social and psychological traits (Orbach, 1978).

Prenatal Development

Determination of sexual characteristics begins at conception. When a woman's ovum (the female reproductive cell with 23 single chromosomes) is fertilized by a sperm cell (the male reproductive cell with 23 single chromosomes), the resulting union is expected to produce the characteristic human cell with a total of 46 chromosomes (23 chromosome pairs). Of these 23 pairs only 1 pair controls the genetic sex of the offspring (Rathus, 1983). Geneticists have long been aware that the woman's ovum possesses only an X chromosome for sex, while the man's sperm cell may contain either an X or Y. When an X-bearing sperm cell fertilizes the X-bearing ovum, the genetic pattern is established for a female offspring (XX). When a Y-bearing sperm cell fertilizes the X-bearing ovum, the genetic pattern is established for a male (XY). This explanation of the development of sexual characteristics allows one to conclude that the donor of the male sperm cell controls the sex of the offspring and that chromosomes are the determinants of sexual characteristics. While these are basically correct assertions, other factors may mediate the outcome.

Female Viability

Whether the process of fertilization occurs through artificial insemination, in a test tube, or through intercourse, the environment through which the sperm cell must pass to reach the ovum must be considered a factor in sex determination (Rathus, 1983). Genetic researchers have found that the X-bearing sperm appear more viable than the Y-bearing sperm. Physicians note that women who conceive during times when their vaginal environment is likely to be strongly acidic are more likely to produce girls. This suggests that a strongly acidic environment is detrimental to the Y-bearing sperm. Other data support the finding of greater female viability even after birth (Jacklin, 1989). Women have an overall life span expectancy that surpasses men at every age regardless of race. In addition, girls have fewer congenital disorders, are less likely to succumb to sudden infant death syndrome, and are less prone to hyperactivity (Paludi, 1985). Each of these findings indicates a degree of genetically determined strength.

Hormonal Factors in Sex Development

While the normal chromosomal pairing of XX or XY occurs in most cases, there are occasional anomalies in which too many or too few chromosomes connect, resulting in physical differences. The female pattern of development appears to be the standard. While male development needs the secretion of the male hormones from the testes to stimulate the growth and development of the male reproductive system, female development occurs spontaneously, even in the absence of ovaries and their hormonal secretions (Money & Ehrhardt, 1972).

Hormonal factors, then, in addition to chromosomes influence sex development prenatally and after birth. One example of a hormonal condition that results in a male baby being labeled a girl is androgen insensitivity. Although the child is genetically male (XY), his body is insensitive to the hormones his body has produced. This insensitivity prevents the complete development of the male reproductive system and the inhibition of the female development. Studies of androgen-insensitive people who were raised as girls demonstrate that they conform to the general expectations of femininity in our society (Money & Ehrhardt, 1972).

Andrenogential syndrome is another hormonal abnormality. This condition most seriously affects genetically normal female fetuses. Sometimes it occurs when the adrenal gland of the fetus overproduces androgen; some occurrences are due to the mother's taking large doses of androgen. The effect of the excessive androgen is that the external genitalia of the female appear masculine despite the XX chromosome pair. These females may be labeled and raised as boys. Although surgical procedures may be necessary at puberty to facilitate development as a male, these individuals will adjust to the sex designation that they were given at birth (Money & Tucker, 1975). The results of studies of individuals with abnormal genetic or hormonal conditions clearly indicate that biological factors are necessary but not sufficient in producing the characteristics that we attribute to sex. Even in the prenatal period there appears an interaction between physical and social conditions that will be repeated again and again.

Development of Female Characteristics in Infancy and Childhood

After birth there is no greater rate of growth and change than that which occurs during the period we call infancy (0 through 18 months—the period prior to the onset of language; Rathus, 1983). During this stage there have been some well-documented sex-linked characteristics, for example, generally smaller size for girls compared with boys and more advanced skeletal and neurological systems and greater sensitivity to auditory stimuli for girls (Paludi, 1985). However, for the most part, researchers have not assigned a great deal of importance to sex characteristics in many areas of infant learning, for example, habituation, conditioning, bonding. Sex as a factor in physical activity continues, however, to generate high research interest. Nevertheless, few unambiguous results have been found. Sex links that have been found suggest a complex interaction of both biological and social factors. For this reason, some recent investigators have adopted a position that social influences should be interpreted as magnifying existing differences rather than as creating them (Jacklin, 1989).

Interestingly, sex becomes increasingly important as the physical changes of childhood (and adolescence) are examined. Many studies report sex as a factor in performance of motor tasks, but they frequently give the advantage to boys. This assignment of advantage contradicts the fact that girls have more accelerated physical development. It is illogical that biological acceleration may be given as an explanation of girls' rapid acquisition of language skills (Maccoby & Jacklin, 1974) and their ability to excel in fine motor skills, while there remains an expectation of inferior performance in gross motor activities. According to Bem (1981), gender differences in motor performance appear to be influenced by both biological and environmental factors. The low expectations that parents and teachers have with respect to girls' motor performance and the lack of rewards given to girls for such activities apparently combine to produce low motivation and low performance levels for girls in the behaviors that have been societally defined as appropriate for boys.

Expectations of femininity are not limited to the types of behavior that girls are supposed to adopt. For example, underlying the culture's definition of physical femininity is the assumption that feminine translates as physical incompetence, or weakness. Although the population in general is concerned with fitness and honors have been given to women as well as men sports heroes, there remain suspicions about the woman with athletic prowess. The recent example of the Olympic superstar, Florence Griffith-Joyner, demonstrated that media reporters were as much, or even more, interested in discussing her flamboyant dress or designer fingernails as her feats of skill on the track. The message for girls continues to focus concern that sports ability means masculinity.

Adolescent Development

The beginning of adolescence is typically marked by changes in physical development that are part of the passage from childhood to adulthood. These physical changes occur during the stage known as pubescence, which is the period of rapid growth that culminates in puberty, or sexual maturity and reproductive capacity.

Pubescence technically begins when the hypothalamus signals the pituitary gland to release the hormones known as gonadotrophins. This usually occurs during the adolescents' sleep a year or so before any of the physical changes associated with pubescence appear (Schowalter & Anyan, 1981). The exact factors that activate the hypothalamus are not determined. However, researchers (Frisch, 1984; Katchadorian, 1977; Tanner, 1962) have argued that the hypothalamus monitors adolescents' body weight and releases the necessary hormones when the body is of sufficient weight. In the United States, the age when puberty is reached has steadily decreased, with the trend now leveling off. Most adolescent girls in the United States begin pubescence at approximately 11 years of age and reach the end of their growth by 17. Their height spurt starts between 9.5 and 14.5 years. Girls typically mature on the average of two years earlier than boys. Data indicate that in most cultures the age at which girls begin to menstruate has been dropping steadily for the last several centuries, illustrating the "secular trend."

During adolescence girls and boys undergo common physical changes. For example, their lymphatic tissues decrease in size. Also during adolescence, both girls and boys lose vision due to rapid changes in eyes between the ages of 11 and 14, and the facial structure of adolescent girls and boys changes dramatically during pubescence. During this period, the hairline recedes and the facial bones mature in such a way that the chin and nose become prominent. Adolescents' weight nearly doubles during pubescence. Boys typically weigh 25 pounds more than girls as a result of their higher proportion of muscle-to-fat tissue. There is considerable overlap in the distributions, however (Marshall, 1981; Petersen & Taylor, 1980). By the time they are 15, adolescents have lost 20 deciduous teeth. The number of bone masses during pubescence drops from approximately 350 to less than 220 as a result of epiphyseal unions (Petersen & Taylor, 1980).

The sequence of events in the maturation of girls' sexual and reproductive anatomy is not universally predictable, yet maturation does proceed in distinct developmental stages: growth of breasts, growth of pubic hair, body growth, menarche, underarm hair, oil- and sweat-producing glands (Katchadorian, 1977). For adolescent girls a significant aspect of this maturational experience is menarche. Researchers indicate that girls may be ambivalent about menarche and its meaningfulness to them varies depending on the information they have received (Ruble & Brooks-Gunn, 1982).

The age at which puberty is reached in adolescent girls has a considerable impact on girls' behavior during adolescence. Research has generally indicated that the impact of early or late puberty for girls is not favorable (Clausen, 1975; Eichorn, 1963; Gunn & Petersen, 1984) and generally poses a source of anxiety and embarrassment. These concerns affect the development of girls' self-concept and identity.

Girls who mature early usually date earlier and more often express less self-confidence than girls who reach puberty at a later age. They also express dissatisfaction with their bodies, feel isolated from other girls their own age who have not reached puberty, and make lower grades (Blyth, Simmons & Zakin, 1985). Furthermore, early maturing adolescent girls have imposed upon them sexual responsibilities that they are not ready to accept, considering the fact that their intellectual, social, and emotional maturity lags behind their physical maturity. Follow-up studies have reported that by adulthood, early maturing girls exhibit a high level of cognitive mastery and coping skills as a result of their experiences throughout adolescence (Livson & Peskin, 1980).

Adolescent girls who mature later tend to be more tense, have lower self-esteem, and are more actively attention-seeking than earlier-maturing girls. Once menarche is reached, however, these feelings of low self-esteem diminish.

The advantages of early or late maturation depend on the communication that exists between adolescent girls and their adult caretakers (Clausen, 1975). Girls who have had adults discuss with them the emotional and social ramifications of early or late puberty adjust more successfully to their physical maturation than girls whose family has less time to invest in assisting them with coping with puberty. Blyth et al. (1985) pointed out the need to consider the school environment in relation to specific body image dimensions, especially a youth culture that supports an ideal of thinness in women. In the United States, girls are considered most feminine if they meet the cultural ideal (large breasts, but generally thin). Adolescent girls, more so than boys, are concerned about body size and image. They are more concerned with the social appeal of their appearance (Schlesier-Stropp, 1984). Many girls are, in fact, obsessed with their efforts to match the ideal of physical femininity, illustrated by the incidence of eating disorders, dieting behavior, and surgical procedures developed to "correct" faulty anatomy (Boskind-Lohdal, 1976; Bruch, 1978; Duncan, 1985; Tolmach & Scherr, 1984; Travis, this volume).

Most importantly, research does indicate that the normal developmental process of pubescence and puberty is being viewed negatively by adolescent girls. Certainly the socialization agents contribute to adolescent girls' perceptions about their bodies.

Abnormal Development of the Female Sexual and Reproductive System

While for the majority of adolescent girls physical development proceeds normally, some girls are faced with considerable ordeals as a result of chromosomal sex abnormalities that affect their sexual development. Some girls inherit an XO genetic pattern instead of an XX pattern. This condition is referred to as Turner's syndrome. It is caused by an abnormal division of X and Y chromosomes on the 23rd pair at the time of conception (Higham, 1980).

Girls with Turner's syndrome have only one normal X chromosome; the other X is missing (thus represented by an O). At birth, girls with Turner's syndrome have genitals that look identical to XX girls; thus they are labeled girls. However, XO girls do not have normal ovaries as a result of missing an X chromosome. Consequently, they will not menstruate at adolescence nor will they develop breasts. Their bodies do not produce the estrogen necessary for the development of their secondary sex characteristics during adolescence.

Girls with Turner's syndrome are intellectually normal, but have several physical abnormalities. Typically they remain short in stature and have stubby fingers as well as unusually shaped mouths and ears. They have a shieldlike chest with incompletely developed breasts. Girls who have been given estrogen treatments do look more "normal" in appearance.

COGNITIVE DEVELOPMENT

Over the years researchers have attempted to define areas of cognitive abilities that differ for girls and boys, women and men. Their success with this task has been minimal. No widespread differences exist on tests of general intelligence, learning and memory, or mathematics. Indeed, few areas have been found for which the abilities of girls are clear and consistently related to gender across cultural and ethnic groups (Jacklin, 1989). Despite this fact, interest persists and controversy abounds as researchers examine and attempt to explain the gender/ cognitive relationship. While the examinations and the explanations themselves may have been scientifically rigorous, a great deal of contention and suspicion of biological investigations persists due to past attempts to define women as inferior based on mental capacities and traits (Shields, 1975). Even now minor empirical differences appear to many to be distorted and exaggerated in favor of men and to the distinct disadvantage of women (Lips, 1988). The notion that cognitive abilities of girls and women may be explained by purely biological bases continues to be challenged (Safir, 1986), even though evidence for biological influences such as hormonal levels has been demonstrated (Resnick, Gottesman, Berenbaum & Bouchard, 1986). On the other hand, support for an explanation of experiential influences on girls' cognitive development has also increased (Bloch, 1987; Jahoda, 1986; M.H. Matthews, 1986a).

Cognitive Abilities of Girls

Among the cognitive traits that have been believed to differ based on sex, Maccoby and Jacklin (1974) found that gender differences were clearly present in verbal ability, spatial perception, and arithmetic reasoning. Based on their extensive review of the existing studies, the data indicated that girls surpassed boys in verbal ability. On average, girls begin to vocalize at an earlier age than boys, are more responsive to their mothers' speech, and demonstrate more adeptness at verbal tasks (Hyde, 1981; Maccoby & Jacklin, 1974). While some studies indicate that girls also surpass boys on tests of perceptual speed and accuracy (Antill & Cunningham, 1982), boys have consistently been found superior in tasks of spatial perception (Connor & Serbin, 1985; Linn & Petersen, 1985; M. H. Matthews, 1986b). This advantage has been used to explain the dearth of women experiencing success in fields such as engineering. Yet, when girls' performance in math surpasses boys in several areas, it has been dismissed as due to girls' better behavior (Benbow & Stanley, 1983).

Researchers who study cognitive abilities do not always concentrate on such basic skills as verbal, mathematics, and spatial perception; more complex behavior may also be evaluated in terms of gender. Shaffer (1989) reviewed a number of studies focused on complex cognitive functioning and found girls were more responsive to infants, less demanding, and more likely to respond to parents' social overtures. Boys were more willing to take risks, more vulnerable to reading disabilities and speech defects, and more receptive to rough-and-tumble play. Despite the findings of consistency across groups, caution must be advised before extrapolating to individuals. In many areas, the differences may be, in part, explained by expectations or socialization. The results of group data may be totally inappropriate when applied to any individual girl.

When Hyde (1981) reexamined the cognitive abilities of girls compared with boys, she found that while there were consistent differences, they were quite small. Her research suggested that the attempt to determine cognitive abilities for an individual should best be conducted on that individual and not for the sex group. Tobias (1982) suggested that the differences that exist may actually result from socialization and the expectations that the girls have for their performance. This contention is supported by research that demonstrated that women college students could be quickly trained to perform as well as men in various visual-spatial tasks (Stericker & LeVesconte, 1982).

Much of the research on how children develop concepts, organize information, develop memory, and solve problems has not addressed gender-role relationships at all. Should we, then, conclude that no relationships exist? Making such an assumption in the face of the complexities of advanced cognitive behavior is undoubtedly insupportable. Instead, we must recognize that cognitive abilities are developed as part of the total functioning of girls. As a partner with the other characteristics and abilities, there will be influences both subtle and obvious based on biological structures and on social functioning. Research with people from various parts of the world has already demonstrated a relationship among thinking, language, and culture. Recent investigations also suggest that disadvantageous circumstances in environment or experience may have a demonstrable effect of attitudes toward learning and styles of interacting with other people (Rutter, 1985). Extrapolating from these general findings to understand the development of cognitive skills of girls leads us to expect that there will be an interaction of cognitive functioning with socialization experiences in ways that are not yet fully understood. However, the implications may be found in girls' responses and use of computers (Kiesler, Sproull & Eccles, 1985), their choices of careers (Reid & Stephens, 1985; see also chapter 17), and other expectations and applications of cognitive skills to social and behavioral interactions.

Adolescent Thought and Socialization

This interaction between cognition and socialization is most apparent in adolescence. Adolescents gain insight into their own behavior as well as the behaviors of others. They have a heightened ability for abstract, hypothetical reasoning. As a consequence of adolescents' ability to take account of others' thoughts and their preoccupation with their own, a type of egocentrism develops. Adolescents assume that other people are as interested in, and fascinated by, them and their behavior as they are themselves. There is thus a failure to distinguish between their personal concerns and the opinions of others. They conclude that other people are as accepting or as rejecting and critical as they are of themselves. They worry about having their inadequacies discovered by other people. This assumption about the opinions of people in their environment is referred to as the imaginary audience (Elkind, 1967). This is an audience for adolescents in that they feel they are the focus of attention; it is imaginary, however, in that other individuals are actually not that concerned with the adolescent's thoughts.

It is common for adolescents to use this imaginary audience as an internal sounding board for mentally adopting a variety of roles, behaviors, and attitudes. The imaginary audience also explains why adolescent girls are self-conscious about their clothing and body image, spend hours viewing themselves in front of mirrors, and feel painfully on display.

While absorbed with their own feelings, adolescents frequently believe that their emotions are unique and that such intense feelings have never been experienced by other people, certainly not their teachers and parents. This belief in their uniqueness becomes expressed as a subjective story they tell themselves about their special qualities. This subjective story is referred to by Elkind (1967) as the personal fable. Evidence of this personal fable is present in the diaries adolescents keep, in which they express their feelings of isolation.

These two aspects of egocentrism create an obstacle for adolescents in learning to understand other individuals' perspectives. Furthermore, the belief in their uniqueness gets translated into a conviction that they are not subject to the dangers suffered by others. Consequently, they may avoid using seat belts, drive too fast, binge and then purge, or dispense with using contraceptives, all out of the conviction that "nothing bad will happen to me."

This egocentrism does tend to fade when adolescents have the role-taking opportunities that will help to replace the imaginary audience with a real one and the subjective fable with an objective story. This usually occurs by the time they are 16 or 17. Adolescent girls may not be given such role-taking opportunities because of stereotypic beliefs about girls' becoming argumentative, independent, and assertive. Furthermore, the media and other socialization agents reinforce personal fables and imaginary audiences for adolescent girls through their romanticizing thinness, facial "make-overs," and fairy tale relationships.

Cultural Concerns and Issues

Thus, girls' and women's development must be viewed as taking place within a well-defined cultural and social context. During the past few decades increasing attention has been given to identifying and understanding these definitions. In recent years there has been a concerted effort to extend our understanding of the female experience beyond the presumed limits of white, middle-class contexts to investigate gender-role definitions that operate within Asian, black, and Hispanic American communities (Educators of Women of Color Collective, in preparation). Recently researchers have begun to identify normative patterns of behavior within a variety of social class conditions. These many worlds of girls and women are important for consideration if a complete understanding of the factors that influence developmental processes is to be established.

An important concern of researchers interested in understanding the processes that lead to gender-role development in girls is the use of the assumption of universality. Study after study repeats the fatal flaw by issuing conclusions about developmental processes that influence "girls or women," when in fact only one group, white girls or white women, has been observed. Serious consideration is certainly due the suggestion that there are often significant differences in the socialization experiences of ethnic minority girls. The choice to ignore the differences and to pretend that universality is the rule appears increasingly unacceptable. On the other hand, a total rejection of applicability of findings across cultural and/or racial groups is also unsound. A reasonable solution may be found in the recognition that various degrees of duality exist in the socialization process for ethnic minority girls. Minority group girls, like white girls in our society, are socialized to accept various expectations and roles for which parents, community institutions, and others prepare them (Lott, 1987; Reid, 1981). Girls, regardless of race, are expected to be interested in babies, to develop verbal skills, to be more nurturant, quieter, and more disciplined than boys. While these and many other similarities in girls' experiences may be identified, we must also recognize the differences for children in ethnic communities. The recognition includes understanding that the differences profoundly impact the way the lives of these girls evolve (Paludi, 1988). Each ethnic minority community has its unique set of expectations that has developed from a history, culture, and experience in this country. Typically, racism is an important component of that expectation. For its own survival and self-satisfaction each community will socialize its girls to meet the demands of growing up as an Asian or black or Native American or Hispanic woman. Care must be taken, therefore, in research or discussion to remember that female socialization is not necessarily a homogeneous process that all girls undergo. Efforts must be made to explicate the similarities and the unique differences of the process for girls with different experiences and not to refer to girls and women of color collectively (DeFour & Paludi, 1988).

Researchers must document the diversity of girls' and women's experiences and not reify an essentialist argument about gender-role identity (Fine, 1985).

REFERENCES

Antill, J. K., & Cunningham, J. D. (1982). Sex differences in performance on ability tests as a function of masculinity, femininity, and androgyny. *Journal of Personality and Social Psychology, 42*, 718–728.

Bandura, A., & Walters, R. (1963). *Social learning and personality development.* New York: Holt, Rinehart, & Winston.

Baruch, G. K., & Barnett, R. C. (1986). Fathers' participation in family work and children's sex-role attitudes. *Child Development, 57*, 1210–1223.

Basow, S. (1992). *Gender stereotypes and roles* (3rd ed.). Pacific Grove, CA: Brooks/ Cole.

Bem, S. L. (1981). Gender schema theory: A cognitive account of sex typing. *Psychological Review, 88*, 354–364.

Bem, S. L. (1983). Gender schema theory and its implications for child development: Raising gender-aschematic children in a gender-schematic society. *Signs, 8*, 598–616.

Benbow, C. P., & Stanley, J. C. (1983). Sex differences in mathematical reasoning: More facts. *Science, 222,* 1029–1031.

Bloch, M. N. (1987). The development of sex differences in young children's activities at home: The effect of the social context. *Sex Roles, 16,* 279–301.

Blyth, D., Simmons, R. G., & Zakin, D. F. (1985). Satisfaction with body image for early adolescent females: The impact of pubertal timing within different school environments. Special Issue: Time of maturation and psychosocial functioning in adolescence: I. *Journal of Youth and Adolescence, 14,* 207–225.

Boskind-Lohdal, M. (1976). Cinderella's stepsisters: A feminist perspective on anorexia nervosa and bulimia. *Signs, 2,* 120–146.

Bronstein, P., & Quina, K. (1988). *Teaching a psychology of people.* Washington, DC: American Psychological Association.

Bruch, H. (1978). *The golden cage: The enigma of anorexia nervosa.* Cambridge: Harvard University Press.

Carr, P. G., & Mednick, M. T. (1988). Sex role socialization and the development of achievement motivation in black preschool children. *Sex Roles, 18,* 169–180.

Casenave, N. A. (1979). Middle-income black fathers: An analysis of the provider role. *Family Coordinator, 27,* 583–592.

Clausen, J. (1975). The social meaning of differential physical and sexual maturation. In S. Dragastin & G. Elder (Eds.), *Adolescence in the life cycle* (pp. 25–47). Washington, DC: Hemisphere Press.

Connor, J. M., & Serbin, L. A. (1985). Visual-spatial skill: Is it important for mathematics? Can it be taught? In S. Chipman, L. Brush, & D. Wilson (Eds.), *Women and mathematics: Balancing the equation.* Hillsdale, NJ: Erlbaum.

Connor, J. M., Serbin, L. A., & Ender, R. A. (1978). Responses of boys and girls to aggressive, assertive, and passive behaviors of male and female characters. *Journal of Genetic Psychology, 133,* 59–69.

DeFour, D. C., & Paludi, M. A. (1988, March). *Integrating the scholarship on women of color and ethnicity into the psychology of women course.* Workshop presented at the Association for Women in Psychology, Bethesda, MD.

Delk, J. L., Madden, R. B., Livingston, M., & Ryan, T. T. (1986). Adult perceptions of the infant as a function of gender labelling and observer gender. *Sex Roles, 15,* 527–534.

Dickerson, D. P. (1982). *The role of black females in selected children's fiction.* Unpublished manuscript, Howard University, Washington, DC.

Doyle, J. A., & Paludi, M. A. (1990). *Sex and gender* (2nd ed.). Madison, WI: William C. Brown.

Duncan, P. (1985). The effects of pubertal timing on body image, school behavior, and deviance. Special Issue: Time of maturation and psychosocial functioning in adolescence: I. *Journal of Youth and Adolescence, 14,* 227–235.

Educators of Women of Color Collective. (in preparation). *The psychology of women: Enhancing sociocultural awareness.* Albany: SUNY Press.

Eichorn, D. (1963). Biological correlates of behavior. *Yearbook of the National Society for the Study of Education, 62,* 4–61.

Elkind, D. (1967). Egocentrism in adolescence. *Child Development, 38,* 1025–1034.

Fine, M. (1985). Reflections on a feminist psychology of women: Paradoxes and prospects. *Psychology of Women Quarterly, 9,* 167–183.

Freudinger, P., & Almquist, E. (1978). Male and female roles in the lyrics of three genres of contemporary music. *Sex Roles*, *4*, 51–65.

Frisch, R. (1984). Fatness, puberty, and fertility. In J. Gunn & A. M. Petersen (Eds.), *Girls at puberty*. New York: Plenum.

Gunn, J., & Petersen, A. (Eds.). (1984) *Girls at puberty: Biological, psychological and social perspectives*. New York: Plenum.

Hall, M., & Keith, R. A. (1964). Sex role preferences among children of upper and lower class. *Journal of Social Psychology*, *62*, 101–110.

Halliday, J., McNaughton, S., & Glynn, T. (1985). Influencing children's choice of play activities at kindergarten through teacher participation. *New Zealand Journal of Educational Studies*, *20*, 48–58.

Higham, E. (1980). Variations in adolescent psychohormonal development. In J. Adelson (Ed.), *Handbook of adolescent psychology*. New York: Wiley.

Hill, M. (1988). Child rearing attitudes of black lesbian mothers. In Boston Lesbian Psychologies Collective (Eds.), *Lesbian psychologies: Explorations and challenges*. Urbana: University of Illinois Press.

Hyde, J. S. (1981). How large are cognitive gender differences? A meta-analysis using w^2 and d. *American Psychologist*, *36*, 892–901.

Jacklin, C. N. (1989). Female and male: Issues of gender. *American Psychologist*, *44*, 127–133.

Jacklin, C. N., & Maccoby, E. E. (1983). Issues of gender differentiation. In M. D. Levine, W. B. Carey, A. C. Crocker, & P. T. Gross (Eds.), *Developmental-behavioral pediatrics*. Philadelphia: W. B. Saunders.

Jahoda, G. (1986). A cross-cultural perspective on developmental psychology. *International Journal of Behavioral Development*, *9*, 417–437.

Katchadorian, H. (1977). *The biology of adolescence*. San Francisco: Freeman.

Kiesler, S., Sproull, L., & Eccles, J. S. (1985). Pool halls, chips, and war games: Women in the culture of computing. *Psychology of Women Quarterly*, *9*, 451–462.

Kohlberg, L. (1976). Moral stages and moralization: The cognitive-development approach. In T. Lickona (Ed.), *Moral development and behavior*. New York: Holt, Rinehart, and Winston.

Linn, M. C., & Petersen, A. C. (1985). Emergence and characterization of gender differences in spatial ability: A meta-analysis. *Child Development*, *56*, 1479–1498.

Lips, H. M. (1988). *Sex and gender: An introduction*. Mountain View, CA: Mayfield.

Livson, N., & Peskin, H. (1980). Perspectives on adolescence from longitudinal research. In J. Adelson (Ed.), *Handbook of adolescent psychology*. New York: Wiley.

Lockheed, M. E., & Hall, K. P. (1976). Conceptualizing sex as a status characteristic and applications to leadership training strategies. *Journal of Social Issues*, *32*, 111–124.

Lott, B. (1987). *Women's lives: Themes and variations in gender learning*. Monterey, CA: Brooks/Cole.

Maccoby, E. E., & Jacklin, C. N. (1974). *The psychology of sex differences*. Stanford: Stanford University Press.

Marshall, J. (1981). *The sports doctors fitness book for women*. New York: Delacorte.

Matlin, M. W. (1993). *The psychology of women* (2d ed.). Orlando, FL: Harcourt, Brace, & Jovanovich.

Matthews, W. S. (1975, May). *Sex differences in the fantasy play of young children.*

Paper presented at the meeting of the New Jersey Psychological Association, Somerset, NJ.

Matthews, M. H. (1986a). Gender, graphicacy and geography. *Educational Review, 38,* 259–271.

Matthews, M. H., (1986b). The influence of gender on the environmental cognition of young boys and girls. *Journal of Genetic Psychology, 147,* 295–302.

Mayes, S., & Valentine, K. (1979). Sex-role stereotyping in Saturday morning cartoon shows. *Journal of Broadcasting, 23,* 41–50.

McArthur, L. Z., & Eisen, S. V. (1976). Achievements of male and female storybook characters as determinants of achievement behavior by boys and girls. *Journal of Personality and Social Psychology, 33,* 467–473.

McGhee, P. E., & Frueh, T. (1980). Television viewing and the learning of sex-role stereotypes. *Sex Roles, 6,* 179–188.

Money, J., & Ehrhardt, A. A. (1972). *Man and woman: Boy and girl.* Baltimore: Johns Hopkins University Press.

Money, J., & Tucker, P. (1975). *Sexual signatures: On being a man or a woman.* Boston: Little, Brown.

Mussen, P., Conger, J., & Kagen, J. (1963). *Child development and personality.* New York: Harper & Row.

Newman, B. M., & Newman, P. R. (1987). *Development through life.* Homewood, IL: Dorsey.

Newson, J., & Newson, E. (1968). *Four years old in an urban community.* Harmondsworth, England: Pelican Books.

Orbach, S. (1978). *Fat is a feminist issue.* New York: Berkeley.

Paludi, M. A. (1985). Sex and gender similarities and differences and the development of the young child. In C. McLouglin & D. F. Gullo (Eds.), *Young children in context: Impact of self, family, and society in development.* Springfield, MA: Charles C. Thomas.

Paludi, M. A. (1988, October). *Discussant's comments: Childhood.* Paper presented at the Gender Roles through the Lifespan Conference, Muncie, IN.

Paludi, M. A., & Gullo, D. F. (1986). Effect of sex labels on adults' knowledge of infant development. *Sex Roles, 16,* 19–30.

Parelius, A. P., & Parelius, R. (1978). *The sociology of education.* Englewood Cliffs, NJ: Prentice-Hall.

Petersen, A., & Taylor, B. (1980). The biological approach to adolescence. In J. Adelson (Ed.), *Handbook of adolescent psychology.* New York: Wiley.

Piaget, J. (1947). *The psychology of intelligence.* London: Routledge & Kegan Paul.

Price-Bonham, S., & Skeen, P. (1982). Black and white fathers' attitudes toward children's sex roles. *Psychological Reports, 50,* 1187–1190.

Quay, L. C., & Jarrett, O. S. (1986). Teachers' interactions with middle-and lower SES preschool boys and girls. *Journal of Educational Psychology, 78,* 495–498.

Rathus, S. A. (1983). *Human sexuality.* New York: Holt, Rinehart, & Winston.

Reid, P. T. (1979). Racial stereotyping on television. A comparison of the behavior of both black and white television characters. *Journal of Applied Psychology, 64,* 465–471.

Reid, P. T. (1981). Socialization of black female children. In P. Berman & E. Ramey (Eds.), *Woman: A developmental perspective* (pp. 137–156). Washington, DC: NIH Publication No. 82-2298.

Reid, P. T., & Stephens, D. (1985). The roots of future occupations in childhood: A review of the literature on girls and careers. *Youth and Society, 16*, 267–288.

Reid, P. T., Tate, C. S., & Berman, P. W. (1989). Preschool children's self-presentations in situations with infants: Effects of sex and race. *Child Development, 60*, 710–714.

Resnick, S. M., Gottesman, I. I., Berenbaum, S. A., & Bouchard, T. J. (1986). Early hormonal influences on cognitive functioning in congenital adrenal hyperplasia. *Developmental Psychology, 22*, 191–198.

Romer, N., & Cherry, D. (1980). Ethnic and social class differences in children's sex-role concepts. *Sex Roles, 6*, 245–263.

Rubin, J. Z., Provenzano, F. J., & Luria, Z. (1974). The eye of the beholder: Parents' views on sex of newborns. *American Journal of Orthopsychiatry, 44*, 512–519.

Ruble, D., Balaban, T., & Cooper, J. (1981). Gender constancy and the effects of sex-typed televised toy commercials. *Child Development, 52*, 667–673.

Ruble, D., & Brooks-Gunn, J. (1982). A developmental analysis of menstrual distress in adolescence. In R. C. Freedman (Ed.), *Behavior and the menstrual cycle.* New York: Marcel Dekker.

Russo, N. F. (1976). The motherhood mandate. *Journal of Social Issues, 32*, 143–153.

Rutter, M. (1985). Family and school influences on cognitive development. *Journal of Child Psychology and Psychiatry, 26*, 683–704.

Safir, M. P. (1986). The effects of nature or of nurture on sex differences in intellectual functioning: Israeli findings. *Sex Roles, 14*, 581–590.

Samelson, F. (1978). From "race psychology" to "studies in prejudice": Some observations on the thematic reversal in social psychology. *Journal of the History of the Behavioral Sciences, 14*, 65–78.

Schlesier-Stropp, B. (1984). Bulimia: A review of the literature. *Psychological Bulletin, 95*, 247–257.

Schowalter, J., & Anyan, W. (1981). *Family handbook of adolescence.* New York: Knopf.

Sedney, M. A. (1989). Conceptual and methodological sources of controversies about androgyny. In R. K. Unger (Ed.), *Representations: Social constructions of gender.* Amityville, NY: Baywood.

Serbin, L. A., O'Leary, D. D., Kent, R. N., & Tonick, J. J. (1973). A comparison of teacher response to the preacademic and problem behavior of boys and girls. *Child Development, 44*, 796–804.

Shaffer, D. R. (1989). *Developmental psychology: Childhood and adolescence* (2nd ed.). Pacific Grove, CA: Brooks/Cole.

Shields, S. (1975). Functionalism, Darwinism, and the psychology of women: A study in social myth. *American Psychologist, 30*, 739–754.

Smith, P. A., & Midlarsky, E. (1985). Empirically derived conceptions of femaleness and maleness: A current view. *Sex Roles, 12*, 313–328.

Stericker, A., & LeVesconte, S. (1982). Effect of brief training on sex-related differences in visual-spatial skill. *Journal of Personality and Social Psychology, 43*, 1018–1029.

Sternglanz, S. H., & Serbin, L. (1974). Sex role stereotyping in children's television programs. *Developmental Psychology, 10*, 710–715.

Tanner, J. (1962). *Growth at adolescence.* Oxford: Blackwell.

Ten Houten, W. D. (1970). The black family: Myth and reality. *Psychiatry, 33*, 145–173.

Tobias, S. (1982, January). Sexist equations. *Psychology Today*, pp. 14–17.

Tolmach, R., & Scherr, R. (1984). *Face value*. Boston: Routledge & Kegan Paul.

Unger, R. K. (1981). Sex as a social reality: Field and laboratory research. *Psychology of Women Quarterly, 5*, 645–653.

Waite, B., & Paludi, M. A. (1987). *Gender role stereotypes present in rock music videos*. Paper presented at the Midwestern Psychological Association, Chicago, IL.

Wallston, B. S., & Grady, K. E. (1985). Integrating the feminist critique and the crisis in social psychology: Another look at research methods. In V. E. O'Leary, R. K. Unger, & B. S. Wallston (Eds.), *Women, gender, and social psychology*. Hillsdale, NJ: Erlbaum.

Williams, J. E. (1982). An overview of findings from adult sex stereotype studies in 25 countries. In R. Rath, H. S. Asthana, D. Sinha, & J. B. H. Sinha (Eds.), *Diversity and unity in cross-cultural psychology*. Lisse, Netherlands: Swets & Zeitlinger.

7

Women in the Middle and Later Years

Claire Etaugh

This chapter examines the major characteristics and experiences of middle-aged and older women. To do so, we should first define what is meant by "middle age" and "old age." In fact, there is no firm consensus. Definitions given by economists, psychologists, and sociologists variously refer to the middle years as beginning anywhere between the ages of 25 and 45 and as ending somewhere between 54 and the end of one's work life (Giele, 1982b). Clearly, the boundaries of the middle and later years are quite flexible. No one biological or psychological event signals the beginning of middle or old age (Neugarten & Datan, 1974). Rather, there are a number of life events that often occur during these years, including marriage, childrearing, employment, grandparenting, retirement, and physical changes. It is important to realize that these events are not experienced by everyone, nor do they occur at the same age or in the same sequence (Brooks-Gunn & Kirsh, 1984). This chapter focuses on some of these key events in the lives of women in the middle and later years. We will look at physical changes, sex roles, family roles and relationships, and participation in higher education and the labor force.

PHYSICAL CHANGES

Physical Appearance

Physical appearance begins to change in midlife (Rossman, 1980; Whitbourne, 1985). The hair becomes thinner and grayer. Weight increases until about age 50 and declines somewhat after that. Fat becomes redistributed, decreasing in the face, legs, and lower arms and increasing in the abdomen, buttocks, and upper arms. Starting at about age 40, the discs between the spinal vertebrae begin to compress, resulting in an eventual loss in height of one to two inches. Bones become more brittle and porous, especially in women, sometimes resulting in the collapse of vertebrae and the appearance of a "dowager's hump." The skin becomes drier and, along with the muscles, blood vessels, and other tissues, begins to lose its elasticity. Wrinkles appear, and age spots may develop. Skin that has been exposed to the sun is affected most, particularly in light-skinned individuals (Selmanowitz, Rizer & Orentreich, 1977).

Double Standard of Aging

How do women react to the changes in physical appearance just described? In our youth-oriented society, the prospect of getting older generally is not relished by either sex. For women, however, the stigma of aging is greater than it is for men. This phenomenon, labeled the double standard of aging (Sontag, 1979), has been described this way:

Aging has traditionally been for women an unenviable prospect. Her most socially valued qualities, her ability to provide sex and attractive companionship and to have children and nurture them, are expressed in the context of youth, which is endowed with physical beauty and fertility. As she ages, she is seen as less physically attractive and desirable, and her reproductive and nurturant functions are no longer relevant . . . . Traditionally women have not been encouraged to develop those qualities that often improve with age, such as intellectual competence. (Williams, 1987, pp. 476–477)

On the other hand, as Sontag (1979) notes: " 'Masculinity' is identified with competence, autonomy, self-control—qualities which the disappearance of youth does not threaten. Competence in most of the activities expected from men, physical sports excepted, increases with age" (p. 464).

Thus, the same wrinkles and gray hair that may enhance the perceived status and attractiveness of an older man may be seen as diminishing the attractiveness and desirability of an older woman. Middle-aged women themselves are more critical of the appearance of middle-aged women than are men and women of other age groups (Nowak, 1977). Concern with one's appearance is characteristic of black as well as white women of middle age (Alston & Rose, 1981).

Mortality and Illness

In 1920, life expectancy for a woman was 54.6 years, one year longer than that for a man. By 1979, the difference between the sexes had increased to 7.8 years, although it has decreased slightly since then. In 1988, life expectancy was 78.9 for white women and 72.1 for men; the corresponding figures for black women and men were 73.8 and 65.1 (U.S. Bureau of the Census, 1990). Because women live longer than men, the ratio of female to males increases with age. In 1986, there were 83 men for every 100 women between the ages of 65 and 69 years. However, there were only 40 men for every 100 women 85 and over (U.S. Senate, 1987–1988). Both biological and environmental explanations have been proposed to account for the sex difference in longevity. Genetic and hormonal factors have been cited as increasing females' resistance to certain diseases, including cardiovascular disease (Turner, 1982; Woodruff-Pak, 1988). Differences in the behaviors and life-styles of women and men are thought to be even more critical in determining sex differences in longevity. Cigarette smoking, more common in men than women, is responsible for some of the female-male mortality difference (Turner, 1982). Since 1960, however, as the proportion of women smokers has increased, lung cancer mortality rates in older women have gone up (Kart, Metress & Metress, 1988; Nathanson & Lorenz, 1982). Deaths resulting from accidents, suicide, and cirrhosis of the liver, which are more prevalent among males, are attributed to behaviors such as aggression, risk-taking, and alcohol consumption, which are more socially encouraged in males (Turner, 1982). The overrepresentation of males in dangerous occupations is another environmental variable cited to explain the sex difference in longevity. Still another contributing factor may be the more frequent use of health services by women (Kart et al., 1988).

Among women 45–64 years of age, the leading cause of death is cancer, followed by heart disease, cerebrovascular accidents, and pulmonary diseases. Men have a higher mortality rate than women in each of these categories. The mortality rates for nonwhite women are greater than those for white women for all major causes of death (U.S. Bureau of the Census, 1990). It may be that nonwhite women have less access to health services or are exposed to more hazardous working conditions (DeLorey, 1984).

While death rates are higher for men, women have higher rates of reported illness at all ages, with black women reporting more illness than white women. Compared with men, middle-aged and older women have higher rates of arthritis and rheumatism, diabetes, hypertension, osteoporosis, and visual impairments. Men are more likely to have respiratory problems, hernias, and hearing impairments (Edinburg, 1982; Kart et al., 1988). Women of all ages are more likely than men to report that they limited their activities or went to bed because of illness (Nathanson & Lorenz, 1982). Men, on the other hand, are more likely to report limitation of major work activities resulting from chronic conditions (Turner, 1982). Are women actually ill more frequently than men? Older men are more likely than women to deny signs of illness (Turner, 1982). Furthermore, women are more likely to express fear and worries, to be sensitive to symptoms of illness, and to get physical examinations (Nathanson & Lorenz, 1982). These findings suggest that women may be more apt to report illness and to seek treatment for it. Such factors would tend to exaggerate estimates of actual sex differences in illness.

Menopause

Menopause is defined as the cessation of menstruation. It is generally said to have occurred when no menstrual periods have occurred for a full year (Woods, 1982). Typically, the months preceding the beginning of menopause are marked by increasing irregularity of the menstrual cycle and variations in the quantity of menstrual flow (Voda & Eliasson, 1983). For American women, the average age of menopause is approximately 50 years (Archer, 1982; Friederich, 1982).

Menopause occurs because of the decline in the number of ovarian follicles (egg-producing cells), which results in a decline in the production of both estrogen and progesterone (Archer, 1982). Some estrogen continues to be produced after menopause by the adrenal glands and fat cells (Archer, 1982; Millette & Hawkins, 1983).

There is considerable disagreement concerning the frequency and severity of physical symptoms associated with menopause. The most commonly reported symptom is the hot flash, characterized by a sudden feeling of warmth, reddening of the skin, and occasional perspiration (Voda & Eliasson, 1983). Estimates of the prevalence of hot flashes range from 30 to 93% of menopausal women (Nathanson & Lorenz, 1982; Woods, 1982). The vaginal lining becomes thinner, and vaginal lubrication decreases, which may lead to painful sexual intercourse (Voda & Eliasson, 1983). Headaches, fatigue, joint pains, and tingling sensations are other physical symptoms that are occasionally reported (Woods, 1982). It should be kept in mind, however, that anywhere between 16 and 80% of women studied have reported having no menopausal symptoms (DeLorey, 1984; Woods, 1982).

The most serious physical consequence of menopause is osteoporosis, an excessive loss of bone tissue in older adults that results in the bones becoming thinner, brittle, and more porous (Whitbourne, 1985). Fractures are more likely to occur, causing not only decreased mobility but even death. For example, about 12% of hip fracture victims die of complications (Culliton, 1987).

At least 15 million people in the United States have osteoporosis (Silberner, 1987). Women are at greater risk than men, particularly in the first 8 to 10 years after menopause, when bone mass decreases sharply. Total skeletal mass decreases by 20 to 30% in the 20 years following menopause (Heaney, 1987). Thin white women, particularly those with fair skin and hair, are at greatest risk for osteoporosis. Other risk factors include a family history of osteoporosis, early menopause, cigarette smoking, excessive consumption of alcohol, caffeine and protein, low calcium intake, corticosteroid use, and lack of exercise (Culliton, 1987; Heaney, 1987). The National Institute of Health recommends consumption of 1000 milligrams of calcium a day for all adults and 1500 milligrams for postmenopausal women in order to suppress bone loss (Culliton, 1987).

Estrogen, another key factor in retarding bone loss after menopause, may be even more critical than calcium (Riis, Thomsen & Christiansen, 1987). Estrogen is the most widely used treatment for menopausal symptoms, not only retarding bone loss, as noted above, but alleviating hot flashes and vaginal dryness (Friederich, 1982; Voda & Eliasson, 1983). Furthermore, it may reduce mortality from cardiovascular disease in postmenopausal women (Culliton, 1987). Nevertheless, evidence accumulating since the mid-1970s indicates that estrogen replacement therapy also increases the risk of blood clots and uterine cancer (Archer, 1982; DeLorey, 1984; Voda & Eliasson, 1983). Currently, because of these risks, estrogen is less frequently prescribed, the doses used are smaller, and it is sometimes combined with progesterone, which may minimize negative side effects (Archer, 1982; DeLorey, 1984; Friederich, 1982). Unfortunately, recent research indicates that this combination therapy may increase the risk of breast cancer (Kolata, 1989). However, a new treatment for osteoporosis involving the drug etidronate combined with calcium appears to be safer and even more effective than hormone therapy (Altman, 1990).

In addition to the physical symptoms sometimes associated with menopause, it is popularly believed that menopausal women also are more likely to display such psychological symptoms as depression, irritability, or mood swings. There is no evidence, however, that these or other psychological symptoms are more prevalent among menopausal women (Archer, 1982; Lennon, 1987; Nathanson & Lorenz, 1982; Perlmutter & Bart, 1982). Even if some women do show heightened psychological distress during the menopausal years, this cannot be attributed solely to biological processes. Changes in social roles that occur in midlife may be largely responsible for increased distress (Lennon, 1987; McKinlay, McKinlay & Brambilla, 1987). Women not only are confronting their own aging during this time, but also may be coping with the illness or death of a spouse, divorce or separation, difficult teenagers, children who are preparing to leave home, and/or aging parents who increasingly require care (McKinlay et al., 1987; Voda & Eliasson, 1983).

A woman who expects menopause to be unpleasant may focus upon its negative aspects (Perlmutter & Bart, 1982). But most middle-aged American women minimize the significance of menopause. In a classic series of studies done in the 1960s, Neugarten and Datan (1974) found that women in their mid-40s to mid-50s viewed menopause as only a temporary inconvenience. Many looked forward to menopause as marking the end of menstruation and childbearing. Interestingly, younger women had more negative views of menopause than did middle-aged and older women. More recent research confirms that middle-aged women generally have positive attitudes toward menopause and do not view it as an illness (Black & Hill, 1984; Frey, 1981; Millette, 1981).

Sexuality

Changes in sexual physiology occur with aging. Less muscle tension develops during sexual arousal, and orgasmic contractions decrease in number and intensity. Although clitoral response apparently does not change with age, we have already seen that lowered estrogen levels lead to thinning and shrinking of the vaginal wall and decreased vaginal secretions. These conditions can result in painful intercourse (Masters, Johnson & Kolodny, 1985).

Research on the sexuality of postmenopausal women has produced inconsistent results. While some studies indicate a decline in sexual interest and the capacity for orgasm during these years, others have found the opposite pattern (Masters et al., 1985). Clearly, changes in sexual physiology and hormonal levels are not the only factors determining female sexuality in the middle and later years.

The extent of sexual activity in middle-aged women is strongly influenced by past sexual enjoyment and experience (Luria & Meade, 1984). Williams (1987) points out a number of reasons postmenopausal women may show increased sexual interest. One reason is freedom from fear of pregnancy, a factor that probably is particularly salient for older cohorts of women for whom highly effective birth control methods were not available during their fertile years. A second reason cited by Williams is increased marital satisfaction during the "empty nest" years. Rubin (1979), in a study of midlife women, found that most reported greater sexual interest and pleasure with increasing age. Similarly, a survey of about 1,800 middle-class women over age 50 found 91% to be interested in sex and 84% to be coitally active (Corby & Brecher, 1984).

Most studies have found that although sexual activity continues well into old age for both women and men, the overall frequency of activity declines. This decrease results from a number of factors, including health problems, lack of a partner, and cultural stereotypes that view sexuality among the elderly in a negative light (Masters et al., 1985). Because older women are much more likely than men to become widowed (see discussion later in this chapter) and because available men tend to seek out younger women, older women are much more likely than men to be without a partner.

It is important to keep in mind that the information reported here on sexuality in middle-aged and older women is derived from studies of women who grew up when attitudes toward female sexuality were much less permissive and women's sexual behavior was more restricted. In recent years, sexual behaviors and attitudes of women have become increasingly liberal (Hunt, 1974). Thus, as today's young women move into midlife and beyond, their patterns of sexual behavior may differ somewhat from those of today's middle-aged and older women.

SEX ROLES IN MIDLIFE

As both women and men move into the middle and later years, research indicates that they often become more androgynous; that is, they are more likely to display both feminine and masculine psychological characteristics. Women in many societies, including our own, appear to become more assertive, independent, and accepting of aggressive and egocentric feelings, while men seem to become less domineering and more receptive to feelings of nurturance and affiliation (Gutmann, 1975, 1977; Lowenthal, Thurnher & Chiriboga, 1975;

Neugarten & Associates, 1964). Gutmann (1975, 1977) has labeled this shift the "normal unisex of later life." He attributes the change to the decline of the "parental imperative." Gutmann believes that sex-role differences are heightened in young adulthood because of parenting responsibilities. Mothers specialize in the role of nurturer and fathers in the role of provider. When children are grown, parents can express the other-sex characteristics that were repressed earlier.

A variety of other explanations have been proposed for the shift to greater androgyny in midlife, ranging from women's increased participation in the labor force (McGee & Wells, 1982) to changes in the balance of the sex hormones (Rossi, 1980). A variety of life experiences can influence changes in sex-role behavior, and not everyone becomes more androgynous with age (Hyde & Phillis, 1979; Sinnott, 1982). Both androgynous and more traditionally feminine women may show good mental health in middle age. A key factor appears to be the fit between a woman's personality and her chosen life-style (Livson, 1981).

FAMILY ROLES AND RELATIONSHIPS

Marriage

For most women and men, marriage is viewed as the most natural and desirable marital status (Duberman, 1974). Fully 94% of all American women marry at some time in their lives (U.S. Bureau of Census, 1990).

Marital satisfaction typically is high for women in the early years of marriage (Campbell, Converse, & Rodgers, 1976). By middle age, however, men appear to be more satisfied with their marriages than are women (Lowenthal et al., 1975; Rhyne, 1981; Veroff & Feld, 1970). Additionally, marriage appears to be more beneficial to men than to women (Bernard, 1972; Peplau & Gordon, 1985). For example, married men enjoy better mental health than married women, while unmarried women (including the never-married, divorced, and widowed) have better mental health than their male counterparts (Gove, 1972; Gove & Geerken, 1977; Radloff, 1975). Why is marriage more stressful for women than for men? For one thing, marriage entails a greater loss of autonomy and independence for women (Frieze, Parsons, Johnson, Ruble, & Zellman, 1977). Gove (1972) suggests several other factors. First, a married man has two primary sources of gratification—his family and his work. A married woman who does not work, however, may have no alternative source of gratification to turn to if her family roles are unfulfilling. In addition, women who are full-time homemakers may be frustrated by the monotony, low status, and lack of structure of the housewife role. Even if a woman is employed, she may well be a victim of sex discrimination in the workplace and find herself in a menial, low-paying job.

Furthermore, women still do most of the child care and housework even if they are employed (Berardo, Shehan & Leslie, 1987; Douthitt, 1989; Maret &

Finlay, 1984; Nyquist, Slivken, Spence & Helmreich, 1985; Pleck, 1985). Estimates of time spent on housework range from 3.2 to 4.8 hours per day for employed wives compared to 1.1 to 1.7 hours for employed husbands (Abdel-Ghany & Nichols, 1983; Lawrence, Draughn, Tasker & Wozniak, 1987; Robinson, 1977; Walker & Woods, 1976).

Motherhood

The fertility rate (that is, the average number of births a woman will have in her lifetime based on present birthrates) declined in the United States throughout the early 20th century, reaching a low point of 2.2 births during the depression years of the late 1930s. The "baby boom" following World War II peaked in the late 1950s, when the fertility rate reached 3.7. After that, the fertility rate gradually dropped to 1.8 in the mid-1970s, where it has remained since. Hispanic women have the highest fertility rate, followed in descending order by black women and white women (U.S. Bureau of the Census, 1988, 1990).

Women not only are having fewer children, but also are having them later. Between 1960 and 1988, the percentage of ever-married women between 20 and 24 years of age with no children grew from 24% to 42%. For 25-to-29-year-old ever-married women, the percentage who were childless grew during this period from 13% to 29%. Even among 30-to-34-year-olds, who are approaching the end of their childbearing years, 17% had no children in 1988, compared with only 8% in 1970 (U.S. Bureau of the Census, 1975, 1990). As in the case of delayed marriage, this trend may indicate that many women have decided not only to postpone motherhood, but to remain childless.

Why are more women choosing to have no children? Career and income factors often are key considerations in making this decision (Silka & Kiesler, 1977). In some instances, having grown up in a less-than-ideal family environment also may be involved. One study, for example, found that women who decided early (even before marriage) not to have children reported more psychological distance and incompatibility between themselves and their parents and less warmth in their families when they were growing up (Houseknecht, 1979).

Despite the fact that more women are deciding not to have children, the majority do become mothers. In 1988, for example, 90% of all ever-married American women between the ages of 40 and 44 had had at least one child (U.S. Bureau of the Census, 1990). Motherhood still is considered to be a central component of a woman's life, a concept that has been labeled the "motherhood mandate" (Russo, 1979). This mandate is so powerful that couples who choose to remain child-free are often perceived as selfish, immature, poorly adjusted, and unhappy (Peterson, 1983; Veevers, 1973).

Motherhood can be extremely fulfilling, although it is often stressful as well. In a recent study, 90% of parents said that if they could relive their lives, they would have children again (Yankelovich, 1981). Yet the ɩ ɩrth of the first child can create considerable strain. The new mother is expecteɹ to be the infant's primary caretaker, a time-consuming and exhausting job for which she usually has no formal preparation. The new child places an added economic burden on the couple as well and to some extent disrupts the husband-wife relationship. Indeed, married couples without children report greater happiness and marital satisfaction than do married couples with children (Campbell et al., 1976). Studies of marital satisfaction over the life span indicate that satisfaction is highest for young married couples with no children. Satisfaction drops after the birth of the first child and is at its lowest during the years when children are preschoolers and again when they are teenagers. As children get older, marital happiness begins to increase again. It continues to grow after the children have left home, almost reaching the peak level of the early "honeymoon" years (Anderson, Russell & Schumm, 1983; Antonucci, Tamir & Dubnoff, 1980; Campbell, 1981). This latter finding appears to contradict the popular notion that women become depressed when their children leave home (the so-called empty nest syndrome). Some women do react negatively to the departure of children; they tend to be women who were extremely child-centered, developing few other interests or extrafamilial activities during their lives (Bart, 1971; Lehr, 1984). Most women, however, are not distressed by the departure of their children. In fact, a number of studies indicate that women whose children have left home are happier, less depressed, and more satisfied with their marriages than women of similar age with a child living at home (Glenn, 1975; Radloff, 1975, 1980).

Overall, does motherhood contribute to a woman's sense of happiness and well-being? Research indicates that it does not (Baruch, Barnett & Rivers, 1983; Campbell et al., 1976; Glenn & McLanahan, 1981; Veroff, Douvan & Kulka, 1981). Even among widows between 60 and 75 years old, having children was found to enhance life satisfaction only slightly (Beckman & Houser, 1982). Baruch (1984) suggests that one reason for these somewhat surprising findings is that the rewards of parenting experienced by some are counteracted by the disappointments and frustrations experienced by others.

Relationships with Adult Children and Aging Parents

Middle-aged adults are often referred to as the "caught" or "squeeze" generation because of the responsibilities that they assume both for their adolescent and young adult children and for their aging parents (Lang & Brody, 1983; Stueve & O'Donnell, 1984). Middle-aged women carry out most of the caregiving and support functions. Families tend to be linked through their female members, who have closer ties with each other than with male members (Troll & Bengtson, 1982; Troll, 1987). Middle-aged and older women are more likely than men or younger women to worry about the well-being of their children, husbands, parents, and other family members (Turner, 1982). Additionally, they report more family conflicts and stresses than do men (Lehr, 1984).

Middle-aged women are more likely than men to use their adult children as confidants (Hagestad, 1984). Middle-aged mothers expect more interaction and help from their daughters than from their sons (Wood, Traupmann & Hay, 1984). At the same time, more middle-aged parents are providing assistance and support for the increasing number of young adults who are staying at home or returning home for financial reasons or following divorce (Turner, 1982).

Middle-aged women also maintain ties with, and provide care for, their elderly parents. About three-quarters of older adults see at least one of their adult children once a week or more (Aizenberg & Treas, 1985). The extent of assistance provided may range from no help at all (either because none is needed or because it is provided by others) to around-the-clock care including household maintenance, transportation, cooking, shopping, and personal and medical care (Aizenberg & Treas, 1985; Lang & Brody, 1983). Again, it is the daughter or daughter-in-law who typically provides such services (Horowitz, 1985; Stone, Cafferata & Sangl, 1987). Demographic changes in recent years appear to be increasing the parent-care responsibilities of middle-aged women. More parents are living well into old age, and their caregiving children themselves are becoming old. Furthermore, as the birthrate declines, there are fewer siblings to share the burden of the care. Finally, middle-aged women are increasingly likely to be employed, adding to their list of competing roles and responsibilities (Lang & Brody, 1983; Stueve & O'Donnell, 1984).

Grandmotherhood

The stereotyped portrayal of a grandmother is often that of an elderly, white-haired woman providing treats for her young grandchildren (Hagestad, 1985; Robertson, 1977). However, grandmothers do not fit into any one pattern. While approximately 75% of Americans over age 65 are grandparents (Harris & Associates, 1975), some people become grandparents as early as their late 20s (Burton & Bengtson, 1985). Many middle-aged grandmothers are in the labor force and may also have responsibilities for caring for their elderly parents (Troll, 1980). Thus, they may have less time to devote to grandparenting activities.

As noted earlier, the ties between family generations are maintained largely by women. One example is the finding that grandmothers tend to have warmer relationships with their grandchildren than do grandfathers. Grandmothers appear to be especially close to the daughters of their daughters (Hagestad, 1985).

Many different grandparenting styles have been identified. Neugarten and Weinstein (1964) described five types. The formal grandparent provides occasional treats and baby-sitting and maintains a constant interest in the grandchild, but does not offer childrearing advice. The funseeker grandparent has an informal, playful relationship with the grandchild. The surrogate parent, typically a grandmother, takes care of the grandchild when the mother is employed. The reservoir of family wisdom, typically a grandfather, dispenses skills or resources. The distant figure is benevolent, but sees the grandchild only infrequently on holidays and special occasions.

More recently, Robertson (1977) has developed a different classification of grandparenting styles, based on a study of 125 grandmothers. The apportioned type has high social and personal expectations of the grandmother role. She is concerned about doing what is morally right for her grandchildren (the social aspect) and also emphasizes indulging them (the personal aspect). The symbolic type is primarily concerned with the moral or social aspect, but not the personal one. The individualized type emphasizes the personal aspect but not the moral one. Finally, the remote type places little emphasis on either the social or personal aspects of grandparenthood.

Still another way of categorizing grandparents, offered by Cherlin and Furstenberg (1985), is based on the extent to which grandparents exchange services, help, or chores with their teenaged grandchildren, and the extent to which they exert influence (i.e., discipline, advice) over them. Grandparents with a high degree of both exchange and influence are labeled influential; those high only on exchange are called supportive; those high only on influence are referred to as authoritative. Grandparents who are low in both areas are called passive if they see the grandchild at least once or twice a month and are called detached if contact is less frequent.

A slightly different approach is taken by Kivnick (1983), who examined the meaning of grandparenthood among a group of grandparents, most of them women. Five dimensions of grandparenthood emerged: (1) centrality, in which grandparenthood was central to grandparents' lives; (2) valued elder, involving passing on family and cultural traditions; (3) immortality through clan, involving feelings of immortality achieved through descendants; (4) reinvolvement with personal past, in which grandparents relived their earlier lives and identified with their own grandparents; and (5) indulgence, characterized by attitudes of lenience and indulgence toward grandchildren.

Differences in grandparenting styles are determined by many factors. Age is one of these. Formal (Neugarten & Weinstein, 1964) and passive/detached (Cherlin & Furstenberg, 1985) types are more likely to be found among older (over age 65) grandparents, whereas funseeker (Neugarten & Weinstein, 1964) and influential (Cherlin & Furstenberg, 1985) types are more common in younger grandparents. The effect of becoming a grandmother at a very young age is illustrated in a study of black grandmothers (Burton & Bengtson, 1985). Those who became grandmothers in their late 20s and 30s often were reluctant to accept the role, unlike the women who became grandmothers in their 40s and 50s.

The grandparenting role appears to vary somewhat among racial and ethnic groups, although no consistent patterns have emerged. Bengtson (1985) reported that black and white grandparents were very similar in activities and attitudes. Compared with these two groups, Mexican-American grandparents had more contact with their grandchildren and reported more satisfying relationships with them. Cherlin & Furstenberg (1985), on the other hand, found marked differences in the styles of black and white grandparents, with blacks much more likely to assume an authoritative or influential role. This was true whether the grandchildren were living in one-parent or two-parent homes. Black grandparents also were much more likely than whites to have raised children other than their own and to have maintained contact with nonrelated "grandchildren" (Bengston, 1985).

Divorce

An increasing number of American women and men are experiencing divorce, single parenting, and remarriage (Hetherington & Camara, 1984; Hetherington, Stanley-Hagan & Anderson, 1989). The ratio of divorced to married people increased from 47 per 1,000 in 1970 to 133 per 1,000 in 1988 (U.S. Bureau of the Census, 1990). The divorce rate for black families is approximately twice that of white families (McNett, Taylor, & Scott, 1985). While there are indications that the divorce rate leveled off in the 1980s, it is estimated that as many as 60% of women who were in their 30s in 1985 eventually will divorce (Norton & Moorman, 1987). The rising divorce rate has been largely responsible for an increase in the number of one-parent households, 90% of which are headed by the mother. In 1984, 44% of black families, 23% of Hispanic families, and 13% of white families were headed by women (National Commission, 1986). Between 1970 and 1986, the percentage of children living with only one parent doubled from 12% to 24%. In 1988, 13% of children under the age of 18 were living with a divorced or separated mother, and under 3% with a divorced or separated father. The comparable figures for 1970 were 8% and less than 1% (U.S. Bureau of the Census, 1990). Of those individuals who divorce, about 75% of women and nearly 85% of men remarry. Approximately half of these remarriages occur within three years after the divorce (Cherlin, 1981).

As Bee (1987) notes, reactions to divorce vary considerably. In one study of adults who had divorced 10 to 15 years earlier, 13% of women and 20% of men described their divorce as "relatively painless," and 40% of both sexes reported it to be "stressful but bearable," while 27% of women and 16% of men described it as "traumatic, a nightmare" (Albrecht, 1980). Women who are more dependent, more traditionally oriented, and older have greater difficulty coping with the change in role from that of married to divorced person (Brown & Manela, 1978; Chiriboga, 1982; Chiriboga, Roberts & Stein, 1978; Granvold, Pedler & Schellie, 1979; Hetherington, Cox & Cox, 1982).

Divorced women experience stress in several areas. For one thing, divorced persons in our society are perceived in an unflattering light: they are considered to be less stable, less responsible, less reliable, less satisfied, and less well adjusted than married individuals (Etaugh & Malstrom, 1981; Etaugh & Petroski, 1985; Etaugh & Stern, 1984; Etaugh & Study, 1989). Divorced women (and men) do, in fact, frequently experience emotional upheaval right before the divorce and during the following year (Albrecht, 1980; Kolevson & Gottlieb, 1983). They report feeling more anxious, depressed, angry, rejected, and incompetent (Hetherington & Camara, 1984; Hetherington et al., 1982).

There are practical problems for divorced women as well. Financial burdens are increased, as are the responsibilities of running a household (Hetherington et al., 1982; Weiss, 1979). Income drops sharply for women with children following marital dissolution. A recent national study (Weiss, 1984) found that income was reduced by approximately one-third for middle-income mothers and by about one-fourth for lower-income mothers. Since the mother usually is the custodial parent, she must take on not only the major responsibilities of raising her children and supporting them financially, but also any household responsibilities formerly carried out by her husband. Consequently, role overload is a frequent problem (Hetherington et al., 1982). In addition, social life often is curtailed. Mothers may feel isolated from adult contacts, especially if they are not employed. Problems in parent-child relationships also may occur initially. Hetherington and her colleagues (1982) found that in the year following divorce, parents communicated less well with their children, were less affectionate, and were more inconsistent in discipline than were married parents. Mothers of sons experienced more problems than mothers of daughters. By the end of the second year following the divorce, the various emotional, economic, household, social, and parent-child stresses had diminished, and most parents and children had adapted reasonably well to their lives. Relationships between divorced mothers and their sons still were problematic six years after the divorce, however (Hetherington, 1989).

Support from family and friends is important in helping both women and men adjust to divorce (Cherlin & Furstenberg, 1986; Colletta, 1979; Hetherington et al., 1982; Weiss, 1975). Having a supportive, intimate relationship also enhances feelings of life satisfaction in the years following divorce (Spanier & Furstenberg, 1986).

Widowhood

Despite the increasing divorce rate, most marriages are terminated not by divorce, but by the death of a spouse. Women are much more likely to become widowed than are men, since women not only have a longer life expectancy but also tend to marry men older than themselves. As of 1988, there were 11.2 million widows but only 2.3 million widowers in this country, a ratio of about five to one. About 66% of women over the age of 75, but only 24% of men the same age are widowed (U.S. Bureau of the Census, 1990). Remarriage rates are much higher for widowers than for widows. Widowed men over 65, for example, are eight times more likely to remarry than are widows of the same age (Carter & Glick, 1976). One reason for the higher remarriage rate of widowers is that unmarried older women greatly outnumber unmarried older men. In 1988, for instance, there were 27 unmarried men aged 65 and over for every 100 unmarried women in that age category (U.S. Bureau of the Census, 1990). Furthermore, since men tend to marry women younger than themselves, the pool of potential mates expands for an older man but shrinks for an older woman.

A woman's reaction to widowhood depends upon many factors, including her age, the degree of forewarning of the spouse's death, and her financial, social, and personal resources. Compared with the young widow, the older widow is more likely to be financially secure, to have no child care responsibilities, to have friends in similar circumstances, and to be more psychologically prepared for the death of herself and her spouse (Treas, 1983). Studies comparing the mental and physical health of older widows and older married women generally have not found any differences between these groups (Heyman & Gianturco, 1973; Pihlblad & Adams, 1972). Younger widows, however, appear to experience greater difficulties than older widows in coping with their situation (Ball, 1976–1977). In addition to the reasons mentioned above, one reason for the greater distress experienced by young widows may be the greater likelihood that the husband's death was unexpected. In a longitudinal study of widows and widowers younger than 45 years of age, Parkes and Weiss (1983) found that those persons whose spouses died with little or no forewarning had greater difficulty accepting the reality of the death and felt more anger and guilt than those who had knowledge of the impending death.

Widowhood often results in a substantial reduction in financial resources for women, not only because the husband's income ceases, but also because considerable expenses may be incurred during the husband's final illness (Barrett, 1977; Thompson, 1980). Elderly women, especially those living alone, are more likely than elderly men to live in poverty. Older minority women are in even more dire financial straits than white women (Hess & Waring, 1983; Lott, 1987; Markson & Hess, 1980).

Loneliness is one of the greatest problems of widowhood. Most research has found that widowhood increases social isolation (Barrett, 1977). Among widows, loneliness is related to having few social supports (Lopata, Heinemann, & Baum, 1982; Rook, 1984). While support from their children may enhance the psychological well-being of widows (McGloshen & O'Bryant, 1988), social contact with friends and neighbors has an even more positive impact (Peplau, Bikson, Rook & Goodchilds, 1982).

The importance of economic, social, and personal resources in a woman's adaptation to widowhood has been shown in a series of studies by Lopata (1973, 1975, 1979, 1980). She classified widows in terms of their degree of reengagement in social activities. At one extreme was the active, engaged woman, who initiated changes and retained control of her life after her spouse's death. She was likely to have a greater income, a higher educational level, and more friends than other groups of widows. Another type of widow lived in an essentially sexsegregated world, often in an ethnic community. She frequently continued to remain involved with her neighbors, relatives, and church group. At the other extreme was the widow who became a social isolate. She often had a low educational level and had married a man of similar status upon whom she became quite dependent. Lacking adequate financial resources and the skills needed to successfully reengage in social activities after her husband's death, she became withdrawn and isolated.

Evidence from a large number of studies indicates that men suffer more than women from the death of a spouse, as measured by incidence of psychological depression, psychiatric disorders, physical illness, death rates, and suicide rates (Stroebe & Stroebe, 1983). Moreover, death rates of widowed men who remarry are lower than those of men who do not, whereas death rates do not differ for women who do or do not remarry (Helsing, Szklo & Comstock, 1981). Why are widows better able to cope with the death of a spouse? Stroebe and Stroebe (1983) suggest that social supports serve as critical buffers against the stresses of widowhood. They note that women are more apt both to admit a need for support and to have developed broad social networks with friends and relatives.

It is important to note that our knowledge of widows has been obtained primarily from older women, most of whom have had traditional marriages. When the young women of today become widows, they will be more likely to have had a college education and occupational experience than the current population of widows, better preparing them for a healthy adjustment to widowhood (Perlmutter & Hall, 1985).

Singlehood

The average age at first marriage for women has increased from 20.6 in 1970 to 23.3 years in 1988 (U.S. Bureau of the Census, 1990). Moreover, in the age group in which women and men have typically married (20–24 years old), the percentage of never-married women increased sharply from 36% in 1970 to 61% in 1988. Over the same period of time, the percentage of never-married women of ages 30–34 increased from 6% to 16% (U.S. Bureau of the Census, 1990). The percentage of never-married black women is even higher than that for white women at most ages (Braito & Anderson, 1983). These trends suggest not only that women are postponing marriage, but that an increasing number of them may never marry.

What are the reasons for this change in marriage patterns? One explanation is that the growth of educational opportunities for women has given them alternatives to the traditional life pattern and that more women are delaying their roles as wife (and mother) in order to pursue educational and career goals. Another factor is the greater incidence and acceptance of unmarried couples living together (Van Dusen & Sheldon, 1976).

Society's attitudes toward those who remain single is changing as well. In 1957, 80% of Americans labeled those who do not marry as "sick," "neurotic," or "immoral"; by 1981, only 25% felt this way (Yankelovich, 1981). Negative stereotypes still persist, however. Middle-aged people who have never married are perceived as less sociable, less likable, less attractive, and less well adjusted than middle-aged married individuals (Etaugh & Malstrom, 1981; Etaugh & Petroski, 1985; Etaugh & Stern, 1984), although they are not viewed as less professionally competent (Etaugh & Foresman, 1983; Etaugh & Riley, 1983).

To be sure, there are some disadvantages to the single life. American society is couples-oriented, and the single person may feel left out and lonely (Baruch et al., 1983; Loewenstein et al., 1981; Cargan & Melko, 1982; Parlee, 1979).

There are a number of advantages to being single, however. These include personal freedom, opportunities for career development, and the availability of privacy (Edwards, 1977; Stein, 1975). Another frequently mentioned advantage of being a single woman is a sense of self-sufficiency and competency (Donelson, 1977). Single middle-aged women, compared with married women, view themselves as more independent and assertive, and they place greater value on personal growth and achievement (Baruch et al., 1983).

Singlehood appears to be a more advantageous state for women than for men. Compared with single men, single women are happier (Campbell, 1975) and have better mental health (Gove, 1972). Furthermore, single women have higher levels of education, occupational status, and earnings than do married women, whereas this pattern is reversed for men (Hudis, 1976; Spreitzer & Riley, 1974; Treiman & Terrell, 1975). Among single women themselves, life satisfaction is associated with being healthy, not being lonely, living with a female housemate, having some intimate and many casual friendships, and being highly involved with work (Loewenstein et al., 1981). Additionally, single women holding high-status jobs have greater feelings of mastery and pleasure than those in lower-status jobs (Baruch et al., 1983).

About 5% of all adults over the age of 65 have never been married (U.S. Bureau of the Census, 1990). They are not especially lonely in old age, and their life satisfaction is similar to that of married older adults. They are more positive than widowed or divorced older adults, who have undergone the experience of losing a spouse (Gubrium, 1974). In this sense, being single in old age may be advantageous.

Women in Higher Education

We have seen that women are marrying later, delaying childbearing, and having fewer children. In other words, they are spending less time in traditional family roles. At the same time, women are becoming more involved in roles outside the family, particularly the roles of student and paid worker (Van Dusen & Sheldon, 1976). Let us first examine women's increasing participation in higher education.

Historically, women have been less likely to enroll in college and to complete degrees than men, but the difference between the sexes has been decreasing since 1950 (Bianchi & Spain, 1983). Women's enrollments in higher education have increased at a faster rate than men's since the 1970s, and by 1980 over half of all college students were women (U.S. Bureau of the Census, 1990). Much of the enrollment increase for women has occurred in the older age groups, particularly age 25 and older (Randour, Strasburg & Lipman-Blumen, 1982). Nearly 42% of the college population is now older than age 25, and 57% of these older students are women (U.S. Bureau of the Census, 1990). Since the 1960s, minority women have improved their educational attainments. Asian

American women have the highest college graduation rates among women, followed by whites, blacks, Hispanic, and American Indian women (Daniel, 1987).

There are several possible explanations for women's greater participation in higher education in recent years. Young women of traditional college age (18 to 24) are postponing marriage and motherhood, giving them more time to attend school or work before getting married and starting a family (Bianchi & Spain, 1983). Older returning women students may resume their education for a variety of reasons depending upon their marital and family status, occupational status, and financial needs. The reentry woman may be a middle-class woman taking courses for personal fulfillment, but she is increasingly likely to be a lower-income single parent seeking better support for her family or a single woman preparing for career advancement (Holliday, 1985).

Reentry women must overcome a number of obstacles. Cross (1981) categorizes these barriers into three types: situational (e.g., cost, time constraints, home and/or job responsibilities); institutional (e.g., course scheduling problems, difficulty in transferring course credits earned many years ago, financial aid policies that favor full-time students); and dispositional (e.g., low self-confidence, feeling awkward in classes with younger students).

Despite these barriers to learning, not only are more women enrolling in institutions of higher education, but more of them are completing degrees at every level. In 1987, more than half of all bachelor's and master's degrees and over one-third of all doctoral degrees were earned by women (U.S. Bureau of the Census, 1990).

Certain majors remain popular with women students: home economics, library science, health professions, education, foreign languages, and fine and applied arts. More than half of the master's degrees and over one-third of the doctoral degrees earned by women are in the field of education (Randour et al., 1982). Still, more women have been moving into traditionally male fields. Between 1971 and 1987, the percentage of bachelor's degrees awarded to women increased in agriculture from 4 to 31%; in architecture, from 12 to 37%; in life sciences, from 29 to 49%; in business and management, from 9 to 47%; in computer and information sciences, from 14 to 35%; in engineering, from less than 1 to 14%; and in physical sciences, from 14 to 28% (U.S. Bureau of the Census, 1990). Women have made inroads into the traditionally male-dominated professional fields of law, medicine, and dentistry, as well. In 1987, 40% of all law degrees were earned by women, compared with only 5% in 1970. During the same period of time, the proportion of medical degrees awarded to women increased from 8 to 32%, and the percentage of dentistry degrees from less than 1 to 24% (U.S. Bureau of the Census, 1990).

Women in the Labor Force

Women's participation in the labor force has increased dramatically during this century. In 1900, only 20% of women were in the labor force (Bernard,

1981). By 1988, this figure had risen to 57% (as compared with 76% of men), and women constituted 45% of the total labor force (U.S. Bureau of the Census, 1990). Employment rates are higher among black women than white women, with Hispanic and American Indian women having the lowest rates (Almquist & Wehrle-Einhorn, 1978; Nieva & Gutek, 1981; U.S. Bureau of the Census, 1990).

Since the 1960s, the largest increase in women's labor force participation has been among 25-to-34-year-olds, the age range when most women are bearing and rearing young children. Historically, women were least likely to work during these years (Van Dusen & Sheldon, 1976). In 1960, 36% of women 25–34 years old were in the labor force; by 1988, this figure had risen to 73% (U.S. Bureau of the Census, 1990; U.S. Department of Labor, 1983).

What are the reasons for women's increasing participation in the labor force? For one thing, their rising educational levels have given them access to more attractive, higher-paying jobs. In addition, service occupations expanded after World War II. These jobs—including teacher, nurse, librarian, social worker, and clerical worker—have traditionally attracted a high proportion of female workers. The supply of young, single women who had filled these positions in the past was not large enough to keep up with the growing demand for female labor. As a result, married women were increasingly drawn into the work force. Other factors leading to women's greater labor force participation include rising divorce rates, declining birthrates, the lessening of housework demands, and changing sex-role attitudes that made it more socially acceptable for married women and those with children to work (Nieva & Gutek, 1981; Smith, 1979; Van Dusen & Sheldon, 1976). It is not always easy to tell whether a particular factor is a cause of increased employment or an effect of it, however. For example, employed women have fewer children than women who are not employed (Moore & Hofferth, 1979). Is this because women with fewer children are more likely to decide to work or because working women decide to have fewer children? Both factors appear to be involved.

Certain factors increase the likelihood that a woman will work. One factor is financial need: women with no husbands or with husbands who are unemployed or have low incomes are more likely to work than are women who have husbands with high earnings. A second factor is the age of a woman's children: women with school-age children are more likely to be employed than those with preschoolers (Moen, 1985; Pfeffer & Ross, 1982; Smith, 1979).

Recent statistics illustrate how these marital and family characteristics influence labor force participation in women. In 1988, 73% of 35-to-44-year-old married women with husbands present were in the labor force, compared with 82% of never-married, divorced, separated, and widowed women. In the same year, 73% of married mothers with 6-to-17-year-old children were employed, as compared with 57% of married mothers with preschoolers (U.S. Bureau of the Census, 1990). For divorced mothers, the comparable figures were 84% and 70%. Even married women with infants under one year of age are participating in the labor force in unprecedented numbers: 52% of them were employed in 1988 (U.S. Bureau of the Census, 1990).

The labor force participation rates of black mothers are higher than those of white mothers, with Hispanic mothers having the lowest rates (National Commission, 1986; U.S. Bureau of the Census, 1990). Married black mothers, in particular, are more likely to be employed than their white counterparts, especially when the youngest child is of preschool age. For single mothers, however, this relationship is reversed, with white mothers more apt to be employed (Hayghe, 1986).

Not only are women majoring in traditionally male fields and joining the work force in increasing numbers, but they are moving into occupations traditionally dominated by men. From 1962 to 1982, the percentage of women bartenders grew from 11 to 50%, and the percentage driving buses rose from 12 to 47%. Other jobs showing an increase in the proportion of women during this period include engineers, from 1 to 6%; mail carriers, from 3 to 17%; physicians, from 6 to 15%; and insurance agents, from 10 to 26% (Serrin, 1984). Between 1979 and 1986, the percentage of women working as accountants and auditors grew from 34 to 45%; as lawyers, from 10 to 15%; as computer programmers, from 28 to 40%; and as managers and administrators, from 22 to 29% (U.S. Bureau of the Census, 1987).

Nevertheless, most women work in jobs that are highly sex-segregated (that is, dominated by members of their own sex). Of 420 different occupations listed by the U.S. Department of Labor, 80% of all women work in only 25 of them (Ferraro, 1984). In 1988, women comprised 99% of all secretaries, 97% of child-care workers, 96% of domestic workers, 95% of registered nurses, 85% of librarians and elementary school teachers, and 83% of file clerks and food servers (U.S. Bureau of the Census, 1990). About half of all employed women were in clerical and service occupations (including private household work) in 1985. Black women were somewhat more likely to hold such jobs (55% of black women workers) than were Hispanic women (51%) or white women (47%; National Commission, 1986).

One reason for occupational segregation may be "initial assignment segregation," in which women and men with equal entry-level skills are channeled into different jobs based on their sex (Ferraro, 1984). For example, although women are more likely than men to have so-called white-collar jobs, men's white-collar jobs tend to be the better-paying and higher-status professional, administrative, or scientific occupations. Women's white-collar jobs, on the other hand, are more likely to be lower-paying, dead-end clerical positions (Kahl, 1983).

Historically, women have earned much less than men. In 1960, women working full-time earned an average of 61¢ for every dollar earned by men. This figure remained virtually unchanged for the next 20 years. Women have made gains in pay in the 1980s, but they still lag behind men. Difficult as it is to believe, the average female college graduate earns less than the average male high school graduate (U.S. Bureau of the Census, 1990). In 1988, women who were employed full-time averaged 70% of men's pay (Women's Research & Education Institute, 1990). The difference in earnings of women and men is smaller for younger age groups than for older ones. In 1988, women between the ages of 25 and 34 earned nearly 78% of the wages of men in that age group. By comparison, 35-to-44-year-old women made 68% of the wages of similar-aged men, while women of ages 55 to 64 earned only 62% of men's wages (Women's Research & Education Institute, 1990). These sex differentials in salary apply to both white and nonwhite women. Since minority women earn approximately 10 to 16% less than white women, they are the lowest paid of all groups (National Commission, 1986).

Male-female salary discrepancies are not due simply to the fact that women are concentrated in lower-paying jobs and are more likely than men to have experienced a work interruption. Even after statistically adjusting for sex differences in age, education, type of occupation, and prior work experience, approximately 40 to 50% of the wage gap between the sexes remains, suggesting the presence of sex discrimination (Bianchi & Spain, 1983; Ferraro, 1984; U.S. Bureau of the Census, 1987).

Although the Equal Pay Act of 1963 outlawed separate pay scales for women and men doing the same work, some employers got around the law simply by reclassifying certain jobs (Barrett, 1979). More recently, the issue of "equal pay for equal work" has been replaced by the concept of "equal pay for comparable work." Supporters of "comparable worth," also known as "pay equity," believe that women and men should receive comparable salaries for jobs that require equivalent overall effort, skill, responsibility, and working conditions. Some recent court decisions and state laws have supported efforts to adopt comparable worth policies. For example, in 1987 the state legislatures of Connecticut and Oregon and the city of San Francisco appropriated $11 million, $22.6 million, and $35 million, respectively, for pay equity adjustments ("Pay Equity," 1987). In sum, over $450 million worth of pay equity adjustments were made or appropriated between 1979 and 1989 (National Committee on Pay Equity, 1989).

Are working women more satisfied with their lives than full-time homemakers? The answer to this question is not clear. Some studies have found that working women have better psychological health than nonworking women (Ferree, 1976; Gove & Geerken, 1977; Kessler & McCrae, 1981; Northcott, 1981; Welch & Booth, 1977). Others, however, find no differences in psychological well-being between the two groups (Aneshensel, Frerichs, & Clark, 1981; Newberry, Weissman & Myers, 1979; Wright, 1978). A major reason for the apparent contradiction in research findings is that a woman's well-being depends not just on her employment status but, as we have seen, on many other factors, such as her marital status and the presence of children in the home. For single women with no children at home, a clear association has been found between employment and better mental health (Warr & Parry, 1982), probably because employment is a major source of role satisfaction for such women (Gove, 1972). For married women with children at home, however, life satisfaction and happiness are no greater for the employed woman than for the full-time homemaker (Warr & Parry, 1982). It may be that the psychological and social rewards provided by outside employment are offset by the strains of juggling the multiple and often conflicting demands of the roles of wife, mother, and worker (Elman & Gilbert, 1984; Sheehan, 1984; Yogev, 1981). We have already seen that even when a woman is employed, she still has the major responsibility for both childrearing and household chores. Among employed mothers, the maternal role appears to be a greater source of stress than the role of paid worker (Barnett & Baruch, 1985; Johnson & Johnson, 1977). As women move into middle age and approach the "empty nest" period of life when children leave home, women who work outside the home once again are found to have better mental health and higher levels of self-esteem than homemakers (Baruch et al., 1983; Birnbaum, 1975; Coleman & Antonucci, 1983; Powell, 1977). Employment at this time in a woman's life may be beneficial because it directs attention away from concerns about physical health, marital dissatisfaction, and the launching of children (Coleman & Antonucci, 1983).

Another factor affecting the well-being of employed women in addition to their marital and parental status is the importance they attach to their job. A recent study found that career-oriented women who were employed reported greater self-esteem and life satisfaction than those who were not employed. For women who were not career-oriented, however, employment was not related to self-esteem or life satisfaction (Pietromonaco, Manis & Markus, 1987).

In a recent comprehensive review of the evidence concerning the effects of paid employment on women's mental and physical health, Repetti, Matthews, and Waldron (1989) concluded that women's employment does not have an overall negative effect on health. They noted that employment appears to improve the health of unmarried women and married women who have positive attitudes toward employment. Increased social support from supervisors and coworkers appears to be an important mediator of the beneficial health effects of employment.

Retirement

Much of what we know about the effects of retirement is based on studies of men. One reason for this is that, until recently, a relatively small proportion of women spent their adult lives in the labor force. In addition, it has been assumed that retirement is a less critical event for women than for men because of women's greater involvement in family roles. Research indicates, however, that female retirees were just as committed to their work as were male retirees (Atchley, 1976; Streib & Schneider, 1971) and that retirement from the labor force has important consequences for women (George, Fillenbaum & Palmore, 1984; Szinovacz, 1982).

Women are more likely than men to retire for voluntary reasons, whereas men are more apt to retire for involuntary reasons, such as mandatory retirement or ill health (George et al., 1984; Gratton & Haug, 1983; Szinovacz, 1983). Reasons for women's retirement include the retirement of one's husband and his health status (Shaw, 1984). Professional women and those who are self-employed are less likely than other women to retire early (Prentis, 1980; Shaw, 1984). Retirement income is an important factor in the decision to retire for both women and men. Not surprisingly, those with Social Security or pension coverage are more likely to retire (Gratton & Haug, 1983; Shaw, 1984).

Both sexes typically adjust well to retirement (Gratton & Haug, 1983), although women may take longer to get adjusted (Atchley, 1976; Szinovacz, 1983). One reason for this may be that women are not under the same social pressures to be employed as are men. Those women who have chosen to work, whether out of financial need or commitment to their job, therefore may find it more difficult to stop working (Szinovacz, 1983). Retirement has both negative and positive effects on women and men. Negative effects include increased psychosomatic symptoms and decreased income (George et al., 1984). Retired women are more likely than retired men to report that their incomes are inadequate (Atchley, 1976). This reflects the fact that women's retirement income typically is only about one-half that of men's (Bentsen, 1984). Women's concentration in low-paying jobs and their often interrupted or delayed work careers result in smaller retirement benefits. In 1986, retired women received annual monthly Social Security benefits of $380, compared with $495 for men ("Most Depend," 1986). In addition, women are less likely than men to be covered by private pension plans ("Most Depend," 1986; O'Rand & Henretta, 1982). Only 20% of retired women received pensions in 1983, averaging $243 a month, compared with 43% of men, who averaged $473.

On the positive side, retired women and men spend more time in personal hobbies and increase their interactions with friends (George et al., 1984; Holahan, 1981). Retired women, particularly unmarried ones, are more involved with friends and neighbors than are retired men or lifelong housewives (Depner & Ingersoll, 1982; Fox, 1977). For both sexes, a high level of life satisfaction in retirement generally is associated with having good health, adequate income, and a high activity level (Atchley, 1982).

Future Directions

Women's life patterns have been changing throughout this century, but the pace of change has been particularly rapid in the past 25 years. Women increasingly are choosing nontraditional family roles: remaining single, getting divorced, deciding not to have children. Even when choosing traditional family roles, women are delaying entry into these roles and are spending less time in them (Van Dusen & Sheldon, 1976). Additionally, more women are getting a college education and spending a significant number of years in the labor force. Long and Porter (1984) note that the midlife period, in particular, often is marked by a number of transitions that may include changes in family life, in labor force participation, and in the emphasis given to women's many roles. Much of the previous research on women in the middle and later years has focused on attempts to answer which life pattern is most healthy or satisfying for women: marriage or singlehood, employment or nonemployment. As Giele (1982a) points out, this rather simplistic approach has not proved to be very fruitful because of the increasing complexity and variability of women's life patterns today. Newer research is beginning to look at the linkages between work and family and how these are integrated at different stages in the life cycle of the woman and her family. In addition, instead of looking only at such broad outcomes as happiness or life satisfaction, newer research is focusing on various components of well-being, as well as on styles and mechanisms of coping and adapting.

It is important to remember that as each generation of women matures and grows older, it encounters a different set of conditions and experiences. Our current information about women in the middle and later years is based on the lives of women who grew up in circumstances very different from those of today's young women. As Abu-Laban (1981) notes, if current trends involving family life, sexuality, reproductive freedom, and labor force participation continue, older women of the future are likely to increase their occupational prestige and economic independence, as well as enhance their opportunities for a variety of rewarding interpersonal relationships.

NOTE

The author wishes to thank Margaret Carter, Andrea Etaugh, and Harold Rosenberg for providing valuable comments on earlier drafts of this chapter.

REFERENCES

Abdel-Ghany, M., & Nichols, S. Y. (1983). Husband/wife differentials in household worktime: The case of dual earner families. *Home Economics Research Journal*, *12*, 159–167.

Abu-Laban, S. I. (1981). Women and aging: A futurist perspective. *Psychology of Women Quarterly*, *6*, 85–98.

Aizenberg, R., & Treas, J. (1985). The family in late life: Psychological and demographic considerations. In J. E. Birren & K. W. Schaie (Eds.), *Handbook of the psychology of aging* (2nd ed., pp. 169–189). New York: Van Nostrand Reinhold.

Albrecht, S. L. (1980). Reactions and adjustments to divorce: Differences in the experience of males and females. *Family Relations*, *29*, 49–68.

Almquist, E. M., & Wehrle-Einhorn, J. L. (1978). The doubly-disadvantaged: Minority women in the labor force. In A. H. Stromberg & S. Harkess (Eds.), *Women working* (pp. 63–88). Palo Alto, CA: Mayfield.

Alston, D. N., & Rose, N. (1981). Perceptions of middle-aged black women. *Journal of General Psychology*, *104*, 167–171.

Altman, L. K. (1990, July 12). New therapy shown to fight bone loss in elderly. *New York Times*, pp. A1, B8.

Anderson, S., Russell, C., & Schumm, W. (1983). Perceived marital quality and family life cycle categories: A further analysis. *Journal of Marriage and the Family, 45*, 127–138.

Aneshensel, C., Frerichs, R., & Clark, V. (1981). Family roles and sex differences in depression. *Journal of Health and Social Behavior, 22*, 379–393.

Antonucci, T., Tamir, L. M., & Dubnoff, S. (1980). Mental health across the family life cycle. In K. W. Back (Ed.), *Life course: Integrative theories and exemplary populations*. American Association for the Advancement of Science Selected Symposium No. 41. Boulder, CO: Westview Press.

Archer, D. (1982). Biochemical findings and medical management of the menopause. In A. M. Voda, M. Dinnerstein, & S. R. O'Donnell (Eds.), *Changing perspectives on menopause* (pp. 39–48). Austin: University of Texas Press.

Atchley, R. C. (1976). Selected psychological and social differences among men and women in later life. *Journal of Gerontology, 31*, 204–211.

Atchley, R. C. (1982). The process of retirement: Comparing women and men. In M. Szinovacz (Ed.), *Women's retirement* (pp. 153–168). Beverly Hills: Sage.

Ball, J. F. (1976–1977). Widow's grief: The impact of age and mode of death. *Omega, 7*, 307–333.

Barnett, R. C., & Baruch, G. K. (1985). Women's involvement in multiple roles and psychological distress. *Journal of Personality and Social Psychology, 49*, 135–145.

Barrett, C. J. (1977). Women in widowhood. *Signs, 2*, 856–868.

Barrett, N. S. (1979). Women in the job market: Occupations, earnings and career opportunities. In R. E. Smith (Ed.), *The subtle revolution: Women at work* (pp. 32–61). Washington, DC: Urban Institute.

Bart, P. B. (1971). Depression in middle-aged women. In V. Gornick & B. K. Moran (Eds.), *Women in sexist society* (pp. 163–186). New York: Basic Books.

Baruch, G. (1984). The psychological well-being of women in the middle years. In G. Baruch & J. Brooks-Gunn (Eds.), *Women in mid-life* (pp. 161–180). New York: Plenum.

Baruch, G., Barnett, R., & Rivers, C. (1983). *Life prints: New patterns of love and work for today's women*. New York: McGraw-Hill.

Beckman, L. J., & Houser, B. B. (1982). The consequences of childlessness for the social-psychological well-being of older women. *Journal of Gerontology, 37*, 243–250.

Bee, H. L. (1987). *The journey of adulthood*. New York: Macmillan.

Bengtson, V. L. (1985). Diversity and symbolism in grandparental roles. In V. L. Bengtson & J. F. Robertson (Eds.), *Grandparenthood* (pp. 11–25). Beverly Hills: Sage.

Bentsen, S. K. (1984). Old age financial security—or insecurity? In *Women, work and age: Policy challenges*. Ann Arbor: University of Michigan, Institute of Gerontology.

Berardo, D. H., Shehan, C. L., & Leslie, G. R. (1987). A residue of transition: Jobs, careers, and spouses' time in housework. *Journal of Marriage and the Family, 49*, 381–390.

Bernard, J. (1972). *The future of marriage*. New York: World.

Bernard, J. (1981). *The female world*. New York: Free Press.

Bianchi, S. M., & Spain, D. (1983). *American women: Three decades of change* (Report No. CDS-80-8). Washington, DC: Bureau of the Census.

Birnbaum, J. A. (1975). Life patterns and self-esteem in gifted family-oriented and career-committed women. In M. Mednick, L. W. Hoffman, & S. Tangri (Eds.), *Women and achievement: Social and motivational analysis* (pp. 396–419). New York: Halsted Press.

Black, S. M., & Hill, C. E. (1984). The psychological well-being of women in their middle years. *Psychology of Women Quarterly, 8*, 282–292.

Braito, R., & Anderson, D. (1983). The ever-single elderly woman. In E. W. Markson (Ed.), *Older women* (pp. 195–225). Lexington, MA: Lexington.

Brooks-Gunn, J., & Kirsh, B. (1984). Life events and the boundaries of midlife for women. In G. Baruch and J. Brooks-Gunn (Eds.), *Women in mid-life* (pp. 11–30). New York: Plenum.

Brown, P., & Manela, R. (1978). Changing family roles: Women and divorce. *Journal of Divorce, 4*, 315–328.

Burton, L. M., & Bengtson, V. L. (1985). Black grandmothers. In V. L. Bengtson & J. F. Robertson (Eds.), *Grandparenthood* (pp. 61–77). Beverly Hills: Sage.

Campbell, A. (1975, May). The American way of mating: Marriage sí, children only maybe. *Psychology Today*, pp. 39–42.

Campbell, A. (1981). *The sense of well-being in America*. New York: McGraw-Hill.

Campbell, A., Converse, P. E., & Rodgers, W. L. (1976). *The quality of American life*. New York: Russell Sage.

Cargan, L., & Melko, M. (1982). *Singles: Myths and realities*. Beverly Hills: Sage.

Carter, H., & Glick, P. C. (1976). *Marriage and divorce: A social and economic study* (rev. ed.). Cambridge: Harvard University Press.

Cherlin, A. J. (1981). *Marriage, divorce, and remarriage*. Cambridge: Harvard University Press.

Cherlin, A., & Furstenberg, F. F. (1985). Styles and strategies of grandparenting. In V. L. Bengtson & J. F. Robertson (Eds.), *Grandparenthood* (pp. 97–116). Beverly Hills: Sage.

Cherlin, A., & Furstenberg, F. F. (1986). *The new American grandparent: A place in the family, a life apart*. New York: Basic Books.

Chiriboga, D. A. (1982). Adaptation to marital separation in later and earlier life. *Journal of Gerontology, 37*, 109–114.

Chiriboga, D. A., Roberts, J., & Stein, J. A. (1978). Psychological well-being during marital separation. *Journal of Divorce, 2*, 21–36.

Coleman, L. M., & Antonucci, T. C. (1983). Impact of work on women at midlife. *Developmental Psychology, 19*, 290–294.

Colletta, M. D. (1979). Support systems after divorce: Incidence and impact. *Journal of Marriage and the Family, 41*, 837–846.

Corby, N., & Brecher, E. (1984). *Love, sex, and aging*. Mt. Vernon, NY: Consumer's Union.

Cross, K. P. (1981). *Adults as learners*. San Francisco: Jossey-Bass.

Culliton, B. (1987). Osteoporosis re-examined: Complexity of bone biology is a challenge. *Science, 235*, 833–834.

Daniel, R. L. (1987). *American woman in the 20th century*. San Diego, CA: Harcourt Brace Jovanovich.

DeLorey, C. (1984). Health care and midlife women. In G. Baruch & J. Brooks-Gunn (Eds.), *Women in mid-life* (pp. 277–301). New York: Plenum.

Depner, C., & Ingersoll, B. (1982). Employment status and social support: The experience of the mature woman. In M. Szinovacz (Ed.), *Women's retirement* (pp. 61–76). Beverly Hills: Sage.

Donelson, E. (1977). Becoming a single woman. In E. Donelson & J. Gullahorn (Eds.), *Women: A psychological perspective* (pp. 228–246). New York: Wiley.

Douthitt, R. A. (1989). The division of labor within the home: Have gender roles changed? *Sex Roles, 20*, 693–704.

Duberman, L. (1974). *Marriage and its alternatives*. New York: Praeger.

Edinburg, G. M. (1982). Women and aging. In C. C. Nadelson & M. T. Notman (Eds.), *The woman patient: Vol 2. Concepts of femininity and the life cycle* (pp. 169–194). New York: Plenum.

Edwards, M. (1977). Coupling and recoupling vs. the challenge of being single. *Personnel and Guidance Journal, 55*, 542–545.

Elman, M. R., & Gilbert, L. A. (1984). Coping strategies for role conflict in married professional women with children. *Family Relations, 33*, 317–327.

Etaugh, C., & Foresman, E. (1983). Evaluations of competence as a function of sex and marital status. *Sex Roles, 9*, 759–765.

Etaugh, C., & Malstrom, J. (1981). The effect of marital status on person perception. *Journal of Marriage and the Family, 43*, 801–805.

Etaugh, C., & Petroski, B. (1985). Perceptions of women: Effects of employment status and marital status. *Sex Roles, 12*, 329–339.

Etaugh, C., & Riley, S. (1983). Evaluating competence of women and men: Effects of marital and parental status and occupational sex-typing. *Sex Roles, 9*, 943–952.

Etaugh, C., & Stern, J. (1984). Person perception: Effects of sex, marital status and sex-typed occupation. *Sex Roles, 11*, 413–424.

Etaugh, C., & Study, G. G. (1989). Perceptions of mothers: Effects of employment status, marital status, and age of child. *Sex Roles, 20*, 59–70.

Ferraro, G. A. (1984). Bridging the wage gap. *American Psychologist, 39*, 1166–1170.

Ferree, M. (1976). Working-class jobs: Housework and paid work as sources of satisfaction. *Social Problems, 23*, 431–441.

Fox, J. H. (1977). Effects of retirement and former work life on women's adaptation in old age. *Journal of Gerontology, 32*, 196–202.

Frey, K. A. (1981). Middle-aged women's experience and perceptions of menopause. *Women and Health, 6*, 25–36.

Friederich, M. (1982). Aging, menopause, and estrogens: The clinician's dilemma. In A. M. Voda, M. Dinnerstein, & S. R. O'Donnell (Eds.), *Changing perspectives on menopause* (pp. 335–345). Austin: University of Texas Press.

Frieze, I. H., Parsons, J. E., Johnson, P. B., Ruble, D. N., & Zellman, G. L. (1977). *Women and sex roles: A social psychological perspective*. New York: W. W. Norton.

George, L. K., Fillenbaum, G. G., & Palmore, E. (1984). Sex differences in the antecedents and consequences of retirement. *Journal of Gerontology, 39*, 364–371.

Giele, J. (1982a). Future research and policy questions. In J. Giele (Ed.), *Women in the middle years: Current knowledge and directions for research and policy* (pp. 199–240). New York: Wiley-Interscience.

Giele, J. (1982b). Women in adulthood: Unanswered questions. In J. Giele (Ed.), *Women in the middle years: Current knowledge and directions for research and policy* (pp. 1–35). New York: Wiley-Interscience.

Glenn, N. D. (1975). Psychological well-being in the postparental stage: Some evidence from national surveys. *Journal of Marriage and the Family, 37,* 105–109.

Glenn, N. D., & McLanahan, S. (1981). The effects of offspring on the psychological well-being of older adults. *Journal of Marriage and the Family, 43,* 409–422.

Gove, W. R. (1972). The relationship between sex roles, marital status and mental illness. *Social Forces, 51,* 34–44.

Gove, W. R., & Geerken, M. R. (1977). The effect of children and employment on the mental health of married men and women. *Social Forces, 56,* 66–76.

Granvold, D. K., Pedler, L. M., & Schellie, S. G. (1979). A study of sex role expectancy and female postdivorce adjustment. *Journal of Divorce, 2,* 383–393.

Gratton, B., & Haug, M. R. (1983). Decision and adaptation: Research on female retirement. *Research on Aging, 5,* 59–76.

Gubrium, J. F. (1974). Marital desolation and the valuation of everyday life in old age. *Journal of Marriage and the Family, 35,* 107–113.

Gutmann, D. L. (1975). Parenthood, key to comparative study of the life cycle. In N. Datan & L. Ginsberg (Eds.), *Life span development psychology: Normative life crisis* (pp. 167–184). New York: Academic Press.

Gutmann, D. L. (1977). The cross-cultural perspective: Notes toward a comparative psychology of aging. In J. E. Birren & K. W. Schaie (Eds.), *Handbook of the psychology of aging* (pp. 302–326). New York: Van Nostrand Reinhold.

Hagestad, G. O. (1984). Multi-generational families, socialization, support and strain. In V. Garms-Homolova, E. M. Hoerning, & D. Schaeffer (Eds.), *Intergenerational relationships* (pp. 105–114). Lewiston, NY: C. J. Hogrefe.

Hagestad, G. O. (1985). Continuity and connectedness. In V. L. Bengtson & J. F. Robertson (Eds.), *Grandparenthood* (pp. 31–47). Beverly Hills: Sage.

Harris, L., & Associates. (1975). *The myth and reality of aging in America.* New York: National Council on Aging.

Hayghe, H. (1986). Rise in mothers' labor force activity includes those with infants. *Monthly Labor Review, 109*(2), 43–45.

Heaney, R. P. (1987). Prevention of osteoporotic fracture in women. In L. V. Avioli (Ed.), *The osteoporotic syndrome: Detection, prevention and treatment* (2nd ed. pp. 67–90). Orlando, FL: Grune & Stratton.

Helsing, K. J., Szklo, M., & Comstock, G. W. (1981). Factors associated with mortality after widowhood. *American Journal of Public Health, 71,* 802–809.

Hess, B., & Waring, J. (1983). Family relationships of older women: A women's issue. In E. W. Markson (Ed.), *Older women: Issues and prospects* (pp. 227–251). Lexington, MA: Lexington Books.

Hetherington, E. M. (1989). Coping with family transitions: Winners, losers, and survivors. *Child Development, 60,* 1–14.

Hetherington, E. M., & Camara, K. A. (1984). Families in transition: The processes of dissolution and reconstitution. In R. D. Parke (Ed.), *Review of child development research: Vol 7. The family* (pp. 398–439). Chicago: University of Chicago Press.

Hetherington, E. M., Cox, M., & Cox, R. (1982). Effects of divorce on parents and children. In M. Lamb (Ed.), *Nontraditional families* (pp. 233–288). Hillsdale, NJ: Erlbaum.

Hetherington, E. M., Stanley-Haga.. M., & Anderson, E. R. (1989). Marital transitions: A child's perspective. *American . ·chologist, 44*, 303–312.

Heyman, D. K., & Gianturco, D. T. (1973). Long-term adaptation by the elderly to bereavement. *Journal of Gerontology, 28*, 359–362.

Holahan, C. K. (1981, August). *Activity involvement in aging women: Career pattern and retirement*. Paper presented at the meeting of the American Psychological Association, Los Angeles.

Holliday, G. (1985). Addressing the concerns of returning women students. In N. J. Evans (Ed.), *Facilitating the development of women* (pp. 61–73). San Francisco: Jossey-Bass.

Horowitz, A. (1985). Sons and daughters as caregivers to older parents: Differences in role performance and consequences. *Gerontologist, 25*, 612–617.

Houseknecht, S. K. (1979). Timing of the decision to remain voluntarily childless: Evidence for continuous socialization. *Psychology of Women Quarterly, 4*, 81–96.

Hudis, P. M. (1976). Commitment to work and family: Marital status differences in women's earnings. *Journal of Marriage and the Family, 38*, 267–278.

Hunt, M. (1974). *Sexual behavior in the 1970's*. Chicago: Playboy Press.

Hyde, J. S., & Phillis, D. E. (1979). Androgyny across the lifespan. *Developmental Psychology, 15*, 334–336.

Johnson, C. L., & Johnson, F. A. (1977). Attitudes toward parenting in dual career families. *American Journal of Psychiatry, 134*, 391–395.

Kahl, A. (1983). Characteristics of job entrants in 1980–1981. *Occupational Outlook Quarterly, 27*, 18–26.

Kart, C. S., Metress, E. K., & Metress, S. P. (1988). *Aging, health and society*. Boston: Jones & Bartlett.

Kessler, R., & McCrae, J. (1981). Trends in the relationship between sex and psychological distress: 1957–1976. *American Sociological Review, 46*, 443–452.

Kivnick, H. Q. (1983). Dimensions of grandparenthood meaning: Deductive conceptualization and empirical derivation. *Journal of Personality and Social Psychology, 44*, 1056–1068.

Kolata, G. (1989, August 2). Menopause hormone linked to breast cancer. *New York Times*, pp. 1, 21.

Kolevson, M. S., & Gottlieb, S. J. (1983). The impact of divorce: A multivariate study. *Journal of Divorce, 7*, 89–98.

Lang, A. M., & Brody, E. M. (1983). Characteristics of middle-aged daughters and help to their elderly mothers. *Journal of Marriage and the Family, 45*, 193–202.

Lawrence, F. C., Draughn, P. S., Tasker, G. E., & Wozniak, P. H. (1987). Sex differences in household labor time: A comparison of rural and urban couples. *Sex Roles, 17*, 489–502.

Lehr, U. (1984). The role of women in the family generation context. In V. Garms-Homolova, E. M. Hoerning, & D. Schaeffer (Eds.), *Intergenerational relationships* (pp. 125–132). Lewiston, NY: C. J. Hogrefe.

Lennon, M. C. (1987). Is menopause depressing? An investigation of three perspectives. *Sex Roles, 17*, 1–16.

Livson, F. B. (1981). Patterns of personality development in middle-aged women: A longitudinal study. In J. Hendricks (Ed.), *Being and becoming old* (pp. 133–140). Farmingdale, NY: Baywood.

Loewenstein, S. F., Bloch, N. E., Campion, J., Epstein, J. S., Gale, P., & Salvatore, M. (1981). A study of satisfactions and stresses of single women in midlife. *Sex Roles*, *7*, 1127–1141.

Long, J., & Porter, K. (1984). Multiple roles of midlife women: A case for new directions in theory, research, and policy. In G. Baruch & J. Brooks-Gunn (Eds.), *Women in mid-life* (pp. 109–159). New York: Plenum.

Lopata, H. (1973). *Widowhood in an American city*. Cambridge, MA: Schenkman.

Lopata, H. Z. (1975). Widowhood: Societal factors in life-span disruption and alternatives. In N. Datan & L. H. Ginsberg (Eds.), *Life-span developmental psychology: Normative crises* (pp. 217–234). New York: Academic Press.

Lopata, H. Z. (1979). *Women as widows: Support systems*. New York: Elsevier-North Holland.

Lopata, H. Z. (1980). The widowed family member. In N. Datan & N. Lohman (Eds.), *Transitions of aging* (pp. 93–118). New York: Academic Press.

Lopata, H. Z., Heinemann, G. D., & Baum, J. (1982). Loneliness: Antecedents and coping strategies in the lives of widows. In L. A. Peplau & D. Perlman (Eds.), *Loneliness* (pp. 310–326). New York: Wiley.

Lott, B. L. (1987). *Women's lives: Themes and variations in gender learning*. Monterey, CA: Brooks/ Cole.

Lowenthal, M., Thurnher, M., & Chiriboga, D. (1975). *Four stages of life*. San Francisco: Jossey-Bass.

Luria, Z., & Meade, R. G. (1984). Sexuality and the middle-aged woman. In G. Baruch & F. Brooks-Gunn (Eds.), *Women in mid-life* (pp. 371–397). New York: Plenum.

Maret, E., & Finlay, B. (1984). The distribution of household labor among women in dual-career families. *Journal of Marriage and the Family*, *46*, 357–364.

Markson, E. W., & Hess, B. (1980). Older women in the city. *Signs*, *5*, (Suppl.), 127–141.

Masters, W. H., Johnson, V. E., & Kolodny, R. C. (1985). *Human sexuality* (2nd ed.). Boston: Little, Brown.

McGee, J., & Wells, K. (1982). Gender typing and androgyny in later life: New direction for theory and research. *Human Development*, *25*, 116–139.

McGloshen, T. H., & O'Bryant, S. L. (1988). The psychological well-being of older, recent widows. *Psychology of Women Quarterly*, *12*, 99–116.

McKinlay, J. B., McKinlay, S. M., & Brambilla, D. (1987). The relative contributions of endocrine changes and social circumstances to depression in mid-aged women. *Journal of Health and Social Behavior*, *28*, 345–363.

McNett, I., Taylor, L., & Scott, L. (1985). Minority women: Doubly disadvantaged. In A. G. Sargent (Ed.), *Beyond sex roles* (2nd ed., pp. 226–232). St. Paul, MN: West.

Millette, B. (1981). Menopause: A survey of attitudes and knowledge. *Issues of Health Care in Women*, *3*, 263–276.

Millette, B., & Hawkins, J. (1983). *The passage through menopause: Women's lives in transition*. Reston, VA: Reston.

Moen, P. (1985). Continuities and discontinuities in women's labor force activity. In G. H. Elder (Ed.), *Life course dynamics: Trajectories and transitions, 1968–1980* (pp. 113–155). Ithaca, NY: Cornell University Press.

Moore, K. A., & Hofferth, S. L. (1979). Women and their children. In R. E. Smith

(Ed.), *The subtle revolution: Women at work* (pp. 125–157). Washington, DC: Urban Institute.

Most depend on social security. (1986, March 20). *New York Times*, p. 8.

Nathanson, C., & Lorenz, B. (1982). Women and health: The social dimensions of biomedical data. In J. Giele (Ed.), *Women in the middle years: Current knowledge and directions for research and policy* (pp. 37–87). New York: Wiley-Interscience.

National Commission on Working Women and Wider Opportunity for Women. (1986). *An overview of minority women in the work force*. Washington, DC: Author.

National Committee on Pay Equity. (1989). *Pay equity in the public sector 1979–1989*. Washington, DC: Author.

Neugarten, B. L., & Associates. (1964). *Personality in middle and later life*. New York: Atherton.

Neugarten, B. L., & Datan, N. (1974). The middle years. In S. Arieti (Ed.), *American Handbook of Psychiatry: Vol. 1* (2nd ed., pp. 592–608). New York: Basic Books.

Neugarten, B. L., & Weinstein, K. (1964). The changing American grandparent. *Journal of Marriage and the Family, 26*, 197–204.

Newberry, P., Weissman, M. M., & Myers, J. K. (1979). Working wives and housewives: Do they differ in mental status and social adjustment? *American Journal of Orthopsychiatry, 49*, 282–291.

Nieva, V. F., & Gutek, B. A. (1981). *Women and work: A psychological perspective*. New York: Praeger.

Northcott, H. (1981). Women, work, health and happiness. *International Journal of Women's Studies, 4*, 268–276.

Norton, A. J., & Moorman, J. E. (1987). Current trends in marriage and divorce among American women. *Journal of Marriage and the Family, 49*, 3–14.

Nowak, C. (1977). Does youthfulness equal attractiveness? In L. Troll, J. Israel, & K. Israel (Eds.), *Looking ahead: A woman's guide to the problems and joys of growing old* (pp. 59–64). Englewood Cliffs, NJ: Prentice-Hall.

Nyquist, L., Slivken, K., Spence, J. T., & Helmreich, R. L. (1985). Household responsibilities in middle-class couples: The contribution of demographic and personality variables. *Sex Roles, 12*, 15–34.

O'Rand, A., & Henretta, J. C. (1982). Midlife work history and retirement income. In M. Szinovacz (Ed.), *Women's retirement* (pp. 25–44). Beverly Hills: Sage.

Parkes, C. M., & Weiss, R. S. (1983). *Recovery from bereavement*. New York: Basic Books.

Parlee, M. B. (1979, October). The friendship bond. *Psychology Today*, pp. 43–54.

Pay equity victories. (1987, Summer). *Pay Equity Newsnotes*, p. 1.

Peplau, L. A., Bikson, T. K., Rook, K. S., & Goodchilds, J. D. (1982). Being old and living alone. In L. A. Peplau & D. Perlman (Eds.), *Loneliness* (pp. 327–347). New York: Wiley.

Peplau, L. A., & Gordon, S. L. (1985). Women and men in love: Gender differences in close heterosexual relationships. In V. E. O'Leary, R. K. Unger, & B. S. Wallston (Eds.), *Women, gender and social psychology* (pp. 257–291). Hillsdale, NJ: Erlbaum.

Perlmutter, E., & Bart, P. (1982). Changing views of "The Change": A critical review and suggestions for an attributional approach. In A. M. Voda, M. Dinnerstein, & S. R. O'Donnell (Eds.), *Changing perspectives on menopause* (2nd ed., pp. 187–199). Austin: University of Texas Press.

Perlmutter, M., & Hall, E. (1985). *Adult development and aging.* New York: Wiley.

Peterson, R. A. (1983). Attitudes toward the childless spouse. *Sex Roles, 9,* 321–332.

Pfeffer, J., & Ross, J. (1982). The effects of marriage and a working wife on occupational and wage attainment. *Administrative Science Quarterly, 27,* 66–80.

Pietromonaco, P. R., Manis, J., & Markus, H. (1987). The relationship of employment to self-perception and well-being in women: A cognitive analysis. *Sex Roles, 17,* 467–477.

Pihlblad, T., & Adams, C. (1972). Widowhood, social participation and life satisfaction. *Aging and Human Development, 3,* 323–330.

Pleck, J. H. (1985). *Working wives/working husbands.* Beverly Hills: Sage.

Powell, B. (1977). The empty nest, employment, and psychiatric symptoms in college-educated women. *Psychology of Women Quarterly, 2,* 35–43.

Prentis, R. S. (1980). White-collar working women's perception of retirement. *Gerontologist, 20,* 90–95.

Radloff, L. (1975). Sex differences in depression: The effects of occupation and marital status. *Sex Roles, 1,* 249–265.

Radloff, L. S. (1980). Depression and the empty nest. *Sex Roles, 6,* 775–781.

Randour, M. L., Strasburg, G. L., & Lipman-Blumen, J. (1982). Women in higher education: Trends in enrollments and degrees earned. *Harvard Educational Review, 52,* 189–202.

Repetti, R. L., Matthews, K. A., & Waldron, I. (1989). Employment and women's health. *American Psychologist, 44,* 1394–1401.

Rhyne, D. (1981). Bases of marital satisfaction among men and women. *Journal of Marriage and the Family, 43,* 941–955.

Riis, B., Thomsen, K., & Christiansen, C. (1987). Does calcium supplementation prevent postmenopausal bone loss? *New England Journal of Medicine, 316,* 173–177.

Robertson, J. F. (1977). Grandmotherhood: A study of role conceptions. *Journal of Marriage and the Family, 39,* 165–174.

Robinson, J. P. (1977). *How Americans use time.* New York: Praeger.

Rook, K. S. (1984). The negative side of social interaction: Impact on psychological well-being. *Journal of Personality and Social Psychology, 46,* 1097–1108.

Rossi, A. S. (1980). Aging and parenthood in the middle years. In P. B. Baltes & O. G. Brim, Jr. (Eds.), *Life-span development and behavior: Vol. 3* (pp. 137–205). New York: Academic Press.

Rossman, I. (1980). Bodily changes with aging. In E. W. Busse & D. G. Blazer (Eds.), *Handbook of geriatric psychiatry* (pp. 125–146). New York: Van Nostrand Reinhold.

Rubin, L. B. (1979). *Women of a certain age: The midlife search for self.* New York: Harper & Row.

Russo, N. F. (1979). Overview: Sex roles, fertility, and the motherhood mandate. *Psychology of Women Quarterly, 4,* 7–15.

Selmanowitz, V. J., Rizer, R. I., & Orentreich, N. (1977). Aging of the skin and its appendages. In C. E. Finch & L. Hayflick (Eds.), *Handbook of the biology of aging* (pp. 496–509). New York: Harcourt Brace Jovanovich.

Serrin, W. (1984, November 25). Experts say job bias against women persists. *New York Times,* pp. 1, 18.

Shaw, L. B. (1984). Retirement plans of middle-aged married women. *Gerontologist, 24,* 154–159.

Sheehan, C. L. (1984). Wives' work and psychological well-being: An extension of Gove's social role theory of depression. *Sex Roles, 11*, 881–899.

Silberner, J. (1987). Osteoporosis: Most answers yet to come. *Science News, 131*(8), 116.

Silka, L., & Kiesler, S. (1977). Couples who choose to remain childless. *Family Planning Perspective, 9*, 16–25.

Sinnott, J. D. (1982). Correlates of sex roles of older adults. *Journal of Gerontology, 37*, 587–594.

Smith, R. E. (1979). The movement of women into the labor force. In R. E. Smith (Ed.), *The subtle revolution: Women at work* (pp. 1–29). Washington, DC: Urban Institute.

Sontag, S. (1979). The double standard of aging. In J. H. Williams (Ed.), *Psychology of women: Selected readings* (pp. 462–478). New York: Norton.

Spanier, G. B., & Furstenberg, F. F. (1986). Remarriage and reconstituted families. In M. B. Sussman & S. K. Steinmetz (Eds.), *Handbook of marriage and the family* (pp. 419–434). New York: Plenum.

Spreitzer, E., & Riley, L. F. (1974). Factors associated with singlehood. *The Journal of Marriage and the Family, 36*, 533–542.

Spreitzer, E., Snyder, E., & Larson, D. (1975). Age, marital status and labor force participation as related to life satisfaction. *Sex Roles, 1*, 235–247.

Stein, P. (1975). Singlehood: An alternative to marriage. *Family Coordinator, 24*, 489–505.

Stone, R., Cafferata, G. L., & Sangl, J. (1987). Caregivers of the frail elderly: A national profile. *Gerontologist, 27*, 616–626.

Streib, G. F., & Schneider, C. J. (1971). *Retirement in American society: Impact and process*. Ithaca, NY: Cornell University Press.

Stroebe, M. S., & Stroebe, W. (1983). Who suffers more: Sex differences in health risks of the widowed. *Psychological Bulletin, 93*, 279–301.

Stueve, A., & O'Donnell, L. (1984). The daughter of aging parents. In G. Baruch & J. Brooks-Gunn (Eds.), *Women in mid-life* (pp. 203–225). New York: Plenum.

Szinovacz, M. (1982). Introduction: Research on women's retirement. In M. Szinovacz (Ed.), *Women's retirement* (pp. 13–21). Beverly Hills: Sage.

Szinovacz, M. E. (1983). Beyond the hearth: Older women and retirement. In E. W. Markson (Ed.), *Older women: Issues and prospects* (pp. 93–120). Lexington, MA: Lexington Books.

Thompson, G. (1980). Economic status of late middle-aged widows. In N. Datan & N. Lohman (Eds.), *Transitions of aging* (pp. 133–139). New York: Academic Press.

Treas, J. (1983). Aging and the family. In D. S. Woodruff & J. E. Birren (Eds.), *Aging: Scientific perspectives and social issues* (2nd ed., pp. 94–109). Monterey, CA: Brooks/Cole.

Treiman, D. J., & Terrell, K. (1975). Sex and the process of status attainment: A comparison of working men and women. *American Sociological Review, 40*, 174–200.

Troll, L. E. (1980). Grandparenting. In L. W. Poon (Ed.), *Aging in the 1980's: Psychological issues* (pp. 475–481). Washington, DC: American Psychological Association.

Troll, L. E. (1987). Gender differences in cross-generation networks. *Sex Roles, 17*, 751–766.

Troll, L. E., & Bengtson, V. (1982). Intergenerational relations throughout the life span. In B. B. Wolman (Ed.), *Handbook of developmental psychology* (pp. 890–911). Englewood Cliffs, NJ: Prentice-Hall.

Turner, B. F. (1982). Sex-related differences in aging. In B. B. Wolman (Ed.), *Handbook of developmental psychology* (pp. 912–936). Englewood Cliffs, NJ: Prentice-Hall.

U.S. Bureau of the Census. (1975). *Fertility expectations of American women: June 1974.* (Current Population Reports, Series P-20, No. 271). Washington, DC: U.S. Government Printing Office.

U.S. Bureau of the Census. (1987). *Male-female differences in work experience, occupation, and earnings: 1984.* (Current Population Reports, Series P-70, No. 10). Washington, DC: U.S. Government Printing Office.

U.S. Bureau of the Census. (1988). *Fertility of American women: June 1987.* (Current Population Reports, Series P-20, No. 427). Washington, DC: U.S. Government Printing Office.

U.S. Bureau of the Census. (1990). *Statistical abstract of the United States: 1990* (110th ed.). Washington, DC: U.S. Government Printing Office.

U.S. Department of Labor. (1983). *Time of change: 1983 handbook on women workers* (Bulletin 298). Washington, DC: U.S. Government Printing Office.

U.S. Senate Special Committee on Aging. (1987–1988). *Aging America: Trends and projections.* Washington, DC: U.S. Department of Health and Human Services.

Van Dusen, R. A., & Sheldon, E. B. (1976). The changing status of American women: A life cycle perspective. *American Psychologist, 31,* 106–116.

Veevers, J. E. (1973). Voluntarily childless wives: An exploratory study. *Sociology and Social Research, 57,* 356–366.

Veroff, J., Douvan, E., & Kulka, R. A. (1981). *The inner American: A self portrait from 1957–1976.* New York: Basic Books.

Veroff, J., & Feld, S. (1970). *Marriage and work in America: A study of motives and roles.* New York: Van Nostrand Reinhold.

Voda, A. M., & Eliasson, M. (1983). Menopause: The closure of menstrual life. In S. Golub (Ed.), *Lifting the curse of menstruation* (pp. 137–156). New York: Haworth.

Walker, K. E., & Woods, M. E. (1976). *Time use: A measure of household production of family goods and services.* Washington, DC: American Home Economics Association.

Warr, P., & Parry, G. (1982). Paid employment and women's psychological well-being. *Psychological Bulletin, 91,* 498–516.

Weiss, R. S. (1975). *Marital separation.* New York: Basic Books.

Weiss, R. S. (1979). *Going it alone: The family life and social situation of the single parent.* New York: Basic Books.

Weiss, R. S. (1984). The impact of marital dissolution on income and consumption in single-parent households. *Journal of Marriage and the Family, 46,* 115–127.

Welch, S., & Booth, A. (1977). Employment and health among married women with children. *Sex Roles, 3,* 385–397.

Whitbourne, S. (1985). *The aging body.* New York: Springer-Verlag.

Williams, J. H. (1987). *Psychology of women: Behavior in a biosocial context* (3rd ed.). New York: W. W. Norton.

Women's Research & Education Institute. (1990). *The American woman 1990–91: A status report.* New York: Norton.

Wood, V., Traupmann, J., & Hay, J. (1984). Motherhood in the middle years: Women and their adult children. In G. Baruch & J. Brooks-Gunn (Eds.), *Women in mid-life* (pp. 227–244). New York: Plenum.

Woodruff-Pak, D. (1988). *Psychology and aging*. Englewood Cliffs, NJ: Prentice-Hall.

Woods, N. (1982). Menopausal distress: A model for epidemiologic investigation. In A. M. Voda, M. Dinnerstein, & S. R. O'Donnell (Eds.), *Changing perspectives on menopause* (pp. 220–238). Austin: University of Texas Press.

Wright, J. D. (1978). Are working women *really* more satisfied? Evidence from several national surveys. *Journal of Marriage and the Family, 40*, 301–313.

Yankelovich, D. (1981). *New rules*. New York: Random House.

Yogev, S. (1981). Do professional women have egalitarian marital relationships? *Journal of Marriage and the Family, 43*, 865–871.

8

Theories of Female Personality

Phyllis A. Katz, Ann Boggiano, and Louise Silvern

They told the story the other way around (Adam forfeits ribs: Eve is born)—
Obvious irony. Everyone knew that women do the bearing; men are born.
—Jong, 1971, p. 91

Assume that you are in an intimate theater watching a strange pantomine between two people. The individuals acting are wearing hoods, masks, and costumes that make them completely unrecognizable to the audience. One is somewhat shorter and moves gracefully. The other is more vigorous and occupies more space on the stage. At one point the two sit down upon a bench and begin interacting. The taller one sits down first, occupying more than half the bench while the other tries to find space to sit down. The shorter one, who seems to understand the taller one, then tries to communicate nonverbally with the first one. In the middle of each gesture, however, the taller one responds either by looking away with disinterest or by interrupting the communication.

What are you, as a spectator, willing to conclude (if anything) about this interaction? The assumptions that most people would make demonstrate the pervasiveness of gender in our construction and interpretation of social reality. As we will elaborate in this chapter, the pervasiveness of the gender construct gives rise to many complex issues involved in theorizing about female personality.

Note that the only distinguishing cues mentioned in the hypothetical scene were the heights, types of movement, and interaction styles of the two individuals. Without discussing other possible stimulus differences (such as voice or speech style), most spectators would still assume (1) that the characters differ in gender, (2) that the shorter one is female, and (3) that whatever personality differences are exhibited within this brief episode are probably attributable to the assumed gender differences. Notice also that such assumptions and attributions are far from atypical in our everyday lives, whether or not we proclaim ourselves personality theorists.

As scientists, we are trained to understand the overlap in statistical distributions of traits. Nevertheless, we also manifest strong biases to perceive and magnify sex differences (what Hare-Mustin & Maracek, 1988, label ''alpha bias'') even when they have not been substantiated. Early personality theorists have exhibited such biases and dealt with them in a variety of ways. For some the bias was so strong that gender attributions were treated as not requiring additional explanations. Others regarded perceived gender differences as ''noise'' in their theories, an annoying variability. Consequently, many focused only on males and assumed that female behavior represented relatively minor variations from a supposedly universal male norm. Others assumed that female behavior, which differed too much from the male norm, was essentially deviant, a function of irrationality or other negative attributions. (As Henry Higgins laments in ''My Fair Lady,'' ''Why can't a woman be more like a man?'')

The major purpose of this chapter is to consider how women have been conceptualized by personality theorists and to trace these trends historically. In so doing, we will attempt to demonstrate how political concepts about women and gender differences have played a major role in what earlier theorists regarded as a simple, objective, scientific enterprise. The political influences are particularly apparent when popular personality theories of psychology are examined in terms of whether they originated before or after the women's movement. Interestingly, if not surprisingly, both the assumptions made about gender and the gender of most of the theorists differ during these two periods.

There have been numerous controversies about what constitutes an appropriate designation of the construct of ''personality.'' For the purposes of the present chapter, we chose to define it rather broadly and inclusively. Thus, when we refer to personality, we mean those global patterns of behavior that are organized, learned, relatively stable, that are most apparent in the social and affective domains, and that appear to distinguish individuals. We recognize that the construct of personality is itself an interpretation of complex observations involving multiple interactions of organismic and situational characteristics. This learning over time is often referred to as the ''socialization'' process. Theorists have often categorized these observations in terms of more specific constructs such as personality structure, dynamics, and content. The role of gender may well differentially impact these various subcategories of personality.

Psychological theory serves a variety of functions, including global goals such as the understanding and prediction of individual behavior and explanations of a variety of group phenomena. Of the theories employed in psychology, personality theories have often been the most all-encompassing in their attempts to explain complex human behavior. These theories have also been influential in guiding research. Perhaps even more significantly, they have influenced generations of clinical practitioners in their treatment of males and females, an influence that has been decisive even in the absence of acceptable scientific evidence. Irrespective of whether or not these theories are susceptible to scientific test, they provide clinicians with conceptual categories, values about what constitutes healthy functioning, and preferred modes of intervention (Barlow, 1981; Giorgi, 1970; Mahrer, 1978). This is one of the reasons we chose to focus this chapter upon the political implications of personality theories. Both constructionist philosophers of science (Habermas, 1971; Polanyi & Prosch, 1975) and some psychologists (Polkinghorne, 1983) have come to recognize that the "neutrality stance" presumed by earlier social scientists was inaccurate and that values invariably play a role in scientific and especially psychological inquiry. Nevertheless, there is no parallel in psychology for the impact of both acknowledged and unacknowledged gender biases embedded in personality theory.

Because of these previously held beliefs and values, there may be those who would question why a specific focus upon female personality is needed at all. Isn't an emphasis on human personality sufficient? Unfortunately not, because "human" has been too often synonymous with "male." Whether particular theories are, in fact, equally applicable to both sexes appears to us to be essentially an empirical issue. Interestingly, this empirical generalizability has not been forthcoming for theories that have focused upon males as the human prototype.

The problem of how to deal with gender differences in personality has been of concern to feminist scholars as well (Hare-Mustin & Maracek, 1988). Politically, findings of gender differences can always be interpreted against women in an unequal society. Nevertheless, many investigators are unwilling to adopt a stance of ignoring differences (what Hare-Mustin & Maracek call "beta bias") for fear of ignoring what may be very special, important, and non-universal for women.

This chapter will selectively review how various personality theories have constructed female personality in the context of these issues. An exhaustive review would require a volume of its own. In our review, our discussion will deal with four questions that would seem quite simple except for the complicated role of biases and values. These questions are:

1. Do the personalities of males and females differ in significant and meaningful ways? (A constructionist's phrasing of this question would be, How much have theorists and investigators focused upon gender differences?)

2. What are the major dimensions of personality involved in these differences?

3. What factors may account for observed personality differences of males and females? (Biology, socialization, and sexism are the three most frequently discussed.)

4. What are the implications of these differences for research, treatment, and further development of theory?

However one is inclined to answer these questions, there appears to be general agreement, at least among theorists within the past 15 years, that gender is a major organizing factor in personality development. Theorists have exhibited great variability, however, in considerations of which aspects of gender are most salient in this process (e.g., the biological correlates, the social stimulus aspects, or the social stratification system), and what dimensions of personality are, in turn, most affected. While it seems clear that these interactions are robust and complex, no agreement appears to exist as to their form. We will be presenting some of these concepts in our review of the various theories.

Theorists prior to the Women's Movement were not uninterested in female personality. In fact, Freud's attribution of gender differences to anatomy ("anatomy is destiny") remains one of the clearest, if unsupported, hypotheses of the biological position. As previously noted, the perspective used by earlier theorists viewed males as central and females as "other" (see de Beauvoir, 1952, for an elegant elaboration of this argument). Early theories about achievement motivation (McClelland et al., 1953) were a prime example of how women were ignored. Human nature was essentially male nature.

A paper written in 1972 by Carlson demonstrates the frustration women were beginning to express about this state of affairs, as the Women's Movement trickled into psychology. She notes: "Revolutions often provide the contexts for introducing basic intellectual reforms. In this sense the social impact of the new feminism may provide the occasion for introducing some long overdue changes in psychology's construction of human nature" (p. 17).

While she cautions the reader against reacting in ideological terms, she describes the relative neglect of women as an object of study as well as the lack of attention then being given to what she referred to as "distinctively feminine" concerns and experiences such as love, altruism, and intimacy. In order to progress, she called for the development of new research paradigms, different emphases that dealt with women's issues, and increasing the number of female investigators. She was one of the earliest to assess the state of personality theory and its relation to women at the start of the seventies. Her conclusion:

Current theoretical orientations in personality . . . despite major controversies concerning the kinds of constructs and observations deemed relevant—are united in presenting a general, universalistic (and largely masculine) account of personality. Thus, the problem of accounting for feminine deviations from universal principles has been almost equally embarrassing to (and ignored by) all major theorists. A genuinely adequate theory of personality will need to draw from many existing formulations [of] those problems and insights which could provide a comprehensive view of total human functioning. (p. 29)

Clearly, there have been dramatic changes over the last decade and a half. This chapter will trace what progress has been made toward these still-laudable goals.

A concern with the implications of different theoretical approaches requires an initial consideration of the "data" about gender differences—the "facts" that are the raw material for theoretical construction. It is well beyond our present task to discriminate these "facts" from the theories that provide terms for conceptualizing and focusing upon them (Polanyi & Prosch, 1975; Toulmin, 1983). Our more limited goal will be to review briefly current opinion about the "facts" of gender differences and to demonstrate the salience of differences of their interpretation.

EMPIRICAL RESEARCH EXAMINING GENDER DIFFERENCES

Intellectual Functioning

What gender differences in the extant literature have been investigated and documented? This list is seemingly endless and insatiable. Even now, a considerable portion of manuscript submissions to *Sex Roles*, for example, focuses on sex differences. While differences in intellectual functioning may not be considered critical to an understanding of "personality" differences per se, any empirical work or cultural stereotypes affirming the relative superiority of one gender's intellectual functioning may be expected to form a backdrop that differentially influences factors that have traditionally been within the domain of personality. These include self-esteem, feelings of competence, need to dominate, feelings of deference, and the general milieu of social expectations that confront males and females.

Early work in this field demonstrates the vagaries of trying to establish sex differences. Research demonstrations of gender differences in intelligence were frequently published in the late 19th and early 20th centuries. Deaux and Kite (1987) noted that male psychologists of that period concluded that women were inferior to men in intellectual functioning. In direct contrast to these conclusions, however, female researchers who subsequently investigated these claims by surveying the same relevant literature concluded that unadulterated bias and/or poor methodology had accounted for the appearance that women were intellectually inferior (Woolley, 1910). Subsequent scrutiny of differences in performance across a wide variety of intellectual tasks led Hollingsworth to state that gender differences, if any, were random and meaningless with regard to overall mental functioning (Hollingworth, 1918).

Later work in this area was guided by the assumption that there were no gender differences in intellectual functioning (or at least no differences favoring females). Perhaps the perspective that males and females were comparable in intellectual functioning prompted the decision made by Binet and Terman, in their development of a "standardized" intelligence test, to eliminate questions on which females as a group scored higher than males. Yet, as Jacklin (1987) has pointed out, one wonders if the same procedure would have ensued had males scored higher.

Although contemporary researchers have concurred with the conclusion that no viable evidence exists documenting gender differences in general intellectual functioning, researchers have more recently investigated potential gender differences in more circumscribed cognitive abilities. After their influential review of the relevant literature, Maccoby and Jacklin (1974) found evidence for male superiority in mathematical and visual/spatial abilities and female relative superiority in verbal skills.

These findings generated a burgeoning interest focusing on gender differences in math aptitude. This line of research exemplifies how the same ostensible findings can yield very different interpretations.

One viewpoint is represented by Benbow and Stanley (1983), who concluded that the significantly higher scores obtained by males on the mathematics subtest of the Scholastic Aptitude Test used for college admissions represent biological gender differences in math aptitude. Findings of gender differences in visual/spatial ability also have been taken as support for this viewpoint, although there has been debate over the existence and magnitude of these differences (Caplan, MacPhearson & Tobin, 1985).

While findings regarding mathematical aptitude have been fairly consistent, a contrasting interpretation of them was proposed by Eccles and Jacobs (1986). These latter researchers have pointed out that (1) SAT scores reflect acquired skills rather than aptitude per se, (2) motivational and personality factors (e.g., test anxiety, confidence level) affect test results markedly, (3) teachers spend relatively more class time teaching mathematics to boys in comparison with girls, and (4) different experiences and kinds of extracurricular activities of males versus females are likely to facilitate the development of mathematical skills in males. Furthermore, based on their own findings, Eccles and Jacobs (1986) concluded that social and attitudinal variables influence students' grades and enrollment in mathematics courses to a greater extent than do differences in math aptitude. Moreover, they argued that gender differences in mathematical ability or achievement are largely a result of gender differences in math anxiety, adults' and students' own gender-stereotyped beliefs and expectations, and values placed on math.

Sometimes the issue is not only one of interpretation, but how meaningful the obtained gender difference actually is. Thus, Deaux and Kite (1987) have argued, for example, that even if biologic differences exist in spatial ability, this ability accounts for no more than 5% of the variance in mathematical performance. Consistent with this argument, Linn and Petersen (1985) found that gender differences in spatial task performance often reflect the particular type of task used in testing more than the aptitude underlying differences in performance on a given task. Interestingly, a recent analysis (Linn & Hyde, 1988) suggests that gender differences in both verbal and mathematical skills have declined so much that they may now be negligible.

Contemporary thinking about gender differences in this area is similar to contextual views expressed about cognitive development generally (Fischer &

Silvern, 1985). Such an approach emphasizes the embeddedness of factors and views task performance within a context of social and affective conditions. It can be argued, then, that obtained gender-related differences in verbal or mathematical performance cannot unequivocally be attributed to innate biological differences without at least equal consideration being given to the role of differential socialization experiences. Interestingly, recent meta-analyses of sex differences in cognitive skills indicate that females are performing better relative to males than was true in earlier studies (Becker & Hedges, 1984; Rosenthal & Rubin, 1982). Indeed, the fact that gender differences seem to be diminishing (Linn & Hyde, 1988) attests to the significance of socialization in this area. While such caution has not always been employed, the search for alternative causes and interpretations represents good science.

Social Behavior

A considerable amount of empirical work has focused on gender differences in the development and adult manifestations of social behaviors. Males and females have exhibited differential and predictable responses within a variety of social contexts. Reviews of hundreds of studies examining a wide variety of social behaviors have produced the following conclusion: social behaviors that reliably differentiate males from females include aggression, sensitivity to nonverbal cues, conformity, and helping behavior (Maccoby & Jacklin, 1974; Eagly, 1987). Assuming that there are gender-related propensities to behavior in certain situations, the critical questions that follow (analogous to the intellectual area) have to do with the magnitude of the differences and how they are interpreted.

With regard to gender differences in aggressive behavior, a meta-analytic review presented by Eagly and Steffen (1986) indicates that, on the average, men are somewhat more likely to behave in an aggressive way than are women. As these investigators point out, however, a number of important factors need to be taken into account to interpret this gender difference adequately. First, gender differences in aggression are much smaller for adults than for children (Hyde, 1986). Second, these differences are less pronounced than differences in other social behaviors, such as helping and nonverbal behaviors. Third, gender differences in aggressive responses are not only relatively small on average but also not consistent across studies of different aspects of aggression. For example, differences in verbal aggression sometimes go in the other direction (Frodi, Macaulay & Thome, 1977). On the other hand, males are vastly overrepresented on indices of extreme physical aggression, as attested to by crime statistics regarding homicides and other violent crimes.

Subjects' concerns about the consequences of aggression often predict aggressive behaviors. For instance, females are more likely than males to report anxiety and guilt about others' suffering due to aggressive behavior and are also more likely to be concerned about harm to others. Indeed, for females the affective reaction of guilt/anxiety and concern about harm were the most significant predictors of aggression. Finally, the tendency for males to be more aggressive than females was significantly more pronounced when the situation provided opportunity for physical, rather than psychological, forms of aggression, as reflected in the differential crime statistics. These examples suggest that gender differences depend partially upon the potential for guilt and the potential for physical versus verbal aggression in a situation.

Thus, one can conclude that (1) there are gender differences in aggression, (2) these are relatively small in laboratory studies, and (3) these differences depend on both socializational and situational factors.

Turning to gender differences in helping behavior, a review of meta-analyses suggests, perhaps counterintuitively, that males are more likely to provide help to others than females (Eagly, 1986). Eagly noted that, for the most part, the studies upon which the conclusion was based concern situations in which strangers are the recipients of the assistance. Moreover, the research conducted generally addresses short-term assistance as opposed to ongoing, long-term modes of support. While information about helping within intimate relationships is not as readily available in experimental contexts, one would expect differences in the opposite direction. Indeed, sociological research on families suggests, for example, that it is most often daughters, rather than sons, who care for aging parents (Brody, 1986). Moreover, the child development literature suggests that mothers provide more nurturance to children than do fathers (Lamb & Lamb, 1976).

Even within experiments, however, gender differences across studies appear to depend largely on contextual factors. These factors include the perceived danger in a situation, whether the assistance was public, and whether others were also accessible to help. As Eagly notes, helping strategies in short-term encounters, particularly if physical danger is a potential issue, are consistent with the prescribed male gender role of behaving in a "chivalrous" or heroic way. If helping is defined as long-term nurturing behavior, the patterns are clearly different, as noted above. Additional research is needed to examine the range of ways in which males versus females behave altruistically toward others. Moreover, long-term relationships, as well as short-term encounters, need to be looked at in future meta-analytic examinations.

A third documented social behavior differentiating males and females is in the area of small group behavior. A review of the relevant literature indicates both that (1) males are somewhat more influential than females in studies of small group interactions conducted in laboratories and other contexts (e.g., juries) but that these differences are relatively small; and (2) females are more likely to conform to, and be persuaded by, males in the few studies that report significant differences as a function of gender (Eagly, 1983).

A meta-analytic review of this literature shows that females are more easily influenced than males (Eagly & Carli, 1981). Consistent with this, high femininity was found to be associated with susceptibility to conformity pressure (Bem, 1974). Again, however, several caveats are in order with regard to interpreting these results. First, more traditional masculine than feminine content was used in the influence induction of these studies. Second, gender of the researcher appears to be an important factor influencing data outcome. Eagly (1983), for example, states that 79% of the authors reporting influence effects were male, and male authors reported larger sex differences than did female authors. The correlation between sex of investigator and effect size of the reported sex difference was .41 (with larger effects reported by male authors). Even if not entirely an artifact, the finding that women are more affected by others' beliefs and values can be evaluated either positively or negatively. The typical implication has been negative—females are more capable of being "fooled." Alternatively, Langer (1989) has noted that sensitivity to social cues may be more adaptive in certain contexts than insensitivity.

A final social behavior given careful scrutiny by several investigators centers on gender differences in nonverbal behaviors. A number of compelling components of nonverbal behaviors have been examined, with several striking conclusions. First, as noted in Hall's (1978) review, females show more ability in decoding nonverbal cues or interpreting the meaning of others' messages. Of interest is the finding that gender differences are greatest when the task involves the decoding of facial cues. Second, females are more able than males to send nonverbal messages effectively (Hall, 1984). Third, within social situations females are more apt than males to exhibit positive affect by means of facial cues (e.g., smile) and gaze more at others than do males. In addition, women display more "immediate" (Mehrabian, 1969) or supportive behaviors toward others than males do, for example, more head nodding, forward leaning, and expressiveness.

The implications of these kinds of nonverbal behaviors for affecting others' sense of self are perhaps best understood in light of research findings reported by Word, Zanna, and Cooper (1974). These findings show that increased frequency of immediate nonverbal responses (i.e., head nodding, forward leaning, gazing) has been found to produce more competent behaviors on the part of their recipients. Competence was measured by observers' evaluations. It could be argued, then, that the interactive style of females often enhances others' self-esteem and sense of efficacy. It should be noted that unlike the data on gender differences in conformity, gender differences on the part of researchers, that is, male versus female authors, do not significantly account for the pattern of data obtained with regard to gender differences in nonverbal behaviors.

Similar findings with regard to females' competence in an affective domain have been obtained by researchers investigating task-oriented versus social-emotional behaviors in small groups (Anderson & Blanchard, 1982; Carli, 1982). These results indicate that males are more task-oriented in small group sessions, that is, oriented toward problem-solving behavior, whereas females are more competent in the social and expressive domain by inducing a positive affect and atmosphere among members of the group.

Gender differences in communication and relationship style often have been noted in the domain of marital and family relationships, as well as in the more artificial small groups that have been studied more rigorously. Researchers and clinicians have noted that wives are more able and motivated than are husbands to engage in emotionally expressive, self-disclosing communication within marriages (Markman & Kraft, 1989). At least in distressed marriages husbands more often fail to notice or respond to their partners' negative affect, often withdrawing or seeking impersonal instrumental solutions to emotional difficulties (Floyd & Markman, 1983; Notarius & Pelligrini, 1987). At the level of autonomic functioning there is some evidence that men may find it more difficult to regulate arousal in the face of affectively charged communication (Notarius & Johnson, 1982) and that such high arousal predicted declines in marital satisfaction measured three years later. Markman and Kraft (1989) concluded that men's greater difficulty with communication in marriage contributes to considerable distress and anger on the part of women and ultimately to a distressed marital relationship cycle.

In sum, then, it appears that females have developed better skills in decoding the feelings of others (and perhaps their own). This may in part account for their greater ability to empathize and to communicate emotional support (Reisman, 1990). Furthermore, women's nonverbal skills in understanding and effectively responding to others in a way that enhances others' self-esteem may underlie both males' and females' willingness to self-disclose more to females than to males. For example, women's same-sex relationships were characterized by more intimacy and disclosure than men's, but men looked to women partners for such intimacy (Reisman, 1990).

These data, taken together, suggest a greater sense of empathy or relatedness on the part of females that may be one of the most significant dimensions of female personality.

Trait Descriptions

The research described above centered on gender differences in intellectual performance or social behaviors demonstrated in laboratory experiments. An alternative approach to investigating gender differences in personality is the assessment of one's own and others' traits. Have males and females, for example, differed in how they ascribe traits to themselves and/or others? Over the past 15 years a number of different kinds of inventories have been developed to assess such trait patterns, and these have been widely used. Bem developed a Sex Role Inventory (BSRI) on the basis of sex-typed "socially desirable" traits, that is, traits that are desirable or normative for males versus females (Bem, 1974), whereas Spence, Helmreich, and Stapp (1974) developed the Personal Attributes Questionnaire (PAQ) to tap traits or characteristics that are more typical (i.e., descriptive) of one sex compared with the other. In contrast to earlier assessment techniques that treated masculinity-femininity as a bipolar dimension, both of these inventories reflected a "dualistic" view of masculinity/femininity, that is, that two basic dimensions may coexist to some degree in every person.

Bem's scale taps whether a person sees himself or herself as having clusters of traits as mostly feminine or masculine, high on both (i.e., androgynous), or low on both (undifferentiated). The two clusters of masculine and feminine traits have been likened to concepts of agency versus community. Agency is directed toward self-accomplishment, achievement, and assertiveness (a task orientation), whereas communion reflects more sensitivity toward others (associo-emotional orientation). Bakan (1966) and others have suggested, of course, that agency is more associated with masculinity and community with femininity.

The findings obtained by Spence and colleagues using the PAQ have demonstrated that these two gender-related clusters (which they prefer now to term warmth/expressiveness versus instrumentality) emerged in regard to both individual self-descriptions and stereotypic conceptions of others. Moreover, in a cross-cultural study covering 30 countries, Williams and Best (1982) found evidence that these different characteristics were predictably ascribed to males and females. Males were generally perceived as more dominant, autonomous, aggressive, and active and as having a high need for achievement; whereas females were viewed as more concerned with nurturance, affiliation, and deference and were perceived as less active. Gender-related trait ascriptions, then, appear to correspond with social behaviors reported by investigators.

Psychopathology

Gender differences are even more impressive in psychological symptomatology than in the areas previously discussed. Marked differences have been found in both frequency and content of maladjustment for both children and adults. The gender trends obtained depend largely on age.

The developmental literature suggests that between infancy and adolescence boys are considerably more at risk for displaying psychopathology than are girls (Eme, 1979), whereas a reverse gender difference appears in adulthood (Regier et al., 1988; Silvern & Katz, 1986). At the grade school level, for example, the preponderance of children in special classes for those with emotional problems are boys, and a majority of these exhibit "acting out" types of symptoms, that is, poor impulse control, physical aggressiveness, very short attention span, and so on (Achenbach, 1982; Achenbach & Edelbrock, 1981). Much has been written about this syndrome, with some investigators suggesting that boys have particular difficulty adapting to female teachers and their expectations regarding classroom behavior (Biller, 1974; Gold & Reis, 1982; Sexton, 1969). A recent study by two of the present authors (Silvern & Katz, 1986) assessed a variety of etiologic hypotheses regarding sex differences in these kinds of behaviors, taking sex roles into account. In that study we found that for both boys and girls, their sex-role patterns were related to the type of mental health problems they exhibited. Externalizing or conduct disorder problems were associated with stereotypically masculine self-concepts in boys. High femininity in girls was associated with higher levels of internalizing or personality problems, such as shyness, anxiety, and so on.

Sex roles play a part in adult psychopathology as well, and both masculinity and femininity have their hazards. Acting out behavior continues to predominate in males over the life span, as attested by gender differences in rates of violent crimes, antisocial personality disorders, and substance abuse, whereas women have higher rates of affective and somatization disorders (Regier, et al., 1988). Strickland (1988) notes that psychiatric diagnosis may be influenced by sex-role bias and that diagnoses are often linked to conformity or lack of conformity to traditional sex roles.

Variations in interpretations of gender differences are very much in evidence. Let us take as an example the frequently documented finding that women are twice as likely to suffer from depression as men (Dusek, 1987). Almost every imaginable type of explanation has been offered for this gender difference, ranging from the hormonal predisposition theory (Akiskal, 1979), long accepted by physicians, to the possibility that the phenomenon is an artifact attributable either to women's greater verbalization about these symptoms or to clinicians' bias in diagnosis (Phillips & Segal, 1969). The fact that women have less power than males has also been suggested as an explanation for the high rate of depression in women (Nolen-Hoeksema, 1987; Herschfield & Cross, 1982). An interesting finding that has not been as widely popularized as differences in depression rates is that men have a higher incidence of successful suicides (Strickland, 1988). Achievement-oriented instrumentality is not invariably positive.

None of the various explanations for gender differences in feelings of depression has yet received unambiguous support, and a study by Ingram, Cruet, Johnson, and Wisnicki (1988) offers a good example of how newer methodology may help rule out earlier, widely held, but perhaps erroneous, assumptions. Ingram et al. (1988) looked specifically at the role of two potential variables in depression: self-described gender role and degree of self-focus upon emotions. These investigators argued that a greater propensity to direct attention inward in response to a negative event may trigger a depressive response. Women are more likely to think negatively about themselves when focusing on interpersonal relationships than men are (Boggiano & Barrett, 1991), and Ingram and his colleagues found that women and men did, indeed, differ in their self-focusing responses. Of particular interest, however, was a study in which both sex and sex role were varied; when this was done, the effects of sex were not significant—males and females did not differ in initial depression levels, self-focused attention, or response to experimentally induced failure. Since this study was conducted with a college sample, the one population where gender differences in level of depression have not been found, this particular finding may have limited generalizability (Nolen-Hoeksema, 1987). Nevertheless, of particular significance is the fact that significant differences on all of these factors were found for those subjects (both males and females) who described themselves as feminine on the Bem Sex Role Inventory. Those who described themselves as masculine (whether male or female) showed less inward-directed negative affect and more hostility than feminine subjects under conditions where self-focusing was not made salient. In explaining their findings, the authors suggest that either (1) females are more vulnerable to depression because they are more likely to have feminine personalities and to self-focus more (i.e., they have an "affective expressive schema") or (2) males are more insulated from depression because they are more likely to have masculine personalities and are more able to avoid self-focusing in response to aversive stimuli (i.e., they have an "affective repressive schema"). Men may more frequently use distraction as a strategy to distance themselves from aversive stimuli (Nolen-Hoeksema, 1987).

The idea of an "affective repressive schema" is particularly interesting in view of the "masculinity model" (Kelly & Worell, 1977) espoused by some to explain the seeming advantages to mental health associated with masculinity. Results of several meta-analyses (Whitley, 1983; Bassoff & Glass, 1982) have found that masculine and androgynous individuals tend to have more positive scores on self-esteem and self-reported adjustment scales than those who describe themselves as lower in masculinity (e.g., feminine and undifferentiated individuals). Indeed, the effect size related to femininity is considerably less than that for masculinity. These findings may well be due to the mediating response of the "affective repressive schema" posited by Ingram et al. (1988). Dusek (1987) also notes that most studies have utilized only single measures of adjustment, generally those involving the very traits that are ordinarily associated with masculinity, such as achievement and independence. Adams and Scherer (1985) found considerable overlap between measures of masculinity and self-efficacy, with the latter variable accounting for apparent relationships between masculinity and self-esteem. Thus, Dusek argues that the stronger effect size associated with masculinity may well be an artifact. Indeed, when more feminine adjustment measures have been included, such as sociability and congeniality, effect sizes were higher with femininity (Flaherty & Dusek, 1980).

It is somewhat ironic to note, despite subsequent demonstrations of possible artifacts and incomplete experimental designs, how quickly published gender differences are interpreted as a masculine advantage. Assertiveness and self-confidence are often taken as the criteria of psychological health at a measurement level, just as such masculine strengths are valued culturally. In most research concerning adults, nurturance, emotional expressiveness, intimate communication, and so on are ignored as indications of health, just as criminality and conduct disorder are ignored as indications of pathology in favor of depression and low self-esteem. The emphasis is particularly paradoxical in this case because of the long tradition of psychodynamic theory, suggesting that it is healthier to express than repress. Nevertheless, if the women are the affect expressers, they are deemed less healthy. It is also noteworthy that the more males self-disclose or express feelings of dejection, the more negatively they are evaluated relative to females.

Summary

This section has summarized findings of gender differences in a number of areas related to personality. Meta-analyses revealed that there have been a few consistent gender differences obtained, although in many cases the effect sizes are relatively small. The research designs are often confounded or incomplete, and various interpretations have been posited. As research improves (e.g., use of meta-analyses), supposed differences appear to diminish.

How much of a difference has been documented depends on one's perspective. Perhaps the most adequate way to assess the question of the significance of these differences would be to look at the ratio of positive to negative findings. This is not possible, however, since most negative findings never see the light of day. Negative findings are not typically published in journals, unless they are deemed "meaningful" in some way.

THEORETICAL MODELS USED TO INTERPRET GENDER DIFFERENCES IN PERSONALITY

There have been three major types of theories that have focused upon why males and females may differ in personality patterns. The first type has emphasized the role of biological factors, including the possible behavioral effects of genetic, hormonal, and morphological factors. The second type has emphasized the significance of differential socialization for boys and girls as they mature and/or an adult milieu that maintains differential expectations and treatment in a wide variety of areas. A third type, emerging more recently, has focused upon the role of sexism as the major underlying factor involved in sex differences in personality. Although this last type of theory could be subsumed under the category of socialization, its emphasis is sufficiently different to warrant separate discussion. Its focus has been upon the structural aspects of society, which, in turn, influence both individual socialization and most adult activity.

Biologically Based Theories

Theories emphasizing biological factors have long been and continue to be espoused. In one sense beliefs that behavioral differences are attributable to biological causes appear to flow quite naturally from a gender category system defined by a biological dichotomy. In another sense, however, unsupported assumptions about the biological underpinnings of gender differences are good exemplars of transductive reasoning, which Piaget (1928) describes as typical of preschoolers. Essentially, it can be seen in the belief that when two people differ in certain respects (e.g., genitals), they must also differ on other dimensions as well (e.g., behavior). The biological assumption sometimes goes even further, suggesting that all these differences have a common cause. We are not suggesting here that there may not be meaningful, biologically based gender differences that underlie some of the previously discussed personality differences—these are empirical questions—but only that the logic involved in formulating such hypotheses is not inherently unassailable.

Another problem that arises in evaluating the adequacy of evidence for biological positions in this area is political, perhaps unnecessarily so. To the lay public, biological causes appear to be more fundamental and unchangeable than psychological ones. Thus, feminists may be justifiably concerned that biological findings may be used against women, much in the way that such findings have hindered the cause of racial equality. Often, as was illustrated in earlier sections, it is not only the accuracy of a documented difference but both the interpretation and the power of the interpreter that can be potentially damaging. Take the case of hormonal differences between men and women. Women's greater variability has been used to buttress charges of emotional instability. Of course, men are also affected by hormones, and one former president of the American Psychological Association suggested that antitestosterone pills be taken by male leaders to reduce war (Clark, 1971). If men were more hormonally variable rather than women, however, it would probably be argued that because they were more flexible and more in touch with themselves and their social environment, they were thus better suited by "nature" to fill important leadership positions. If it were simply an issue of the difference itself, why hasn't it been proposed, for instance, that women are better suited for elective office because their greater longevity makes it less likely that they will die while in office?

The best-known advocate of a biological approach to personality is, of course, Sigmund Freud. His oft-cited dictum that "anatomy is destiny" may be the most global statement of this position (Freud, 1964). While this position might certainly have some validity in, say, a society that practices female infanticide, most contemporary theorists assume that this position, at the very least, needs further elaboration and is missing needed mediating variables. Freud's positions tell us less about female personality than about Victorian males' thought processes. Although medically trained, he assumed that genital differences were the primary determinant of personality differences in females and males. Women were considered to feel inferior, to be more vain, and to be less ethical than their male counterparts because they develop weaker superegos and gender identities during the Oedipal stage. Because girls were presumed automatically and universally to feel castrated and to develop penis envy upon comparing their own anatomy with that of boys, girls were not expected to experience as much of the anxiety about future castration, which motivates strict impulse control or superego development in boys. That is, girls experience themselves as having "less to lose" from impulsive or taboo behavior. Similarly, girls were presumed to identify less completely and more ambivalently with their own gender and so sometimes enviously to seek to take on men's characteristics. Moreover, this incomplete resolution of the Oedipal stage, which was itself due to anatomy, was thought to have even further consequences. Without a sufficiently mature resolution, women were presumed to be more likely to manifest the wishes associated with pre-Oedipal stages. Such wishes would include dependency, which Freud linked to expressions of infantile oral stage drives.

This classical Oedipal explanation of gender differences has been dismissed in many critiques (Chodorow, 1978; Horney, 1967; Shafer, 1974), and these ideas have been sufficiently discussed that they need not be further pursued here. It is, however, worth noting that in the not too far distant past, such concepts provided the theoretical terms through which therapists have interpreted patients' ambitions and marital dissatisfactions as signs of penis envy and immaturity.

Even a "datum" so irrefutable as anatomical differences must be interpreted before it can enter meaningfully into psychological theory. It is the meaning of anatomical differences that is at issue, and this meaning inevitably reflects social context and values. In this regard it is useful to examine the contrast between Freud's and Chodorow's (1974, 1978) psychoanalytic versions of gender differences in personality because both give importance to anatomy. Chodorow basically has agreed with Freud that many (but not necessarily all) girls experience penis envy, some ambivalence and less rigidity in gender identity, and more pre-Oedipal wishes. In terms of their potential influence on gender equality and social practice, however, the influence of these two theorists could not be more different.

Chodorow argued that penis envy symbolizes girls' frustrated experience of the disadvantages of being female in this society. According to her, girls first develop a secure sense of femaleness, then experience restrictions, and finally, during the Oedipal stage, the anatomical difference comes to stand for dissatisfaction with being female in this society. (See also Horney, 1967.) Such envy would not be so common in a different social context that provided different meanings to anatomy.

In regard to men's firmer endorsement of their gender role, Chodorow emphasizes biological sex but attributes the differences to the biological similarity of mothers and their daughters. Chodorow has argued that for girls, gender identity is emotionally compatible with maintaining the emphatic, preverbal attachment to mother as the primary caretaker. Young boys, however, must reassure themselves of their difference from the caretaker in order to affirm their masculinity. In the course of this, a reactive insistence on differentness from mother is sometimes necessary. Masculinity is initially experienced through identifying oneself as different and separate. This early, unconscious need is subsequently manifested in males' greater concern with maintaining gender-role distinctions (see, e.g., Silvern & Katz, 1986; Maccoby & Jacklin, 1974; Johnson, 1975 for relevant empirical findings). Thus, Chodorow suggests that males are more likely than females to become excessively restricted in their insistence of gender-consistent behavior, due to the biological difference between themselves and their early caretakers. In dramatic contrast to Freud, Chodorow views this as a disadvantage to males, not female immaturity. Additionally, in contrast to Freud, the importance of biology for Chodorow is socially mediated. She notes that if more fathers shared in early caretaking, boys would not need to sacrifice continuity in identity nor defensively to construct an identity based on separation and differences among people.

Chodorow further suggests that in the course of establishing their gender difference from the primary caretaker in the pre-Oedipal period, young boys often become threatened by the experience of the preverbal empathic bonds that characterize early attachment. In the process of self-other differentiation, separateness and a focus on an autonomous self become dominant. Consequently, at later stages the boys' access to empathy and dependency feelings may become too dangerous a reminder of earlier feelings of union with an opposite-sex caretaker. Again, Freud's position is reversed. A male's more complete suppression of "pre-Oedipal" longings and memories is seen not as "mature" but as unfortunate, depriving him of a more richly empathic and interdependent relationship between a fully differentiated self and others. Again, it is because of social arrangements that give mothers the dominant role in early childrearing that boys' and girls' anatomies produce different destinies.

Most contemporary approaches that focus on biology have been much less global than the psychoanalytically oriented theorists and more closely associated with nonclinical research. One widely researched area, for example, has been on the effects of prenatal hormones on sex differences. Studies in this area are of two kinds: (1) experimental work with nonhuman species and (2) studies of individuals who were abnormally exposed to gonadal hormones in utero, either because of genetic defects or medications their mothers took while pregnant. Both of these groups are, of course, problematical with regard to generalizability but are often the only plausible techniques for investigating these issues.

A review by Hines (1982) concludes that research with a wide variety of nonhuman species (rats, mice, hamsters, guinea pigs, cattle, rhesus monkeys) partially supports the model that the perinatal presence of different patterns of estrogens and androgens produces differences in genital structure, patterns of behavior, and discernible changes in areas of the brain. Evidence also exists that prenatal exposure to androgens influences differentiation of human genitalia as well (Money & Ehrhardt, 1972). Evidence for effects on human behavior, however, have been much less clear-cut and harder to find. Moreover, even when such differences are obtained, it is hard to assess whether they are primarily attributable to hormonal differences in the uterine environment or to the special attention and abnormal status associated with children who are born with such conditions. In most cases the physical abnormalities themselves (e.g., girls born with masculinized genitalia) can account for the few positive findings obtained. Although Hines is hopeful in this review that methodological advances may make it possible to relate specific aspects of sexually dimorphic behavior to specific hormones in humans, the research she presents suggests that very few, if any, gender differences in personality have been shown to be so related. It should be noted that hormonal influences may involve a "threshold effect," and thus even clear-cut findings from clinical groups may not imply that similar relationships will be found in a normal population.

A more recent review (Hood, Draper, Crockett & Petersen, 1987) dealing with the effects of biological influences upon sex differences in development comes to an even less positive conclusion. These authors, surveying a broader literature, make a number of interesting points. They note that in all studies of human gender differences, the biological aspects of gender are completely confounded with its social and psychological factors. The process of physical sex differentiation clearly involves genes and hormones. The evidence relating these, either directly or indirectly (e.g., through differences in brain organization), is much less clear-cut. With regard to brain structures themselves, they conclude that "brain organization of males and females are more similar than they are different" (p. 62). Moreover, they note that even when sex differences are found, the magnitude tends to be small. For example, while some consistent differences in spatial ability have been found (e.g., in mental rotation tasks, see Linn & Petersen, 1985), these differences disappear after only one training trial (Krauss, 1985; Willis, 1985). Hood et al. (1987) also note that a significant part of brain development occurs after birth, in the context of consistent and pervasive environmental differences for boys and girls (Katz, 1983). Because of this they suggest it is necessary to consider an alternative causal pattern, namely that "the effects of differential experience could accumulate to produce slight differences in brain development and test performance" (p. 63).

What emerges from these reviews, then, is the sense that current conceptualizations about the biological underpinnings of behavioral gender differences are very different from earlier ones. Evidence to date is far from persuasive that biological factors are the primary determinants of such differences. Moreover, the notion that such factors are immutable appears equally untenable.

Socialization Theories

Considerably more psychological attention has been devoted to positions that have espoused the significance of socialization in gender differences in personality.

One of the most widely discussed developmental theories has been concerned with moral development (Kohlberg, 1969). Moral behavior clearly constitutes one significant aspect of personality since it is typically regarded as indicative of stable, underlying patterns. In one sense Kohlberg's emphasis upon cognitive factors makes it less of a socialization theory than, say, the work of the social learning investigators (Bandura, 1986). His work is of particular interest to this chapter, however, because it originally ignored the issue of gender differences, but his findings have been reinterpreted and his theory expanded by Gilligan (1982) to include what we regard as meaningful dimensions of possible gender differences. There is, therefore, an interesting analogy here to our previous discussion of Freud and Chodorow.

In his classic study of 10- to 17-year-old males, Kohlberg suggested that the ability to reason about moral dilemmas followed a predictable developmental sequence. The first level addressed by Kohlberg is presumed to occur between 6 and 11 years of age and is designated the "preconventional" level. Most characteristic of this level of moral reasoning is a fear of punishment and external constraints. Children at this level suggest that it is wrong to engage in immoral behavior mostly because one can get caught. Beginning in early adolescence, children enter what Kohlberg labeled as the "conventional" stage, where the roles of authority and convention are emphasized. Concern is expressed over appearance, that is, what people will think of particular behaviors. In late adolescence, development makes possible the cognitive capacity to reason in postconventional ways. At this latter developmental level (which is not reached by everyone), justice and principle become the overriding concerns in solving moral dilemmas, such as whether it is all right to steal an overpriced drug to save a spouse's life. Within each of the three levels there are additional stages presumed to be indicative of increasing cognitive maturity.

Considerable research generated by this theory suggests that the sequence postulated and subsequently elaborated has some validity. Nevertheless, its gender universality has been questioned because of apparent gender differences in results. Girls often score at "lower" developmental levels than do boys.

Gilligan (1982) was one of the first investigators to draw attention to sex differences in moral reasoning that did not devalue female behavior. (It should be recalled that Freud and many of his psychoanalytic disciples believed that women had weaker "superegos" and were, thus, less prone to moral behavior.) Gilligan suggested in her book, *In a Different Voice*, that there might be two parallel developmental courses in moral reasoning, one that focuses upon justice principles and individual rights (more closely associated with males) and another that puts greater emphasis on caring and relationships (more associated with females). Kohlberg maintained that the two were not philosophically equivalent and that justice was, in fact, the "higher" stage (Kohlberg, 1981).

Gilligan's position has certainly struck a chord with feminists, although considerable controversy exists regarding the magnitude and significance of obtained gender differences in moral reasoning (Walker, 1984). It is the opinion of the present writers that this controversy is not completely on target, since neither Gilligan's original position nor subsequent elaborations suggest that the two types of orientations are exclusively associated with each sex. It has, in fact, been demonstrated that both types of orientations are present and available to most adults and that they each can be elicited under appropriate conditions. Nevertheless, boys are more likely to select the justice orientation, whereas girls are more likely to select care orientations. According to Gilligan and Wiggins (1987), the developmental roots of these orientations can be traced to two experiences in infancy, the perception of powerlessness (justice) and early attachment (caring). While these are both universal experiences, our sex-role socialization practices may well channel boys' attention to the powerlessness aspects and the subsequent need to remediate these earlier feelings, whereas girls' attachment experiences focus more upon the importance of relationships rather than individual rights, when the two appear to be in conflict. For a variety of reasons, the relatedness aspect of female personality has been either ignored historically or evaluated negatively (e.g., "lower" developmental level). In a world where competition and violence threaten our existence, it behooves us to concentrate considerably more attention on the positive facets of this relatedness, as well as upon its developmental origins.

Some socialization theories have focused more on adult behavior rather than developmental origins. Based on an impressive array of studies, Eagly (1987) has developed a theory termed social-role theory, which implicates compliance to gender-role expectations as the major determinant of males' versus females' differing social behaviors. Social behaviors that depict males versus females are, according to Eagly, a result of prescribed social roles that stem from family life and occupational settings and produce the "content" of gender-role prescribed behaviors. Unique communal aspects of the female cluster of traits may derive to a large extent from the role played by women in the family, whereas the agentic set of traits can be assumed to derive from the role males play in society and in the work force. Indeed, as noted recently by Ruble (1988), males versus females continue to have distinctly different functions and responsibilities in the home and workplace (Eccles & Hoffman, 1984; Ruble, Cohen & Ruble, 1984). For example, while more than half of women in America are presently in the labor force, women still account for almost all nurses and secretaries, while males represent most engineers and architects. The maintenance of different roles held by males versus females in families and societies would appear to perpetuate differences in traits people ascribe and even prescribe to the two genders. Interestingly, Eagly argues that adult social roles are more directly relevant to gender differences in social behaviors than prior socialization experiences or biological factors.

A related theoretical perspective assumes that while social roles are significant determinants of beliefs about different "personality traits" of males and females (and help to maintain such beliefs), early socialization practices and experiences are also of critical importance (Ruble, 1988). From this vantage point differential treatment by parents (and other socialization agents such as teachers and peers) shapes personality characteristics of boys and girls from very early on (Katz, 1979; Block, 1983; Fagot, 1984; Lamb, Easterbrooks & Holden, 1980). Indeed, within the first 24 hours of a child's life parents see their boys as more alert and stronger than their daughters, whereas their daughters are perceived to be softer, more finely featured, and less attentive than boys (Rubin, Provenzano & Luria, 1974). Infants are also treated differently by strangers as a consequence of their assigned gender labels (Seavy, Katz & Zalk, 1975). These differing perceptions and expectations appear to have marked effects with regard to differential treatment of children, particularly for fathers. Fathers perceive information about their children in more stereotyped ways than mothers, and these perceptions extend to differential behaviors directed at daughters versus sons. For example, boys are generally stimulated more often by their fathers and engage in more gross motor play, and fathers offer more stereotypic toys to their children (Maccoby & Jacklin, 1974). Moreover, more positive reactions and attention on the part of parents are directed to children when they behave in sex-appropriate as opposed to sex-inappropriate ways (Fagot, 1978). Ruble concludes that the evidence clearly points to pressure for children to behave in sex-appropriate ways, with boys receiving more pressure and fathers particularly prone to extend such pressure. In addition, as noted previously, teachers and other socializing agents respond very differently to girls versus boys in other settings (Eccles-Parsons, 1983); for example, parents and teachers expect girls to exhibit the helpless response pattern (Dweck & Leggett, 1988) to a greater extent than boys (Boggiano & Barrett, 1991). These early experiences may lead to the development of gender-related traits that, in turn, may direct and perpetuate the entry of males versus females into differing social roles in the family and work force.

A third group of researchers considering determinants of gender-related traits have developed the self-in-relation theory, which posits that early socialization experiences account for gender-related characteristics (Miller, 1984). This theory assumes that the relational self is the core self-structure in women. The self, according to this perspective, is experienced in a way not addressed by psychoanalytic or traditional developmental theories. Previous theorists have emphasized the critical importance of separation from the mother and others as one develops in order to form a mature, separate identity (Erikson, 1963; Levinson, 1978; Mahler, Pine & Berman, 1975). According to Erikson (1963), characteristics of independence and autonomy are deemed valuable, and true intimacy and relational trust are not possible until the closure of identity is experienced. The self-in-relation theory provides a distinctly different emphasis on the processes of development by assuming that relatedness is the primary and basic goal of development. Moreover, autonomy is assumed to develop only within the context of a capacity for relating. Thus, in direct contrast to previous theories, self as an autonomous being is subsumed and dependent on relational competence.

From this perspective even at a very early stage, the infant develops an internal representation of self that reflects a relationship between self and caretakers. The formation of self depends on "being in relation," to use Miller's term (1984), and a sense of well-being is presumed to occur only as the infant and caretaker move dynamically in an emotional relationship that promotes positive emotional interplay between self and caretaker. Not only does the caretaker attend to the infant, but the infant has an effect on both the caretaker and the dynamics of their emotional relationship. The development of the self then is seen in this view as inseparable from a reciprocal, ongoing, emotional interplay between the self and caretaker.

The primary thrust of the theory, then, is the importance of early emotional interactions that form the underpinnings of all subsequent emotional relationships and connections with others. These theorists, thus, underscore the notion that the interplay—attending to the needs of the caretaker and reciprocally being attended to—does not produce fusion or a sense of merger with the other.

The self-in-relation theory provides a model that attempts to account for the heightened empathic competence in women that stems from the early mother-daughter relationship (see Eisenberg & Lennon, 1983, for a review of gender differences in empathy). Although the self in a relationship is, of course, part of development for both males and females, it is believed that females are more apt to be encouraged to "feel as the other feels" (Miller, 1984, p. 3), whereas boys are discouraged in this activity. As development progresses, females are motivated to feel related and connected with others and are less threatened by closeness. Indeed, self-esteem itself for females is assumed to be derived from feelings that they are part of relationships and play a nurturing role in them. Moreover, a feminine sense of effectiveness and competence is seen as based on the quality of emotional connectedness—"agency in community"—as opposed to an agentic versus a communal orientation.

The socialization theories described above clearly point to pressure on males and females over the life span to behave in sex-appropriate ways. Theoretical and empirical analyses of the social role perspective and socialization practices suggest that the prescription of agency for males and communal qualities for females is alive and well. Yet what is heartening about recent theorizing is that there is a burgeoning amount of research concerned with the maintenance of relatedness, a cluster of characteristics previously devalued (Broverman et al., 1972).

For instance, the implication of the development of self-in-relation theory and the research by Gilligan and her associates are far-reaching. The central point raised by these theorists is the value placed on relatedness. Virtually all of the "female" documented social behaviors described in this chapter bear directly or indirectly on relatedness. The outcome of socializing emphases placed on females to maintain relationships and to be emotionally attuned to others (Surrey, 1985) has typically been negatively perceived as dependency, deference, or acquiescence. The devaluation of this central orientation of women may well put them at risk for depression, since an integral part of their identity is often degraded. If their self-esteem is, indeed, based on relatedness and yet this aspect of self is labeled and responded to in negative ways by society, it follows that females would feel quite negatively about themselves. Indeed, they may feel worthless and inferior (in Freudian terms) and experience feelings of self-blame and powerlessness (Nolen-Hoeksema, 1987). Unless feelings of relatedness and connectedness are experienced, feelings of depression may develop, which, in turn, may exacerbate relationship conflict. Moreover, attempts at expressing nurturance and empathy in the workplace, which values competitiveness and isolated ambitiousness, would be extremely difficult and may produce heightened anxiety in women. Indeed, the expression of nurturance in the workplace may be defined by employers as immature submissiveness and approval seeking.

These negative connotations would consequently thwart cooperation and harmony among coworkers in occupational settings. Clinicians also may regard the continued desire to be in reciprocally fulfilling relationships as dependent and actively discourage this basic goal. (See Westkott's, 1986, argument that the expectation that females should be caring and empathic may perpetuate male privilege and promote female subservience, however.)

The shift in socialization theories suggests the need for new models of self in which the developmental areas of relatedness and caring provide a fruitful pathway for researchers. For example, if self-esteem for females is tied in an integral manner to relatedness, future researchers may find that analyzing agentic versus communal qualities on traditional self-esteem scales may yield higher self-esteem for feminine sex-typed and androgynous types than the masculinity model described above suggests. Moreover, applications of these theoretical assumptions to clinical practice may produce dramatically different outcomes for clients whose identity is tied to reciprocal relatedness.

Sexism as a Theoretical Focus

Feminist researchers have brought yet a different perspective to the realm of female personality theory, both in critiquing and reconstructing earlier writing and in attending more to previously neglected or underinvestigated variables that are more strongly associated with women (Fine, 1985). Feminist theorists have also been inclined to attribute most previously obtained gender differences to a political, economic, and social system that has traditionally discriminated against women for centuries. It has been argued (Schaef, 1981) that much of what seems distinctive about women is shared by other low-power groups. This would include such traits as greater sensitivity to social cues, less expressed aggression, higher deference, and better knowledge and understanding of the group in power than that group has of them. (Henry Higgins's sister, Henrietta, would lament, if given the chance to write it, ''Why can't a man understand a woman?'') Thus, according to many recent feminist theorists, gender differences in personality are most explainable in terms of deep structural organizations of a society that has systematically condoned and practiced sexism.

Psychology is only one of many areas that are being changed by feminist thought. Feminist historians, for example, have noted the distortions and omissions that have occurred in our understanding of the past because of male historians' essentially ignoring the world of women (Eisler, 1987). A burgeoning field of women's studies has demonstrated comparable trends in almost all known academic fields in the humanities and social sciences.

Within the social sciences the formation of journals such as *Sex Roles* in 1975, the *Psychology of Women* in 1976, and *Gender and Society* in 1987 has given researchers new forums in which to publish and consolidate research in the field. Much of this research has been feminist-oriented in that attention has been given to research areas seldom seen before in other traditional journals, such as menstruation, menopause, sexual harassment, and other fairly unique aspects of the female experience.

Another aspect of feminist theory that has differed from more traditional views about gender is its contextual approach, that is, the recognition that traditional laboratory research is often inaccurate because it ignores the very contexts that are most psychologically relevant for women (Sherif, 1979; Parlee, 1979; Wallston & O'Leary, 1981). For an example of this, see our discussion above regarding gender differences in helping behavior.

According to some feminists (MacKinnon, 1987), one of the primary reasons for women's behaving differently than men has to do with male dominance and, particularly, living under the constant shadow of physical assault and sexual exploitation. MacKinnon, a law professor, believes that even feminists have not yet fully appreciated the degree of misogyny and sexual sadism that underlie gender inequality. Gender in her view is primarily ''an inequality of power, a social status based on who is permitted to do what to whom. . . . Inequality comes first; differences come after'' (p. 8). Feminist lawyers have adopted such views because of the seeming ineffectiveness of sex equality laws to obtain for most women decent job opportunities, reasonable physical security, and dignity. The communalities in women's personalities, then, would be attributable to their similar social status.

The threat of exposure to violence has led to a relatively new area of research focusing upon victimization. Given that violence can profoundly influence social, emotional, and cognitive development, it would seem appropriate to ask whether some gender differences in personality could be associated with gender differences in incidence of victimization.

Although all methods for studying incidence rates of violence are flawed to some extent (Gelles, 1987; Widom, 1988), conclusions drawn across multiple studies do suggest that women are victimized more often than are men and that large numbers of women are affected (Dobash & Dobash, 1979; Finkelhor, 1984; Gelles, 1987). For example, estimates of sexual abuse against girls cluster between 12 and 19% (Finkelhor, 1984), although Russell (1986) found 38%. In contrast, boys are abused much less often, and such abuse is rarely intrafamilial and is often in conjunction with a girl victim (Finkelhor, 1984). The most accepted estimates suggest that 12% of women are victims of spousal abuse every year (Straus & Gelles, 1986) and that at least 30% of all women are battered at least once during adult life (Straus, Gelles & Steinmetz, 1980). Marital violence results in injury almost exclusively for women (Greenblat, 1983), and wife-to-husband violence is usually retaliatory or in self-defense (Saunders, 1986). While some recent estimates (Strickland, 1988) suggest that almost 2 million wives are beaten by their husbands in any one year, abuse often begins before marriage, with 38% of college women reporting battering by dates (Cate, Henton, Koval, Christopher & Lloyd, 1982). Finally, there is rape. This is overwhelmingly, but not exclusively, a female experience. In different studies between 8 and 15% of college women disclosed that they were raped, and at least one-third of battered women have been raped by the batterer (Hanneke, Shields & McCall, 1986). Startlingly, when all forms of rape, sexual abuse, and sexual harassment are combined, only 8% of women have *never* been assaulted (Russell, 1986).

The consequences of violence to personality are difficult to study with precision. It is difficult to disentangle other confounding environmental influences, and different studies employ diverse methods, making it difficult to integrate findings. Moreover, most of the literature has not employed adequate control groups. At this point in the relatively new development of this literature, however, there are certain areas of consensus that are pertinent to the issue of gender differences in personality. Effects that are widely agreed on include low self-esteem, clinical levels of depression, compliance or lack of assertiveness, feelings of low control or helplessness, strong fear reactions to threatening situations, vulnerability to medical illness, and a sense of needing to hold one's aggressiveness in check because of a fear of being overwhelmed. The eerie thing about this list is its considerable overlap with personality traits, already discussed, that have been the focus of studies about gender differences in personality and/or that are intrinsic to gender-role stereotypes.

A particular irony should be mentioned. Child abuse may have a special relationship to the development of dissociative disorders (Briere, 1984). These disorders are exactly the sort that Freud focused on in his women patients. Freud's early "seduction hypothesis" may have been completely accurate in attributing the problems that these women had to the sexual abuse to which girls were frequently subjected during his time. When Freud later rejected the seduction hypothesis, he attributed the peculiarities of these women to their own wish-fulfilling, irrational fantasies (i.e., the theory of "infantile sexuality"), and he turned to hypotheses about women's biologically based inferiority, in part to explain women's psychological disturbance. By critically de-emphasizing the importance of victimization, Freud introduced a tradition of theorizing about female personality while ignoring what was done to women. (Freud's later acceptance of his earlier-developed seduction hypothesis, however, has received much recent attention.)

It is puzzling, however, as to why the literature on violence has not been better integrated with the literature on gender differences in personality. This may be due to a general societal denial of the extent and importance of violence. It may also be as disquieting now as it was in Freud's time to inquire as to whether certain female characteristics represent an accommodation to maltreatment.

There is little question that the sexism-feminist perspective has and continues to contribute much to our knowledge base about women.

SUMMARY AND IMPLICATIONS

We have focused the previous discussion on possible gender differences in the structure and components of personality. This focus was not determined by a belief that gender is necessarily the most significant influence upon personality, but rather because the gender construct has been and continues to be intertwined both theoretically and politically with personality theory.

Personality theory has served important functions in psychology and psychiatry, as noted earlier in this chapter. In the research area these theories have suggested which areas are worthy of scientific attention and which are not. In the clinical area such theories have served to direct therapeutic attention to areas labeled "pathology" and to influence therapeutic interpretations and modification of behavior. In view of this, it is quite disheartening to note that a perusal of theories promulgated prior to the mid-1960s shows that most either ignored or devalued women. Except for a few investigators (Chodorow, 1974, 1978; Horney, 1967), theorists of the psychodynamic persuasion posited views that suggested women were generally inferior to men in their level of development, their morality, their strength, and their sexuality and were more prone to pathology. While adhering to a biological explanation of gender differences, most early analytic writers focused primarily on children's perceptions of, and responses to, the superiority of male genitalia. A biological view that was not misogynist could just as readily have focused upon the role of female expectancies concerning pregnancy and birth. This issue goes beyond the "womb envy" posited by a few early female theorists. Anticipation of maternity is a uniquely female experience that may well have extremely significant ramifications for female personality. Except for Erikson's (1963) ideas about "inner space," however, almost no research attention has been devoted to such variables. Clinically, Freud could understand a woman's desire for children only by transforming it into male terms, that is, a desire for a penis.

Our reading of the empirical work attempting to substantiate gender differences in personality suggests that it is necessary to proceed with caution. The use of improved statistical techniques such as meta-analyses appears to have had a conservative influence on acceptance of gender differences. Many findings cited several years ago have not held up under more sophisticated statistical scrutiny. Even when they have, differences appear smaller than earlier investigators assumed. Moreover, the advent of more female investigators has been associated with a much broader range of interpretations regarding the meaning of obtained differences.

Despite these provisos, we believe that the findings suggest that there are some meaningful differences in a few enduring dimensions intrinsic to personality. It was noted even in Aristotle's time that women are more compassionate (Book 9 of the *History of Animals*, Chapter 1, cited in Miles, 1935, p. 700). Women as a group do appear to be more nurturant, more interested in intimacy and connectedness, more expressive, and more empathic and responsive to others. These traits and behaviors can be conceptualized as forming a cluster labeled "relatedness" by theorists at the Stone Center. For a number of reasons previously alluded to, this constellation has been either neglected in research or negatively valued. These traits have often, for example, been viewed as "dependency'' (negative) or as contributing to the underpinning of psychopathology. It has only been since women have found their voice that the valence and importance of these factors have been changing. We hope that continuing concern with the development and maintenance of relatedness will be extended to males as well so that the various voices will be in better harmony.

Our emphasis upon gender differences was not intended to obscure the very considerable variability that exists among women and girls. Gender-role socialization practices differ with socioeconomic level, race, ethnicity, and culture (Katz, 1987). Gender differences are never absent. It is because of this pervasiveness that it becomes extremely difficult to disentangle biological, social, and structural explanations. Redundancy abounds in all areas. As Unger notes (1989), the meaning of gender is constantly altered by social context.

We feel that feminist-oriented theories of personality hold the most promise for the near future. One of their strengths is the focus upon previously neglected variables that may help us to better understand female personality. They are also helping us to reanalyze and reinterpret a multitude of older findings, as well as developing new research paradigms designed to better illuminate the female experience.

REFERENCES

Achenbach, T. M. (1982). *Developmental psychopathology*. New York: Wiley.

Achenbach, T. M., & Edelbrock, C. S. (1981). Behavioral problems and competencies reported by parents of normal and disturbed children aged four through sixteen. *Monographs for the Society for Research in Child Development*, *46* (1), Serial No. 188.

Adams, C. A., & Scherer, M. (1985). Sex role orientation and psychological adjustment: Implications for the masculinity model. *Sex Roles*, *12*, 1121–1128.

Akiskal, H. S. (1979). A biobehavioral approach to depression. In R. A. Depue (Ed.), *The psychobiology of the depressive disorders: Implications for the effects of stress* (pp. 409–437). New York: Academic Press.

Anderson, L. R., & Blanchard, P. N. (1982). Sex differences in task and social-emotional behavior. *Basic and Applied Social Psychology*, *3*, 109–139.

Bakan, D. (1966). *The duality of human existence: An essay on psychology and religion*. Chicago: Rand McNally.

Bandura, A. (1986). *Social foundations of thought and action: A social cognitive theory*. Englewood Cliffs, NJ: Prentice-Hall.

Barlow, D. H. (1981). On the relation of clinical research to clinical practice: Current issues, new directions. *Journal of Consulting and Clinical Psychology*, *49*, 147–155.

Bassoff, E., & Glass, G. (1982). The relationship between sex roles and mental health: A meta-analysis of twenty-six studies. *Counseling Psychologist*, *10*, 105–112.

Becker, B. J., & Hedges, C. V. (1984). Meta-analysis of cognitive gender differences: A comment on an analysis by Rosenthal and Rubin. *Journal of Educational Psychology*, *76*, 583–587.

Bem, S. L. (1974). The measurement of psychological androgyny. *Journal of Consulting and Clinical Psychology*, *42*, 155–162.

Benbow, C. P., & Stanley, J. C. (1983). Sex differences in mathematical reasoning ability: More facts. *Science, 222,* 1029–1031.

Biller, H. B. (1974). Paternal and sex-role factors in cognitive and academic functioning. In J. K. Cole & R. Dienstbier (Eds.), *Nebraska symposium on motivation* (pp. 83–123). Lincoln: University of Nebraska Press.

Block, J. H. (1983). Differential premises arising from differential socialization of the sexes: Some conjectures. *Child Development, 54,* 1335–1354.

Boggiano, A. K., & Barrett, M. (1991). Strategies to motivate helpless and mastery-oriented children: The effects of gender-based expectancies. *Sex Roles, 51,* 435–442.

Briere, J. (1984). *The effects of childhood sexual abuse on later psychological functioning: Defining a post-sexual abuse syndrome.* Paper presented at the Third National Conference on Sexual Victimization of Children, Washington, DC.

Brody, E. M. (1986). Parent care as a normative family stress. The Donald P. Kent Memorial Lecture. *Gerontologist, 25,* 19–29.

Broverman, J. K., Vogel, S. R., Broverman, D. M., Clarkson, F. E., & Rosencrantz, P. S. (1972). Sex role strategies: A current appraisal. *Journal of Social Issues, 28,* 59–78.

Caplan, P. J., MacPhearson, G. M., & Tobin, P. (1985). Do sex-related differences in spatial abilities exist? *American Psychologist, 40,* 786–799.

Carli, L. L. (1982). *Are women more social and men more task oriented? A meta-analytic review of sex differences in group interaction, reward allocation, coalition formation, and cooperation in the Prisoner's Dilemma game.* Unpublished manuscript, University of Massachusetts, Amherst.

Carlson, R. (1972). Understanding women: Implications for personality theory and research. *Journal of Social Issues, 28* (2), 17–32.

Cate, R. M., Henton, J. M., Koval, J., Christopher, F. S., & Lloyd, S. (1982). Premarital abuse: A social psychological perspective. *Journal of Family Issues, 3,* 79–90.

Chodorow, N. (1974). Family structure and feminine personality. In M. S. Rosaldo & L. Lamphere (Eds.), *Woman, culture & society* (pp. 43–66). Stanford, CA: Stanford University Press.

Chodorow, N. (1978). *The reproduction of mothering: Psychoanalysis and the sociology of gender.* Berkeley: University of California Press.

Clark, K. B. (1971). Pathos of power: A psychological perspective. *American Psychologist, 26,* 1047–1057.

Deaux, K., & Kite, M. E. (1987). Thinking about gender. In B. B. Hess & M. M. Ferree (Eds.), *Analyzing gender: A handbook of social science research.* Newbury Park, CA: Sage.

de Beauvoir, S. (1952). *The second sex.* New York: Random House.

Derlega, V. J., Durham, B., Gochel, B., & Sholes, D. (1981). Sex differences in self-disclosure: Effects of topic content, friendship and partner's sex. *Sex Roles, 7,* 433–477.

Dobash, R. E., & Dobash, R. (1979). *Violence against wives.* New York: Free Press.

Dusek, J. B. (1987). Sex roles and adjustment. In D. B. Carter (Ed.), *Current conceptions of sex roles and sex typing* (pp. 211–222). New York: Praeger.

Dweck, C. S., & Leggett, E. L. (1988). Social/cognitive approach to motivation and personality. *Psychological Review, 95* (2), 256–273.

Eagly, A. H. (1983). Gender and social influence: A social psychological analysis. *American Psychologist*, *38*, 971–981.

Eagly, A. H. (1986). Some meta-analytic approaches to examining the validity of gender-difference research. In J. Hyde & M. C. Linn (Eds.), *The psychology of gender: Advances through meta-analysis* (pp. 159-177). Baltimore: Johns Hopkins University Press.

Eagly, A. H. (1987). *Sex differences in social behavior: A social-role interpretation.* Hillsdale, NJ: Erlbaum.

Eagly, A. H., & Carli, L. L. (1981). Sex of researchers and sex-typed communications as determinants of sex differences in influenceability. A meta-analysis of social influence studies. *Psychological Bulletin*, *90*, 1–20.

Eagly, A. H., & Steffen, V. J. (1986). Gender and aggressive behavior: A meta-analytic review of the social psychological literature. *Psychological Bulletin*, *100*, 309–330.

Eccles, J. S., & Hoffman, L. W. (1984). Socialization and the maintenance of a sex segregated labor market. In H. W. Stevenson & A. E. Siegel (Eds.), *Research in child development and social policy* (Vol. 1). Chicago: University of Chicago Press.

Eccles, J. S., & Jacobs, J. E. (1986). Social forces shape math attitudes and performance. *Signs*, *11* (21), 367–380.

Eccles-Parsons, J. (1983). Expectancies, values, and academic behaviors. In J. T. Spence (Ed.), *Achievement and achievement motives*. San Francisco: Freeman.

Eisenberg, N., & Lennon, R. (1983). Sex differences in empathy and related capacities. *Psychological Bulletin*, *94* (1), 100–131.

Eisler, R. (1987). *The chalice and the blade*. New York: Harper & Row.

Eme, R. F. (1979). Sex differences in childhood psychopathology. *Psychological Bulletin*, *86*, 574–593.

Erikson, E. (1963). *Childhood and society*. New York: W. W. Norton.

Fagot, B. I. (1978). The influence of sex of child on parental reactions to toddler children. *Child Development*, *49*, 459–465.

Fagot, B. I. (1984). Teacher and peer reactions to boys' and girls' play styles. *Sex Roles*, *11*, 691–762.

Fine, M. (1985). Reflections on a feminist psychology of women: Paradoxes and prospects. *Psychology of Women Quarterly*, *9*, 167–183.

Finkelhor, D. (1984). *Child sexual abuse*. New York: Free Press.

Fischer, K. W., & Silvern, L. (1985). Stages and individual differences in cognitive development. *Annual Review of Psychology*, *36*, 613–648.

Flaherty, J., & Dusek, J. (1980). An investigation of the relationship between psychological androgyny and components of self-concept. *Journal of Personality and Social Psychology*, *38*, 984–992.

Floyd, F., & Markman, H. (1983). Observational biases in spouse observations. Toward a cognitive/behavioral model of marriage. *Journal of Consulting and Clinical Psychology*, *51*, 450–457.

Freud, S. (1964). Some psychical consequences of the anatomical distinction between the sexes. In J. Strackey (Ed. & Trans.), *The standard edition of the complete psychological works of Sigmund Freud* (pp. 243–260). London: Hogarth Press. (Original work published 1925.)

Frodi, A., Macaulay, J., & Thome, P. R. (1977). Are women always less aggressive than men? A review of the experimental literature. *Psychological Bulletin, 84* (4), 634–660.

Gelles, R. J. (1987). *Family violence.* Beverly Hills: Sage.

Gilligan, C. (1982). *In a different voice: Psychological theory and women's development.* Cambridge: Harvard University Press.

Gilligan, C., & Wiggins, G. (1987). The origins of morality in early childhood relationships. In J. Kagan & S. Lamb (Eds.), *The emergence of morality.* Chicago: University of Chicago Press.

Giorgi, A. (1970). *Psychology as a human science.* New York: Harper & Row.

Gold, D., & Reis, M. (1982). Male teacher effects on younger children: A theoretical and empirical consideration. *Sex Roles, 8,* 493–514.

Greenblat, C. (1983). Physical force by any other name . . . Quantitative data and the politics of family violence research. In D. Finkelhor, R. J. Gelles, G. T. Holating, & M. Straus (Eds.), *The dark side of families: Current family violence research.* Beverly Hills: Sage.

Habermas, J. (1971). *Knowledge and human interests.* (J. Shapiro, Trans.). Boston: Beacon Press.

Hacker, M. H. (1981). Blabbermouths and class: Sex differences in self-disclosure in same-sex and cross-sex friendship dyads. *Psychology of Women Quarterly, 5,* 385–401.

Hall, J. A. (1978). Gender effects in decoding nonverbal cues. *Psychological Bulletin, 85,* 845–875.

Hall, J. A. (1984). *Nonverbal sex differences: Communication, accuracy and expressive style.* Baltimore: Johns Hopkins University Press.

Hamilton, M. C. (1988). Using masculine generics: Does generic He increase male bias in the user's imagery? *Sex Roles, 19* (11/12), 785–799.

Hanneke, C. R., Shields, N. M., & McCall, G. J. (1986). Assessing the prevalence of marital rape. *Journal of Interpersonal Violence, 1* (3), 350–362.

Hare-Mustin, R. T., & Maracek, J. (1988). The meaning of difference. *American Psychologist, 43* (6), 455–464.

Herschfield, R. M., & Cross C. K. (1982). Epidemiology of affective disorders. *Archives of General Psychiatry, 39,* 35–46.

Hines, M. (1982). Prenatal gonadal hormones and sex differences in human behavior. *Psychological Bulletin, 92* (1), 56–80.

Hoffman, M. L. (1977). Sex differences in empathy and related behaviors. *Psychological Bulletin, 84,* 712–722.

Hollingworth, L. S. (1918). Comparison of the sexes in mental traits. *Psychological Bulletin, 15,* 427–432.

Hood, K. E., Draper, P., Crockett, L. J., & Petersen, A. C. (1987). The ontogeny and phylogeny of sex differences in development: A biopsychosocial synthesis. In D. B. Carter (Ed.), *Current conceptions of sex roles and sex typing: Theory and research* (pp. 49–77). New York: Praeger.

Horney, K. (1967). Inhibited femininity: Psychoanalytical contribution to the problem of frigidity. In H. Kelman (Ed.), *Feminine Psychology* (pp. 71–83). New York: W.W. Norton. (Original work published 1926.)

Hyde, J. S. (1986). Gender differences in aggression. In J. S. Hyde & M. C. Linn (Eds.), *The psychology of gender: Advances through meta-analysis* (pp. 51–66). Baltimore: Johns Hopkins University Press.

Ingram, R. E., Cruet, D., Johnson, B. R., & Wisnicki, K. S. (1988). Self-focused attention, gender, gender role, and vulnerability to negative affect. *Journal of Personality and Social Psychology, 55* (6), 967–978.

Jacklin, C. N. (1987). Feminist research and psychology. In C. Farnham (Ed.), *The impact of feminist research in the academy* (pp. 95–107). Bloomington: Indiana University Press.

Jacklin, C. N. (1989). Female and male: Issues of gender. *American Psychologist, 44* (2), 127–133.

Jacklin, C. N., DiPietro, J. A., & Maccoby, E. E. (1984). Sex-typing behavior and sex-typing pressure in child/parent interaction. *Archives of Sexual Behavior, 13* (5), 413–425.

Johnson, M. (1975). Fathers, mothers, and sex-typing. *Sociological Inquiry, 45*, 15–26.

Jones, J. M. (1972). *Prejudice and racism*. Reading, MA: Addison-Wesley.

Jones, J. M. (1988). Racism in black and white: A bicultural model of reaction and evolution. In P. A. Katz & D. A. Taylor (Eds.), *Eliminating racism: Profiles in controversy* (pp. 117–135). New York: Plenum.

Jong, E. (1971). *Half-lives*. New York: Holt, Rinehart, & Winston.

Katz, P. A. (1979). The development of female identity. *Sex Roles, 5*, 155–178.

Katz, P. A. (1983). Development of racial and sex-role attitudes. In R. L. Leahy (Ed.), *The child's construction of social inequality* (pp. 41–78). New York: Academic Press.

Katz, P. A. (1987). Variations in family constellation: Effects on gender schemata. In L. S. Liben & M. Signorella (Eds.), *Children's gender concepts. New directions in child development*, No. 38 (pp. 39–56). San Francisco: Jossey-Bass.

Katz, P. A. (1988). Children and social issues. *Journal of Social Issues, 44* (1), 193–209.

Kelly, J. A., & Worell, J. (1977). New formulations of sex roles and androgyny: A critical review. *Journal of Consulting and Clinical Psychology, 45*, 1101–1115.

Kohlberg, L. (1964). The development of moral character and ideology. In M. Hoffman & L. Hoffman (Eds.), *Review of child development research*, Vol. 1 (pp. 383–432). New York: Russell Sage.

Kohlberg, L. (1969). *Stages in the development of moral thought and action*. New York: Holt, Rinehart, & Winston.

Kohlberg, L. (1981). *Essays on moral development: Vol. 1, The philosophy of moral development, moral stages and the idea of justice*. New York: Harper & Row.

Krauss, I. K. (1985, August). *Rotating a spatial image: The sex by angle interaction*. Paper presented at the annual meeting of the American Psychological Association, Los Angeles.

Lamb, J. E., Easterbrooks, M. A., & Holden, G. A. (1980). Reinforcement and punishment among preschoolers: Characteristics, effects and correlates. *Child Development, 51*, 1230–1236.

Lamb, M., & Lamb, V. (1976). The nature and importance of the father-infant relationship. *Family Coordinator, 25*, 379–385.

Langer, E. (1989). *Mindfulness*. Reading, MA: Addison-Wesley.

Levinson, D. (1978). *The seasons of a man's life*. New York: Knopf.

Linn, M., & Hyde, J. (1988). *Gender mathematics and science*. Sections of this paper were presented at a symposium entitled, Sex-related differences in spatial ability:

Recent meta-analyses and future directions, at the convention of the Society for Research in Child Development, Baltimore, 1987.

Linn, M. C., & Petersen, A. C. (1985). Emergence and characterization of sex differences in spatial ability: A meta-analysis. *Child Development, 56*, 1479–1498.

Maccoby, E. E., & Jacklin, C. N. (1974). *The psychology of sex differences.* Standford, CA: Stanford University Press.

MacKinnon, C. A. (1987). *Feminism unmodified: Discourses on life and law.* Cambridge: Harvard University Press.

Mahler, M., Pine, F., & Berman, A. (1975). *The psychological birth of the human infant: Symbiosis and individuation.* New York: Basic Books.

Mahrer, A. B. (1978). *Experiencing: A humanistic theory of psychology and psychiatry.* New York: Brunner/Mazel.

Markman, H., & Kraft, S. A. (1989). Dealing with gender differences in marital therapy. *Behavior Therapist, 12*, 51–56.

McClelland, D. C., Atkinson, J. W., Clark, R. A., & Lowell, E. L. (1953). *The achievement motive.* New York: Appleton-Century-Crofts.

Mehrabian, A. (1969). Some referents and measures of nonverbal behavior. *Behavioral Research Methods & Instrumentation, 1*, 203–207.

Miles, C. (1935). Sex in social psychology. In C. Murchinson (Ed.), *Handbook of social psychology* (pp. 683–797). Worcester, MA: Clark University Press.

Miller, J. B. (1984). The development of women's sense of self. *Work in progress*, No. 12. Wellesley, MA: Stone Center Working Papers Series.

Money, J., & Ehrhardt, A. A. (1972). *Man & woman: Boy & girl.* Baltimore: Johns Hopkins University Press.

Nolen-Hoeksema, S. (1987). Sex differences in unipolar depression: Evidence and theory. *Psychological Bulletin, 101* (2), 259–282.

Notarius, C. I., & Johnson, J. (1982). Emotional expression in husbands and wives. *Journal of Marriage and the Family, 44*, 483–489.

Notarius, C. I., & Pelligrini, D. S. (1987). Differences between husbands and wives: Implications for understanding marital discord. In K. Hahlweg & M. Goldstein (Eds.), *Understanding major mental disorders: The contribution of family inter-action research.* New York: Family Process Press.

Parlee, M. B. (1979). Psychology and women. *Signs, 5*, 121–133.

Phillips, D., & Segal, B. (1969). Sexual status and psychiatric symptoms. *American Sociological Review, 34*, 58–72.

Piaget, J. (1928). *Judgment and reasoning in the child.* New York: Harcourt, Brace.

Polanyi, M., & Prosch, H. (1975). *Meaning.* Chicago: University of Chicago Press.

Polkinghorne, D. (1983). *Methodology for the human sciences: Systems of inquiry.* Albany: University of New York Press.

Regier, D. A., Boyd, J. H., Burke, J. D., Rae, D. S., Myers, J. K., Kramer, M., Robins, L. N., George, L. K., Karno, M., & Locke, B. Z. (1988). One-month prevalance of mental disorders in the United States. *Archives of General Psychiatry, 45*, 977–986.

Reisman, J. M. (1990). Intimacy in same-sex friendships. *Sex Roles, 23*, 65–72.

Rosenkrantz, P. S., Vogel, S. R., Bee, H., Broverman, I. K., & Broverman, D. M. (1968). Sex-role stereotypes and self-concepts in college students. *Journal of Consulting Clinical Psychology, 32*, 287–295.

Rosenthal, R., & Rubin, D. B. (1982). Further meta-analytic procedures for assessing cognitive gender differences. *Journal of Educational Psychology, 74*, 708–712.

Rossi, A. (1983). *Seasons of a woman's life*. Amherst: Social Demographic Research Institute of the University of Massachusetts.

Rubin, J. S., Provenzano, F. J., & Luria, Z. (1974). The eye of the beholder: Parents' views on sex of newborns. *American Journal of Orthopsychiatry, 5*, 353–363.

Ruble, D. N. (1988). Sex-role development. In M. H. Bornstein & M. E. Lamb (Eds.), *Developmental psychology: An advanced textbook* (pp. 411–460). Hillsdale, NJ: Erlbaum.

Ruble, T. L., Cohen, R., & Ruble, D. N. (1984). Sex stereotypes: Occupational barriers for women. *American Behavioral Scientist, 27*, 339–356.

Russell, D. (1986). *The secret trauma: Incest in the lives of girls and women 20–37*. New York: Basic Books.

Saunders, D. G. (1986). When battered women use violence: Husband abuse or self-defense? *Violence and Victims, 1*, 47–60.

Schaef, A. W. (1981). *Women's realities: An emerging female system in a white male society*. New York: Harper & Row.

Seavy, C. A., Katz, P. A., & Zalk, S. R. (1975). Baby X: The effect of gender labels on adult responses to infants. *Sex Roles, 1* (2), 103–109.

Sexton, P. C. (1969). *The feminized male*. New York: Random House.

Shafer, R. (1974). Problems in Freud's psychology of women. *American Psychoanalytic Association Journal, 22*, 469–485.

Sherif, C. W. (1979). Bias in psychology. In J. A. Sherman & E. T. Beck (Eds.), *The prism of sex: Essays in the sociology of knowledge* (pp. 93–133). Madison: University of Wisconsin Press.

Silvern, L., & Katz, P. A. (1986). Gender roles and adjustment in elementary-school children: A multidimensional approach. *Sex Roles, 14* (3/4), 181–202.

Spence, J. T., Helmreich, R., & Stapp, J. (1974). The Personal Attributes Questionnaire: A measure of sex-role stereotypes and masculinity-femininity. *JSAS Catalog of Selected Documents in Psychology, 4*, 43 (MS No. 617).

Straus, M., & Gelles, R. J. (1986). Societal change and change in family violence from 1975 to 1985 as revealed by two national surveys. *Journal of Marriage and the Family, 48*, 465–479.

Straus, M. A., Gelles, R. J., & Steinmetz, S. K. (1980). *Behind closed doors: Violence in the American family*. Garden City, NY: Anchor/Doubleday.

Strickland, B. R. (1988). Sex-related differences in health and illness. *Psychology of Women Quarterly, 12*, 381–399.

Surrey, J. L. (1985). Self-in-relation: A theory of women's development. *Work in Progress*. Wellesley, MA: Stone Center Working Paper Series.

Thompson, C. (1964). *Interpersonal psychoanalysis*. (M. R. Green, Ed.). New York: Basic Books.

Toulmin, S. (1983). *The uses of argument*. London: Cambridge University Press.

Unger, R. (1989). *Representations: Social constructions of gender*. Amityville, NY: Baywood.

Walker, L. J. (1984). Sex differences in the development of moral reasoning: A critical review. *Child Development, 55*, 677–691.

Wallston, B. S., & O'Leary, V. E. (1981). Sex and gender make a difference: The differential perceptions of women and men. *Review of Personality and Social Psychology*, *2*, 9–41.

Westkott, M. (1986). *The feminist legacy of Karen Horney*. New Haven: Yale University Press.

Whitley, B. E. (1983). Sex role orientation and self-esteem: A critical meta-analytic review. *Journal of Personality and Social Psychology*, *44*, 765–778.

Widom, C. (1988). Sampling biases and implications for child abuse research. *American Journal of Orthopsychiatry*, *58* (2), 260–270.

Williams, J. E., & Best, D. L. (1982). *Measuring sex stereotypes: A thirty-nation study*. Newbury Park, CA: Sage.

Willis, S. L. (1985). Towards an educational psychology of the older adult learner: Intellectual and cognitive bases. In J. E. Birren & K. W. Schaie (Eds.), *Handbook of the psychology of aging* (2nd ed., pp. 818–846). New York: Van Nostrand Reinhold.

Woolley, H. T. (1910). A review of the recent literature on the psychology of sex. *Psychological Bulletin*, *7*, 335–342.

Word, C. H., Zanna, M. P., & Cooper, J. (1974). The nonverbal mediation of self-fulfilling prophecies in interracial interaction. *Journal of Experimental Social Psychology*, *10*, 109–120.

Part IV
Women's Bodies and Minds

9

Women and Health

Cheryl Brown Travis

Women's health status; their access to, and utilization of, health care; the quality of health care for women; and related public policies are significantly shaped by the social and political status of women. The major thesis of this chapter is that health is always a social as well as a biomedical phenomenon, a thesis that can be extended to a wide variety of women's health issues (Travis, 1988a, 1988b). In addition to an overview of health status, four topics are covered in detail: cesarean birth, abortion, AIDS, and health among women in developing countries.

HEALTH STATUS

Sex Differences

Sex differences in health status as well as health behavior have important implications for health services planning, prevention, and improved quality of care. Even relatively "simple" indicators of health status, such as mortality and morbidity, can be reviewed as reflections of social structures.

Sex differences in health status are easily documented. Life expectancy has favored females since 1950, as illustrated in Figure 1. Women have had a six- to seven-year advantage for most years, and this advantage continues at age 65, with only slight reduction. There is some suggestion that women have a biological advantage over men, reflected in these statistics. However, racial differences typically have exceeded sex differences, with black females reaching parity with white males only as recently as the 1960s. Black women continue to have a

Figure 1
Life Expectancy at Birth

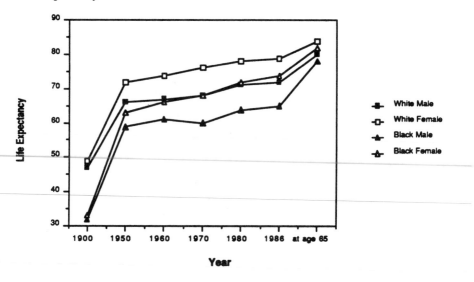

Source: National Center for Health Statistics (1988b).

Table 1
Leading Causes of Death

1. Heart Disease	6. Pneumonia / Influenza

2. Malignant Neoplasms
    (a. respiratory)   (c. stomach)
    (b. colorectal)   (d. breast)
	7. Diabetes Mellitus

	8. Suicides
3. Accidents	
	9. Chronic Liver Disease / Cirrhosis
4. Stroke	
5. Chronic Obstructive Lung Disease	10. Atherosclerosis

Source: National Center for Health Statistics (1988b).

shorter life expectancy than white women, and black men have a significantly shorter life expectancy than each of these groups. Sex differences in causes of death also consistently favor females, while continuing to reveal racial differences. Leading causes of death, listed in Table 1, have remained relatively stable over recent decades, with heart disease heading the list. It is important to note that heart disease is the leading cause of death in the United States, by a large margin, and this is true regardless of sex or race. Therefore, heart disease is not

Figure 2
Causes of Death

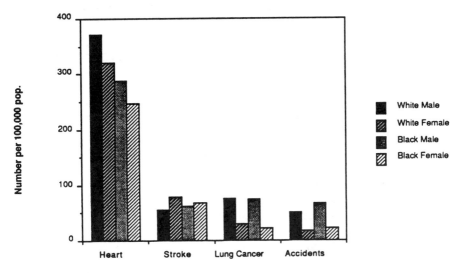

Note: Leading causes of death are crude rates for all ages. It is important to note that heart disease is a leading cause of death for women as well as men.

Source: National Center for Health Statistics (1988b).

just something of relevance to men. In fact, more women are hospitalized for hypertension and hypertensive heart disease than are men. These facts make it clear that research on various types of interventions, such as bypass surgery, and prevention programs should be examined in terms of efficacy, safety, and cost-effectiveness for both women and men. Research programs, especially those funded by federal programs, should incorporate women subjects. Examination of sex and race patterns in leading causes of death reveals some important differences, illustrated in Figure 2. White males have a higher rate of death from heart disease, rates are uniformly higher among whites of both sexes. It has been suggested that sex differences in lung cancer can probably be traced almost entirely to differences in cigarette smoking; however, males have more occupational exposure to toxins that also play a significant role in lung cancer and lung disease (e.g., coal mining). Nevertheless, sex differences do not always favor women, and women have consistently higher rates of death from stroke, partly as a function of their longer life expectancy.

Other indicators of health status, such as disability days, physician visits, and surgical procedures all suggest that sex differences in mortality are only part of the story. Women, on the average, have more physician visits than men, and women are more likely to be admitted to hospitals and to utilize more days of hospital care. About 16 million men receive inpatient hospital care each year, while about 23 million women become hospital inpatients. Only part of this difference is accounted for by labor and delivery (approximately 4 million deliveries each year). There continue to be dramatic differences in numbers and rates of surgical procedures each year as well, with about 9 million operations on men and about 17 million operations on women.

Women are more likely to receive care for a number of metabolic disorders than are men. For example, about 1.6 million women are hospitalized annually for diabetes mellitus, the vast majority of whom are over 65. Perhaps as a precursor to this condition, women are almost twice as likely as men to be hospitalized for obesity. However, a number of metabolic and nutritional disorders among women also reflect severe malnutrition, with nearly half a million women hospitalized annually for various forms of anemia, protein or caloric malnutrition, or related nutritional deficiencies, a rate that is about 70% higher than that observed among men (National Center for Health Statistics [NCHS], 1988b).

Diseases of the musculoskeletal system and connective tissue constitute another area where women may be at particular risk. Compared to men, women are at three times the risk for lupus (a blood disease affecting connective tissue) and rheumatoid arthritis. Osteoporosis, loss of bone calcium and density, is two to three times as common among women as men. Fractures of the hip, often associated with osteoporosis, are similarly more common among women than men, with about 200,000 women versus 74,000 men hospitalized annually. Among individuals over 65, this is a life-threatening event, and a significant proportion of deaths associated with fractures come from conditions of osteoporosis and related fractures. Obviously, as the general population ages, the incidence of osteoporosis and related fractures will increase.

Fractures commonly associated with osteoporosis are fractures of the hip, forearm, humerus, and pelvis. Consequences of hip fracture are particularly serious. The average length of hospital stay is about three weeks, and at least for the first year following the fracture, mortality is increased 12% to 20% (Cummings et al., 1985). Vertebral fractures are less frequent, but may often produce permanent deformity in the vertebrae that largely account for the kyphosis or "Dowager's hump" posture. Unfortunately, in severe cases vertebral fracture may occur from even minor stresses, such as coughing or sneezing.

In addition to age and sex as important variables in the incidence of osteoporosis, race, body build, activity patterns, and even geography are important. For example, white women have almost twice as many hip fractures as black women (Farmer, White & Brody, 1984). This may be partially due to limitations in access to health care among blacks or other biases in case identification. However, it is true that bone mass is generally greater among blacks of both sexes. There are also impressive geographic variations in the incidence of hip fracture, as illustrated in Figure 3. Diet may be a significant aspect of these geographic patterns.

Diet and exercise appear to be reasonable avenues for preventing osteoporosis.

Figure 3
Rates of Hip Fracture

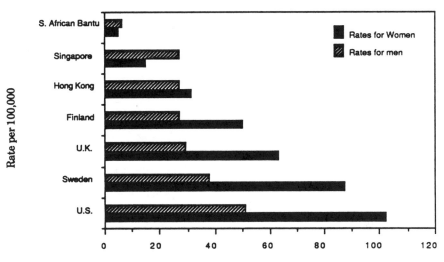

Note: Rates of hip fracture are age adjusted. Geographic variations are probably due to actual morbidity and to the availability of care and health registries.

Based on data from Cummings et al. (1985).

A lifelong high level of calcium intake contributes to an overall higher bone density at menopause. Research is mixed concerning the effects of calcium supplements, but some studies do indicate a benefit, and it has been estimated that women over 50 require about 1,500 mg of calcium per day.

One explanation for sex differences in health status is that women simply have greater biomedical morbidity, combined with the fact that they live somewhat longer than men and are thus more subject to degenerative diseases associated with aging. A significant aspect of care also involves reproductive health. Procedures to assist delivery, cesarean section, diagnostic dilation and curettage, and other gynecological procedures account for about 5 million operations among women. The high incidence of breast cancer also accounts for some of the higher utilization of health care by women. Women have an astonishingly high rate of breast cancer; nearly 1 woman in 11 will have breast cancer at some time in her life.

A variety of social and behavioral explanations have also been proposed to account for sex differences (Verbrugge, 1982; Meininger, 1986). For example, it has been suggested that women are socialized to seek help from others, including physicians. Women tend to be less tolerant of symptoms, and acknowledgment of ailments is consistent with feminine sex roles. Additionally, women tend to have more positive beliefs about the efficacy of medical care. Finally, women's roles often allow for more flexibility of schedule and the option to make office visits. Estimates are that about half of sex differences in care patterns are a function of differing medical needs of women and men; however, the other half appears to be based on a social construction of gender and health (Verbrugge & Steiner, 1984).

Quality of Care

Beyond questions of sex differences, quality of care emerges as an important issue for women and health. Feminists have argued that physicians contribute to the lower status of women by recapitulating the sexist provisions of the larger social system and that the medical system has colluded in the social construction of women as weak and helpless (Corea, 1977; Dreifus, 1977; Fee, 1983). Specific effects of these sexist practices have been hypothesized to include (1) under-diagnosis, (2) misdiagnosis, (3) overmedication, and (4) unnecessary use of intrusive technology. Issues surrounding psychotropic drug prescriptions and gynecological surgery are briefly reviewed here to illustrate some of the problems involving quality of care.

Underdiagnosis and misdiagnosis may contribute to the overmedication of women, particularly with psychotropic drugs. Although morbidity explains most of the variance in who gets psychotropic drugs, gender also appears to play a role (Verbrugge, 1982). Even when the relevant signs, symptoms, and diagnoses are controlled, small, but consistent, sex differences persist in national trends (Verbrugge & Steiner, 1985). Stereotypes regarding women as helpless and overly emotional may also contribute to the misdiagnosis of legitimate biomedical problems as psychogenic (Fidell, 1980). Once a mental health diagnosis has been made and a psychotropic drug prescribed, women may receive only limited biomedical examination and related health status checks, such as blood pressure evaluation (Verbrugge, 1984).

Approximately 62% of all visits to physicians are drug visits; that is, pre-scriptions for one or more drugs are provided, and about 10% of these drug visits involve one or more psychotropic drugs (NCHS, 1983). A wide variety of diagnostic conditions, in addition to mental disorder, may be treated with psychotropic drugs. In addition to prescriptions for frank mental disorders, a wide variety of conditions may also be treated with psychotropic drugs, including somatic complaints such as stomach pains, headaches, insomnia, palpitations, and so on. Chronic conditions and illnesses may also benefit from treatment with psychotropics, for example, cardiovascular diseases, diabetes mellitus, and mul-tiple sclerosis. In addition to psychotropic effects, these drugs also have muscle relaxant qualities and serve as effective antiemetics.

Thus, sex differences in the use of psychotropic drugs are partly related to treatment for mental disorder, but are also related to sex differences in other types of symptoms and illnesses. For example, since women outlive men, more women than men are likely to receive psychotropics to treat symptoms of senility.

The extent to which the labeling of older women as senile is shaped by negative stereotypes about women and aging is a matter of speculation.

Absolute numbers of psychotropic prescriptions, rate of prescriptions per 1,000 office visits, and long-term use patterns all indicate that women are more likely than men to receive psychotropic prescriptions. Approximately twice as many women (31%) as men (15%) will use some type of psychotropic drug during a given 12-month period (Parry, 1968).

Women receive roughly 53 million prescriptions for psychotropics annually, whereas men receive only about 26 million. The rate (per 100 office visits) of prescriptions is also higher for women (8%) than men (6%). Long-term data suggest that sex differences may be even larger. One five-year study period revealed that 15% of women receiving a psychotropic in 1970 also received one in 1974, whereas this was true for only 7% of men (Cooperstock, 1978). These data indicate that once women receive psychotropic drugs, there is a tendency for prescriptions to be continued and use patterns to be extended over periods of several years.

Explanations for these differences include both person and situation variables (Smith, 1977; Verbrugge, 1982). Mental health status is a significant factor. Women do receive relatively high rates of diagnosis for depression, anxiety, and psychoneurotic reactions. The fact that men are most likely to be hospitalized for drug dependence probably also contributes to a lower prescription rate for men. However, it is not until after age 45 that sex differences in the rates of prescriptions become most apparent. This pattern suggests that it is the medicalization of menopause that also contributes significantly to differential prescription patterns.

A radical analysis of this prescription pattern suggests an additional hypothesis, namely, that prescription of psychotropic drugs represents a form of social control. At precisely the point in life when child care obligations are reduced, career options come to fruition, and political savvy can be engaged, women are eased into senior citizen status with the help of tranquilizers and sedatives.

System-level explanations focus on the medicalization of stress, research methods, economic incentives, and social acceptance of chemical comforts. The medicalization of stress reflects a general preference to locate causes for events in individuals rather than situational factors. This contributes to a perception that problems can be strictly delineated and treated within a set prescription. Additionally, it is apparent that the pharmaceutical industry has a significant financial interest in maintaining this perception of stress and how to treat it.

Advertisements for psychotropic drugs in medical journals often depict a female patient (Seidenberg, 1971; Prather & Fidell, 1975). These advertisements complement the gender stereotypes that abound in medical education. Medical students learn that basic elements of the female personality consist of narcissism and masochism (Weiss, 1977, 1984). Women's physical complaints may be perceived as originating from essential features of femininity and as reflecting concerns of the "worried well."

Other features of medical care that have been seriously challenged as representing questionable care involves gynecological care, particularly gynecological surgery. About 65% of the 30 million surgical procedures performed annually in the United States are performed on women. Obstetrical and gynecological surgery is the most frequent category among women and accounts for more than a third of all procedures. Substantial growth has characterized gynecological surgery, especially hysterectomy. In 1965, 427,000 hysterectomies were performed in the United States, while in 1984 665,000 were recorded (NCHS, 1987). Hysterectomy is now the most frequent major surgery in the United States. Do these statistics represent the best of modern medical care? Or do they reflect simplistic medical traditions that equate women's problems and women themselves with their reproductive functions (Ehrenreich & English, 1977)? It is certainly the case that public perceptions of a considerable amount of women's behavior, especially troublesome or emotional behavior, continue to be associated with women's reproductive physiology (Unger, 1979). This perception is reaffirmed to some extent in medical education as well (Weiss, 1977).

Indicators for hysterectomy include gynecological structure, function, and disease processes (Amirikia & Evans, 1979; Bunker, McPherson & Henneman, 1977). Major diagnostic categories that precede hysterectomy are cancer, endometrial hyperplasia, fibroids, endometriosis, and prolapse. The most common diagnostic category is fibroids (benign fibrous growths). Cancer and potentially precancerous conditions, such as endometrial hyperplasia, constitute the most infrequent categories. About 21% of cases are not assignable to one of these major categories and may reflect a variety of symptoms and conditions, such as disorders of menstruation (NCHS, 1987).

These surgeries are not without risk, and it has been estimated that the death rate for healthy 40-year-old women would be 5 deaths in 10,000, while the rate for 50-year-old women with mild hypertension might be as high as 75 in 10,000 (Bunker et al., 1977). Death is usually due to thromboembolism (Amirikia & Evans, 1979). However, surgeons typically consider hysterectomy relatively safe.

The psychological impact of hysterectomy has received only limited analysis. One hypothesis is that hysterectomy may precipitate depression or other mental disorders. Another hypothesis is that women who tend to somaticize psychological conflict are more likely to be recommended for surgery, with the result that gynecological complaints will be replaced by, for example, urinary complaints, producing the same number of physician visits, special procedures, medications, and associated health care costs.

Reactions to any hospitalization, loss of control, and the trauma of any major surgery may provoke anxiety, depression, and anger. These deserve attention as part of the decision-making process, informed consent, and aftercare. These decisions are not simply medical decisions (Polivy, 1974), and women's sense of womanhood, femininity, and self should be psychologically secure, especially before an elective hysterectomy. Research on the long-term psychological implications of hysterectomy is fraught with confounds and limitations. No convincing data exist to suggest that hysterectomy in and of itself produces comprehensive mental dysfunction. However, it does appear that women who have had episodes of clinical depression prior to surgery are at risk for similar problems following surgery (Martin et al., 1980).

Given the risks of hysterectomy, it is particularly important to evaluate the possibility that many are performed for elective conditions where no disease pathology exists and where alternative, nonsurgical treatment is available. Detailed analyses of several sources of data consistently indicate that approximately 25% of all hysterectomies are elective and that over the past decade, this percentage may have even increased (Travis, 1985; Travis, Perkins & Phillippi, 1988). Estimates of benefits from these elective procedures indicate that gains in life expectancy are minimal (Bunker et al., 1977). Prophylactic hysterectomy performed basically to avoid risks of pregnancy, childbirth, and cancer will on average produce a net gain of roughly two weeks in life expectancy. On average, elective hysterectomy does not even produce a significant cost savings in health care expenses in standard gynecological/contraceptive care or potential costs of cancer care. The questionable value of elective hysterectomy has not been a matter for discussion only among feminists, but has also received critical and systematic analysis from congressional agencies, with the general conclusion that elective hysterectomies do not encompass acceptable standards of professional practice (Korenbrot et al., 1981).

The limited data presented here for psychotropic drug prescriptions and gynecological surgery demonstrate the complexity of the field. The issues of quality of care and health care policy are evidenced in a variety of contexts. The following sections present two problem areas that have long been focal points in the feminist criticism of women and health, abortion and cesarean surgery. Additionally, two problem areas that have only recently been identified are reviewed from feminist perspectives, AIDS and health among women in developing countries.

ABORTION

The first socially acceptable justification for birth control and abortion in the United States was based on concerns for overpopulation, limited resources, and the generally high reproductive rate among the lower classes. Thus, it was the concern for maintaining social order and perhaps the sense of upper-class obligation to protect the fragile health of lower-class women and children that found broad-based social and political support. When birth control of any sort, let alone abortion, was advocated as a woman's right to self-determination, extensive political and legal forces were engaged to repress the movement.

Margaret Sanger, the first American full-time advocate of women's reproductive rights, was strongly influenced by labor movements (Direct-Actionists, Industrial Workers of the World, otherwise known as Wobblies, Marxian Socialists, and Trade Unionists). In her own account she saw her work as emerging from the development of a new faith, made up of scoffers, rebels, revolutionists, anarchists, and socialists of all shades (Sanger, 1931).

Currently, provisions for information on contraception and assistance in birth control are mandated in the United States by various provisions of the Public Health Services Act and Social Security Act. These include maternal and child health programs, Medicaid, Family Planning Services and Population Research. Funds are designated for public information and education, delivery of services, training of health care personnel, and research. Although these laws require services, assignment of health care personnel, and expenditure of funds for prenatal care and hospital delivery, the law has not been interpreted as also requiring services and health care for women who choose abortion. Issues that continue to be debated, legislated, and adjudicated involve provision of services to minors and advertising.

The 1973 Supreme Court decision legalizing abortion (*Roe v. Wade*, 410 U.S. 113) was ultimately decided on the merits of arguments pointing out that the Constitution guarantees certain areas of personal privacy. Thus, the principle of a woman's right to self-determination and control of her body has not been legally affirmed in the United States.

Legal judgment about reproductive decisions gets especially tricky when adolescents are involved. Since approximately 1 million adolescents will become pregnant each year, this is no small problem. The crux of the matter has revolved around the access to counseling and abortion services for teens and the manner in which services are delivered. Whether adolescents can reach competent decisions regarding sexual behavior, contraception, and reproduction has been the subject of only limited research (Melton, 1987; Lewis, 1987; Interdivisional Committee on Adolescent Abortion, 1987). This, however, has not restrained legislative and legal bodies, including the Supreme Court, from generating a number of psychological assumptions as the basis for requiring parental notification and consent for adolescent access to these services (Melton & Russo, 1987).

Incidence and Epidemiology

The incidence of legal abortion increased from 600,000 in 1973 to just over a million in 1983, with relatively constant numbers in more recent years. Approximately 75% of abortions occur within the first nine weeks of gestation, and most of these occur on an outpatient basis, with less than 10% conducted for hospital inpatients. Only a very small percentage occur later than a gestation period of 16 weeks, with a substantial number of these cases induced because of neonatal death or other traumas. Most women are now able to obtain abortions within their own state of residence, a major change that followed the 1973 legalization of abortion.

Utilization of abortion differs dramatically by race, with abortion ratios for whites recorded as consistently below that of all others. This difference reflects the effects of a number of diverse variables, including limited access to counseling, health care, and family planning services, as well as styles of female-male relationships. Additionally, the lower socioeconomic standing of most minorities may mean an unplanned pregnancy has less impact on career, job aspirations, or income.

The impact of legal abortion on fertility rates and population growth is less than the impact of family planning and contraceptive programs. The overall reduction in births is substantial, however, and has been estimated to be approximately 20% (Frejka, 1985; Forrest, 1984). This indicates that abortion typically is not viewed by most women, or even in most countries, as a means of contraception or family planning. However, in industrialized countries where abortion is legal, such as the United States, USSR, Japan, and Israel, most women will have one abortion at some time during their fertile years (Forrest, 1984). Among developing countries with legal abortion and where rates are reliably reported, such as South Korea, China, and Singapore, a similar pattern of one or two abortions during reproductive years is common (Forrest, 1984).

In addition to the impact on population growth, legal abortion also appears to have a favorable impact on overall infant health. Large-scale studies indicate that legalization of abortion is followed by reduced neonatal and infant mortality, fewer cases of low birth weight, a decrease in preterm births, and lower rates of Down's syndrome (Hansen, 1978; Joyce, 1987). These benefits are likely to be especially apparent among teen pregnancies, because the problems of fetal and infant death, low birth weight, and preterm births are most frequent in this age group.

Finally, an important health effect of legal abortion is a dramatic decline in abortion-related deaths. In the years between 1975 and 1982, mortality from induced abortion declined 89% while the decline in mortality associated with pregnancy and contraception declined 35% (Rosenberg & Rosenthal, 1987). Thus, legal abortion has a significant impact on life and death for women. The relative risk of death from early abortions (gestation under nine weeks) is minimal and is currently estimated at one maternal death per 500,000 abortions (NCHS, 1988b).

Public Opinion

Public opinion is often referenced as the justification for public policy and the legal status of abortion. Therefore, it is particularly interesting to examine public opinion data, with the understanding that they are elusive and subject to a number of confounds. Difficulties in measuring opinions include the fact that questionnaire context can significantly shape responses (Schuman, Presser & Ludwig, 1981). Sample size and methods of selection are relevant as well. Even the general format of study instruments can be critical. For example, general or theoretical questions about abortion can elicit quite different responses than those recorded for evaluations based on specific case histories, with opinions typically more favorable when subjects are presented with specific cases (Wright & Rogers, 1987).

Arguments bolstered by claims of public opinion support have been particularly salient among speakers referencing a new moral majority or religious right. It appears that there is little evidence for a newly politicized religious right. Data from the National Opinion Research Corporation General Social Surveys from 1972 through 1980 show that, while religious conviction has been a basis for differentiating respondents on social issues, neither the degree of disagreement nor the balance of support for antiabortion positions has increased (Mueller, 1983). This is true for positions on abortion, sexual preference, and women's liberation.

Surveys conducted in 1965, 1970, and 1975 as part of the National Family Surveys indicate that substantial liberalization occurred during that decade (Jones & Westoff, 1978). Annual surveys between 1972 and 1980, involving approximately 1,500 subjects each year, revealed that increasingly favorable opinions regarding abortion were also recorded among black respondents (Combs & Welch, 1982). Further, the General Social Surveys from the National Opinion Research Center between 1965 through 1984 indicate that while there may be some differences of opinion among males and females, these are slight. In fact, gender plays a very minimal role in attitudes about abortion (Granberg & Granberg, 1985).

It is possible that heated debates may arise over abortion when, in fact, the energizing issues are quite different for the opposing parties. When presented as an issue of civil rights and self-determination, abortion may be less objectionable to some. Issues of individual privacy and restraint of government intrusiveness are also commonly acceptable. However, as long as mistaken beliefs regarding the reasons for abortion, that is, sexual promiscuity, remain unaddressed, opposition may be highly rigid.

Large-scale studies have found some consistent differences among those who support or oppose abortion. Factors that do account for variations in opinion include religiosity, educational level, and rural residence. There also appear to be some differences of opinion among blacks and whites, typically with white respondents more favorable than blacks (Combs & Welch, 1982; Hall & Ferree, 1986). In their review of General Social Surveys between 1972 and 1984, Hall and Ferree (1986) used multivariate regression to account for differences in opinion. When socioeconomic status, religiosity, and southern culture were controlled, racial differences were still apparent. The exact reason for this could not be determined on the basis of questionnaire data.

A few small-scale studies do suggest some interesting potential for different perspectives among women and men. Even though these studies are based on small samples and are short-term, they raise some points for reflection. To the extent that women and men do hold differences of opinion about abortion, these appear to be whether abortion is seen as a global issue of gender role and social rights for women or as an issue linked with sexuality, sex guilt, and control of sexual behavior. Among college student samples, women are more likely to see abortion as a global issue of gender roles, while men who hold negative opinions are more likely to see abortion as related to sexual promiscuity and to have relatively higher sex guilt than those with favorable opinions (Finlay, 1981; Allgeier, Allgeier & Rywick, 1981; Hall & Ferree, 1986).

Decision Making and Psychological Consequences

Little research of scientific quality is available regarding abortion decisions or individual differences in this process. Women become pregnant at all ages under all circumstances, and no simple statement is possible regarding their experiences. However, a few findings may be of interest. For example, locus of control appears to affect the latency between receiving a confirmation of pregnancy and subsequent decisions to obtain an abortion. Women having lower internal locus of control scores tend to delay the decision to abort (Dixon, Strano & Willingham, 1984). Teens also appear to delay decisions to abort, and mid-pregnancy abortions, as opposed to first trimester, tend to be more common among this group (Joseph, 1985). A strong involvement with the sexual partner also appears to complicate the decision process (Friedlander, Kaul & Stimel, 1984).

Reasons for seeking an abortion typically include strong work commitment, unreadiness for parenthood, financial difficulties, and absence of a steady partner (Friedlander et al., 1984; Faria, Barret & Goodman, 1985). Whether the decision process does or should involve the male partner has been addressed only peripherally. The role of a male partner certainly appears to make a difference to the women involved; however, one study found that only 41% of women seeking an abortion consulted their partners (Faria et al., 1985).

Age and racial status also appear to have an impact. Among black teens who had carried a pregnancy to term, many viewed pregnancy and parenthood as a way to gain adulthood (Falk, Gispert & Baucom, 1981). Thus, in some respects pregnancy and parenthood may reflect a desire for individuation, greater sense of control, and a generally enhanced social status. Although it is unlikely that these outcomes will, in fact, follow early pregnancy and parenthood, the motivation nevertheless is relevant.

An important issue with respect to teen pregnancy is the need for information about, and availability of, contraceptives. Some researchers feel the data indicate a need for more information at an earlier age (Joseph, 1985). However, at least one study of pregnant black teens found that the vast majority knew of contraceptive methods, but simply did not use them (Landry, Bertrand, Cherry & Rice, 1986).

Beyond the question of who makes what decisions, a broad perspective suggests that here, as in other aspects of our social system, sexism has shaped the problem of unintended pregnancy. Anxiety over female sexuality, the view that females need protection and socialization while males do not, the expectation that females will be the primary caretakers for their families, and so on have changed but little in recent decades. The adequacy of education, counseling, and services for sexual health, contraception, and abortion, as well as parenting, is greatly biased in focusing almost exclusively on young women. A consequence is to continue a sexist division of expectations, communication, and intimate relationships that tends to place the burden for planning, decision making, and family on the female, while simultaneously excluding the male and to some extent dehumanizing him (Chilman, 1985).

Research on coping with abortion is particularly sensitive to a number of methodological problems. Consequently, conclusions are general and provide little analysis of specific cases or coping responses. Methodological problems are apparent in the typical age range included in coping studies, often mixing subjects in their teens and women in peak childbearing years, as well as women in late childbearing years. Assessment instruments have included open-ended interviews, structured questionnaires, formal personality measures, and actual health care records. When both subjective and objective measures are compared, there is often little correlation among them (Robbins, 1979). Married and single patients may be recruited as subjects, and there is often no distinction regarding the circumstances leading to the abortion, for example, terminations due to marginal social or economic circumstances as opposed to terminations for the health of the mother or antenatal diagnosis of genetic or developmental defects. Further, the point at which coping or mood is assessed varies dramatically. Some studies report results from questionnaires administered during the first hour of recovery, while others involve follow-ups of three months to a year or longer. Serious problems also arise due to sample attrition, with some studies losing as much as 80% of the initial sample to follow-up (Adler, 1976). Nevertheless, a few general observations are possible.

Few women find the decision to terminate a pregnancy an easy one, and many indicate that nonjudgmental counseling is helpful (Handy, 1982). Attitudes prior to the abortion are good predictors of reactions to the experience. Those who initially favor principles supporting abortion generally report continued favorable opinions and most often a sense of relief (Eisen & Zellman, 1984; Lazarus, 1985; Major et al., 1985). Even early studies immediately following legalization of abortion, a period when social support might be low, indicate that consequences appear to be benign (Shusterman, 1976). Although relatively few studies have focused on minority women, findings among Mexican-American (Eisen & Zellman, 1984) and among black women (Robbins, 1979) suggest that minority women are most often satisfied with their decision and seldom experience serious negative reactions.

However, some women do experience negative reactions involving depressed mood, guilt, anxiety, and occasionally serious clinical stress responses. Data on the proportion of women susceptible to negative reactions may be partially biased by the fact that many health care providers, both medical and counseling personnel, often expect women to have negative reactions and may subtly impose demand characteristics on the women (Baluk & O'Neill, 1980). In any case, studies indicate that 5 to 10% of women will have negative reactions (Friedman, Greenspan & Mittleman, 1974; Jacobsson & Solheim, 1975; Lazarus, 1985).

Favorable coping is correlated with positive attitudes toward abortion and strong social support from family, partner, or other social groups (Bracken, Hachamovitch & Grossman, 1974; Moseley et al., 1981; Robbins & DeLamater, 1985). Women with serious problems following abortion tend to be those who have weak social support and who have a history of previous emotional and mental health problems (Payne et al., 1976; Lazarus, 1985). The best predictor of emotional status following abortion is general adaptation and coping prior to abortion (Belsey et al., 1977).

These findings generally apply to elective procedures and are only partially relevant to cases of spontaneous miscarriage, perinatal death, or abortions conducted for genetic defects. Typically, these pregnancies are very much wanted, and pregnancy interruption in these cases often constitutes an emotional hammer blow and a grief process similar to that in deaths of important others. Research on these issues suggests a much more complicated phenomena (Herz, 1984; Leon, 1986, 1987).

Clearly, abortion encompasses psychological, social, and political elements. In this case, health is much more a social than a biomedical phenomenon. Cesarean surgery is another case study that illustrates these principles.

CESAREAN

The view that pregnancy and birth are illnesses requiring careful medical supervision has been a major point of conflict between feminists and the medical profession. The American College of Obstetricians and Gynecologists has adopted the view that labor and delivery are dangerous events requiring careful supervision by trained medical personnel. Feminists argue that the medicalization of pregnancy and birth has had important negative effects on the physical well-being of both mothers and infants, as well as impeding healthy psychological responses to mothering (Oakley, 1980). Feminists have attacked authoritarian medical systems as simultaneously a reflection of male fears of female reproduction and unconscious desires to assume those powers.

Points of conflict include, but are not limited to, the appropriate location for first-stage labor, artificial rupture of membranes, use of oxytocin to induce or speed labor, prohibitions on intake of food during labor, the number of pelvic examinations, use of anesthesia, maternal position during delivery (the lithotomy position), use of forceps, episiotomy, necessity for internal fetal monitoring, and the frequency of cesarean surgery.

Nevertheless, medical control of childbirth has steadily increased, and virtually all births in the United States now occur in a hospital setting, with only a few alternative birthing centers available in most areas. Hospital policies have traditionally imposed limitations on access to the mother's support network, re-

Figure 4
Number of Cesarean Deliveries, 1977–1986 (in thousands)

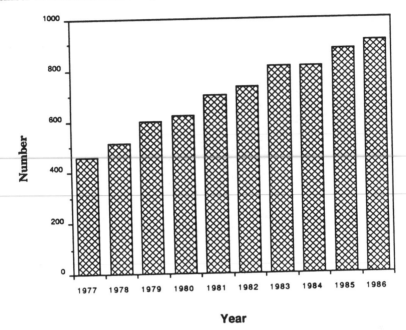

Year

Source: National Center for Health Statistics (1988a).

stricted movement, induced labor, monitored, and probed in invasive procedures. Efforts to promote patient preparation for birth and the inclusion of partners in the birthing process have been strongly influenced by economic pressure on hospitals to attract patients. Hundreds of articles are published annually in medical journals of both clinical and research focus. However, articles in medical journals that assess self-management during pregnancy, for example, exercise and strength training during pregnancy, are rare (Hall & Kaufmann, 1987).

Incidence and Indicators

Increasing use of technology in childbirth is particularly evident in the increasing incidence of surgical deliveries. The number of cesarean births has doubled over the last decade, as illustrated in Figure 4. In 1977 there were 455,000 cesarean deliveries, while in 1986 there were 906,000. The rate has also dramatically increased, from 214 per 100,000 population in 1977 to 378 per 100,000 in 1986. To put it more dramatically, in 1986 there were approximately 4 million births in the United States, 24%, or nearly 1 million, of these were by cesarean. Although a greater number of cesareans are performed among white women than women from racial minorities, the percent of live births in each group with cesarean delivery is regularly higher for minority women (about 26% compared with 19% among whites).

A variety of indicators may be the basis for surgical intervention. Marieskind (1979) suggests that the demand for perfect birth outcomes and increased malpractice suits may be significant social psychological factors in the equation as well. However, most indicators involve the prior health status of the mother, such as epilepsy, diabetes, or myocardial infarction. An active herpes II condition may also warrant cesarean. Conditions associated with the pregnancy itself may also come into play, for example, eclampsia, a condition of high blood pressure and edema that can precipitate seizures and sometimes death of mother and infant. In addition, size, position, and general health conditions of the fetus are considered, and cesarean is often recommended for cephalopelvic disproportion, breech presentation, or twins.

Antenatal assessment by ultrasound and doppler methods also often produce warnings about the probable physiological vigor of the fetus and the ability to undergo the stresses of labor and delivery. For example, reduced flow velocity of umbilical arteries may give warnings that a fetus is likely to be unduly stressed during labor. The volume of amniotic fluid can also be assessed. The most frequent indicator in this category is nonstress testing that monitors fetal heart rate response to contractions (Eden et al., 1988).

Another major factor is the general practice of automatically repeating cesarean sections for subsequent deliveries. This practice inflates the annual number of cesareans and has been recently questioned. Physicians are beginning to recommend a ''trial of labor'' among many women with previous cesarean surgery, and studies indicate that 70%–80% of these women can have normal deliveries in later pregnancies (Duff, Southmayd, & Read, 1988; Phelan, Clark, Diaz, & Paul, 1987; Stovall, Shaver, Solomon & Anderson, 1987).

However, the progress of labor and the response of the fetus to labor are probably the most frequent indicators for cesarean. Dystocia, failure to progress, is one of the more common indicators in this category (Boyd, Usher, McLean & Kramer, 1988). With increasing reliance on electronic fetal monitoring, fetal heart rate reactivity has been a major indicator as well. When spontaneous decelerations occur independently of uterine contractions, the fetus is presumed to be in distress and probably receiving inadequate supplies of oxygen.

It appears that to some extent technology begets technology and that early interventions seem to increase the probability that other interventions will become necessary at a later point in the birth process. Thus, the use of some technologies may be iatrogenic effects of interventions that take place at some prior time.

The increased use of electronic fetal monitoring (EFM) may be one example of this phenomenon. When first introduced, electronic fetal monitoring was indicated for women at risk for complications because of prior existing health conditions or early antenatal monitoring of the fetus. Without adequate assessment of outcomes and effects, electronic fetal monitoring has become standard practice for all deliveries.

When there are no prior indicators for risk, fetal monitoring appears to be associated with increased incidence of cesarean section. A reanalysis of data published elsewhere (Ott, 1981) indicates that when there were no antepartum or intrapartum risk factors, monitoring was associated with a 37% rate of cesarean section as opposed to a rate of 21% under the same conditions, but without fetal monitoring.

Labeling—a cognitive, rather than a technological, factor—may also play an important role in the decision process. If antepartum risk factors exist, such as diabetes, almost all deliveries will be by cesarean, regardless of EFM indicators recorded during the labor (Ott, 1981). Thus, once a woman is labeled at risk, the probability of a cesarean section is very high, regardless of the actual progress of labor.

An associated factor may be the increased classification of dystocia. Dystocia, difficult childbirth, may indicate inappropriate fetal position, disproportion, or failure for labor to progress (uterine inertia, failure to dilate, or sluggish progress of fetus through the birth canal). Effacement and dilation of the cervix typically requires 11 to 14 hours on a first delivery. Once dilation of 10 centimeters is reached, the fetus should be delivered within two hours or less. Progress through these stages can be influenced by a number of factors: atmosphere of the labor room, presence of a labor coach, labor position, analgesics, and so on. However, when progress is slow, physicians may be more ready to suspect strictly medical-physiological factors rather than social-psychological ones. Thus, when the fetus is within normal weight ranges and in an orientation suitable for vaginal delivery, slow progress is likely to be attributed to some unforeseen or undiagnosed complication requiring surgical intervention.

Estimates of unnecessary cesarean procedures vary, suggesting that between 1 and 2% are unjustified (Ott, 1981; Jessee et al., 1982). However, cesarean due to "failure to progress" may be significantly shaped by the patience of the attending staff and the expectations of the woman herself. Cesareans performed for fetal distress indicated by EFM probably have a higher proportion of questionable cases and may be as high as 24%. These conclusions have been reached by peer review of patient charts (Jessee et al., 1982) and by review of actual monitor strips (Ott, 1981). The role of EFM in this case is primarily due to misclassification of patient signs on the printout.

There is considerable variation in the incidence of cesarean delivery, and this suggests the possibility of differing standards. In addition, patient and hospital characteristics for cesarean delivery show some interesting differences (Goldfarb, 1984). Hospitals with neonatal intensive care units or a medical teaching status have higher rates of cesarean. If technology is available, it tends to be used. Insurance coverage is also a major factor, and women having group insurance plans such as Blue Shield, Blue Cross, workmen's compensation, or Medicaid are more likely to receive cesarean procedures than women who are self-insured or without insurance. Thus, the ability to pay is a significant factor. Additionally, women aged 30–35 are more likely to have a cesarean procedure than either younger or older women. This, of course, is a critical fact for women who plan to delay parenthood. Patient case mix is also relevant, and those hospitals with higher proportions of case complications do perform more cesareans.

These issues of practice variation and medical decision making have been of some concern to the National Institutes of Health, and a number of recommendations on cesarean delivery were established in recent consensus development programs. However, the impact of these recommendations on actual practice appears to be quite limited (Kosecoff, Kanouse, Rogers, McClosky, Winslow & Brook, 1987).

Concerns that some cesareans might be avoided if different procedures were followed have led some medical researchers to recommend "active management of labor." Essentially, this involves early diagnosis of labor, careful monitoring of cervical dilation, and use of oxytocin to maintain cervical and uterine activity. A Canadian study found that "active management of labor" was associated with fewer cesareans, reduced percentage of births with forceps, and fewer labors lasting more than 12 hours (Akoury, Brodie, Caddick, McLaughin & Pugh, 1988). A similar London study of 1,000 actively managed births also found reduced cases of cesarean delivery with no increase in perinatal mortality (Turner, Brassil & Gordon, 1988). These data are confounded by the fact that physicians preselect those patients assigned to active management, and differences in patient characteristics might well alter results. A prospective randomized assignment of subjects (women in their first pregnancy) to standard treatment or active management found no significant effects on the incidence of cesarean (Cohen, O'Brien, Lewis & Knuppel, 1987).

Outcomes and Effects

Initial demand for increased technology was based on the assumption that mortality and morbidity would be reduced, and these have come to be the criterion measures for evaluation. However, infant mortality in the United States does not compare particularly favorably with rates in other developed countries, where births are associated with less technology. Japan, Sweden, Finland, and several other countries have lower infant mortality rates than the United States (NCHS, 1988b). Infant mortality per 1,000 live births is approximately 6.6 for Japan, Sweden, and Finland in 1982, while that for the United States is approximately 11.6 (NCHS, 1988b).

Other measures of outcomes also suggest equivocal results. Surgical delivery is justified by improved medical outcomes for the infant and mother, reflected in reduced cerebral palsy, seizures, and other neurological signs. When acute or traumatic conditions prevail, surgical delivery may significantly increase the likelihood of survival, for example, in the case of a breech presentation (Tejani, Verma, Shiffman & Chayen, 1987). However, research problems make general conclusions difficult, particularly when researchers persist in use of idiosyncratic measurement and presentation of results (Jakobi, Weissman & Paldi, 1987).

Some long-term studies suggest that the benefits of cesarean delivery are questionable. One three-year comparison of perinatal death and neonatal seizures for a Dublin hospital (the control) and a Dallas hospital with three to four times the rate of cesarean section found no difference in perinatal death, and the incidence of seizures was twice as high in the Dallas hospital (O'Driscoll, Foley, MacDonald & Stronge, 1988). Surveillance of cerebral palsy and cesarean section for over a decade in Australia found no decrease in cerebral palsy, although cesareans significantly increased during the study period (Stanley & Watson, 1988).

Infant well-being may also be shaped by factors not easily measured. These are sometimes referred to as "soft" outcomes (Nadelson, 1978). A woman's sense of mastery, assertiveness, and agency, which may or may not be enhanced during labor and delivery, may well affect postpartum depression, difficulties in maternal or paternal infant bond, difficulties in mother-father relationship, or developmental problems in the baby (Oakley, 1983).

Consequences of cesarean birth include psychological, behavioral, and developmental factors, as well as standard biomedical effects. Marieskind (1982) concludes that psychological costs can be dramatic, involving feelings of inadequacy, guilt, regret, and hostility toward the infant. Apparently any risk condition that becomes relevant during labor and delivery tends to increase anxiety following delivery and also to lead to more negative perceptions of the newborn (Blumberg, 1980). Data indicate that mothers may continue to have feelings of depression and negative mood a month or more following delivery (Gottlieb & Barrett, 1986).

Physician attitudes about cesareans are probably quite important and can be partly inferred from the fact that although it is a major surgical procedure, it is called a cesarean section. This clean label may have major effects on decision making and follow-up care. For example, common psychological reactions to major surgery may be ignored, and patients' emotional reactions may be judged as incidental (Oakley, 1983). Additionally, issues of quality assurance and surgical review may be more casual.

Conditions during cesarean procedures can vary dramatically from emergency cases to planned cesareans, in type of anesthesia, and in presence of the partner. In fact, there are some data to indicate that it is the presence (or absence of the partner) that is critical to the woman's experience of the cesarean (Mercer, Hackley & Bostrom, 1983; Cranley, Hedahl & Pegg, 1983). The effects of partner presence have not been well researched and deserve particular attention. This point is especially important, because medical personnel may view a husband's presence with a good deal of skepticism.

Behavioral observations of cesarean mother-infant interactions on the first visit indicate that these mothers handle their infants less than mothers with normal deliveries (Tulman, 1986). This may be partly due to the fact that cesarean infants, even those delivered with minimal anesthesia, tend to exhibit depressed behavioral activity for several weeks following birth. Interestingly, this effect is magnified when the cesarean father is present. However, long-term follow-up suggests that some of these effects may dissipate with time. A survey of first-graders entering Baltimore city schools found that children delivered by cesarean had typical scores on standard achievement tests, and they and their parents expected average or better school performance (Entwisle & Alexander, 1987).

Adjustment to cesarean motherhood can be difficult for many women, who feel they have failed in their reproductive roles. Disappointment and lingering doubts about the newborn's health can be compounded by the prolonged physical recovery period, pain, discomfort, and fatigue associated with cesarean delivery. Social support is critically important at these times, particularly those networks that are already well grounded and operational (Hobfoll, Nadler & Leiberman, 1986). Social support groups formed specifically for cesarean mothers can have significant positive effects. Women in cesarean support groups report that the groups provide information, role models, and an opportunity to help others (Lipson & Tilden, 1980; Lipson, 1981). Typically, participants feel such groups are positive forces for postpartum adjustment and motherhood.

Issues of knowledge, assertiveness, and informed consent are central to the phenomenon of hi-tech births. Medical care utilization and decision making are areas where knowledge of basic information, procedures, and standards of practice is the most important source of power available to the woman patient. Unfortunately, many women may have only a vague understanding of the factors that shaped their birth experience. For example, a survey of recent mothers that assessed their knowledge of informed consent and assertive behaviors during labor found that both were associated with normal delivery, while cesarean delivery was associated with lack of knowledge and passive behavior (Morford & Barclay, 1984).

Significant features of birth and delivery are obviously shaped by expectations, labels, and access to information. These same factors are perhaps even more relevant to a new health issue for women, AIDS.

ACQUIRED IMMUNODEFICIENCY SYNDROME

Acquired immunodeficiency syndrome (AIDS) was first recognized and formally reported to health registries in spring of 1981. Within six years, AIDS had been reported in 109 countries, and by March 1988, 55,315 cases had been reported in the United States alone. Compared with other world regions (Africa, Europe, Asia, and Oceania), the United States has by far the highest number of reported cases (Mann, 1987). As of spring 1992, 230,000 cases had been reported (Centers for Disease Control, 1992) requiring an estimated expenditure of $16 billion for direct health care costs (Eickhoff, 1988), and approximately 54,000 of these will die of AIDS in that year (Hatziandreu, Graham & Stoto, 1988).

Epidemiology

Worldwide estimates of human immunodeficiency virus (HIV) infection range from 5 to 10 million, with the prediction that in the next five years 10–30% will develop AIDS (Mann, 1987). The reported incidence is very much a function of access to, and utilization of, health care services and disease registries as well as the actual prevalence of disease. Surveillance and reporting in developing countries are especially problematic, and it may well be that HIV infection is an underlying factor in the high incidence of opportunistic infections and respiratory disease in developing countries. Spot sampling in a few countries in Africa suggests that the HIV infection rate may be increasing from approximately 5% of the adult population to 8–10% among younger age groups (Ronald et al., 1988).

Data from developing countries suggest a behavioral path for transmission that differs from that in the United States. Approximately equal rates of infection among males and females have been observed, and multiple sexual partners appear to be the only clearly identified risk factor. Apparently prostitution is one related pathway; this may be more or less true for any country where sexual and economic freedom of women is severely restricted. However, maternal transmission to the fetus or newborn may also be a major factor. Early marriage and pregnancy as well as frequent pregnancies complicate this risk pathway.

Case surveys based on registries maintained by the U.S. Centers for Disease Control indicate that by March 1988, over 55,315 AIDS cases have been identified in the United States, 4,199 of them women (Allen, 1988). Early symptoms are often those of pneumonia or related respiratory disease. Women represent about 6.7% of all cases in the United States; a third of these women are 20–29 years old, a younger age pattern than that observed for AIDS among men; and over 50% are black women (Guinan & Hardy, 1987). States having the highest proportion of female cases are New Jersey, Connecticut, Puerto Rico, Florida, Rhode Island, and New York. Factors that constitute highest risk for these women are intravenous drug use and heterosexual contact with a person at risk for AIDS. Heterosexual contact includes prostitution and also contact with bisexual males or contact with males having multiple partners. Artificial insemination is also a possible transmission pathway for AIDS.

Epidemiological features of AIDS among women suggest that it is partly related to women's social and economic status. In particular, being a young black female invokes relatively greater risk for educational drop-out, drastically reduced earning potential, and limited access to social assistance agencies, with subsequent prostitution and drug abuse. Early data from New York suggest that intravenous drug use is the primary pathway of HIV infection among women and that approximately 40% of the women at risk are infected (Joseph, 1988). It has been suggested that targeting of prostitutes for intervention strategies may be an important component of health care policy (Rosenberg & Weiner, 1988).

Policy and Planning

Public policy and intervention/prevention strategies are only now becoming formalized. Past experience with public reactions and overreactions to other sexually transmitted diseases, such as syphilis, suggest that fears (whether well founded or not) will influence policy (Brandt, 1988). Historical lessons also suggest that rational-educational strategies for behavior change will require substantial time to become effective, if at all. Furthermore, social conventions and attitudes tend to be at odds with many of the policy recommendations under consideration, for example, advertising of condoms (Osborn, 1988). Programs for mandatory testing or restriction of infected individuals unfortunately may be deemed appropriate measures in some communities (Loewy, 1988). It is, in fact, these quick-fix solutions that public officials appear most comfortable in advocating, even though mandatory testing of selected groups would have little or no impact on the spread of disease (Joseph, 1988).

There is also evidence of poor communication between scientists and policymakers, with the result that budgets are set and revised without appropriate guidance on some points (Stoto, Blumenthal, Durch & Feldman, 1988). Estimated federal expenditures for AIDS in 1986 were $274 million, partially funded through the U.S. Public Health Service (85%) and the Department of Defense (15%); however, it has been suggested that the appropriate level of funding is closer to $1 billion annually (Hatziandreu, Graham & Stoto, 1988).

Other issues that emerge involve planning for health care needs of AIDS patients and those with AIDS-related complex (ARC). Treatment has been organized only for acute care, but current insurance and payment systems make acute care extremely expensive. The possibility of having local, decentralized patient management centers in the community will eventually have to be considered (Shulman & Mantell, 1988). Whether there are sufficient health care personnel capable of providing direct primary care to AIDS patients is another serious problem (Cotton, 1988). The question also becomes one of not only "who shall live," but "who shall pay" (Joseph, 1988).

Related issues involve professional quandaries regarding risks to health care providers. Although the American College of Physicians and the Infectious Diseases Society jointly subscribe to the ethical principle that all individuals deserve humane care, including those with AIDS (Eickhoff, 1988), it is also the case that anonymous surveys of health care workers indicate that 50% would transfer to another unit if regularly assigned to care for an AIDS patient (Wormser, Joline, Sivak, & Arlin, 1988). Initial anecdotal reports of refusal to treat were followed by official policy of some physicians to screen patients for HIV status and refuse to treat positive cases (Bayer, 1988). Discretionary assignment of cases and thus indirect refusal to treat are more often the option of physicians, while nurses, technicians, aides, and other floor personnel may be forced to assume more exposure.

Risk to health care workers of AIDS infection, though low, is not zero. To date, eight workers have been reported in whom HIV infection may have been acquired from occupational exposure, seven of whom were women who had had needle stick accidents (Wormser et al., 1988). Apparently such accidents, though preventable, are not rare, and over 1,000 health care workers have reported a history of accidental inoculation with infected materials (Gerberding, 1988). One survey reported that 36% of medical staff had been exposed to contaminated needles (Link, Feingold, Charap, Freeman & Shelov, 1988). Recommendations for reducing risk have included better physician-patient communication and complete history taking, increased screening of hospital patients belonging to high-risk groups, and measures to ensure the confidentiality of patients (Eickhoff, 1988).

The fact that AIDS has been identified as a disease of homosexual men has probably affected diagnosis and screening strategies, provisions for treatment, prevention, and development of policy and planning in general. Although women constitute a small percentage of current cases, some features of health care delivery could be readily modified to improve diagnosis and screening as well as public education and prevention programs where women are concerned. For example, the fact that 80% of female cases are among women of reproductive age constitutes serious health planning and education problems, because AIDS is readily transmitted to the developing fetus.

Heterosexual Risk

Heterosexual transmission of AIDS has been a burning question as awareness of the disease has become more public. To date, about 2% of men and about 29% of women have contracted AIDS through heterosexual contact (Allen, 1988); these rates are likely to go up in the future. Drug use is a major factor confounded with heterosexual contact for both women and men, and contact with a bisexual male is the other major heterosexual risk factor for women. The proportion of black men with AIDS contracted through heterosexual contact is about twice as high as that of white males (Allen, 1988).

It is important to remember that heterosexual transmission may occur under monogamous circumstances as well, and women whose partners were infected through blood transfusion have a relatively high infection rate (10 women out of 55 known to be at risk) (Allen, 1988). Wives of hemophiliac men are also at risk, and their risk may increase as the disease progresses. Estimates vary regarding exactly what the risk is for these women, with some studies suggesting an infection rate of 10% or less (Jason, McDougal & Dixon, 1986; Kreiss, Kitchen & Prince 1985) and others suggesting a rate closer to 20% (Padian, Marquis, & Francis, 1987).

These transmission rates are forecasts of serious problems over the next five years, the time period thought typical for the development of AIDS. There are 20,000 cases of hemophilia in the United States, a substantial percentage among adult males. The rate of HIV infection varies with the severity of bleeding disorder, and it is thought to be more likely among individuals who received treatment of blood products before the currently available factor was submitted to adequate protection measures. The rate of infection overall for hemophiliacs is estimated to be 33–92% for hemophilia-A patients and 14–52% for patients with hemophilia-B (Stehr-Green, Holman, Jason, & Evatt, 1988). The wives of these patients are at special risk, because they are likely to have repeated exposure. Sexual practices among such couples may have dramatic interplay with their relationship, trust, and loyalty as well as adaptation to ill health. Failure to use condoms or follow relatively safe sexual practices is often reported among these couples. These acts reflect the desire to communicate total acceptance of the individual and also may serve to deny the risk of disease.

The implications of these data for behavioral science and the real life context of sexual decision making are only beginning to be explored (Ehrhardt, 1988). Popular assumptions that infection can be transmitted only through taboo behaviors (bisexuality, homosexuality, intravenous drug use) make it less likely that the average person will think it appropriate or necessary to follow even simple protection measures. HIV infection should certainly also have an impact on women's reproductive choices such as use of contraceptives and choices regarding abortion if the woman does become pregnant. A related question will also involve the expenditure of public funds for abortions among infected women. Since federal policy does not at present include exceptions for rape or incest, it will be interesting to see the impact of AIDS on funding policy.

Sexual activity patterns among adolescents of all genders are an additional behavioral correlate related to transmission of infection that has implications for future planning. Will sex and masculine status continue to be strongly linked? Will sex and love continue to be intertwined with tests of female commitment? Will sex continue to be seen as acceptable only when it ensues from irrational impulse?

Other social trends and problems also deserve attention. As more females and children enter the homeless population, they are likely to experience increased risk for entry into drug cultures and prostitution. These individuals may very well have limited access to care, partly because they are to some extent migratory.

Thus, it is apparent that AIDS is not a problem limited to a unique subpopulation. Women and children are at risk through a number of behavioral pathways and conditions of social status. Policy issues involve planning for funding of research, providing for care, access to care among impoverished and migratory groups, training of professional health care providers, and management of risk within health care professions. Long-term problems of prevention involve ingrained values and attitudes about gender, sexuality, and relationships.

WOMEN IN DEVELOPING COUNTRIES

Women in developing countries experience a health status that is partly a reflection of their residence in developing countries and partly a reflection of their status as women. Although life expectancy for women in developing countries is typically one or two years longer than that of men, life expectancy in general is quite low and often less than 55 years. For example, in Afghanistan life expectancy is 37 for males and 37.8 for females, perhaps the lowest in the world (United Nations [UN], 1984). Life expectancy is typically lower among residents of rural areas, and mortality rates are actually higher for female children in many countries, such as Turkey, Afghanistan, and Iran (U.S. Census, 1985c).

Sex comparisons within developing countries indicate that sexism makes a significant contribution to mortality and morbidity among women. For example, the incidence of anemia and malnutrition following periods of famine is likely to be higher among females than males, extending to children as well as adults. Utilization of care has also been observed to differ for girl and boy children, with parents less likely to take girl children to clinics (Waldron, 1987).

Women's health is closely integrated with their social, political, and economic status in general. For example, women constitute no more than a third of all paid workers in Mexico, Peru, Bolivia, Egypt, Algeria, Chad, Iran, or Saudia Arabia (U.S. Census, 1985a). In Mexico, where women constitute about 28% of the work force, most are employed as domestics (Seager & Olson, 1986). Similar patterns of women working in services, as opposed to technical or professional occupations, exist in Indonesia, Malaysia, South Korea, and the Philippines (U.S. Census, 1985b). The other most common occupational activity among Asian women is production work, especially in garment and electronics assembly (U.S. Census, 1985b).

Women's economic status is further complicated by migration trends among male workers. There is major migration from rural areas to cities in almost all developing countries; in Africa and Asia, most of this is of male workers, in many instances leaving women to care for their children and maintain rural households alone. Some of this migratory behavior is international as well, and industrialized countries, such as Canada, West Germany, and the United States, attract a significant number of workers from Mexico, Pakistan, India, and Malaysia. Since in many of these countries women do not have the right to own or inherit land, these trends offer little opportunity for women to establish independent means of subsistence. The fact that rural dwellers of either sex typically have lower opportunities for education and overall lower literacy means that women have limited prospects of changing their status. For example, in North African countries (Algeria, Egypt, Morocco, Tunisia) fewer than 20% of rural women are literate, while roughly 40% of rural men are literate (U.S. Census, 1985a, 1985c).

Pregnancy and Birth

World statistics indicate that a half million women die each year in pregnancy and birth, the vast majority occurring in developing countries (Royston & Lopez, 1987). In fact, the leading cause of death for women in most developing countries

Figure 5
Rates of Maternal Mortality (per 100,000 live births)

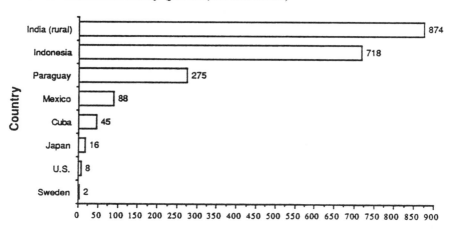

Based on data from Royston and Lopez (1987).

is pregnancy and childbirth. Sex differences in life expectancy in developing countries are largely explained by reproductive risks to women. In the United States only about 2% of all deaths are associated with pregnancy and childbirth, compared with approximately 20% in Egypt and Indonesia (Stein & Maine, 1986).

Areas with the highest number of cases of maternal mortality lie among those countries within the southern Asia region, such as India, Bangladesh, and Pakistan (Royston & Lopez, 1987). Rates (per 100,000 live births) are probably highest in Africa, but are difficult to document due to poor civil registries and biases in access to, and utilization of, hospital care. Rates are also compounded by high fertility, especially in Africa, where for many countries women can expect on average to have 8–10 pregnancies, resulting in 6 live births. Figure 5 illustrates rates of maternal mortality for some countries.

Precipitating causes of maternal death include failed abortions and ectopic pregnancies, hemorrhage, and sepsis. Sometimes death is intertwined with preexisting chronic health problems, such as hepatitis. Additionally, deaths are partly explained by pandemic poor health due to parasitic and infectious disease, the particular burden imposed by reproduction when overall health status has been compromised, and limited access to health care and adequate sanitation.

Deaths are also partly explained by the sociocultural patterns of young age at marriage and the cumulative effects of frequent pregnancy, anemia, and malnutrition. In Africa nearly 75% of all births are to females under 20, whereas in Europe the comparable figure is 15% (Ferguson, 1987). The Food and Agricultural Organization (FAO) acknowledges that the heavy burden of agricultural work that falls to women is often a major factor in their protein and energy requirements (Food & Agricultural Organization [FAO]/World Health Organization [WHO], 1985). These nutritional requirements may be met on only a marginal basis at best. Since pregnant women in developing countries seldom have the possibility of reducing physical activity levels, many suffer from chronic undernourishment. The added costs of pregnancy and lactation, compounded by poor quality of diet and chronic parasitic disease and diarrhea, can produce serious risks to women's health.

The fact that polygyny is practiced to some degree in almost all countries in Africa and the eastern Mediterranean, as well as India, suggests another socio-cultural factor. The loss of one woman from the household may not have very large psychological implications, because the male's dependency and comfort needs can be met by other females. Additionally, the loss of one woman may not have very large economic implications, resulting in somewhat less motivation to protect women's health.

Governmental support for family planning and access to contraception and to abortion are also major factors in maternal and child mortality. Direct and strong support is available for family planning in China, India, Thailand, Indonesia, and Mexico, while moderate or indirect support is available in many African countries. However, a number of countries provide no support or have active prohibitions on family planning; Saudi Arabia, Libya, Niger, Romania, and Argentina fall in this category. Regardless of official support, many women do not have ready access to contraceptive assistance, and less than 15% of women in most African countries use contraception, in contrast, for example, with France at the highest use of 82% (Seager & Olson, 1986).

Access to legal and safe abortion is a related feature of public policy affecting maternal mortality. In almost no developing country is abortion available on the basis of the woman's request, and it is illegal in a number of them. It is permitted only if the woman's life is endangered or the woman's health is seriously compromised in selected other countries. Rates of abortions per 1,000 women of reproductive age are typically low, even among developed countries, such as the United States, where the abortion rate is about 3%, or Sweden, where it is only 2% (Seager & Olson, 1986).

Infectious and Parasitic Disease

Approximately a third of all deaths in the world are due to infectious and parasitic diseases, and a major portion of these occurs in developing countries, particularly in Africa and Southeast Asia (Hakulinen, Hansluwka, Lopez & Nakada, 1986). The nature of the problem can be better appreciated when lists of leading causes of death are reviewed. Tuberculosis, malaria, measles, leprosy, tetanus, typhoid, and diarrhea are leading causes of death in developing countries (UN, 1984).

The lack of a safe and adequate water supply for vast portions of the world is a major contributor as well, resulting in thousands of deaths due to diarrhea, enteric fever, and typhoid. Women in developing countries may be particularly at risk for illnesses associated with infections and parasites because, compared with men, women are more likely to be undernourished or anemic.

Parasitic infections are also serious health problems. For example, it is estimated that 700 to 900 million individuals are infected with hookworm (an intestinal parasite) and that intestinal parasites as a group account for 100,000 deaths each year (WHO, 1986a). Even infections having low prevalence, such as trypanosomiasis (sleeping sickness), constitute serious health risks, because they have the potential for epidemic outbreaks with a high mortality rate.

Malaria (a protozoan infection transmitted by mosquito vectors) is estimated to be endemic in 100 countries, with nearly 5 million cases reported annually through formal registries (WHO, 1986c, 1987). However, it is estimated that unreported cases in Africa alone might well reach 98 million (WHO, 1986c). Unfortunately, the primary forms appear to be gaining resistance to chloroquine, the treatment drug of choice, and several species of the mosquito vectors are acquiring resistance to insecticides (WHO, 1986b).

Schistosomiasis is probably the major waterborne parasitic infection of public health significance, producing disease in a number of organ systems, primarily the intestines and liver. It is endemic in 74 countries, ranging from the eastern Mediterranean, across most of Africa, and the eastern coast of Latin America. It is estimated that 20% of the population in these countries are infected (WHO, 1986a). Since it is waterborne, water development projects, permanent water impoundments, and year-round irrigation programs can increase the prevalence of schistosomiasis from a seasonal to a perennial problem. For example, egg counts among Egyptian children before and after the completion of the Aswan dams revealed a dramatic increase in the number of infected children. Similar measurements before and after the creation of Lake Volta in Ghana revealed an increase from 7% to 90% of children infected with schistosomiasis (WHO, 1986a). The potential impact of water development projects is indeed a major one. With the assistance of foreign aid programs, 50,000 small dams were constructed in Mali over a three-year period, 20 dam projects were scheduled for one region of Kenya, and 120 have been scheduled for Ghana.

Women and children are more likely to be at risk from schistosomiasis and similar parasitic infections because of their roles as agricultural workers involved in watering and caring for livestock in rivers and water impoundments, irrigation, collection of home drinking water, and laundry. All these are activities that involve prolonged exposure.

Toxic Substances

Technological innovations in agriculture and industry among developing countries have been dramatic, producing significant economic growth and improved health. However, these innovations carry with them special risks as well (Bauman, 1986). Toxic substances are being introduced, at steadily increasing rates, often in settings where safety standards are not well understood, quality control for chemical production is casual, workers are poorly informed about risks, and emergency response preparedness is minimal. In addition, pandemic poor health and nutrition make entire populations relatively more vulnerable to the effects of toxic substances.

Many developing nations have recognized occupational health hazards associated with industrial expansion, for example, lung disease, heavy metal poisoning, and cancer. Programs are often instituted to improve worker education, use of safety equipment, and environmental monitoring, as, for example, in China (Christiani, 1984). However, exposure to toxic substances in agricultural development has received somewhat less attention. Exposure may occur from direct insult associated with insecticides, herbicides, or fungicides during formulation, application, harvesting, or ingestion of treated crops (Jeyaratnam, 1985).

Chronic and acute exposure to significant levels of agricultural chemicals has been documented for several countries, including India (Kashyap, 1986), Ivory Coast (Kummer & van Sittert, 1986), Pakistan (Rowley et al., 1987), Turkey (Karakaya & Ozalp, 1987), Thailand (Sivaborvorn, Pongpaew, Huangprasert & Chaikitiporn, 1983), Japan (Matsumoto, Murakami, Kuwabara, Tanaka & Kashimoto, 1987), Indonesia, Malaysia, and Sri Lanka (Jeyaratnam, Lun, & Phoon, 1986). Body burdens may show a tenfold increase over time, with symptoms of toxicity occurring in 60% to 70% of workers (Kashyap, 1986). In addition to symptoms of gross toxicity and poisoning, assay techniques have revealed by-products in blood, urine, and fatty tissue. Other tests indicate changes in blood cholinesterase activity, liver enzymes, and cardiac function.

Health effects are not trivial, and there are an estimated 500,000 cases of pesticide poisoning annually, resulting in 10,000 deaths, most found in Third World countries (Sridhar & Ogbalu, 1986; Jeyaratnam, 1982). Periodically, poisoning reaches epidemic proportions. For example, poisoning cases in 21 Pakistan villages were linked to endrin in household sugar supplies ("Acute Convulsions," 1984; Rowley et al., 1987). Treatment of wheat seedlings with the fungicide hexachlorobenzene resulted in an estimated 4,000 cases of toxicity in Turkey, 1956–1961 (Cripps, Gocmen & Peters, 1980). Ingestion of bread made from wheat seedlings treated with methylmercury in Iraq, 1971–1972, resulted in widespread poisoning and increased mortality that could be only indirectly estimated (Greenwood, 1985; Amin-Zaki et al., 1980, 1981; Bakir et al., 1980).

Since the roles of women and children as agricultural workers appear to be increasing, their risks of health effects due to pesticide exposure are probably increasing, especially as the male population migrates to industrialized centers in search of employment. In some developing countries, such as China, Thailand, Turkey, and Tanzania, women make up a significant proportion (sometimes as high as 80%) of the agricultural work force. Women agricultural workers are often exposed to organochlorines and organophosphorous products during pregnancy.

Infants and children may also be at risk because they accompany their mothers into the fields. Nursing infants may additionally be exposed through mothers' milk (Atuma & Okor, 1987; Tojo et al., 1986). Many pesticides and related compounds are lipophilic and may be transferred to suckling infants in breast milk. Contamination of breast milk is almost universal and is indicative of widespread pollution from organics (Travis & Arms, 1987), a finding that has been documented for many countries: Israel (Weisenberg et al., 1985), Iraq (Al-Omar, Tawfiq & Al-Ogaily, 1985), Kenya (Kanja et al., 1986), Nigeria (Atuma & Vaz, 1986), and India (Siddiqui & Saxena, 1985; Ramakrishnan et al., 1985). The most frequently cited contaminant is DDT, often at levels significantly higher than those recommended as tolerable by the World Health Organization (WHO) (Kanja et al., 1986).

SUMMARY

Feminist analyses of women's health reaffirm that "the personal is political." Often what might initially be viewed as biologically impersonal and objective is embedded in a social and political context. Thus, whether an Egyptian woman carries the burden of schistosomiasis, or an Indian woman suffers pesticide poisoning, or a homeless New York woman contracts HIV infection is shaped not only by access to medical care, but also by sociocultural factors. These relationships may appear somewhat more obvious when economic hardship is prevalent, but the same principles are relevant, for example, when middle-class women are tranquilized and sedated through their senior years and when young mothers undergo repeat cesarean surgery.

Since many of the practices and policies of health care are invoked for the welfare and protection of women, it is difficult to submit them to the critical analysis they deserve. Negative effects on women's health often are a de facto consequence rather than an intentional outcome. Frequently, it is simply the basic conceptualization of a problem that is at fault. Thus, the medicalization of pregnancy and birth for the protection of women naturally facilitates the introduction of more and more technology and less and less control by women. The conceptualization of AIDS as a problem for male homosexuals fails to consider the risks for women.

Applications of the basic principle of this chapter to women's health are only now emerging in contemporary research efforts and policy analysis. Central issues and health problems and appropriate research methods are gradually being identified. As these principles and methods are extended to concepts and issues of health in general, we have only to gain.

REFERENCES

Acute convulsions associated with endrin poisoning—Pakistan. (1984). *Morbidity and Mortality Weekly Report*, *33*(49), 687–688, 693.

Adler, N. E. (1976). Sample attrition in studies of psychosocial sequelae of abortion: How great a problem? *Journal of Applied Social Psychology*, *6*(3), 240–259.

Akoury, H. A., Brodie, G., Caddick, R., McLaughlin, V. D., & Pugh, P.A. (1988). Active management of labor and operative delivery in nulliparous women. *American Journal of Obstetrics and Gynecology*, *158*(2), 255–258.

Allen, J. R. (1988). Heterosexual transmission of human immunodeficiency virus (HIV) in the United States. *Bulletin of the New York Academy of Medicine*, *64*(6), 464–479.

Allgeier, A. R., Allgeier, E. R., & Rywick, T. (1981). Orientations toward abortion: Guilt or knowledge? *Adolescence*, *16*(62), 273–280.

Al-Omar, M. A., Tawfiq, S. J., & Al-Ogaily, N. (1985). Organochlorine residue levels in human milk from Baghdad. *Bulletin of Environmental Contamination and Toxicology*, *35*(1), 65–67.

Amin-Zaki, L., Elhassani, S. B., Majeed, M. A., Clarkson, T. W., Doherty, R. A., & Greenwood, M. R. (1980). Methylmercury poisoning in mothers and their suckling infants. *Developments in Toxicology and Environmental Science*, *8*, 75–78.

Amin-Zaki, L., Majeed, M. A., Greenwood, M. R., Elhassani, S. B., Clarkson, T. W., & Doherty, R. A. (1981). Methylmercury poisoning in the Iraqi suckling infant: A longitudinal study over five years. *Journal of Applied Toxicology*, *1*(4), 210–214.

Amirikia, H., & Evans, T. N. (1979). Ten-year review of hysterectomies: Trends, indications, and risks. *American Journal of Obstetrics and Gynecology*, *134*, 431–437.

Atuma, S. S., & Okor, D. I. (1987). Organochlorine contaminants in human milk. *Acta Paediatrica Scandinavica*, *76*(2), 365–366.

Atuma, S. S., & Vaz, R. (1986). A pilot study on levels of organochlorine compounds in human milk in Nigeria. *International Journal of Environmental Analytical Chemistry*, *26*(3-4), 187–192.

Bakir, F., Rustam, H., Tikriti, S., Al-Damluji, S. F., & Shihristani, H. (1980). Clinical and epidemiological aspects of methylmercury poisoning. *Postgraduate Medical Journal*, *56*(651), 1–10.

Baluk, U., & O'Neill, P. (1980). Health professionals' perceptions of the psychological consequences of abortion. *American Journal of Community Psychology*, *8*(1), 67–75.

Bauman, P. (1986). *Chemicals policy in the global environment: A report to the World Commission on Environment and Development*. Washington, DC: Conservation Foundation.

Bayer, R. (1988). AIDS and the duty to treat: Risk responsibility and health care workers. *Bulletin of the New York Academy of Medicine*, *64*(6), 498–505.

Belsey, E. M., Green, H. S., Lewis, S. C., & Beard, R. W. (1977). Predictive factors in emotional response to abortion: King's termination study: IV. *Social Science and Medicine*, *11*(2), 71–82.

Blumberg, N. L. (1980). Effects of neonatal risk, maternal attitude, and cognitive style on early postpartum adjustment. *Journal of Abnormal Psychology, 89*(2), 139–150.

Boyd, M. E., Usher, R. H., McLean, F. H., & Kramer, M. S. (1988). Obstetric consequences of postmaturity. *American Journal of Obstetrics and Gynecology, 158*(2), 334–338.

Bracken, M. B., Hachamovitch, M., & Grossman, G. (1974). The decision to abort and psychological sequelae. *Journal of Nervous and Mental Disease, 158*(2), 154–162.

Brandt, A. M. (1988). AIDS in historical perspective: Four lessons from the history of sexually transmitted diseases. *American Journal of Public Health, 78*(4), 367–371.

Bunker, J. P., McPherson, K., & Henneman, P. L. (1977). Elective hysterectomy. In J. P. Bunker, B. A. Barnes, & F. Mosteller (Eds.), *Costs, risks, and benefits of surgery* (pp. 262–276). New York: Oxford University Press.

Centers for Disease Control. (1992). *HIV/AIDS surveillance: U.S. AIDS cases reported through June 1992.* Atlanta: Centers for Disease Control.

Chilman, C. S. (1985). Feminist issues in teenage parenting. Special Issue: Toward a feminist approach to child welfare. *Child Welfare, 64*(3), 225–234.

Christiani, D. C. (1984). Occupational health in the People's Republic of China. *American Journal of Public Health, 74*(1), 58–64.

Cohen, G. R., O'Brien, W. F., Lewis, L., & Knuppel, R. A. (1987). A prospective randomized study of the aggressive management of early labor. *American Journal of Obstetrics and Gynecology, 157*(5), 1174–1177.

Combs, M. W., & Welch, S. (1982). Blacks, whites, and attitudes toward abortion. *Public Opinion Quarterly, 46*(4), 510–520.

Cooperstock, R. (1978). Sex differences in psychotropic drug use. *Social Science and Medicine, 12B,* 179–186.

Corea, G. (1977). *The hidden malpractice.* New York: Jove.

Cotton, D. J. (1988). The impact of AIDS on the medical care system. *Journal of the American Medical Association, 260*(4), 519–523.

Cranley, M. S., Hedahl, K. J., & Pegg, S. H. (1983). Women's perceptions of vaginal and cesarean deliveries. *Nursing Research, 32*(1), 10–15.

Cripps, D. J., Gocmen, A., & Peters, H. A. (1980). Porphyria turcica. Twenty years after hexachlorobenzene intoxication. *Arch Dermatol, 116*(1), 46–50.

Cummings, S. R., Kelsey, J. L., Nevitt, M. C., & O'Dowd, K. J. (1985). Epidemiology of osteoporosis and osteoporotic fractures. *Epidemiologic Reviews, 7,* 178–208.

Dixon, P. N., Strano, D. A., & Willingham, W. (1984). Locus of control and decision to abort. *Psychological Reports, 54*(2), 547–553.

Dreifus, C. (Ed.). (1977). *Seizing our bodies.* New York: Random House.

Duff, P., Southmayd, K., & Read, J. A. (1988). Outcome of trial of labor in patients with a single previous low transverse cesarean section for dystocia. *Obstetrics and Gynecology, 71*(3), 380–384.

Eden, R. D., Seifert, L. S., Kodack, L. D., Trofatter, K. F., Killam, A. P., & Gall, S. A. (1988). A modified biophysical profile for antenatal fetal surveillance. *Obstetrics and Gynecology, 71*(3, Pt. 1), 365–369.

Ehrenreich, B., & English, D. (1977). Complaints and disorders: The sexual politics of sickness. In C. Dreifus (Ed.), *Seizing our bodies* (pp. 43–56). New York: Random House.

Ehrhardt, A. A. (1988). Preventing and treating AIDS: The expertise of the behavioral sciences. *Bulletin of the New York Academy of Medicine, 64*(6), 506–512.

Eickhoff, T. C. (1988). The acquired immunodeficiency syndrome (AIDS) and infection with the human immunodeficiency virus (HIV). *Journal of Infectious Diseases, 158*(2), 273–290.

Eisen, M., & Zellman, G. L. (1984). Factors predicting pregnancy resolution decision satisfaction of unmarried adolescents. *Journal of Genetic Psychology, 145*(2), 231–239.

Entwisle, D. R., & Alexander, K. L. (1987). Long-term effects of cesarean delivery on parents' beliefs and children's schooling. *Developmental Psychology, 23*(5), 676–682.

Falk, R., Gispert, M., & Baucom, D. H. (1981). Personality factors related to black teenage pregnancy and abortion. *Psychology of Women Quarterly, 5*(Suppl. 5), 737–746.

Faria, G., Barrett, E., & Goodman, L. M. (1985). Women and abortion: Attitudes, social networks, decision-making. *Social Work in Health Care, 11*(1), 85–99.

Farmer, M. E., White, L. R., & Brody, J. A. (1984). Race and sex differences in hip fracture incidence. *American Journal of Public Health, 74*, 1374–1380.

Fee, E. (Ed.). (1983). *Women and health: The politics of sex in medicine.* Farmingdale, NY: Baywood.

Ferguson, J. (1987). Reproductive health of adolescent girls. *World Health Statistics Quarterly, 40*, 211–214.

Fidell, L. S. (1980). Sex role stereotypes and the American physician. *Psychology of Women Quarterly, 4*(3), 313–330.

Finlay, B. A. (1981). Sex differences in correlates of abortion attitudes among college students. *Journal of Marriage and the Family, 43*(3), 571–582.

Food & Agricultural Organization / World Health Organization. (1985). *Energy and protein requirements.* World Health Organization, Technical report series, no. 724.

Forrest, J. D. (1984). The impact of U.S. family planning programs on births, abortions and miscarriages, 1970–1979. *Social Science and Medicine, 18*(6), 461–465.

Frejka, T. (1985). Induced abortion and fertility. *Family Planning Perspectives, 17*(5), 230–234.

Friedlander, M. L., Kaul, T. J., & Stimel, C. A. (1984). Abortion: Predicting the complexity of the decision-making process. *Women and Health, 9*(1), 43–54.

Friedman, C. M., Greenspan, R., & Mittleman, F. (1974). The decision-making process and the outcome of therapeutic abortion. *American Journal of Psychiatry, 131*(12), 1332–1337.

Gerberding, J. L. (1988). Transmission of HIV to health care workers: Risk and risk reduction. *Bulletin of the New York Academy of Medicine, 64*(6), 491–498.

Goldfarb, M. (1984). *Who receives cesareans: Patient and hospital characteristics.* Hospital Cost and Utilization Project Research Note 4, National Center Health Services Research, DHHS publication No. (PHS) 84-3345.

Gottlieb, S. E., & Barrett, D. E. (1986). Effects of unanticipated cesarean section on mothers, infants, and their interaction in the first month of life. *Journal of Developmental and Behavioral Pediatrics, 7*(3), 180–185.

Granberg, D., & Granberg, B. W. (1985). A search for gender differences on fertility-related attitudes: Questioning the relevance of sociobiology theory for understanding social psychological aspects of human reproduction. *Psychology of Women Quarterly, 9*(4), 431–437.

Greenwood, M. R. (1985). Methylmercury poisoning in Iraq. An epidemiological study of the 1971–1972 outbreak. *Journal of Applied Toxicology, 5*(3), 148–159.

Guinan, M. E., & Hardy, A. H. (1987). Epidemiology of AIDS in women in the United States 1981–1986. *Journal of the American Medical Association, 257*(15), 2039–2042.

Hakulinen, T., Hansluwka, H., Lopez, A. D., & Nakada, T. (1986). Global and regional mortality patterns by cause of death in 1980. *International Journal of Epidemiology, 15*(2), 226–233.

Hall, D. C., & Kaufmann, D. A. (1987). Effects of aerobic and strength conditioning on pregnancy outcomes. *American Journal of Obstetrics and Gynecology, 157*(5), 1199–1203.

Hall, E. J., & Ferree, M. M. (1986). Race differences in abortion attitudes. *Public Opinion Quarterly, 50*(2), 193–207.

Handy, J. A. (1982). Psychological and social aspects of induced abortion. *British Journal of Clinical Psychology, 21*(1), 29–41.

Hansen, H. (1978). Decline of Down's syndrome after abortion reform in New York state. *American Journal of Mental Deficiency, 83*(2), 185–188.

Hatziandreu, E., Graham, J. D., & Stoto, M. A. (1988). AIDS and biomedical research funding: Comparative analysis. *Reviews of Infectious Diseases, 10*(1), 159–167.

Herz, E. (1984). Psychological repercussions of pregnancy loss. *Psychiatric Annals, 14*(6), 454–457.

Hobfoll, S. E., Nadler, A., & Leiberman, J. (1986). Satisfaction with social support during crisis: Intimacy and self-esteem as critical determinants. *Journal of Personality and Social Psychology, 51*(2), 296–304.

Hoppe, R. B. (1984). The case for or against diagnostic and therapeutic sexism. Special Issue: Women and mental health—new directions for change. *Women and Therapy, 3*(3-4), 129–136.

Interdivisional Committee on Adolescent Abortion. (1987). Adolescent abortion: Psychological and legal issues. *American Psychologist, 42*(1), 73–78.

Jacobson, L., & Solheim, F. (1975). Women's experience of the abortion procedure. *Social Psychiatry, 10*(4), 155–160.

Jakobi, P., Weissman, A., & Paldi, E. (1987). Uniform presentation of data concerning cesarean sections. *Acta Obstetricia et Gynecologica Scandinavica, 66*(7), 657–658.

Jason, J. M., McDougal, S., & Dixon, G. (1986). HTLV-III/LAV antibody and immune status of household contacts and sexual partners of persons with hemophilia. *Journal of the American Medical Association, 255,* 212–215.

Jessee, W. F., Nickerson, C. W., & Grant, W. S. (1982). An evaluation of cesarean births in nine PSRO areas. *Medical Care, 20,* 75–84.

Jeyaratnam, J. (1985). Health problems of pesticide usage in the Third World [editorial]. *British Journal of Industrial Medicine, 42*(8), 505–506.

Jeyaratnam, J., de Alwis Seneviratne, R. S., & Copplestone, J. F. (1982). Survey of pesticide poisoning in Sri Lanka. *Bulletin of the World Health Organization, 60*(4), 615–619.

Jeyaratnam, J., Lun, K. C., & Phoon, W. O. (1986). Blood cholinesterase levels among agricultural workers in four Asian countries. *Toxicology Letters, 33*(1-3), 195–201.

Jones, E. F., & Westoff, C. F. (1978). How attitudes toward abortion are changing. *Journal of Population*, *1*(1), 5–21.

Joseph, C. (1985). Factors related to delay for legal abortions performed at a gestational age of 20 weeks or more. *Journal of Biosocial Science*, *17*(3), 327–337.

Joseph, S. C. (1988). Political and social issues surrounding AIDS. *Bulletin of the New York Academy of Medicine*, *64*(6), 506–512.

Joyce, T. (1987). The impact of induced abortion on black and white birth outcomes in the United States. *Demography*, *24*(2), 229–244.

Kanja, L., Skåre, J.U., Nafstad, I., Maitai, C.K., & Laken, P. (1986). Organochlorine pesticides in human milk from different areas of Kenya 1983–1985. *Journal of Toxicology and Environmental Health*, *19*(4), 449–464.

Karakaya, A. E., & Ozalp, S. (1987). Organochlorine pesticides in human adipose tissue collected in Ankara (Turkey) 1984–1985. *Bulletin of Environmental Contamination and Toxicology*, *38*(6), 941–945.

Kashyap, S. K. (1986). Health surveillance and biological monitoring of pesticide formulators in India. *Toxicology Letters*, *33*(1-3), 107–114.

Korenbrot, C., Flood, A. B., Higgins, M., Roos, N., & Bunker, J. P. (1981). *Case Study #15: Elective hysterectomy: Costs, risks, and benefits. Background paper #2: Case studies of medical technologies: The implications of cost-effectiveness analysis of medical technology*. Office of Technology Assessment. Washington, DC: U.S. Government Printing Office.

Kosecoff, J., Kanouse, D. E., Rogers, W. H., McCloskey, L., Winslow, C. M., & Brook, R. H. (1987). Effects of the National Institutes of Health Consensus Development Program on physician practice. *Journal of the American Medical Association*, *258*(19), 2708–2713.

Kreiss, J. K., Kitchen, L. W., & Prince, H. E. (1985). Antibody to human T-lymphotropic virus type III in wives of hemophiliacs. *Annals of Internal Medicine*, *102*, 623–626.

Kummer, R., & van Sittert, N. J. (1986). Field studies on health effects from the application of two organophosphorus insecticide formulations by hand-held ULV to cotton. *Toxicology Letters*, *33*(1-3), 7–24.

Landry, E., Bertrand, J. T., Cherry, F., & Rice, J. (1986). Teen pregnancy in New Orleans: Factors that differentiate teens who deliver, abort, and successfully contracept. *Journal of Youth and Adolescence*, *15*(3), 259–274.

Lazarus, A. (1985). Psychiatric sequelae of legalized elective first trimester abortion. *Journal of Psychosomatic Obstetrics and Gynecology*, *4*(3), 141–150.

Leon, I. G. (1986). Psychodynamics of perinatal loss. *Psychiatry*, *49*(4), 312–324.

Leon, I. G. (1987). Short-term psychotherapy for perinatal loss. *Psychotherapy*, *24*(2), 186–195.

Lewis, C. C. (1987). Minors' competence to consent to abortion. *American Psychologist*, *42*(1), 84–88.

Link, R. N., Feingold, A. R., Charap, M. H., Freeman, K., & Shelov, S. P. (1988). Concerns of medical and pediatric house officers about acquiring AIDS from their patients. *American Journal of Public Health*, *78*, 455–459.

Lipson, J. G. (1981). Cesarean support groups: Mutual help and education. *Women and Health*, *6*(3-4), 27–39.

Lipson, J. G., & Tilden, V. P. (1980). Psychological integration of the cesarean birth experience. *American Journal of Orthopsychiatry*, *50*(4), 598–609.

Loewy, E. H. (1988). AIDS and the human condition. *Social Science and Medicine*, 27(4), 297–303.

Major, B., Mueller, P., & Hildebrandt, K. (1985). Attributions, expectations, and coping with abortion. *Journal of Personality and Social Psychology*, 48(3), 585–599.

Mann, J. M. (1987). Global AIDS situation. *World Health Statistics Quarterly*, 40, 185–192.

Marieskind, H. I. (1979). An evaluation of caesarean section in the United States. Final report to DHEW. Washington, DC: U.S. Government Printing Office.

Marieskind, H. I. (1982). Cesarean section. *Women and Health*, 7(3-4), 179–198.

Martin, R. L., Roberts, W. V., & Clayton, P. J. (1980). Psychiatric status after hysterectomy, a one-year prospective follow-up. *Journal of the American Medical Association*, 244(4), 350–353.

Matsumoto, H., Murakami, Y., Kuwabara, K., Tanaka, R, & Kashimoto, T. (1987). Average daily intake of pesticides and polychlorinated biphenyls in total diet samples in Osaka, Japan. *Bulletin of Environmental Contamination and Toxicology*, 38(6), 954–958.

Meininger, J. C. (1986). Sex differences in factors associated with use of medical care and alternative illness behaviors. *Social Science and Medicine*, 22(3), 285–292.

Melton, G. B. (1987). Legal regulation of adolescent abortion: Unintended effects. *American Psychologist*, 42(1), 79–83.

Melton, G. B., & Russo, N. F. (1987). Adolescent abortion: Psychological perspectives on public policy. *American Psychologist*, 42(1), 69–72.

Mercer, R. T., Hackley, K. C., & Bostrom, A. G. (1983). Relationship of psychosocial and perinatal variables to perception of childbirth. *Nursing Research*, 32(4), 202–207.

Morford, M. L., & Barclay, L. K. (1984). Counseling the pregnant woman: Implications for birth outcomes. *Personnel and Guidance Journal*, 62(10), 619–623.

Morgan, W. M., & Curran, J. W. (1986). Acquired immunodeficiency syndrome: Current and future trends. *Public Health Reports*, 101, 459–465.

Moseley, D. T., Follingstad, D. R., Harley, H., & Heckel, R. V. (1981). Psychological factors that predict reaction to abortion. *Journal of Clinical Psychology*, 37(2), 276–279.

Mueller, C. (1983). In search of a constituency for the "New Religious Right." *Public Opinion Quarterly*, 47(2), 213–229.

Nadelson, C. C. (1978). "Normal" and "special" aspects of pregnancy: A psychological approach. In M. T. Notman & C. C. Nadelson (Eds.), *The woman patient* (pp. 73–86). New York: Plenum Press.

National Center for Health Statistics. (1983). H. Koch: Utilization of psychotropic drugs in office-based ambulatory care: National ambulatory medical care survey 1980 and 1981. Advance Data from Vital and Health Statistics, No. 90. DHHS Pub. No. (PHS) 83-1250. Hyattsville, MD: Public Health Service.

National Center for Health Statistics. (1986). *Health United States 1985*. DHHS Pub. No. (PHS) 86-1232. Washington, DC: U.S. Government Printing Office.

National Center for Health Statistics, R. Pokras & V. Hufnagel. (1987). Hysterectomies in the United States, 1965–1984. *Vital and Health Statistics*, series 13, no. 92.

National Center for Health Statistics. (1988a). Detailed diagnoses and procedures for patients discharged from short-stay hospitals United States, 1986. *Vital and Health Statistics*, series 13, no. 95.

National Center for Health Statistics. (1988b). *Health United States 1987*. DHHS Pub. No. (PHS) 88-1232. Washington, DC: U.S. Government Printing Office.

Oakley, A. (1980). *Women confined*. New York: Schocken Books.

Oakley, A. (1983). Social consequences of obstetric technology: The importance of measuring "soft" outcomes. *Birth, 10*(2), 99–108.

O'Driscoll, K., Foley, M., MacDonald, D., & Stronge, J. (1988). Cesarean section and perinatal outcome: Response from the House of Horne. *American Journal of Obstetrics & Gynecology, 158*(3), 449–452.

Osborn, J. E. (1988). AIDS: Politics and science. *New England Journal of Medicine. 318*(7), 344–347.

Ott, W. J. (1981). Primary cesarean section: Factors related to postpartum infection. *Obstetrics and Gynecology, 57*, 171–176.

Padian, N. Marquis, L., & Francis, D. P. (1987). Male-to-female transmission of human immunodeficiency virus. *Journal of the American Medical Association, 258*, 788–790.

Parry, H. J. (1968). Use of psychotropic drugs by U.S. adults. *Public Health Reports, 83*(10), 799–810.

Payne, E. C., Kravitz, A. R., Notman, M. T., & Anderson, J. V. (1976). Outcome following therapeutic abortion. *Archives of General Psychiatry, 33*(6), 725–733.

Phelan, J. P., Clark, S. L., Diaz, F., & Paul, R. H. (1987). Vaginal birth after cesarean. *American Journal of Obstetrics and Gynecology, 157*(6), 1510–1515.

Phillips, R. N., Thornton, J., & Gleicher, N. (1982). Physician bias in cesarean section. *Journal of the American Medical Association, 248*, 1082–1084.

Polivy, J. (1974). Psychological reactions to hysterectomy: A critical review. *American Journal of Obstetrics & Gynecology, 118*(3), 417–426.

Prather, J., & Fidell, S. (1975). Sex differences in the content and style of medical advertisements. *Social Science and Medicine, 9*(1), 23–26.

Ramakrishnan, N., Kaphalia, B. S., Seth, T. D., & Roy, N. K. (1985). Organochlorine pesticide residues in mother's milk: A source of toxic chemicals in suckling infants. *Human Toxicology, 4*(1), 7–12.

Robbins, J. M. (1979). Objective versus subjective responses to abortion. *Journal of Consulting and Clinical Psychology, 47*(5), 994–995.

Robbins, J. M., & DeLamater, J. D. (1985). Support from significant others and loneliness following induced abortion. *Social Psychiatry, 20*(2), 92–99.

Ronald, A. R., Ndinya-Achola, J. O., Plummer, F. A., Simonsen, J. N., Cameron, D. W., Ngugi, E. N., & Pamba, H. (1988). A review of HIV in Africa. *Bulletin of the New York Academy of Medicine, 64*(6), 480–490.

Rosenberg, M. J., & Rosenthal, S. M. (1987). Reproductive mortality in the United States: Recent trends and methodologic considerations. *American Journal of Public Health, 77*(7), 833–836.

Rosenberg, M. J., & Weiner, J. M. (1988). Prostitutes and AIDS: A health department priority. *American Journal of Public Health, 78*(4), 418–423.

Rowley, D. L., Rab, M. A., Hardjotanojo, W., Liddle, J., Burse, V. W., Saleem, M., Sokal, D., Falk, H., & Head, S. L. (1987). Convulsions caused by endrin poisoning in Pakistan. *Pediatrics, 79*(6), 928–934.

Royston, E., & Lopez, A. D. (1987). On the assessment of maternal mortality. *World Health Statistics Quarterly, 40*, 214–224.

Sanger, M. (1931). *My fight for birth control*. New York: Maxwell Scientific International.

Schuman, H., Presser, S., & Ludwig, J. (1981). Context effects on survey responses to questions about abortion. *Public Opinion Quarterly, 45*(2), 216–223.

Seager, J., & Olson, A. (1986). *Women in the world.* New York: Simon & Schuster.

Seidenberg, R. (1971). Drug advertising and perception of mental illness. *Mental Hygiene, 55*(1), 21–31.

Shulman, L. C., & Mantell, J. E. (1988). The AIDS crisis: A United States Health Care Perspective. *Social Science & Medicine, 26*(10), 979–988.

Shusterman, L. R. (1976). The psychosocial factors of the abortion experience: A critical review. *Psychology of Women Quarterly, 1*(1), 79–106.

Siddiqui, M. K., & Saxena, M. C. (1985). Placenta and milk as excretory routes of lipophilic pesticides in women. *Human Toxicology, 4*(3), 249–254.

Sivaborvorn, K., Pongpaew, P., Huangprasert, S., & Chaikitiporn, C. (1983). Residue of insecticides in Thai vegetable growers. *Journal of the Medical Association of Thailand, 66* (Suppl. 1), 54–57.

Smith, M. C. (1977). Appeals used in advertisements for psychotropic drugs. *American Journal of Public Health, 67*(2), 171–173.

Sridhar, M. K., & Ogbalu, A. I. (1986). Pesticide usage and poisoning in Nigeria. *Journal of the Royal Society of Health, 106*(5), 182–184.

Stanley, F. J., & Watson, L. (1988). The cerebral palsies in Western Australia: Trends, 1968 to 1981. *American Journal of Obstetrics and Gynecology, 158*(1), 89–93.

Stehr-Green, J. K., Holman, R. C., Jason, J. M., & Evatt, B. L. (1988). Hemophilia-associated AIDS in the United States, 1981 to September 1987. *American Journal of Public Health, 78*(4), 439–442.

Stein, A., & Maine, D. (1986). The health of women. *International Journal of Epidemiology, 15*(3), 303–305.

Stoto, M. A., Blumenthal, D., Durch, J. S., & Feldman, P. H. (1988). Federal funding for AIDS research: Decision processes and results in fiscal year 1986. *Reviews of Infectious Diseases, 10*(2), 406–419.

Stovall, T. G., Shaver, D. C., Solomon, S. K., & Anderson, G. D. (1987). Trial of labor in previous cesarean section patients, excluding classical cesarean sections. *Obstetrics and Gynecology, 70*(5), 713–717.

Tejani, N., Verma, U., Shiffman, R., & Chayen, B. (1987). Effect of route of delivery on periventricular/intraventricular hemorrhage in the low-birth-weight fetus with a breech presentation. *Journal of Reproductive Medicine, 32*(12), 911–914.

Tojo, Y., Wariishi, M., Suzuki, Y., & Nishiyama, K. (1986). Quantitation of chlordane residues in mothers' milk. *Archives of Environmental Contamination and Toxicology, 15*(4), 327–332.

Travis, C. B. (1985). Medical decision making and elective surgery: The case of hysterectomy. *Risk Analysis, 5*(3), 241–251.

Travis, C. B. (1988a). *Women and health psychology: Biomedical issues.* Hillsdale, NJ: Erlbaum.

Travis, C. B. (1988b). *Women and health psychology: Mental health issues.* Hillsdale, NJ: Erlbaum.

Travis, C. B., Perkins, M., & Phillippi, R. H. (1988). *Medical decision making: Uniform standards and variations in practice.* Paper presented at the annual meeting of the American Psychological Association, Atlanta.

Travis, C. C., & Arms, A. (1987). The food chain as a source of toxic chemical exposure. In L. B. Lave & A. C. Upton (Eds.), *Toxic chemicals, health, and the environment.* Baltimore: Johns Hopkins University Press.

Tulman, L. J. (1986). Initial handling of newborn infants by vaginally and cesarean-delivered mothers. *Nursing Research, 35*(5), 296–300.

Turner, M. J., Brassil, M., & Gordon, H. (1988). Active management of labor associated with a decrease in the cesarean section rate in nulliparas. *Obstetrics and Gynecology, 71*(2), 150–154.

Unger, R. (1979). *Female and male.* New York: Harper & Row.

United Nations. (1984). *Mortality and health policy.* New York: United Nations.

U.S. Bureau of the Census. (1984a). *Women of the world: Latin America and the Caribbean.* E. M. Chaney, *Women in Development - 1.* Washington, DC: U.S. Government Printing Office.

U.S. Bureau of the Census. (1984b). *Women of the world: Sub-Saharan Africa.* J. S. Newman, *Women in Development - 2.* Washington, DC: U.S. Government Printing Office.

U.S. Bureau of the Census. (1985a). *Women of the world: Near East and North Africa.* M. Chamie, *Women in Development - 3.* Washington, DC: U.S. Government Printing Office.

U.S. Bureau of the Census. (1985b). *Women of the world: Asia and the Pacific.* N. M. Shah, *Women in Development - 4.* Washington, DC: U.S. Government Printing Office.

U.S. Bureau of the Census. (1985c). *Women of the world: A chartbook for developing regions.* E. Jamison, *Women in Development - 5.* Washington, DC: U.S. Government Printing Office.

Verbrugge, L. M. (1982). Sex differences in legal drug use. *Journal of Social Issues, 38*(2), 59–76.

Verbrugge, L. M. (1984). How physicians treat mentally distressed men and women. *Social Science and Medicine, 18*(1), 1–9.

Verbrugge, L. M., & Steiner, R. P. (1984). Another look at physicians' treatment of men and women with common complaints. *Sex Roles, 11*(11-12), 1091–1109.

Verbrugge, L. M., & Steiner, R. P. (1985). Prescribing drugs to men and women. *Health Psychology, 4*(1), 79–98.

Waldron, I. (1987). Patterns and causes of excess female mortality among children in developing countries. *World Health Statistics Quarterly, 40,* 194–210.

Weisenberg, E., Arad, I., Grauer, F., & Sahm, Z. (1985). Polychlorinated biphenyls and organochlorine insecticides in human milk in Israel. *Archives of Environmental Contamination and Toxicology, 14*(5), 517–521.

Weiss, K. (1977). What medical students learn about women. In C. Dreifus (Ed.), *Seizing our bodies.* New York: Vintage Books.

Weiss, K. (Ed.). (1984). *Women's health care: A guide to alternatives.* Reston, VA: Reston.

Weiss, N. S., Szekely, D. R., English, D. R., & Schweid, A. I. (1979). Endometrial cancer in relation to patterns of menopausal estrogen use. *Journal of the American Medical Association, 242*(3), 261–264.

World Health Organization. (1986a). Major parasitic infections: A global review. *World Health Statistics Quarterly, 39*(2), 145–160.

World Health Organization. (1986b). *WHO expert committee on malaria.* World Health Organization, Technical Report Series, no. 735.

World Health Organization. (1986c). World malaria situation 1984. *World Health Statistics Quarterly, 39*(2), 171–205.

World Health Organization. (1987). World malaria situation 1985. *World Health Statistics Quarterly, 40*(2), 142–170.

Wormser, G. P., Joline, C., Sivak, S. L., & Arlin, Z. A. (1988). Human immunodeficiency virus infections: Considerations for health care workers. *Bulletin of the New York Academy of Medicine, 64*(3), 203–215.

Wright, L. S., & Rogers, R. R. (1987). Variables related to pro-choice attitudes among undergraduates. *Adolescence, 22*(87), 517–524.

10

Psychology of Menstruation and Premenstrual Syndrome

Mary Brown Parlee

Research on the psychology of menstruation expanded rapidly during the past two decades.[1] Comprehensive general reviews or collections of research on normal menstrual experiences are provided by Dan (1988); Gannon (1985); Clare (1985); Golub (1983, 1985a); Paige, Magnus, Hahn, and Carrie (1983); Asso (1983); Friedman (1982); Komnenich, McSweeney, Noack, and Elder (1981); Dan, Graham, and Beecher (1980). More selective reviews are also available of menstrual cycle fluctuations in particular domains of psychological functioning, including cognition (Sommer, 1982, 1985; Dan, 1979); emotions (Parlee, 1988; Gannon, 1985; Asso, 1983; Dennerstein & Burrows, 1979; Smith, 1975); sexual behavior (Williams & Williams, 1982); symptoms (Golub, 1985b; Logue & Moos, 1986; Severino & Moline, 1989); bodily activity (Stenn & Klinge, 1972); dream content (Severino, Bucci & Creelman, 1988); sensation and perception (Parlee, 1983); and perceptual-motor/work performance (Sommer, 1973; Redgrove, 1971; Gamberale, 1985; Harlow, 1986). In addition, reviews of research on premenstrual syndromes (PMS) appear in Severino and Moline (1989); Ginsburg and Carter (1987); Abplanalp (1985a, 1985b); Dalton (1982); O'Brien (1987a, 1987b); Osofsky and Blumenthal (1985); Reid and Yen (1981); Reid (1985); Gannon (1985); Fausto-Sterling (1985); Endicott, Halbreich, and Nee (1986); Ablanalp, Haskett, and Rose (1980); Demers, McGuire, Phillips, and Rubinow (1989); Hammarback (1989).

These reviews cover relatively new and rapidly changing research fields, and many of them focus as much on methodological issues as on substantive conclusions about the topics being investigated. (For discussions explicitly focused on methods in menstrual cycle research see also Koeske, 1980a, 1980b, 1981;

Halbreich & Endicott, 1985a; Rubinow & Roy-Byrne, 1984; Parlee, 1973, 1983; Schilling, 1981; Hamilton & Alagna, 1986.)[2] The psychology of menstruation, thus, is a research area still in flux: the facts (even what counts as a "fact" and what is an artifact of an experimental procedure) are inextricably bound up with the research methods used to produce them and with the investigator's assumptions about what questions need to be (and need not be) asked. Summaries of the literature that present clear-cut conclusions as if they are straightforwardly derived from objective data do not, therefore, adequately reflect the current state of scientific research on this topic.

The aim of the present chapter is not to provide a summary and synthesis of unanalyzed research findings derived from varying methodologies, nor is it to review the many excellent methodological critiques of menstrual cycle research presently available. Rather, the aim is to try to extend and sharpen these by identifying and making explicit some of the connections among methods, theoretical questions, and substantive conclusions in research on normal menstrual experiences and on premenstrual syndrome. Recurring themes will be the ways particular methods reflect and reproduce specific assumptions (theories) about menstrual experiences and the ways data inconsistent with these assumptions are consistently treated as methodological problems rather than as a basis for questioning assumptions and developing new theories. Given the centrality of methods in linking theories and data, the discussion is organized around issues typically treated as methodological. It is followed by a brief consideration of some of the social contexts of the research, focusing on some concrete ways the politics of gender is played out in menstrual research.

ISSUES IN PSYCHOLOGICAL RESEARCH ON MENSTRUAL EXPERIENCES

Retrospective Questionnaires versus Prospective Assessment

Do retrospective accounts of experiences throughout the menstrual cycle confirm changes measured prospectively (on a daily basis)? If not, what do these different forms of self-report mean?

Prior to the late 1960s, investigations of psychological changes associated with normal menstruation usually involved daily or near daily assessments of psychological states or actions throughout the cycle (Hollingworth, 1914; Altmann, Knowles & Bull, 1941; Abramson & Torghele, 1961; Benedek & Rubenstein, 1939a, 1939b; Gottschalk, Kaplan, Gleser & Winget, 1962; Ivey & Bardwick, 1968; Kopell, Lunde, Clayton, & Moos, 1969; McCance, Luff, & Widdowson, 1937; Moos et al., 1969; Pierson & Lockhart, 1963). With the publication of the Moos Menstrual Distress Questionnaire (Moos, 1968, 1969), retrospective questionnaires on which women are asked to report menstrual-related changes they experienced during previous cycles (or the previous cycle) began to be more often used in research on normal menstrual changes, as they

Table 1

Methodological Issues in Psychological Research on the Normal Menstrual Cycle

Methodological Issues	Theoretical Questions
1. Retrospective questionnaires vs. prospective assessment	1. Do responses on retrospective questionnaires represent cultural beliefs about menstruation rather than reports of experience: if so, who holds them, how are they acquired, how do they function psychologically and socially?
2. Subject's awareness of the investigator's interest in menstruation	2. How does awareness influence self-reports of experience? How should "awareness" be conceptualized, how treated in designing research?
3. Comparison groups	3. What is the baseline for describing menstrual cycle changes as increase or decrease? What is the psychological significance of menstrual changes in the context of other mood cycles and events?
4. Interpreting correlations between cycle phase and behavior	4. What reinterpretations of published data are justified/required? How is the menstrual cycle influenced by psychological and social processes?
5. Validity of self-report measures of psychological states	5. In what domain(s) of psychological function can menstrual fluctuations be reliably and validly established? (How) can individual differences in patterns of changes be explained?
6. Validity of determination and definition of menstrual cycle phase	6. If definition and assessment of phase were standardized, what behavioral fluctuations can be (have been) clearly demonstrated?
7. Subject population	7. What is the theoretical rationale for selecting S samples that are homogeneous on some dimensions and unknown on others?

previously had been used to investigate premenstrual syndromes (Sutherland & Stewart, 1965; Levitt & Lubin, 1967; Ferguson & Vermillion, 1957; Coppen & Kessel, 1963).

Empirical and theoretical challenges to the interpretation of retrospective self-reports as unambiguous evidence of psychological changes during the cycle soon arose, however (Paige, 1973; Parlee, 1974), and several studies appeared explicitly comparing women's daily self-reports throughout the cycle with their responses on retrospective questionnaires completed at the end of the cycle (AuBuchon & Calhoun, 1985; May, 1976; Markum, 1976; Slade, 1984; Schilling, 1981; Englander-Golden, Chang, Whitmore, & Dienstbier, 1980; Ablanalp, Donnelly, & Rose, 1979; Parlee, 1982a; McFarlane, Martin, & Williams, 1988; Olasov & Jackson, 1987; Rogers & Harding, 1981; Endicott & Halbreich, 1982;

Chisholm et al., 1990). With some exceptions (Schilling, 1981), these studies generally confirmed the earlier finding of McCance et al. (1937) that reports on retrospective questionnaires do not give the same picture of changes during the cycle as do prospective assessments. While the interpretation of this difference is arguable (see Asso, 1983; Endicott & Halbreich, 1982; Ruble & Brooks-Gunn, 1979; Richardson, 1990; for different views of the issues involved), the significance for empirical work of the choice between prospective and retrospective assessment is not.

Many researchers now appear to agree (to assume) that prospective designs are more appropriate for investigating psychological changes throughout the menstrual cycle than are designs that depend upon inferences about changes made from retrospective questionnaire data (Schechter, Bachmann, Vaitukaitis, Phillips & Saperstein, 1989). However, attention to the methodological issue of retrospective versus prospective designs has also led some researchers not simply to abandon retrospective designs but to investigate the meaning of retrospectively obtained data as phenomena in their own right. (The assumption is that if women reliably respond in particular ways to retrospective questionnaires in a scientific investigation, the data they provide have psychological meaning; the question is what such responses mean.) These latter lines of inquiry are important not only for the substantive topics they explore but also for the challenge they implicitly represent to the widespread view that prospective designs are methodologically superior in all contexts to the use of other designs in menstrual research.

When data from retrospective questionnaires about menstruation are conceptualized as something other than accurate self-reports of changes experienced during previous cycles, some investigators have interpreted the questionnaire responses as evidence of socially shared beliefs about menstruation and have examined possible social and psychological functions and correlates of such beliefs. In a series of important papers, Koeske proposed that beliefs about menstrual cycle changes can be studied within the framework of attribution theory in social psychology: observers of a woman's behavior may invoke menstrual beliefs to account for her emotions and actions under circumstances where other types of explanations would also be possible and plausible (Koeske & Koeske, 1975; Koeske, 1978, 1980a). A hypothesized premenstrual "arousability," which by itself lacks specific psychological content, might thereby be given social and psychological meaning through attributional processes that label a woman as "premenstrual" and invoke the cultural beliefs about what this entails. Since her research showed that biological explanations were more likely to be offered to explain women's negative emotions than positive ones, Koeske proposed that this attributional pattern involving the menstrual cycle might be particularly likely to be used when the woman's behavior is "out of role" for women according to prevailing cultural norms (and so is seen as needing explanation in noncultural terms).

In a paper that is a landmark in theoretical development along these lines (see

Parlee, 1988), Laws (1983) further elaborated Koeske's proposal, describing women's interpretations of menstrual cycle changes within the conceptual/empirical tradition of social psychiatry and from an explicitly feminist perspective. She argues that attribution of women's negative experiences and actions to premenstrual tension serves to privatize, naturalize, and medicalize feelings arising from the cultural contradictions of women's roles, feelings that were framed or attributed differently (more politically and with different implications for subsequent action) when feminist analyses of gender relations had greater cultural visibility. (E.g., anger at a husband "because of premenstrual tension" has very different psychological and social meaning than anger at a husband "because he doesn't do his share of the housework" when both wife and husband are employed full-time. When framed biomedically, the woman is regarded as having an illness requiring medical treatment; when framed in terms of a feminist analysis, she thinks she has a grievance—shared with other women—requiring political redress.) Campos and Thurow (1978), on the other hand, focus on the role of bodily processes (bleeding) in shaping women's attributions of menstrual cycle changes and do not develop Koeske's and Laws's suggestion of a link between the attributional pattern and the broader culture. While the interpretation may still be at issue (and is probably the heart of scientific controversy and gender politics in menstrual research), the basic phenomenon identified by Koeske—a selective attribution of negative emotions to the premenstrual phase of the cycle, with external or personality explanations offered at other phases and for positive emotions—has recently been confirmed by Bains and Slade (1988).

Conducting their research on the assumption that women's responses on a retrospective menstrual questionnaire are best conceptualized as "beliefs" and "attitudes" about the cycle (Parlee, 1974; Ruble, 1977), Ruble and Brooks-Gunn and their colleagues have developed a menstrual attitude questionnaire (Brooks-Gunn & Ruble, 1980) to investigate the development of such beliefs among adolescents and college students in the United States (Brooks, Ruble & Clarke, 1977; Clarke & Ruble, 1978; Brooks-Gunn & Ruble, 1980, 1982; Ruble & Brooks-Gunn, 1979, 1982, 1987; see also The Tampax Report, 1981; Stoltzman, 1986; Golub, 1981, 1983). One large-scale study of Finnish adolescents and their mothers involved the use of retrospective questionnaires to assess menstrual-related symptoms and moods (see Widholm, 1979, and earlier papers cited therein), but because it was begun before the importance of the prospective/retrospective issue in menstrual cycle research was clearly documented, the investigators do not indicate how they conceptualize or interpret their data in light of this issue. Prospective ratings have also been used to investigate menstrual cycle changes in symptoms and moods among adolescent girls in the United States (Golub & Harrington, 1981) and Switzerland (Flug, Largo & Prader, 1985), thus permitting a comparison of data from the two methods. In an important series of studies, Rierdan and Koff and their colleagues have used multiple methods in an attempt to understand the interplay of social, biological, and psychological processes at menarche (Rierdan & Koff, 1985; Rierdan, Koff & Flaherty, 1985–1986; Koff, 1983; Koff, Rierdan & Silverstone, 1978; Rierdan, 1983).

Other researchers have used retrospective menstrual questionnaires to investigate the content and distribution of menstrual beliefs among adult women in other cultures (Janiger, Piffenbaugh & Kersh, 1972; Mac & Chang, 1985; Paige, 1987). It is impossible to draw any general conclusions from such data, however, since the theoretical significance of the methodological difference between prospective and retrospective reports has been sidestepped. Thus, investigators have sometimes interpreted questionnaire responses as evidence of cultural beliefs about menstruation and at other times (more frequently) as unambiguous evidence of premenstrual and menstrual symptomotology experienced by women in different cultures.

Also interested in beliefs qua beliefs, some investigators have focused on the ways menstrual beliefs, when they have been made salient in a particular setting, might shape a woman's interpretation of her own experiences. Ruble's (1977) paper reported her now-classic demonstration that when women are experimentally deceived into believing they are premenstrual, they report feeling more of the negative moods and symptoms associated (in the belief system) with the premenstrual phase. In subsequent work Ruble and Brooks-Gunn (1979) proposed a theoretical account of the cognitive function of menstrual beliefs in terms of information-processing mechanisms hypothesized by social psychologists to account for social cognition more generally. They suggest that women's beliefs about premenstrual psychological changes, functioning in concert with such cognitive mechanisms, result in selective labeling and recall of experiences congruent with the beliefs. More recently, AuBuchon and Calhoun (1985) have confirmed Ruble's basic finding under slightly different circumstances, and in their research McFarlane et al. (1988) extend the theoretical discussion of cognitive-processing mechanisms by conceptualizing menstrual cycle data under the rubric of social psychological schema theory. (Hamilton, Alagna & Sharpe, 1985, have developed cognitive theory within yet another tradition for conceptualizing premenstrual syndrome and its treatment.)

While not working explicitly within a social cognition framework, Rodin (1976) also found indirect evidence that beliefs about the menstrual cycle affect the way women interpret their subjective psychological states. She reports that when women who normally experienced premenstrual symptoms were led to attribute experimentally induced anxiety to the menstrual cycle (to label it as a menstrual cycle symptom), the anxiety did not interfere with their performance on a cognitive task to the same degree as it did for women who did not attribute the anxiety to this bodily cause. On the other hand, Fradkin and Firestone (1986) found that women who were informed that their premenstrual symptoms had a biological cause reported more premenstrual negative moods than did women who were informed that the symptoms arose from negative societal myths. Both groups showed more positive interactions with their child (in a laboratory setting) during the premenstrual phase than during the preovulatory phase. These investigations of a potential relationship between attributional patterns (negative psychological states to a biological or a cultural cause) and other actions (cognitive performance or interpersonal actions) represent a potentially fruitful direction for research, but it has to date been relatively little examined.

It is important to notice that the theoretical construct "menstrual beliefs" functions in the research considered in this section in two methodologically distinct ways. One is as an interpretation of data obtained using retrospective menstrual questionnaires (data that are now almost universally acknowledged not to be simply accurate "self-reports" of menstrual cycle changes, although their interpretation may still be arguable). In this usage of the theoretical construct, menstrual cycle beliefs are methodologically assessed through patterns of responses on the closed-ended questionnaires. In the psychological literature, closed-ended questionnaires have almost invariably been used in cross-cultural and at least some of the developmental investigations of menstrual cycle beliefs (summarized in Severino & Moline, 1989; Golub, 1985b; and Ruble & Brooks-Gunn, 1982, respectively). In the other usage of "menstrual beliefs" (Koeske & Koeske, 1975; Rodin, 1976), the specific content of the beliefs is not determined by the investigator. Rather, the research participants' own beliefs about menstrual cycle changes are made salient in the experimental situation through procedures that highlight menstruation or the menstrual cycle (and presumably heighten the participants' awareness of the complex of beliefs associated with it). Here beliefs about menstruation are not operationalized through use of a questionnaire but rather are invoked by the investigator in the interpretation of data gathered with research procedures presumed to bring beliefs into play. Data generated by research procedures of this latter sort, however, are typically not considered to be substantive phenomena in their own right—as evidence regarding the nature and functioning of beliefs about menstruation. Instead, they have beeen conceptualized as a methodological issue: the effects of subjects' awareness of the menstrual cycle focus of the research.

Subjects' Awareness of Menstruation as a Research Focus

Does it matter whether the subjects are aware or not aware that the menstrual cycle is the focus of the research? If so, how is the difference between results obtained with these different methods to be interpreted?

Several investigators have found that not only do women's responses on mood and symptom questionnaires differ depending on whether the data are gathered prospectively or retrospectively, but they also differ, when prospective assessments are used, depending on whether or not the subjects are aware that the menstrual cycle is the research topic (Englander-Golden et al., 1978; Parlee, 1982a; McFarlane et al., 1988; Swandby, 1981; Slade, 1984; Gallant et al., 1991). These researchers have generally concluded that when the menstrual cycle is made salient through the research methods (manner of recruitment, instructions, description of the study in informed consent procedures), the subjects' beliefs about menstruation also become salient and affect the woman's interpretation ("labeling," "attribution," "framing") of the experiences she reports on the daily ratings. (Other investigators, however, believe that the differences between data obtained from subjects who are aware of the menstrual cycle focus of the research and from those who are not are less clear-cut; see, e.g., Asso, 1983.)

In this literature researchers frequently use language that suggests or explicitly says that experimental methods that make menstrual beliefs salient for the subject are less desirable than are methods in which the menstrual focus of the research is disguised from the subjects. Asso (1983), for example, discusses the possibility that activation of menstrual beliefs may "contaminate" or "confound" self-reports of "real" menstrual cycle experience (problematic assumptions underlying this formulation are discussed in Parlee, 1988.) From a point of view that holds that menstrual beliefs "influence" or "distort" self-reports of "actual" experience (a point of view consistent with Ruble and Brooks-Gunn's theoretical formulation as well as Asso's), an ideal menstrual cycle study might be one in which women are unaware of the focus on menstruation. While in some investigations researchers have successfully disguised the menstrual focus of the study from the participants, as a practical matter it is difficult to do this effectively when the research methods involve the kinds of physiological measurements necessary to define cycle phase with reasonable precision. Of the several prospective studies, many of them recent, reporting concurrent measurements of psychological states and physiological indices of the menstrual cycle, none report using methods that prevented the participants from being aware of the purpose of the investigation.

In addition to these practical difficulties, however, the methodological issue of subjects' "awareness" has both demonstrable significance for the empirical results of an investigation and considerable theoretical import. Again, it raises the question of what the data mean in their own right—how are the disparate findings from methods producing or not producing awareness of the menstrual focus of the research to be conceptualized? Is "awareness" just another instance of the distorting or contaminating effects of menstrual beliefs on self-reports of "real" menstrual cycle changes? Is it a source of "noise" in the psychological data, ideally to be dealt with through experimental procedures that eliminate awareness? Or is it a phenomenon, perhaps the phenomenon, in its own right?

It seems reasonable to think that in real life women are aware of the menstrual cycle to different degrees and take it into account in different ways, as they continually interpret (make sense of) their experiences in particular situations. Beliefs about the menstrual cycle are thus part of this interpretation, as Koeske proposed in different language and concepts, and are constitutive of the responses given by women in menstrual cycle research. Mishler (1986) has cogently made a more general argument along these lines, an argument that, if applied to menstrual research, would emphasize that it is not only a woman's beliefs about menstruation that influence her responses on menstrual questionnaires, but also her beliefs and expectations about participating in the research, her reactions and purposes with respect to the investigator and the setting, and other psychological functions involved when she makes her situation and actions meaningful and socially accountable. All this is disregarded, however, when responses on menstrual questionnaires are interpreted as "self-report data"—the meaning of which is unilaterally assigned by the investigator (Cassell, 1982; Parlee, 1992). Although the heart of Mishler's argument as it applies to menstrual cycle research has not been addressed with the seriousness it merits, his substantive and theoretical point that moods, emotions, and symptoms as "reported" on questionnaires represent a convergence of many psychological and social events and processes has, in fact, been partially explored under the rubric of (again) a methodological issue: the use of comparison groups and contexts in menstrual cycle research.

Comparison Groups and Contexts in Menstrual Cycle Research

Are emotional and behavioral cycles found only in menstruating women? How do psychological changes associated with the menstrual cycle compare with psychological changes associated with other cycles and noncyclic events? How do data from comparison groups and data gathered in other contexts affect the interpretation of menstrual cycle data? Perhaps most importantly, what assumptions about the subject matter are embodied in research designs that do not permit these questions to be answered?

Like other research topics in psychology (see, e.g., Shields, 1975), psychological research and writing on menstruation have historically been shaped to some extent by issues and questions in the broader society (Sayers, 1982). When psychological changes associated with the menstrual cycle began to be discussed in the popular media in the United States in the early 1970s (Abplanalp, 1985b; Parlee, 1987; Chrisler & Levy, 1990), some researchers responded to claims that menstruating women were unsuited to positions of public power and responsibility by examining the existing scientific literature and providing new interpretations and new data. Some of this critical work focused on the implied uniqueness of menstruating women, pointing to the possibility that men also appear to show cyclic changes in emotions and behavior (Ramey, 1973) and arguing that recognition of the pervasiveness of cyclic phenomena is necessary for scientific understanding as well as for fairness in the social realm. (This argument was made implicitly by Seward many years ago—Seward, 1944.)

Currently there are several prospective investigations in the literature comparing (in various combinations) changes in moods, emotions, and symptoms in women with spontaneous menstrual cycles, women taking oral contraceptives, and men (Rogers & Harding, 1981; McFarlane et al., 1988; Alagna & Hamilton, 1986; Wilcoxon, Schrader & Sherif, 1976; Vingilis, 1980; Mansfield, Hood &

Henderson, 1989; Gallant et al., 1991). In general, although the findings vary, these data tend to show that spontaneously cycling women do not report emotional changes that are uniquely large or negative when considered in the context of changes reported by other groups of subjects or in relation to other events.

While the scientific import of these data has typically not been further explored, one potentially fruitful line of research is suggested by Procacci et al.'s studies in which fluctuations in pain perception of women with spontaneous menstrual cycles were compared with those of women who were pregnant (Procacci et al., 1972, 1974). Both groups, they found, showed a circatrigenten (near 28-day) cycle in pain perception (see also Richter, 1968). The authors suggest that both the fluctuations in the psychological domain (pain perception) and the menstrual cycle itself are expressions of, or entrained by, a central biological "clock," which continues to influence the timing of psychological fluctuations even when menstrual cycles cease during pregnancy.

Other researchers responded in another way to the implication in popular media coverage and in the scientific literature that the menstrual cycle is uniquely disruptive of emotional and behavioral stability: they compared the magnitude of emotional changes associated with the menstrual cycle with the magnitude of emotional changes evoked in other contexts. Thus menstrually related mood changes have been compared with those associated with the social cycle of the week (Rossi & Rossi, 1977; Rossi, 1980; McFarlane et al., 1988; Mansfield et al., 1989; Gallant et al., 1991), with other noncyclic events in the social environment (Golub, 1976), and with other biological conditions (Schilling, 1981; Brooks-Gunn, 1985).

In a particularly thoughtful reanalysis of Wilcoxon et al.'s (1976) data on the relationships among stressful life events, cycle phase, and moods, Koeske (1980b, 1981) demonstrates empirically that while "stressful life events" and "menstrual cycle phase" are conceptualized as independent variables in the analysis of variance methodology used in the research, they are, in fact, not independent. The premenstrual and menstrual phase of the cycles in Wilcoxon et al.'s no-pill group were strongly associated with two stress points in the college students subjects' lives—midterms and final examinations. The central assumption embedded in the analysis of variance model therefore is incorrect in (at least) this case: the menstrual cycle cannot be conceptualized simply as an "independent variable" since it is itself affected by external events. Put in language that, while familiar, no longer seems quite appropriate to the phenomena (Parlee, 1981), Koeske observes that the menstrual cycle is both an "independent" and a "dependent" "variable."

Critical attention to the methodological issue of comparison groups and contexts therefore leads in different ways to a central theoretical problem in psychological research on the menstrual cycle: how are temporal associations between the menstrual cycle and behavior and/or the menstrual cycle and events in the social environment to be interpreted? What assumptions about how these data are to be interpreted are embedded in particular research designs and procedures for data analysis? These questions have been raised many times in the past 15 years (especially by Koeske), but examination of the methods used and interpretations of data offered in the current research literature indicates they have not been seriously considered despite the increasingly rich body of empirical evidence of their scientific importance.

Interpreting Correlations Between Cycle Phase and Behavior

Most research on the psychological concomitants of the menstrual cycle at this stage in the development of the field can be said to be correlational in the sense that psychological and physiological measures are separately obtained and a temporal association between changes in one kind of variable with changes in the other is sought. (Experiments providing data from which causal inferences can most directly be made, e.g., Kemnitz, Gibber, Lindsay & Eisele, 1989, have not been done in psychological research on the human menstrual cycle, and for ethical reasons it seems likely that if they are ever carried out, it will be with clinical populations only.) Most often, investigators reporting a temporal association between some physiological parameter of the menstrual cycle and some psychological measurement interpret their data by implying a causal relationship in which the cycle causally influences the psychological event or process (Dalvit, 1981). This interpretation of correlational data is the one most compatible with the psychobiological perspective that characterizes most biomedical research. It is an eminently reasonable interpretation and ultimately will be subjected to the most rigorous tests possible.

Some of the data showing temporal associations between the menstrual cycle and behavior, however, clearly require a different interpretation. As Koeske (1980b) noted in her reanalysis of Wilcoxon et al.'s (1976) data and as others have expressed in pointing to the menstrual cycle as an "open system" (Rossi, 1980; McClintock, 1981), the menstrual cycle not only affects but is affected by many social and psychological influences (see also references in Dan, 1988; Paige et al., 1983). Consistent with this more dynamic, systems perspective, there is now a substantial body of data showing social and psychological influences on the menstrual cycle and thereby suggesting potentially fruitful directions of research that does not focus solely on the causal influences of the menstrual cycle (the psychological "consequences" or "impact" of the cycle). Among the socially mediated influences on menstrual cycle physiology are proximity to, and interaction with, other menstruating women (McClintock, 1971; Jarett, 1984); diet (Hill, Garbaczewski, Helman, Huskisson, Sporangisa & Wynder, 1980); exercise (Bullen, Skrinar, Beitins, Von Mering, Turnball & McArthur, 1985, Loucks, 1990); stress (Metcalf, 1983; Chatterton et al., 1985; Matsumoto, Igarashi & Nagaoka, 1968); sexual behavior (Cutler, Preti, Huggins, Erickson & Garcia, 1985; Cutler, Garcia & Krieger, 1979); body fat (Frisch, 1985); breast-feeding (Berman, Hanson & Hellman, 1972); light (Dewan, 1967; Cutler, 1980;

Lin, Kripke, Parry & Berga, 1990); and olfactory cues (Russell, Switz & Thompson, 1980).

Not only do the documented facts of socially and psychologically mediated influences on the menstrual cycle open up new and potentially fruitful lines of research outside a simple biological-cause/psychological-effect model, but also they should serve to correct a widespread, but misleading, interpretation of one widely cited body of research demonstrating a correlation between menstrual cycle phase and behavior. In a series of important investigations Dalton and others have documented a temporal association between particular actions (e.g., commission of a crime, admission to a mental hospital, accidents at work, suicide attempts) and the phase of the menstrual cycle the woman was in when she performed the act (see d'Orban and Dalton, 1980; Parlee, 1982b, for references). Consistently, this research has shown that if a woman has performed the action under investigation, she is significantly more likely to have done so during the premenstrual and menstrual phase of the cycle than during other phases. Although there have been some failures to replicate (Birtchnell & Floyd, 1974; Patel, Cliff & Machin, 1985, report the association between behavior and cycle phase is found only for women with self-reported symptoms of PMS) and some intriguing reversals (Parlee, 1975a; Doty & Silverthorne, 1975), the correlational data of Dalton and others at present represent the strongest evidence available of the existence of a relationship between menstrual cycle phase and behavior. The question is, How are these data to be interpreted?

The correlational data of Dalton and others are cited in the literature in contexts that suggest they are invariably interpreted as evidence of a premenstrual syndrome of negative affect, with the implication or claim that the negative affect was what prompted the woman to commit the particular action. Data reported in some of Dalton's own papers, however, suggest that this interpretation of the temporal association between cycle phase and behavior must be corrected in some cases and, therefore, perhaps in all. Two of Dalton's papers (Dalton, 1960, 1968) contain data that show that the same association between cycle phase and behavior that is found for actions initiated by the woman herself (e.g., commission of a crime) is also found for activities whose timing was not under her control (being involved in a ''passive accident'' at work; taking a nationwide scholastic examination). While women involved in these activities were found, in fact, to be significantly more likely to be in the premenstrual or menstrual phases than in other phases at the time of the event in question, it cannot be the case that a woman's premenstrual state caused her to take a nationally scheduled examination on the day set by the examining board (Dalton, 1968) or be involved in an accident where there was nothing she could have done to avoid it (Dalton, 1960). These data from Dalton (1960, 1968) mean that the usual causal interpretation of the observed correlation between cycle phase and behavior (that the cycle phase causally influenced the behavior) cannot be correct in all cases. In light of the research on social and psychological influences on menstruation, these data suggest the possibility that all of the correlations observed by Dalton and others may be interpretable as the outcome of a common cause (e.g., a stressful event) that influences the timing of both the behavior and the menstrual cycle. (See Parlee, 1975; 1982b, for a more detailed argument.)

This possible interpretation of the correlational data may or may not be correct (that is a matter for empirical investigation), but the reanalysis of Dalton's data, like the reanalysis of Wilcoxon et al.'s data and the evidence of social influences on the menstrual cycle, points to the need for scrupulous caution and considerable conceptual flexibility and openness in formulating research questions and designs and in interpreting correlations between the menstrual cycle and behavior. Regrettably, neither of these qualities of scientific sensibility is at present consistently evident in the psychological literature on menstruation.

Validity of Psychological Measures

Several reviews of the menstrual cycle literature contain large-scale tables with details of the studies under review, including some or all of the following: authors, number of subjects, how cycle phase was determined, psychological measures used, and results (Sommer, 1982, 1985; Parlee, 1983; Gannon, 1985; Severino & Moline, 1989; Asso, 1983; Dennerstein & Burrows, 1979). From these summary tables, as well as from the literature itself, it seems clear that the technical question of the validity of psychological measures used in menstrual cycle research is likely to be more pertinent for some domains of psychological functioning than for others. Psychological measures of sensory-motor performance (e.g., reaction time) are generally part of long methodological and theoretical traditions in psychological research, and while details of the experimental procedure are of great importance for comparing results across studies, the general scientific import of such data has been fairly uncontroversial. Psychological measures of emotions and self-reports of behaviors, on the other hand, are more subject to interpretive disputes and methodological critiques (as illustrated by the debate over the meaning of retrospective "self-reports" of menstrual cycle changes). In part this is because of the very diverse theoretical frameworks that psychologists in the United States bring to research on emotions (e.g., from Plutchick, 1980 to Harre, 1986) and in part because methodologies accepted within the field as necessary for validating these self-report instruments are more elaborate.

In practice, it appears that the question of the validity of psychological instruments has been explicitly raised and explored primarily in prospective research on menstrual fluctuations in emotions and symptoms. For example, Monagle, Dan, Chatterton, DeLeon-Jones, and Hudgens (1986), Webster, Martin, Uchalik, and Gannon (1979), and Stephenson, Denney, and Aberger (1983) have empirically explored the factor structure of Chesney and Tasto's (1975) Menstrual Symptom Questionnaire, while Rogers and Harding (1981) and others have examined the properties of the Moos Menstrual Distress Questionnaire (see also Moos, 1985). Endicott, Nee, Cohen, and Halbreich (1986) have provided external validation of their Premenstrual Assessment Form (PAF) (Halbreich, Endicott, Schachts & Nee, 1982) by showing an empirical association between one pattern of premenstrual changes on the PAF and a lifetime diagnosis of affective disorder.

Other investigators have dealt with the issue by using well-validated self-report instruments already widely used in the psychological literature, thus enabling comparison of responses from subjects in menstrual cycle research with those in other samples and settings. Among the closed-ended self-report instruments that have been widely used in investigations of menstrual cycles are the Profile of Mood States (McNair, Lorr & Droppleman, 1971), the Nowlis Mood Adjective Check List (Nowlis, 1965), the Moos Menstrual Distress Questionnaire, Form T (daily) (Moos, 1985), and the Multiple Affect Adjective Check List (Zuckerman & Lubin, 1965, Lubin et al., 1986). (Hedges, Jandorf & Stone, 1985, discuss the use of these questionnaires more generally.) The Gottschalk-Glesser coding scheme for analyzing the affective content of unstructured samples of speech (Gottschalk et al., 1962) and the Thayer Activation-Deactivation Adjective Check List (Thayer, 1967, 1970) have also been repeatedly used. While some researchers continue to develop their own self-report instruments for investigating menstrual cycle fluctuations in emotions, the scientific benefits of empirically linking these with well-validated self-report instruments that have been used in other investigations seem evident, and the increasingly frequent use of validated self-report instruments represents one form of methodological progress in menstrual cycle research.

On the other hand, it is important to recognize that the question of validity is not simply a technical problem, to be completely resolved through factor analyses or assessments of the interrelationships among different self-report measures and between self-report measures and other behaviors. As Koeske (1980b) has noted in another context, "The fact that some assumptions [about the phenomenon under investigation] have been legitimated within the field by their incorporation into common statistical analyses, standard design, or *accepted measurement procedures* [emphasis added] should not blind us to their presence" (p. 229).

In research on emotional changes associated with the menstrual cycle, the unnoticed assumptions embedded in an accepted measurement procedure—the use of self-report questionnaires to "measure" emotions—are many and consequential for understanding the psychology of menstruation. Among them are (1) that emotions are states within an individual that can be understood/reported without reference to context and registered in units of quantity, (2) that the "magnitude" of an emotion is the most meaningful (or a meaningful) feature of emotional experience, and (3) that methods (administration of questionnaires) that strip the actions of persons from their contexts yield psychologically meaningful information.

Validity of Physiological Measures and Definitions of Cycle Phase

Several methods have been used in psychological research on the menstrual cycle to determine/define the cycle phase during which the psychological measurements or observations were made. Ranging from lesser to greater precision and detail in describing menstrual status in physiological terms, these include reported date of onset of last menstrual period, counting backward from day of menstrual onset (reverse cycle day), basal body temperature, basal body temperature and menstrual onset, basal body temperature and reverse cycle day, urinary levels of gonadal hormone metabolites, and progesterone and estrogen levels (in plasma or in saliva) determined by radioimmunoassay. Gannon (1985) and Steege (1989) reviewed evidence on the strengths and limitations of some of these techniques for assessing cycle phase, emphasizing, in particular, some of the problems inherent in using basal body temperature alone to determine the time of ovulation.

Like the validity of psychological measures, however, the validity of physiological measures and definitions of menstrual cycle phases have both conceptual and technical aspects and require, as well, an informed and healthy appreciation of the empirical complexity of the relationships among neural structures, neurotransmitter receptor sensitivity, and temporal patterning of gonadal steroid hormones (McEwen, 1980, 1988; Cutler & Garcia, 1980). Regrettably, scientific caution and rigor in this domain are not especially notable in social scientists' research and writing about behavior and the menstrual cycle.

Sample Selection

Given differences in cycle length and in variability of cycle length among women of different ages (Presser, 1974; Chiazze, Brazer, Macasco, Parker & Duffy, 1968; Treolar, Boynton, Behn & Brown, 1967; Cutler, Garcia & Krieger, 1979), and differences in psychological significance of menstruation for women of different ages and circumstances (Notman & Nadelson, 1983; Friedman et al., 1980; Rierdan, 1983; Steege, Stout & Rupp, 1985) and given the cycle-influencing stresses that different groups of women, including college students, may be exposed to (Metcalf, 1983; Koeske, 1980b) sample selection is an aspect of methodology with considerable theoretical and substantive significance in menstrual cycle research (Dan, 1988; Koeske, 1981; Parlee, 1981; Haskett & Abplanalp, 1983). Many investigators urging the use of more homogeneous samples of women assume it is endocrinological homogeneity that is desirable in menstrual cycle research. ("There have been . . . [few] . . . studies in which investigators have been able to evaluate symptom intensity during segments of the menstrual cycle which are defined for a group of subjects in an endocrinologically consistent manner" (Schechter et al., 1989, p. 173).) Consistent with the biomedical/psychobiological focus on the menstrual cycle as a cause of behavior and experience, homogeneity in the physiological domain is desirable from that point of view but not necessarily from others. In their research on premenstrual syndromes, Endicott and Halbreich and their coworkers have found that homogeneity at the psychological level (in terms of patterns of distressing symptom and mood changes) can reveal empirical generalizations that would be obscured in a more heterogeneous sample (Endicott et al., 1986), and this may prove true for research on other menstrual experiences as well (Key, Hammond & Strong, 1986; Hammarback & Backstrom, 1989). Again, it is clear that methods for sample selection reflect and embody assumptions about the phenomenon under investigation and so have theoretical and substantive significance. Making these assumptions explicit and subject to empirical examination (as Endicott and Halbreich have done), rather than leaving them unanalyzed, may be one strategy for developing new theories and findings.

PROSPECTIVELY DOCUMENTED CORRELATIONS BETWEEN THE NORMAL MENSTRUAL CYCLE AND PSYCHOLOGICAL FUNCTIONING: FINDINGS, ASSUMPTIONS, AND UNASKED QUESTIONS

Findings

Given the consensus among many researchers on at least some criteria for evaluating research, what does the "best" research currently suggest are the well-documented psychological changes associated with the normal menstrual cycle? That is, applying the criteria implicit in critiques of menstrual cycle research, what has been found in investigations that, at a minimum, are prospective in design, employ direct measures of at least some endocrinological parameters of the menstrual cycle, and involve women with regular, relatively a-symptomatic cycles?

The following prospective investigations contain data on both psychological functioning and concomitant measures of gonadal hormone levels (either in plasma or as reflected in the concentration of metabolites excreted in urine): Schechter et al. (1989); Rubinow et al. (1988); Both-Orthman, Rubinow, Hoban, Malley, and Grover (1988); Sanders, Warner, Backstrom, and Bancroft (1983); Backstrom et al. (1983); Halbreich, Endicott, Goldstein, and Nee (1986); Doty, Snyder, Huggins, and Lowry (1981); Chatterton, Dan, DeLeon-Jones, Hudgens, Haan, Cheesman, and Cheesman (1985); Abplanalp et al. (1979); Komnenich, Lane, Dickey, and Stone (1978); Moos et al. (1969); Persky, Lief, Strauss, Miller, and O'Brien (1978); Gordon, Corbin, and Lee (1986); Hampson (1990a, 1990b); Graham and Glasser (1985); Lahmeyer, Miller, and DeLeon-Jones (1982). Investigations in which normal psychological functioning was assessed in different cycle phases defined in relation to basal body temperature changes include: Gottschalk et al. (1962); Ivey and Bardwick (1968); Paige (1971); Zimmerman and Parlee (1973); Patkai et al. (1974); Little and Zahn (1974);

Parlee (1983); Wuttke, Arnold, Becker, Creutzfeldt, Langenstein, and Tirsch (1986); Broverman, Vogel, Klaiber, Majcher, Shea, and Paul (1981); Kopell et al. (1969); Gong, Garrel, and Calloway (1989). (To update and expand these lists of investigations in what is a very fast moving research field, psychologists will need to search not only the social science data bases with which they usually work but also those that cover biomedical research.)

For the reviewer, this literature poses two problems in addition to the fact that it cuts firmly across traditional disciplinary boundaries. First, it is expanding very rapidly, so any review will necessarily be incomplete by the time it appears in print. Second, it is difficult—and pointless—to describe these complex research findings with simple summaries and conclusions. (It is like the topic "gender differences in cognition," for example, for which careful summaries of research must specify a particular domain of cognition and, within it, must note disparate findings obtained with different measures.)

To date, few general conclusions can be drawn about experiences and actions associated with normal menstruation, and summaries of research about particular domains of psychological function are closely tied to the complexities of the data in a way that resists easy simplification (or should do). It does not make sense in terms of the data, for example, to summarize even menstrual changes in "sensory functioning" (of which there is considerable evidence; see Parlee, 1983) since each sensory modality shows a different pattern, and within each modality different measures may show conflicting or ambiguous findings. It certainly does not advance scientific understanding to press for generalizations that answer "is there premenstrual impairment in sensory functioning?," since the data show at least that this is the wrong question—some sensory modalities show changes around mid-cycle, some during menstruation, some premenstrually. While there are considerable professional pressures on investigators (and perhaps also psychodynamic ones) to present closure and simplicity in their published research, it is necessary to resist premature simplification of the data, summaries and conclusions that force the data to "answer" the wrong questions. Generalizations about research findings and, eventually, deeper understanding of menstrual experiences will emerge from systematic research, but at this stage getting the questions right may be at least as important as trying to fit data to a Procrustean bed of unexamined and possibly unwarranted assumptions.

Assumptions

The empirical question in this research is whether changes in a particular mode of psychological functioning occur in relation to specified parameters of the menstrual cycle. The implicit underlying question revealed by the research methods used is whether the physiological changes of the menstrual cycle play a causal role in producing the psychological changes. The use of methods that provide physiological measures of individual women's menstrual cycles—and invariably only their menstrual cycles—reveals pervasive assumptions about the domain within which explanations of variations in psychological events are to be sought and found. As revealed by the ubiquitous use of self-report question-naires, furthermore, pervasive assumptions about what emotions are and how they can be measured also structure this research.[3] Finally, by measuring pa-rameters of the menstrual cycle and of psychological states at the same time (or by conceptualizing the data this way even if the measurements are not literally simultaneous), investigators reveal the deeply embedded assumption that tem-poral parameters of psychological events of interest coincide with the temporal parameters of biological events of interest (that is, that the psychological event/ state/process of interest is one that occurs roughly "at the same time" as the specified biological event and will change when "underlying" physiology changes).

While these assumptions of psychobiology (or of a biomedical perspective) may be compatible with recognition that social and psychological processes also shape emotions and influence menstrual cycle physiology (see Severino & Mo-line's (1989) discussion of a biopsychosocial model), it is typical of the pro-spective research cited above that the conceptual/methodological focus has been on psychological changes as effects of (only) menstrual cycle physiology. Indeed, the "obviousness" of this conceptual framework and its associated notions of "reality" and "science" is so ideologically powerful that many investigators seem unable to conceive of the possibility of alternatives or to engage in or even to hear the kind of discussions about the constructed, mediated nature of knowl-edge that characterizes most contemporary work in the humanities and in several of the social sciences. While it is certainly the case that any one piece (or tradition) of research can examine only a limited number of measures and that choices will necessarily have to be made to study one set of phenomena rather than another, these practical considerations alone do not account for the dominance of a biomedical perspective in psychological research on the menstrual cycle over other possible approaches that, through their methodologies, embody a different set of assumptions. (See, e.g., Bell, 1987; Brown & Zimmer, 1986a, 1986b; Buckley & Gottlieb, 1988; Dan & Lewis, 1992; Delaney, Lupton & Toth, 1976; Laws, 1983; Logue & Moos, 1988; Martin, 1987; Matria & Mullen, 1978; Notman, 1982; Notman & Nadelson, 1983; Paige & Paige, 1981; Patterson & Hale, 1985; Renik, 1984; Schultz & Koulack, 1980; Severino, Bucci & Creelman, 1988; Sherif, 1980; Snowden & Christian, 1984; Stewart, 1989.)

Unasked Questions

Asking how the menstrual cycle affects (some particular) behavior is to take a biological phenomenon, the menstrual cycle, as the conceptual starting point for research and to delimit the psychological unit to be analyzed in relation only to the biological cycle. This is different from asking how (some particular) behavior is affected by the menstrual cycle because the latter question delimits the psychological phenomenon for analysis in purely psychological terms (Parlee,

1982b). While it seems reasonable to think that emotions and actions of many kinds may be affected by the menstrual cycle, it is obvious they are also affected by a wide range of other phenomena. Research evidence to date suggests it has not been especially productive, empirically, to assume in advance that cultural beliefs about menstruation (focusing on negative psychological changes in the premenstrual phase) can and do correctly identify the particular psychological phenomena that will repay scientific study from a bottom-up perspective (one that starts conceptually with the menstrual cycle and asks only about its "impact" or "consequences").

It is probably significant that one research topic where cumulative scientific progress clearly is being made—mechanisms regulating eating and drinking throughout the reproductive cycle (Gong, Garrel & Calloway, 1989; Bowen & Grunberg, 1990; Lissner et al., 1988)—is one that was reasonably well developed and conceptualized at the psychological level before the question of menstrual cycle influences arose. When this question began to be asked (Dalvit, 1981; Abraham, Beumont, Argall, & Haywood, 1981), the question of menstrual cycle influences could be elaborated within an already evolving theoretical framework and body of research (Kemnitz et al., 1989). This is not the case for most research on the psychological concomitants of the menstrual cycle, however, where the cycle-related research (e.g., on emotions, cognition, social actions) has remained relatively isolated from other psychological research on these phenomena.

The relative isolation of menstrual research from other areas of psychology may be significant for feminists because it appears to have implications for the political goal of being able to empower women through a reconstruction of psychological knowledge about menstruation. This is perhaps clearest in the case of research on menstrual fluctuations in emotions. Asking how the menstrual cycle affects emotions (which is the general form of the question in menstrual research) is not the same as asking how emotions are affected by menstruation because "emotions," as conceptualized and operationalized through specific research methodologies, undergo subtle shift in meaning in the two contexts. In the first question (the psychobiological one), "emotions" are operationalized in such a way that they can be "measured" on self-report questionnaires, data from which can be (are) interpreted without reference to any context other than phase (or some more specific parameter) of the menstrual cycle. "Emotions" in the second kind of question are operationalized in ways that reflect a different conception: emotions as cognitively constituted, intentional (in the philosophical sense of being about something in the world), and socially situated (therefore socially meaningful and interpersonally accountable) (see, e.g., Rorty, 1980; Harre, 1986). In the latter formulation, but not in the former, a conception of the person as agent, as the subject of the emotion, is retained: an agent feels and acts in the social and moral order in the particular ways she or he does for reasons, toward ends that she or he values. In the psychobiological formulation (embodied in questionnaire methods for "measuring" emotions), however, the person is implicitly conceptualized as an automaton whose behaviors are determined by causal processes of various kinds, including the biological (Harre, 1986). Agents, actions, reasons, values—all are rendered invisible by the positivist assumptions and methods of the psychobiological perspective, leaving subjects, behaviors, and responses (which may fluctuate as a "consequence" of, or under the "impact" of, the menstrual cycle).

It is notable that the more radical critiques and reanalyses of menstrual cycle research (those that go beyond urging adherence to criteria for better research from a psychobiological perspective) can be characterized by their resistance to the conception of women as automata. Laws (1983); Laws, Hey, and Eagan (1985); Patterson and Hale (1985); Harlow (1986); Matria and Mullen (1978); Birke (1980); The Boston Women's Health Book Collective (1984); Guinan (1988); Martin (1987); Brown and Zimmer (1986a)—all work in different ways to reclaim the conception of woman as an agent, who acts for reasons in worlds of meaning and value. Research reported in the recent volume edited by Dan and Lewis (1992) exemplifies this perspective. Since the contextual approach necessarily takes into account social institutions and cultural systems, it seems more likely to be relevant to the kinds of self-understanding feminists seek than is research from a psychobiological perspective.

DISTINCTION BETWEEN NORMAL MENSTRUAL EXPERIENCES AND PREMENSTRUAL SYNDROMES

Reviewers of the psychological literature on menstruation writing in the early to mid-1970s did not distinguish between normal menstrual experiences and pathological premenstrual states (e.g., Sommer, 1973; Parlee, 1973; Smith, 1975), nor did the investigators conducting the research or reporters writing about menstruation in the popular media (Chrisler & Levy, 1990). Feminists in the women's health movement in the late sixties and early seventies, however, actively articulated and promoted the idea that women's experiences of menstruation should not be distorted by being assimilated to a medical model of disease (Weideger, 1976; The Boston Women's Health Book Collective, 1984; Matria & Mullen, 1978). This view was eventually adopted by researchers (Dan, 1986, 1988) and reflected in reviews (Friedman, Hurt, Aranoff & Clarkin, 1980) and, explicitly or implicitly, in much of the research from the late 1970s to the present (Halbreich et al., 1982). In an influential editorial in *Psychosomatic Medicine* in 1986, Brooks-Gunn formulated a distinction on which there is now considerable consensus. She proposed that "premenstrual syndrome" be used to refer to a clinically significant condition, while "premenstrual symptoms" should be used to refer to minor negative (possibly annoying but not serious) premenstrual changes.

From a feminist perspective, recognition within science and in the broader culture that uniquely female physiological functioning is not per se associated with psychological pathology represents both theoretical and political progress (Dan, 1988). It underlies the emerging consensus among researchers on the need for clear criteria for defining premenstrual syndrome as an illness and is responsible in part for the concomitant improvement (from any perspective) in quality of the research. Perhaps because the distinction between normal menstrual fluctuations and illness has so recently been "codified" within the scientific research community, however, some of the problematic aspects of the consensus formulation have not been addressed.

If the distinction between pathology and normal premenstrual changes is simply in terms of magnitude (and/or subjective distress accompanying the changes), what are the theoretical or empirical grounds for treating a premenstrual change of particular magnitude as normal or pathological? Does a premenstrual change of a particular magnitude relative to some baseline (and on what theoretical or empirical grounds is this chosen?) have the same psychological/behavioral significance for all women? What kind of data would answer this question? These questions have been recognized to some extent by investigators seeking to identify criteria for defining/diagnosing PMS, but they have so far been answered on a more arbitrary basis than seems appropriate given their scientific importance.

The idea/assumption that PMS represents an exacerbation of normal premenstrual symptoms ("molimina") remains powerful in the biomedical literature and has distorted research questions about normal menstrual experiences. The relative neglect of positive mood items in investigations of normal premenstrual changes, for example, has been noted (Weideger, 1976) and to some degree rectified (Guinan, 1988; Logue & Moos, 1988). It is less clear that more subtle conceptual distortions have also been rectified. Redgrove (1971), for example, found premenstrual improvement in performance on a typing task and interpreted it as evidence that women made an extra effort during this time to overcome the disruptive influences of the premenstrual phase. Yet her data could also be more straightforwardly interpreted as evidence that there are premenstrual improvements in typing performance. (DeMarchi & Tong, 1972, offered a similarly convoluted interpretation of their data.) Apart from popular beliefs about menstruation that privilege assumptions about negative premenstrual changes, there is little scientific evidence to justify the more complicated interpretation, although it is certainly a plausible one that could be subjected to more direct test.

Apart from scattered examples, scientists in at least one well-developed research area (the regulation of ingestive behaviors) clearly have distorted their research questions by maintaining a rigid conceptual focus on the premenstrual phase of the cycle. For example, both Abraham et al. (1981) and Dalvit (1981) collected data on food intake by adult women throughout the menstrual cycle but reported only the data for the premenstrual and menstrual phases. In the relatively large literature on nonhuman animals, however, the greatest changes in food intake are reported to occur around the time of ovulation, when estrogen levels are high, and considerable progress has been made in delineating hormonal and neural mechanisms mediating these changes (Nance, 1983). Data thus were collected but not reported because of powerful and unexamined assumptions about the (unique) psychological significance of the premenstrual phase for

Table 2
Methodological Issues in Research on PMS

1. Retrospective questionnaires vs. prospective assessment	1. Consensus: PMS must be confirmed with prospective ratings
2. Criteria for defining/diagnosing PMS	2. Consensus: DSM-IIIR LLPDD or similar criteria must be used
3. Double-blind placebo-controlled designs in treatment studies	3. Consensus: such designs must be used
4. Placebo effect	4. Consistently found in treatment studies
5. Prevalence estimates for PMS	5. Approximately 3-5% of women seeking treatment for PMS will have prospectively confirmed PMS

women. (Abraham's group has subsequently reported data on human food intake around ovulation, see Lyons et al., 1989.) More recent investigations similarly fail to connect the human and animal research literatures and focus exclusively on premenstrual changes in appetite in women with normal menstrual cycles (Lissner et al., 1988). Such a rigid focus on the premenstrual phase reflects the implicit assumption that normal menstrual changes are simply an attenuated version of PMS, and this assumption is in no way challenged or corrected by distinguishing between premenstrual symptoms and premenstrual syndrome, scientifically important as this distinction has been in some areas of menstrual research.

ISSUES IN RESEARCH ON PREMENSTRUAL SYNDROMES

Retrospective Questionnaires versus Prospective Assessment

Methodological critiques of research on PMS are unanimous and emphatic in urging the need for prospective assessment of mood and symptom changes in defining and/or diagnosing PMS as a clinical condition (Rubinow & Roy-Byrne, 1984; Hamilton & Alagna, 1986; Severino & Moline, 1989). Women's self-referral for treatment of PMS or self-reports of increases in negative symptoms and moods during the premenstrual phase are no longer, by general consensus among researchers, acceptable as the sole means of identifying women who suffer from PMS. Since much of the literature on premenstrual syndrome prior to about 1983 did not employ prospective assessment, careful reviewers note in their descriptions of published data when a study did or did not involve prospective assessment (Severino & Moline, 1989).

Criteria for Defining/Diagnosing PMS

A major step toward achieving some consensus in the research community on how to define PMS for research purposes was the convening of a consensus conference at the National Institute of Mental Health (NIMH) in April 1983. The criteria agreed to at that conference were that there must be a change of at least 30% in the intensity of symptoms measured in days 5–10 of the cycle as compared with the premenstrual phase (6 or fewer days before menstrual onset) and that these changes must be prospectively documented for at least two consecutive cycles. (Severino & Moline, 1989, discuss some ambiguities and problems with these criteria.) Independently, both before and after that conference, individual investigators or research teams with active programs of PMS research proposed and used definitional criteria that were similar to those proposed by the NIMH conferees (Haskett, Steiner & Carroll, 1984; Magos & Studd, 1986; Eckerd, Hurt & Severino, 1989).

In 1984, similar codification of a premenstrual condition for the purposes of clinical diagnosis was initiated by a committee of the American Psychiatric Association, chaired by Robert Spitzer. As described in Severino and Moline (1989)—Severino was a member of the APA committee considering the PMS diagnostic criteria for the diagnosis—the committee after its deliberations was not in agreement on the usefulness or appropriateness of including such a condition within a classification scheme for psychopathology. Despite arguments by many social scientists and biomedical investigators (Schact, 1985; Hamilton & Alagna, 1986), the diagnostic category Late Luteal Phase Dysphoric Disorder was included in an appendix in the DSM-IIIR (Spitzer et al., 1989; Kaplan, 1983). The criteria for diagnosing LLPDD are shown in Table 3. In reconsidering the LLPDD diagnosis for the next edition of the DSM (DSM-IV), the APA established a Work Group charged with reviewing the scientific evidence regarding the condition. The Work Group's literature review comprehensively covers the biomedical literature on PMS and LLPDD (papers based on it are forthcoming in an APA-published book edited by Severino).

Double-Blind Placebo-Controlled Designs in Treatment Studies

A second methodological criterion for assessing PMS research on which investigators also now agree is on the requirement for double-blind, placebo-controlled designs in studies evaluating treatments of PMS. Not only are such designs widely recognized as the only appropriate ones for evaluating treatment effects in general, but they are also agreed to be crucial in PMS research in particular because of the very high rates of placebo effects that have consistently been reported. O'Brien (1987b) has reviewed this literature on PMS treatments and notes that the placebo effects reported range from 43% to 75%.

Placebo Effects

While investigators with active programs of PMS research agree on the existence of placebo effects and the consequent need for placebo-controlled, double-

Table 3

Diagnostic Criteria for Late Luteal Phase Dysphoric Disorder (LLPDD)

A. In most menstrual cycles during the past year, symptoms in B occurred during the last week of the luteal phase and remitted within a few days after onset of the follicular phase. In menstruating females, these phases correspond to the week before and a few days after, the onset of menses. (In nonmenstruating females who have had a hysterectomy, the timing of luteal and follicular phases may require measurement of circulating reproductive hormones.)

B. At least five of the following symptoms have been present for most of the time during each symptomatic late luteal phase, at least one of the symptoms being either (1), (2), (3), or (4):

  1. marked affective lability, e.g., feeling suddenly sad, tearful, irritable, or angry
  2. persistent and marked anger or irritability
  3. marked anxiety, tension, feelings of being "keyed up," or "on edge"
  4. markedly depressed mood, feelings of hopelessness, or self-deprecating thoughts
  5. decreased interest in usual activities, e.g., work, friends, hobbies
  6. easy fatigability or marked lack of energy
  7. subjective sense of difficulty in concentrating
  8. marked change in appetite, overeating, or specific food cravings
  9. hypersomnia or insomnia
  10. other physical symptoms, such as breast tenderness or swelling, headaches, joint or muscle pain, a sensation of "bloating," weight gain

C. The disturbance seriously interferes with work or with usual social activities or relationships with others.

D. The disturbance is not merely an exacerbation of the symptoms of another disorder such as Major Depression, Panic Disorder, Dysthymia, or a Personality Disorder (although it may be superimposed on any of these disorders).

E. Criteria A, B, C, and D are confirmed by prospective daily self-ratings during at least two symptomatic cycles. (The diagnosis may be made provisionally prior to this confirmation.)

Source: American Psychiatric Association (1987).

blind designs in treatment research, the theoretical significance of the undoubted fact of placebo effects has not been addressed. Why do women seem to feel better when they are treated for PMS, almost regardless of what the treatment is? Given that placebo effects are one of the few well-documented and widely agreed upon phenomena in PMS research, the failure of investigators to take them seriously as a substantive finding as well as a methodological caveat for treatment trials would seem to require explanation.

One reason placebo effects in PMS treatments have not received appropriate theoretical consideration may be that, with the exception of a few investigators,

PMS research is now conducted for the most part in isolation from psychological research on normal menstrual experiences. (Relatively few articles in the biomedical literature cite heavily from the social science literature and vice versa.) PMS researchers may simply be unaware of the data and theories in the social science literature on menstruation that might be relevant for explaining placebo effects. However, another reason may be that placebo effects point fairly unambiguously to a set of research questions about PMS that do not involve the concepts and methods familiar to most biomedically trained investigators. (Again, there are exceptions—e.g., Hamilton, Alagna & Sharpe, 1985). While it is understandable that scientists do and prefer research in the traditions in which they have been trained, this does not by itself account for the almost complete neglect of the implications of placebo effects among members of the menstrual cycle research community as a whole (which is constituted not only by individual investigators but also by advisers to funding agencies, conference organizers, and journal editors).

Prevalence Estimates for PMS

Published estimates of the prevalence of PMS in the United States range from 5% to 95%, a range clearly related to the variability of definitions of PMS used by different investigators (O'Brien, 1987a). Since some consensus has emerged among PMS researchers as to the criteria for defining PMS, the prevalence of women with "true" PMS has been reported to be 4.6% (Rivera-Tovar & Frank, 1990). Estimates of the prevalence of PMS that do not refer to the way the phenomenon is defined are impossible to interpret in any scientifically clinically meaningful way, though they may serve some rhetorical purpose in shaping the scientific and public discourses about women and menstruation.

FINDINGS AND UNASKED QUESTIONS IN PMS RESEARCH

Findings

The great variety of hypothesized causes and proposed treatments for PMS are comprehensively summarized in a thoughtful and balanced way by Severino and Moline (1989) and by the APA's LLPDD Work Group (Hurt et al., 1992). Earlier reviews by Green (1982), Reid (1985), and other reviews of the PMS literature cited earlier cover some of the same material. As Severino and Moline's detailed review indicates, the following physiological processes have been hypothesized to be causally involved in PMS: imbalances in ovarian hormones, androgens, prolactin, aldosterone, angiotensin, thyroid hormone, insulin and glucose metabolism, neurotransmitters, circadian rhythms, prostaglandins, pyridoxine (vitamin B6), nutrition, allergic reactions, *candida albicans*, and altered blood rheology. Among the psychosocial causes that have been proposed are social stress and psychological phenomena such as attitudes toward menstruation (conceptualized within both psychodynamic and social psychological frameworks) and personality profiles (as assessed on well-validated psychological instruments such as the State-Trait Anxiety Inventory, the Eysenck Personality Inventory, locus of control, MMPI, and others).

Given the emergent consensus among investigators with active programs of PMS research on criteria for what counts as sound scientific research on this topic, it is now possible to sift and evaluate the very diverse and voluminous literature on the pathophysiology of PMS from a methodologically informed perspective. Examining the most recent and rigorous biomedical research in its comprehensive review, the APA Work Group on the LLPDD diagnosis concluded that investigators have not yet identified a biological marker that differentiates between women with and without prospectively confirmed PMS LLPDD and women who do not meet the criteria for this condition. Severino and Moline (1989), Rubinow (1987), and O'Brien (1987a) also reached this conclusion. To date, they agree, no such markers have been discovered.

Among the proposed treatments for PMS discussed by Severino and Moline have been education and support, exercise, simple dietary changes (increasing meal frequency, limiting caffeine and salt intake), progesterone, estradiol, oral contraceptives, antiestrogen (Tamoxifen), Danazol, testosterone, gonadotropin releasing hormone (GnRH) agonists, ovariectomy, glucocorticoid-synthesis blocker (Trilostane), bromocriptine, thyroid hormone, diuretics and antihypertensives, prostaglandin-related treatments, histamine-related treatments, nutritional supplements (including Vitamin B6, Vitamin E, Vitamin A, and fatty acids—Evening Primrose Oil), psychotherapy, psychoactive agents, and miscellaneous treatments such as over-the-counter medications for PMS, sleep deprivation, light treatment, antibiotics, anticandida treatment, allergy management techniques, biofeedback relaxation techniques, and acupuncture.

The complexities of the data from treatment studies preclude simple summaries or conclusions, but both Severino and Moline (1989) and the APA Work Group report that some treatments (particularly those suppressing ovulation) have shown to be effective in relieving at least some PMS symptoms. However, the American Psychiatric Association's publication, designed for use by psychiatrists reviewing for their board certification examinations, indicates that at present no treatment for PMS has been shown to be more effective than placebo.

Psychobiological research on the causes of PMS and its treatment continues at a rapid pace, however, and as subtypes of PMS become more precisely delineated at the psychological level (Halbreich, Endicott & Nee, 1982) and at the physiological level (Schecter et al., 1989) and patient populations being investigated therefore become more homogeneous, it seems likely to several groups of biomedical researchers that physiological markers and effective biological treatments will be found. Some of these researchers, in fact, have proposed that PMS might serve as a "model" for other affective disorders and so be of considerable general significance in theoretical as well as clinical terms (Rubinow, Hoban, Roy-Byrne, Grover & Post, 1985; Wurtman & Wurtman,

1989; Hamilton, Alagna & Sharpe, 1985; but see also Haskett, Steiner, Osmun & Carroll, 1980).

Rubinow and Schmidt (1989) have recently proposed three different types of models for the relationship between psychological and biological processes in PMS: a sensitization model, a learned helplessness model, and a state-related model. (This latter is more fully elaborated and investigated by Rubinow et al., 1986, and Rubinow et al., 1988.) Hamilton (1981) has also elaborated a model of attention-regulation and moods that may prove fruitful as a framework for menstrual cycle research. By introducing a new and higher level of theoretical discussion into the research literature on PMS, these authors have set the stage for considerably more sophisticated and focused empirical investigations. Future research on these lines should prove of great interest. It is worth noting, however, that the number of investigators actually able to pursue research questions about PMS framed in this way is likely to be relatively small in view of the practical difficulties involved (both financial and in terms of recruitment/access) in obtaining adequately sized samples of women with confirmed PMS. As Latour has noted in his investigations and analyses of science, a scientific claim/assumption becomes increasingly hard to destabilize (to challenge effectively, "test") as the "costs" of entering into that scientific research arena as a credible player go up (Latour, 1987; Latour & Woolgar, 1986).

MENSTRUAL CYCLE RESEARCH AND THE POLITICS OF GENDER

At the most obvious level, the politics of gender takes place in the ideological realm through struggles to control the terms of discourse about women in public forums like newspaper articles, self-help advice in magazines, how-to books, cartoons, greeting cards, and jokes in TV situation comedies, in more specialized forums such as pharmaceutical advertisements in magazines for physicians, in scientific journals and conferences, and in courtrooms. The contest is over the extent to which women (by implication, all women) can be culturally and politically identified as menstruating females subjected by biology to socially disruptive emotional changes. Insofar as women are so identified, the social meaning of women's lives and the emotions that are part of them is ideologically obscured, rendered as part of the "natural" order, which is then offered as a rationalization of the existing social relations of gender (and of class and ethnicity to the extent that these relations are intertwined). As a key site of cultural contestation, discourse about menstruation is and has been a focus of struggle by feminists who have tried in various ways to resist its ideological use by (or to the benefit of) dominant groups (Sayers, 1982; Severino & Moline, 1989, Chapter 2; Parlee, 1989).

As indicated above, feminists have tried during the past 20 years to include positive as well as negative features of menstruation, have challenged the medical profession's prerogative to define what is "normal" for women, have challenged scientists' focus on biological rhythms in women only, have challenged scientists' assertions about menstrual cycle fluctuations in women, and have challenged the scientific claims and popular beliefs that menstrual experiences have only biological causes. Scientific discourse on menstruation has, indeed, been modified to some extent (in ways described above) as a result of these efforts by feminists.[4] However, the success of feminists' struggles to shape the terms of the public discourse about menstruation can perhaps be judged by comparing a 1955 *Reader's Digest* article on premenstrual tension (Greenblatt, 1955) with one on premenstrual syndrome ("Dr. Jekyll and Ms. Hyde") published in *Reader's Digest* almost three decades later (Angier, 1983). Despite a vast increase in the number of research articles and a clear improvement in the scientific quality of research, popular coverage of menstruation seems remarkably unchanged, like, frequently, introductory paragraphs of scientific papers in which the social and clinical significance of menstruation is described. (Typically, the form of a scientific research paper is followed—references are cited apparently documenting claims that are made—but the substance is lacking since the articles cited do not, in fact, contain scientific data supporting the claims.)

At a deeper level, developments in menstrual cycle research over the past two decades provide an illustration of the ways institutional and economic forces support and are supported by popular discourse about women, thereby illustrating more fully the politics of gender and the role of psychological researchers in these political struggles. In brief, the situation at present appears to be that biomedically trained researchers working with a psychobiological perspective have gained primary influence in research on PMS. Under this influence, PMS research appears to be developing along specialized and predictable lines. Though framed and probably experienced by investigators in terms of its clinical relevance (focusing on treatment and relief of distress), this research has the effect of supporting—or at least of not challenging—the dominant ideological construction of women as debilitated or potentially disruptive menstruating females. Social scientists, who in principle might be somewhat more flexible in their choice of research perspective both because of their training and because of the structures of their institutional settings, have gained primary influence in research on the psychology of normal menstrual experiences. While the story of how and why biomedically trained investigators came to have near-hegemony over PMS research is complex, some of the forces involved can at least be identified and described in a preliminary way (Parlee, 1989).

First, this hegemony is in part an unintended and unforeseen (at the individual level) result of the increasing consensus among researchers on the need for greater detail and precision in specification of physiological parameters of the menstrual cycle. Given federal and institutional regulations governing research with human subjects, investigators who need to take blood samples in their research now almost invariably have to do this in collaboration with, or under the auspices or supervision of, a physician. When social scientists collaborate with medically trained investigators, particularly in a hospital/medical school setting, a psychobiological perspective tends to prevail in the research. Even when the individual physician herself or himself might want to address a broader range of research questions than the psychobiological perspective permits, institutional forces (among them the pressure to bring in grant money) tend to shape the research in predictable ways.

Second, as federal funds for basic research became scarcer in the 1980s, other sources of funding, including drug companies, played a relatively larger role in supporting menstrual cycle research. Drug companies are more likely to fund research on PMS than on the normal menstrual experiences; they are more likely to fund PMS research that is directed toward discovering biological causes and treatments than research on the psychological significance of PMS as a social and cultural phenomenon; and they are highly unlikely to fund research involving drugs unless it is conducted by a medically trained investigator. The potentially large market for medications for menstrual cycle–related problems has led drug companies not only to be involved in funding PMS research but also to promote its dissemination through sponsorship of conferences, continuing medical education seminars, press events, and PMS clinics.

Third, reimbursement by insurance companies for treatment of PMS (a practice facilitated by the inclusion of LLPDD as a diagnostic category in the appendix of the DSM-IIIR) coincided with institutional changes in obstetrics/gynecology and in psychiatry to enhance the significance of PMS within the community of practitioner-researchers. As malpractice insurance rates for obstetricians have risen, many obstetrician-gynecologists have been giving up their obstetrics practices and concentrating solely on gynecology. Regardless of the motives of individual physicians, it is the case that a potential pool of "new" patients for gynecologists is represented by women with PMS. Similar structural incentives are at work in psychiatry where attention to PMS as a biologically based mood disorder can be seen as part of the two-decades' old move away from psychodynamic and toward biological treatments (a move that coincided in time with the entry in significant numbers of nonmedically trained professionals into the mental health field). Freestanding and hospital-based PMS clinics have also become profitable in light of insurance company policies on reimbursement for treatment of PMS, and within a hospital/medical school setting, the head of such a clinic may receive professional recognition and nonfinancial rewards when a program of PMS research is carried out in conjunction with the clinical work.

Finally, the 1983 National Institute of Mental Health consensus conference called to formalize criteria for a diagnosis/definition of PMS was organized primarily by biomedical researchers and did not focus on, or address, the cultural and social issues surrounding menstruation that had been identified and discussed by social scientists throughout the previous decade of research. Coming from a federal agency that seemed likely to be involved in future funding of research on this topic, this conference was important in shaping the approach and content of research on PMS toward the biomedical. It culminated a process of separation between biomedical and social science researchers that may have begun as early as the first (1978) conference organized by a group of investigators who subsequently formed the the Society for Menstrual Cycle Research (Dan, Graham & Beecher, 1980). While the first conference was very broadly interdisciplinary in participation and in the work reported, subsequent conferences of the group were dominated by explicitly feminist social scientists, medical researchers, and activists (see Dan, 1988) and were less well attended by traditional biomedical researchers. (The latter are well represented at other kinds of conferences on the menstrual cycle—e.g., The 2nd International Symposium on Premenstrual, Postpartum, and Menopausal Mood Disorders, held in 1987, supported by an educational grant from Ortho Pharmaceutical Co.; see Demers et al., 1989).

The dominance of a biomedical perspective in menstrual cycle research (dominance as indexed by access to large-scale funding, publication outlets, and even media coverage) is a social/cultural phenomenon calling for a cultural analysis within the emerging research communities known collectively as the social studies of science (Knorr-Cetina & Mulkay, 1983). It is still possible, of course, that a psychobiological perspective in menstrual cycle research may prove empirically and theoretically fruitful in the future, and if so, its present prominence will be regarded as unproblematic because it was the "correct" one for discovering the "truth" (Latour, 1987). However, given the large number of methodologically sound (according to criteria of the psychobiological perspective) research studies that have been carried out over the past five years and given the paucity of consistent or compelling results, the continuing, near-exclusive dominance of the biomedical perspective in the face of continuing negative results and anomalies requires explanation. When, on what grounds, will further research from a psychobiological perspective be finally judged to be less fruitful than research from other perspectives that might be/have been carried out? Given the varied ideological, economic, and social forces involved in perpetuating the psychobiological approach, who will decide to pursue other approaches as well? With what resources and with what effects will this decision be carried out?[5]

FEMINISM AND PSYCHOLOGICAL RESEARCH ON THE MENSTRUAL CYCLE

Feminist researchers, both social scientists and medically trained investigators, have played active political roles at the "margins" where scientific research on menstruation articulates with other institutions that powerfully affect women's lives. In particular, feminists have participated in debates about the use of premenstrual syndrome as a legal defense (Wallach & Rubin, 1971; Mulligan, 1983; see also pp. 65–150 in Ginsburg & Carter, 1987) and have been part of the struggle over whether or not to include PMS (or a similar diagnostic category) in the American Psychiatric Association's revisions of the *Diagnostic and Statistical Manual of Mental Disorders* (Hamilton & Alagna, 1986; Kaplan, 1983;

Caplan, McCurdy-Meyers & Gans, 1992; see also account in Severino & Moline, 1989). Most of feminist psychologists' efforts to reconstruct scientific and cultural knowledge and practices surrounding menstruation, however, have been directed toward shaping the content of scientific knowledge and influencing future directions of research.

As Harraway (1989) has argued with respect to women scientists in another field (primatology), feminist psychologists and other social scientists have used many different strategies in their struggle to contest and destabilize the ideological myth that scientific data show women have a biologically based incapacity to exercise economic, political, and cultural power. Some have claimed or have been misread as claiming that women do not, contrary to the myth, experience or show psychological fluctuations during the menstrual cycle; others have advanced scientific arguments to the effect that women's variability is not unique to women or uniquely related to menstruation; others have emphasized cultural contributions to women's specific experiences of the bodily changes of menstruation.

More radically, however, some feminist social scientists and writers have worked outside the relatively narrow limits imposed by the concepts and methods of mainstream U.S. social psychology and psychobiology and have provided a thoroughgoing cultural and political analysis of women's menstrual experiences. In books such as *Seeing Red* (Laws, Hey, & Eagan, 1985), *The Tyrannical Womb* (Birke, 1980), and *Myths of Gender* (Fausto-Sterling, 1985), it is possible to hear the authentic note of authority and outrage that so often accompanied feminist analyses in the late 1960s and early 1970s. This is where the intellectual and emotional creativity of feminist perspectives still resides, and in light of the lack of compelling findings in current psychobiological research, this is where psychological research on menstruation might begin again as psychologists, too, try to develop approaches to understanding women's menstrual experiences that are genuine alternatives to the traditional biomedical approaches (or to social psychological approaches that incorporate many of the same assumptions).

While critiques from every perspective have been plentiful, relatively few feminist social scientists have over the past two decades gone to the heart of the matter by outlining and/or carrying out positive alternatives in research.[6] The challenge for the rest of us (particularly those trained in the relatively narrow, method-driven paradigms of academic psychology; see Danziger, 1985) is to recognize the value of such innovative research and to struggle to create and maintain forms of social organization that promote it (Morawski, 1990). Over the past two decades psychological research on menstrual experiences and on premenstrual syndromes has become much better according to criteria traditionally employed in evaluating psychobiolgial research—and very important and valuable criteria they are. But it is still a long way from providing the kind of comprehensive, full, nuanced picture of women's menstrual experiences that would represent the best possible scientific contribution to this important part of women's lives and to the academic field of the psychology of women.

NOTES

I want to thank Alice Dan, Sharon Golub, David Rubinow, and Barbara Sommer for reading and commenting on an earlier draft of this chapter, and I especially thank Sheryl Gallant and Randi Koeske for detailed and stimulating discussion; none necessarily agrees with the final version but all have made it better.

1. Psychological publications on menstruation increased in number in the United States for several reasons, all of them outcomes of the second phase of the women's movement in the United States. One was the women's health movement, with its drive to reclaim from medical scientists and practitioners the power to name and define women's body-related experiences. A second was the related feminist focus within psychology on women's experiences as central rather than significant only in the ways they differed from men's experiences. Third, political organizing by feminists within professional organizations (including the American Psychological Association) led to changes in what editors and reviewers defined as appropriate subject matter for particular journals, so the psychology of menstruation was no longer regarded as a "clinical" or "applied" subject, unsuitable for publication in journals of "basic research."

2. Among the methodological issues frequently discussed are prospective versus retrospective assessment of self-reported changes during the menstrual cycle; definition and measurement of cycle phases; validity and reliability of self-report measures; subjects' awareness of the menstrual cycle as the focus of research; control/comparison groups; baseline for describing changes as increases or decreases; and sample selection; and, for research on premenstrual syndromes, double-blind, placebo-controlled designs for evaluating treatments; placebo effects; and differentiating premenstrual syndromes from normal menstrual cycle symptoms and experiences.

Discussions directed toward developing shared understandings of what counts as a "good" piece of research on a particular topic are part of any new research enterprise that will later take on more of the characteristics of normal science. In menstrual cycle research this preliminary scientific work is of particular significance for the broader field of the psychology of women as well, since shared methodological criteria that come to be generally endorsed among researchers will crucially shape the content of the knowledge about the psychology of menstruation that can and will be produced. When widely shared methodological criteria are honed and enforced to the point of near-hegemony by the actions of journal reviewers, editors, conference organizers, and consultants to funding agencies, the direction (content) of the research is affected. It becomes more focused, more cumulative, and clearer as to what general conclusions can be drawn from it. It also becomes narrower and more specialized, and investigators using the consensus methodology become more effective in marginalizing other methods and concepts and the subject matter constituted by them.

3. A general characterization of some of the assumptions involved in framing the research question this way has been offered by Koeske, 1985. Taken-for-granted assumptions guiding menstrual cycle research at the conceptual level, she argues, include the following: (1) a focus on context-free factors inside the organism, (2) strong acceptance of the individual differences model, and (3) implicit normative assumptions about "health" and "illness." Taken-for-granted methodological assumptions include (1) a positivistic emphasis on facts and description and (2) a reductionistic, ahistorical, and atomistic approach to scientific problems.

4. It is highly unlikely that a scientific article in 1989 could begin as Abramson and Torghele's did in 1961. A classic of its genre in several respects, their paper in the *American Journal of Obstetrics and Gynecology* opens:

Women are known [note the agentless passive] to suffer at least some inconvenience during certain phases of the reproductive cycle and often with considerable mental and physical distress [no references]. Woman's [*sic*] awareness of her inherent disabilities [what can one say?] is thought [N.B.] to create added mental and at times physical changes in the total body response, and thus there result problems that concern [who?] the physician who must deal with them. (p. 223)

It is true, however, that a 1978 article in the *British Journal of Pharmacology* bears the title "Menstrual Fluctuations in Hearing—Suggestions for Hormone and Drug Monitoring Methods in Man [*sic*]" (Huzzard, 1978, p. 476).

5. In view of the complex issues touched on here, it is necessary to say something about and to the many women who believe/know they suffer from PMS and who have found relief when it has been diagnosed and treated as a disease. Whatever else it is, PMS is surely an illness (Young, 1982): women suffer physical and/or psychological distress, are diagnosed by a professional healer, and are often relieved of their suffering by such treatment. If PMS ultimately turns out not to have a biological basis (and so turns out not to be a disease, following the anthropologists' illness-disease distinction), such a matter of empirical fact would be relevant to women's experiences of PMS only insofar as socially and psychologically based suffering is ideologically devalued and rendered less "real" than illnesses with a biological basis. Research careers and social institutions of various kinds are affected by, and so will try to influence the outcome of, whether or not PMS is regarded as a disease, but women need not be.

6. The scarcity of research that has actually gone beyond the terms of traditional research approaches and critiques of them is telling. This "de-radicalization" of feminist research on menstruation is not unique in feminist psychology, where research generally appears to remain within the basic conceptual and methodological framework of traditional psychology (Henley, 1986a; Fine, 1985; Lykes & Stewart, 1986) despite discussions to the contrary (Lott, 1985).

REFERENCES

Abplanalp, J. M. (1985a). Premenstrual syndrome. *Behavioral Sciences and the Law*, *3*, 103–115.

Abplanalp, J. M. (1985b). Premenstrual syndrome: A selective review. In S. Golub (Ed.), *Lifting the curse of menstruation* (pp. 107–127). New York: Harrington Park Press.

Abplanalp, J. M., Donnelly, A. F., & Rose, R. M. (1979). Psychoendocrinology of the menstrual cycle: I. Enjoyment of daily activities and moods. *Psychosomatic Medicine*, *41*, 587–604.

Abplanalp, J. M., Haskett, R. F., & Rose, R. M. (1980). The premenstrual syndrome. *Psychiatric Clinics of North America*, *3*, 327–347.

Abplanalp, J. M., Livingston, L., Rose, R. M., & Sandwich, D. (1977). Cortisol and growth hormone responses to psychological stress during the menstrual cycle. *Psychosomatic Medicine*, *39*, 158–177.

Abplanalp, J. M., Rose, R. M., Donnelly, A. F., & Livingston-Vaughan, L. (1979).

Psychoendocrinology of the menstrual cycle: II. The relationship between enjoyment of activities, moods, and reproductive hormones.

Abraham, G. E., & Hargrove, J. T. (1980). Effect of vitamin B6 on premenstrual symptomatology in women with premenstrual syndromes: A double-blind crossover study. *Infertility, 3*, 155–165.

Abraham, S. F., Beumont, P.J.V., Argall, W. J., & Haywood, P. (1981). Nutrient intake and the menstrual cycle. *Australian and New Zealand Journal of Medicine, 11*, 210–211.

Abramson, M., & Torghele, J. R. (1961). Weight, temperature changes, and psychosomatic symptomatology in relation to the menstrual cycle. *American Journal of Obstetrics and Gynecology, 81*, 223–232.

Alagna, S. W., & Hamilton, J. A. (1986). Social stimulus perception and self-evaluation: Effects of menstrual cycle phase. *Psychology of Women Quarterly, 10*, 327–338.

Altmann, M., Knowles, E., & Bull, H. D. (1941). A psychosomatic study of the sex cycle in women. *Psychosomatic Medicine, 3*, 158–224.

American Psychiatric Association. (1987). *Diagnostic and Statistical Manual of Mental Disorders* (3rd ed., rev.). Washington, DC: American Psychiatric Association.

Andersch, B. (1983). Bromocriptine and premenstrual symptoms: A survey of double-blind trials. *Obstetrical and Gynecology Survey, 38*, 643–646.

Angier, N. (1983, February). Dr. Jekyll and Ms. Hyde. *Reader's Digest*, pp. 119–123.

Asso, D. (1983). *The real menstrual cycle*. Chichester: Wiley.

AuBuchon, P. G., & Calhoun, K. S. (1985). Menstrual cycle symptomatology: The role of social expectancy and experimental demand characteristics. *Psychosomatic Medicine, 47*, 35–45.

Backstrom, T., Sanders, D., Leask, R., Davidson, D., Warner, P., & Bancroft, J. (1983). Mood, sexuality, and the menstrual cycle. II. Hormone levels and their relationship to the premenstrual syndrome. *Psychosomatic Medicine, 45*, 503–507.

Bains, G. K., & Slade, P. (1988). Attributional patterns, moods, and the menstrual cycle. *Psychosomatic Medicine, 50*, 469–476.

Bell, B., Christie, M., & Venables, P. H. (1975). Psychophysiology of the menstrual cycle. In P. H. Venables and M. J. Christie (Eds.), *Research in psychophysiology*. Chichester: Wiley.

Bell, S. E. (1987). Premenstrual syndrome and the medicalization of menopause: A sociological perspective. In B. E. Ginsburg and B. F. Carter (Eds.), *Premenstrual syndrome* (pp. 151–174). New York: Plenum.

Benedek, T., & Rubenstein, B. B. (1939a). The correlations between ovarian activity and psychodynamic processes: I. The ovulative phase. *Psychosomatic Medicine, 1*, 245–270.

Benedek, T., & Rubenstein, B. B. (1939b). The correlations between ovarian activity and psychodynamic processes: II. The menstrual phase. *Psychosomatic Medicine, 1*, 461–485.

Berman, M. L., Hanson, K., & Hellman, K. L. (1972). Effect of breast-feeding on postpartum menstruation, ovulation and pregnancy in Alaskan Eskimos. *American Journal of Obstetrics and Gynecology, 114*, 524–534.

Birke, L. (1980). The tyrannical womb: Menstruation and menopause. In Brighton Women and Science Group (Eds.), *Alice through the microscope* (pp. 89-107). London: Virago.

Birtchnell, J., & Floyd, S. (1974). Attempted suicide and the menstrual cycle: A negative correlation. *Journal of Psychosomatic Research, 18,* 361–369.

The Boston Women's Health Book Collective. (1984). *The new our bodies, ourselves.* New York: Simon & Schuster.

Both-Orthman, B., Rubinow, D. R., Hoban, M. C., Malley, J., & Grover, G. N. (1988). Menstrual cycle phase related changes in appetite in patients with premenstrual syndrome and in control subjects. *American Journal of Psychiatry, 145,* 628–631.

Bowen, D. J., & Grunberg, N. E. (1990). Variations in food preference and consumption across the menstrual cycle. *Physiology & Behavior, 47,* 287–291.

Brooks, J., Ruble, D. N., & Clarke, A. (1977). College women's attitudes and expectations concerning menstrual-related changes. *Psychosomatic Medicine, 39,* 288–298.

Brooks-Gunn, J. (1985). The salience and timing of menstrual flow. *Psychosomatic Medicine, 47,* 363–371.

Brooks-Gunn, J. (1986). Differentiating premenstrual symptoms and syndromes. *Psychosomatic Medicine, 48,* 385–387.

Brooks-Gunn, J., & Ruble, D. N. (1980). The menstrual attitude questionnaire. *Psychosomatic Medicine, 42,* 503–512.

Brooks-Gunn, J., & Ruble, D. N. (1982). The development of menstrual-related beliefs and behaviors during early adolescence. *Child Development, 53,* 1567–1577.

Broverman, D., Vogel, W., Klaiber, E. L., Majcher, D., Shea, D., & Paul, V. (1981). Changes in cognitive task performance across the menstrual cycle. *Journal of Comparative and Physiological Psychology, 95,* 646–654.

Brown, M. A., & Zimmer, P. A. (1986a). Help-seeking for premenstrual symptomatology: A description of women's experiences. *Health Care for Women International, 7,* 173–184.

Brown, M. A., & Zimmer, P. S. (1986b). Personal and family impact of premenstrual symptoms. *Journal of Obstetric, Gynecologic, and Neonatal Nursing, 15,* 31–38.

Buckley, T., & Gottlieb, A. (Eds.). (1988). *Blood magic: The anthropology of menstruation.* Berkeley, CA: University of California Press.

Bullen, B. A., Skrinar, G. S., Beitins, I. Z., Von Mering, G., Turnball, B. A., & McArthur, J. W. (1985). Induction of menstrual disorders by strenuous exercise in untrained women. *New England Journal of Medicine, 312,* 1349.

Campos, F., & Thurow, C. (1978). Attributions of moods and symptoms to the menstrual cycle. *Personality and Social Psychology Bulletin, 4,* 272–276.

Caplan, P. J., McCurdy-Meyers, J., & Gans, M. (1992). Should "Premenstrual Syndrome" be called a psychiatric abnormality? *Feminism & Psychology, 2,* 27–44.

Carlson, R. (1972). Understanding women: Implications for personality theory and research. *Journal of Social Issues, 28,* 17–32.

Cassell, J. (1982). Does risk-benefit analysis apply to moral evaluation of social research? In T. L. Beauchamp, et al. (Eds.), *Ethical issues in social science research* (pp. 144–162). Baltimore: Johns Hopkins University Press.

Chadwick, M. (1932). *The psychological effects of menstruation.* New York: Nervous and Mental Disease.

Chadwick, M. (1933). *Women's periodicity.* London: Noel Douglas.

Chakmakjian, Z. H. (1983). A critical assessment of therapy for the premenstrual tension symdrome. *Journal of Reproductive Medicine*, 28, 532–538.

Chan, W. Y. (1983). Prostaglandins in primary dysmenorrhea: Basis for the new therapy. In S. Golub (Ed.), *Menarche* (pp. 243–249). Lexington, MA: Lexington Books.

Chatterton, R. T., Dan, A. J., DeLeon-Jones, F. A., Hudgens, G. A., Haan, N. J., Cheesman, S. D., & Cheesman, K. L. (1985). Relationships between the amount of sleep, stress, and ovarian function in women. In K. McKerns & V. Pantic (Eds.), *Neuroendocrine correlates of stress* (pp. 111–124). New York: Plenum.

Chesney, M. A., & Tasto, D. L. (1975). The development of the Menstrual Symptom Questionnaire. *Behavior Research and Therapy*, 13, 237–244.

Chiazze, L., Brazer, F., Macasco, J., Parker, M., & Duffy, B. (1968). The length and variability of the human menstrual cycle. *Journal of the American Medical Association*, 2036, 89–92.

Chisholm, G., Jung, S. O. J., Cumming, E. C., Fox, E. E., & Cumming, D. C. (1990). Premenstrual anxiety and depression—comparison of objective psychological tests with a retrospective questionnaire. *Acta Psychiatrica Scandinavica*, 81, 52–57.

Chrisler, J. C., & Levy, K. B. (1990). The media construct a menstrual monster: A content analysis of PMS articles in the popular press. *Women and Health*, 16, 89–103.

Christiansen, K., & Knussmann, R. (1987). Sex hormones and cognitive functioning in men. *Neuropsychobiology*, 18, 27–36.

Clare, A. W. (1985). Hormones, behavior, and the menstrual cycle. *Journal of Psychosomatic Research*, 29, 225–233.

Clarke, A. E., & Ruble, D. N. (1978). Young adolescents' beliefs concerning menstruation. *Child Development*, 49, 231–234.

Coppen, W. R., & Kessel, N. (1963). Menstruation and personality. *British Journal of Psychiatry*, 109, 711–721.

Cutler, W. B. (1980). Lunar and menstrual phase locking. *American Journal of Obstetrics and Gynecology*, 137, 834–839.

Cutler, W. B., & Garcia, C. R. (1980). The psychoneuroendocrinology of the ovulatory cycle of women: A review. *Psychoneuroendocrinology*, 5, 89–111.

Cutler, W. B., Garcia, C. R., & Krieger, A. M. (1979). Sexual behavior frequency and menstrual cycle length in mature premenopausal women. *Psychoneuroendocrinology*, 4, 297–309.

Dalton, K. (1960). Menstruation and accidents. *British Medical Journal*, 2, 1425–1426.

Dalton, K. (1968). Menstruation and examinations. *The Lancet*, 2, 1386–1388.

Dalton, K. (1982). Premenstrual tension: An overview. In R. C. Friedman (Ed.), *Behavior and the menstrual cycle* (pp. 217–242). New York: Marcel Dekker.

Dalton, K., & Greene, R. (1953). The premenstrual syndrome. *British Medical Journal*, 1016–1017.

Dalvit, S. P. (1981). The effect of the menstrual cycle on patterns of food intake. *American Journal of Clinical Nutrition*, 34, 1811–1815.

Dan, A. J. (1979). The menstrual cycle and sex differences in cognitive variability. In M. Wittig & A. Peterson (Eds.), *Sex-related differences in cognitive functioning* (pp. 241–260). New York: Academic Press.

Dan, A. J. (1980). Free-associative versus self-report measures of emotional changes over the menstrual cycle. In A. S. Dan, E. A. Graham, & C. P. Beecher (Eds.),

The menstrual cycle, Vol. 1: A synthesis of interdisciplinary research (pp. 115–120). New York: Springer.

Dan, A. J. (1981). An Interdisciplinary Society for Menstrual Cycle Research: Creating knowledge from our experiences. In A. Voda & M. Dinnerstein (Eds.), *New perspectives on menopause*. Houston: University of Texas Press.

Dan, A. J. (1986). The law and women's bodies: The case of menstruation leave in Japan. *Health Care for Women International, 6*, 1–14.

Dan, A. J. (1988). The menstrual cycle research. In C. J. Leppa & C. Miller (Eds.), *Women's Health Perspectives: An Annual Review* (Vol. 1, pp. 143–160). Phoenix, AZ: Oryx Press.

Dan, A. J., Chatterton, R. T., Hudgens, G. A., & DeLeon-Jones, F. A. (1992). Rationale and evidence for the role of circadian desynchrony in premenstrual symptoms. In A. J. Dan & L. L. Lewis (Eds.), *Menstrual Health in Women's Lives* (pp. 52–60). Urbana: University of Illinois Press.

Dan, A. J., Graham, E. A., & Beecher, C. P. (Eds.). (1980). *The menstrual cycle, Vol. 1: A synthesis of interdisciplinary research*. New York: Springer.

Dan, A. J., & Lewis, L. L. (Eds.). (1992). *Menstrual health in women's lives*. Urbana: University of Illinois Press.

Danziger, K. (1985). The methodological imperative in psychology. *Philosophy of the Social Sciences, 32*, 301–316.

Dawood, M. Y. (Ed.). (1981). Hormones, prostaglandins, and dysmenorrhea. In M. Y. Dawood (Ed.), *Dysmenorrhea*. Baltimore: Williams & Wilkins.

Delaney, J., Lupton, M. J., & Toth, E. (1976). *The curse: A cultural history of menstruation*. New York: Mentor.

DeMarchi, G. W., & Tong, J. E. (1972). Menstrual, diurnal, and activation effects on the resolution of temporally paired flashes. *Psychophysiology, 9*, 362–367.

Demers, L. M., McGuire, J. L., Phillips, A., & Rubinow, D. R. (Eds.). (1989). *Premenstrual, postpartum, and menopausal mood disorders*. Baltimore: Urban & Schwarzenberg.

Dennerstein, L., & Burrows, G. D. (1979). Affect and the menstrual cycle. *Journal of Affective Disorders, 1*, 77–92.

Dewan, E. M. (1967). On the possibility of a perfect rhythm method of birth control by periodic light stimulation. *American Journal of Obstetrics and Gynecology, 99*, 1016–1019.

Dingfelder, J. R. (1981). Primary dysmenorrhea treatment with prostaglandin inhibitors: A review. *American Journal of Obstetrics and Gynecology, 140*, 874–879.

d'Orban, P. T., & Dalton, J. (1980). Violent crime and the menstrual cycle. *Psychological Medicine, 10*, 353–359.

Doty, R., & Silverthorne, C. (1975). Influence of menstrual cycle on volunteering behavior. *Nature, 254*, 139–140.

Doty, R. L., Snyder, P. J., Huggins, G. R., & Lowry, L. D. (1981). Endocrine, cardiovascular, and psychological correlates of olfactory sensitivity changes during the human menstrual cycle. *Journal of Comparative and Physiological Psychology, 95*, 45–60.

Eagan, A. (1983, October). The selling of premenstrual syndrome. Who profits from making PMS "the disease of the 80s"? *Ms Magazine*, pp. 26–31.

Eckerd, M. B., Hurt, S. W., & Severino, S. K. (1989). Late Luteal Phase Dysphoric

Disorder: Relationship to personality disorders. *Journal of Personality Disorders*, *4*, 338–344.

Endicott, J., & Halbreich, U. (1982). Retrospective reports of premenstrual changes: Factors affecting confirmation by daily ratings. *Psychopharmacology Bulletin*, *18*, 109–112.

Endicott, J., Halbreich, U., & Nee, J. (1986). Mood and behavior during the menstrual cycle. In L. Dennerstein and I. Fraser (Eds.), *Hormones and behavior: Proceedings of the 8th International Congress of the International Society of Psychosomatic Obstetrics and Gynecology* (pp. 113–119). New York: Elsevier.

Endicott, J., Nee, J., Cohen, J., & Halbreich, U. (1986). Premenstrual changes: Patterns and correlates of daily ratings. *Journal of Affective Disorders*, *10*, 127–135.

Englander-Golden, P., Chang, H., Whitmore, M. R., & Dienstbier, R. A. (1980). Female sexual arousal and the menstrual cycle. *Journal of Human Stress*, *6*, 42–48.

Englander-Golden, P., Sonleitner, F. J., Whitmore, M. R., & Corbley, G.J.M. (1986). Social and menstrual cycles: Methodological and substantive findings. In V. L. Olesen & N. F. Woods (Eds.), *Culture, society, and menstruation* (pp. 77–96). Washington, DC: Hemisphere.

Englander-Golden, P., Whitmore, M. R., & Dienstbier, R. A. (1978). Menstrual cycle as focus of study and self-reports of moods and behaviors. *Motivation and Emotion*, *2*, 75–86.

Ernster, V. (1975). Menstrual expressions. *Sex Roles*, *1*, 3–13.

Eston, R. G. (1984). The regular menstrual cycle and athletic performance. *Sports Medicine*, *1*, 431–445.

Fausto-Sterling, A. (1985). *Myths of gender: Biological theories about women and men.* New York: Basic Books.

Ferguson, J. H., & Vermillion, M. B. (1957). Premenstrual tension: Two surveys of its prevalence and a description of the syndrome. *Obstetrics and Gynecology*, *9*, 615–619.

Fine, M. (1985). Reflections of a feminist psychology of women: Paradoxes and prospects. *Psychology of Women Quarterly*, *9*, 167–183.

Fine, M., & Gordon, S. M. (1989). Feminist transformations of/despite psychology. In M. Crawford & M. Gentry (Eds.), *Gender and Thought* (pp. 146–174). New York: Springer-Verlag.

Flug, D., Largo, L. H., & Prader, A. (1985). Symptoms related to menstruation in adolescent Swiss girls: A longitudinal study. *Annals of Human Biology*, *12*, 161–168.

Fradkin, B., & Firestone, P. (1986). Premenstrual tension, expectancy, and mother-child relations. *Journal of Behavioral Medicine*, *9*, 245–259.

Frank, R. T. (1931). The hormonal causes of premenstrual tension. *Archives of Neurological Psychiatry*, *26*, 1053–1057.

Friedman, R. C. (Ed.). (1982). *Behavior and the menstrual cycle.* New York: Marcel Dekker.

Friedman, R. C., Hurt, S. W., Arnoff, M. S., & Clarkin, J. (1980). Behavior and the menstrual cycle. *SIGNS: Journal of Women in Culture and Society*, *5*, 719–738.

Frisch, R. E. (1985). Fatness, menarche, and female fertility. *Perspectives in Biology and Medicine*, *28*, 611–633.

Gallant, S. J., Hamilton, J. A., Popiel, D. A., Morokoff, P. J., & Chakraborty, P. K.

(1991). Daily moods and symptoms: Effects of awareness of study focus, gender, menstrual cycle phase, and day of week. *Health Psychology, 10*, 180–189.

Gamberale, F. (1985). Effects of menstruation on work performance. *Ergonomics, 28*, 119–123.

Gannon, L. R. (1985). *Menstrual disorders and menopause: Biological, psychological and cultural research*. New York: Praeger.

Ginsburg, B., & Carter, B. F. (Eds.). (1987). *Premenstrual syndrome: Ethical and legal implications in a biomedical perspective*. New York: Plenum.

Gise, L. H., Lebovits, A. H., Paddison, P. L., & Strain, J. J. (1990). Issues in the identification of premenstrual syndromes. *Journal of Nervous and Mental Diseases, 178*, 228–234.

Golub, S. (1976). The magnitude of premenstrual anxiety and depression. *Psychosomatic Medicine, 38*, 4–12.

Golub, S. (1981). Sex differences in attitudes and beliefs regarding menstruation. In P. Komnenich, M. McSweeney, J. A. Noack, & S. N. Elder (Eds.), *The menstrual cycle, Vol. 2: Research and implications for women's health* (pp. 129–135). New York: Springer.

Golub, S. (Ed.). (1983). *Menarche: The transition from girl to woman*. Lexington, MA: D.C. Heath.

Golub, S. (Ed.). (1985a). *Lifting the curse of menstruation: A feminist appraisal of the influence of menstruation on women's lives*. New York: Harrington Park Press.

Golub, S. (1985b). Menstrual cycle symptoms from a developmental perspective. In Z. DeFries, R. C. Friedman, & R. Corn (Eds.), *Sexuality: New perspectives* (pp. 251–270). Westport, CT: Greenwood.

Golub, S., & Harrington, D. M. (1981). Premenstrual and menstrual mood changes in adolescent women. *Journal of Personality and Social Psychology, 5*, 961–965.

Gong, E. J., Garrel, D., & Calloway, D. H. (1989). Menstrual cycle and voluntary food intake. *American Journal of Clinical Nutrition, 49*, 252–258.

Goodale, I. L., Domar, A., & Benson, H. (1990). Alleviation of premenstrual syndrome symptoms with the relaxation response. *Obstetrics and Gynecology, 75*, 649–665.

Gordon, H. W., Corbin, E. D., & Lee, P. A. (1986). Changes in specialized cognitive function following changes in hormone levels. *Cortex, 22*, 399–415.

Gottschalk, L., Kaplan, S., Gleser, G., & Winget, C. (1962). Variations in magnitude of emotion: A method applied to anxiety and hostility during phases of the menstrual cycle. *Psychosomatic Medicine, 24*, 300–311.

Graham, E. A., & Glasser, M. (1985). Relationship of pregnanediol level to cognitive behavior and mood. *Psychosomatic Medicine, 47*, 26–34.

Graham, E. A., & Sherwin, B. B. (1987). The relationship between retrospective premenstrual symptom reporting and present oral contraceptive use. *Journal of Psychosomatic Research, 31*, 45–53.

Green, J. (1982). Recent trends in the treatment of premenstrual syndrome: A critical review. In R. C. Friedman (Ed.), *Behavior and the Menstrual Cycle* (pp. 367–396). New York: Marcel Dekker.

Greenblatt, R. B. (1955, May). Pre-menstrual tension: The needless misery. *Reader's Digest*, pp. 36–38.

Greene, R., & Dalton, K. (1953). The premenstrual syndrome. *British Medical Journal, 1*, 1007–1014.

Guinan, M. E. (1988). Women's health: PMS or perifollicular phase euphoria. *Journal of the American Medical Women's Association, 43* (3), 91–92.

Halbreich, U., & Endicott, J. (1985a). The biology of premenstrual changes: What do we really know? In H. J. Osofsky & S. J. Blumenthal (Eds.), *Premenstrual syndrome: Current findings and future directions* (pp. 75–124). Washington, DC: American Psychiatric Press.

Halbreich, U., & Endicott, J. (1985b). Methodological issues in studies of premenstrual changes. *Psychoneuroendocrinology, 10,* 15–32.

Halbreich, U., & Endicott, J. (1985c). Relationship of dysphoric premenstrual changes to depressive disorders. *Acta Psychiatrica Scandinavica, 40,* 535–542.

Halbreich, U., Endicott, J., Goldstein, S., & Nee, J. (1986). Premenstrual changes and changes in gonadal hormones. *Acta Psychiatrica Scandinavica, 74,* 576–586.

Halbreich, U., Endicott, J., & Nee, J. (1982). Premenstrual depressive changes—value of differentiation. *Archives of General Psychiatry, 40,* 535–542.

Halbreich, U., Endicott, J., Schachts, S., & Nee, J. (1982). The diversity of premenstrual changes as reflected in the premenstrual assessment form. *Acta Psychiatrica Scandinavica, 65,* 46–64.

Hamilton, J. A. (1981). Attention, personality, and the self-regulation of mood: Absorbing interest and boredom. *Progress in Experimental Personality Research, 10,* 281–315.

Hamilton, J. A., & Alagna, S. W. (1986). *On premenstrual psychiatric diagnosis: What's in a name?* Paper presented at the 94th annual meeting of the American Psychological Association, Washington, DC.

Hamilton, J. A., Alagna, S. W., & Sharpe, K. (1985). Cognitive approaches to understanding and treating premenstrual depressions. In H. Osofsky & S. Blumenthal (Eds.), *PMS: New findings and future directions* (pp. 69–84). Washington, DC: American Psychiatric Press.

Hamilton, H. A., & Gallant, S. A. (1988). Premenstrual symptom changes and plasma B-endorphin/B-lipotropin throughout the menstrual cycle. *Psychoneuroendocrinology, 13,* 505–514.

Hammarback, S. (1989). The premenstrual syndrome: A study of its diagnosis and pathogenesis. *Acta Obstetricia et Gynecologica Scandinavica,* 1–48.

Hammarback, S., & Backstrom, T. (1989). A demographic study in subgroups of women seeking help for premenstrual syndrome. *Acta Obstetricia et Gynecologica Scandinavica, 68,* 247-253.

Hampson, E. (1990a). Estrogen-related variations in human spatial and articulatory motor skills. *Psychoneuroendocrinology, 15,* 97–111.

Hampson, E. (1990b). Variations in sex-related cognitive abilities across the menstrual cycle. *Brain and Cognition, 14,* 26–43.

Hampson, E., & Kimura, D. (1988). Sex differences and hormonal influences on cognitive brain function. In R. Lewis (Ed.) *Society for Neuroscience Abstracts,* Part I, Vol. 14, p. 595.

Harlow, S. D. (1986). Function and dysfunction: A historical critique of the literature on menstruation and work. *Health Care for Women International, 7,* 39–50.

Harraway, D. (1989). *Primate visions.* New York: Routledge.

Harre, R. (Ed.). (1986). *The social construction of emotions.* New York: Basil Blackwell.

Harrison, W. M., Rabkin, J. G., & Endicott, J. (1985). Psychiatric evaluation of premenstrual changes. *Psychosomatics, 26,* 789–799.

Haskett, R. F., & Abplanalp, J. M. (1983). Premenstrual tension syndrome: Diagnostic criteria and selection of research subjects. *Psychiatry Research*, *9*, 125–128.

Haskett, R. F., Steiner, M., & Carroll, B. J. (1984). A psychoendocrine study of premenstrual tension syndrome: A model for endogenous depression. *Journal of Affective Disorders*, *6*, 191–199.

Haskett, R. F., Steiner, M., Osmun, J. N., & Carroll, B. J. (1980). Severe premenstrual tension: Delineation of the syndrome. *Psychiatry*, *15*, 121–139.

Hedges, S. M., Jandorf, L., & Stone, A. A. (1985). Meaning of daily mood assessments. *Journal of Personality and Social Psychology*, *48*, 428–434.

Henley, N. M. (1986a). *Feminist Psychology and Feminist Theory: Carolyn Wood Sheriff Memorial Lecture (Division 35)*. Washington, DC: American Psychological Association.

Henley, N. M. (1986b). Women as a social problem: Conceptual and practical issues in defining social problems. In E. Seidman & J. Rappaport (Eds.), *Redefining social problems* (pp. 65–79). New York: Plenum.

Henley, N., & Thorne, B. (1975). Sex differences in language, speech, and nonverbal communication: An annotated bibliography. In B. Thorne & N. Henley (Eds.), *Language and Sex: Difference and Dominance* (pp. 375–398). Rowley: Newbury House.

Hill, P., Garbaczewski, L., Helman, P., Huskisson, J., Sporangisa, E., & Wynder, E. L. (1980). Diet, lifestyle, and menstrual activity. *American Journal of Clinical Nutrition*, *33*, 1192–1198.

Hollingworth, L. S. (1914). Functional periodicity: An experimental study of the mental and motor abilities of women during menstruation. *Columbia University contributors to education*, Teachers College series, No. 69.

Hurt, S. W., Schnurr, P. P., Severino, S. K., Freeman, E. W., Gise, L. H., Rivera-Tovar, A., & Steege, J. F. (1992). Late luteal phase dysphoric disorder in 670 women evaluated for premenstrual complaints. *American Journal of Psychiatry*, *149*, 525–530.

Huzzard, M. P. (1978). Menstrual fluctuations in hearing—suggestions for hormone or drug monitoring methods in man. *British Journal of Pharmacology*, *64*, 476.

Ivey, M., & Bardwick, J. M. (1968). Patterns of affective fluctuation in the menstrual cycle. *Psychosomatic Medicine*, *30*, 151–169.

Janiger, O., Piffenbaugh, R., & Kersh, R. (1972). Cross-cultural study of premenstrual syndromes. *Psychosomatics*, *13*, 226–235.

Jarett, L. R. (1984). Psychosocial and biological influences on menstruation: Synchrony, cycle length, and regularity. *Psychoneuroendocrinology*, *9*, 21–28.

Kaplan, M. (1983). A woman's view of DSM-III. *American Psychologist*, *40*, 786–792.

Kemnitz, J. W., Gibber, J. R., Lindsay, K. A., & Eisele, S. G. (1989). Effects of ovarian hormones on eating behaviors, body weight, and glucoregulation in rhesus monkeys. *Hormones and Behavior*, *23*, 235–250.

Key, W. R., Jr., Hammond, D. C., & and Strong, T. (1986). Medical and psychological characteristics of women presenting with premenstrual symptoms. *Obstetrics and Gynecology*, *68*, 634–637.

Knorr-Cetina, K. D., & Mulkay, M. (Eds.). (1983). *Science observed: Perspectives on the social study of science*. Beverly Hills, CA: Sage.

Koeske, R. D. (1978, March). *Menstrual cycle research: Challenge or chuckle?* Paper presented at the Association of Women in Psychology Conference, Pittsburgh.

Koeske, R. D. (1980a). Theoretical perspectives on menstrual cycle research: The relevance of attributional approaches for the perception and explanation of premenstrual emotionality. In A. J. Dan, E. A. Graham, & C. P. Beecher (Eds.), *The menstrual cycle, Vol. 1: A synthesis of interdisciplinary research* (pp. 8–25). New York: Springer.

Koeske, R. D. (1980b). The theoretical/conceptual implications of study design and statistical analysis: Research on the menstrual cycle. In C. Stark-Adamec (Ed.), *Sex roles: Origins, influences, and implications for women* (pp. 217–232). Montreal: Eden Press.

Koeske, R. D. (1981). Theoretical and conceptual complexities in the design and analysis of menstrual cycle research. In P. Komnenich et al. (Eds.), *The menstrual cycle, Vol. 2: Research and implications for women's health* (pp. 54–70). New York: Springer.

Koeske, R. D. (1985). Lifting the curse of menstruation: Toward a feminist perspective on the menstrual cycle. In S. Golub (Ed.), *Lifting the curse of menstruation* (pp. 1–16). New York: Harrington Park Press.

Koeske, R. D., & Koeske, G. F. (1975). An attributional approach to moods and the menstrual cycle. *Journal of Personality and Social Psychology, 31*, 473–478.

Koff, E. (1983). Through the looking glass of menarche: What the adolescent girl sees. In S. Golub (Ed.), *Menarche* (pp. 77–86). Lexington, MA: D.C. Heath.

Koff, E., Rierdan, J., & Silverstone, E. (1978). Changes in representation of body image as a function of menarcheal status. *Developmental Psychology, 14*, 635–642.

Komnenich, P., Lane, M. D., Dickey, R. P., & Stone, S. C. (1978). Gonadal hormones and cognitive performance. *Physiological Psychology, 6*, 115–120.

Komnenich, P., McSweeney, M., Noack, J. A., & Elder, S. N. (Eds.). (1981). *The menstrual cycle, Vol. 2: Research and implications for women's health.* New York: Springer.

Kopell, B. S., Lunde, D. T., Clayton, R. B., & Moos, R. H. (1969). Variations in some measures of arousal during the menstrual cycle. *Journal of Nervous and Mental Diseases, 148*, 180–187.

Lahmeyer, H. W., Miller, M., & DeLeon-Jones, F. (1982). Anxiety and mood fluctuation during the normal menstrual cycle. *Psychosomatic Medicine, 44*, 183–194.

Latour, B. (1987). *Science in action.* Cambridge: Harvard University Press.

Latour, B., & Woolgar, S. (1986). *Laboratory life: The construction of scientific facts* (2nd ed.). Princeton, NJ: Princeton University Press.

Laws, S. (1983). The sexual politics of premenstrual tension. *Women's Studies International Forum, 6*, 19–31.

Laws, S., Hey, V., & Eagan, A. (Eds.). (1985). *Seeing red.* London: Hutchinson.

Levitt, E. E., & Lubin, B. B. (1967). Some personality factors associated with menstrual complaints and menstrual attitude. *Journal of Psychosomatic Research, 11*, 267–270.

Lidz, R. W., & Lidz, T. (1977). Male menstruation: A ritual alternative to the oedipal transition. *International Journal of Psychoanalysis, 58*, 17–31.

Lin, M. C., Kripke, D. F., Parry, B. L., & Berga, S. L. (1990). Night light alters menstrual cycles. *Psychiatry Research, 33*, 135–138.

Lissner, L., Levitsky, D. A., Stevens, J., Strupp, B. J., & Rasmussen, K. M. (1988). Variation in energy intake during the menstrual cycle: Implications for food-intake research. *American Journal of Clinical Nutrition, 48*, 956–962.

Little, B. C., & Zahn, T. P. (1974): Changes in mood and autonomic functioning during the menstrual cycle. *Psychophysiology, 11*, 579–580.

Logue, C. M., & Moos, R. H. (1986). Perimenstrual symptoms: Prevalence and risk factors. *Psychosomatic Medicine, 48*, 388–414.

Logue, C. M., & Moos, R. H. (1988). Positive perimenstrual changes—toward a new perspective on the menstrual cycle. *Journal of Psychosomatic Research, 32*, 31–40.

Lott, B. (1985). The potential enrichment of social/personality psychology through feminist research and vice versa. *American Psychologist, 40*, 155–164.

Loucks, A. B. (1990). Effects of exercise training on the menstrual cycle. *Medicine and Science in Sports and Exercise, 22*, 275–280.

Lubin, B., Zuckerman, M., Hanson, P. G., Armstrong, T., Rinck, C. M., & Seever, M. (1986). Reliability and validity of the MAACL-Revised. *Journal of Psychopathology and Behavioral Assessment, 8*, 103–117.

Lykes, M. B., & Stewart, A. J. (1986). Evaluating the feminist challenge to research in personality and social psychology: 1963–1983. *Psychology of Women Quarterly, 10*, 393–412.

Lyons, P. M., Mira, M., Truswell, A., Vizzard, J., & Abraham, S. F. (1989). Reduction of food intake in the ovulatory phase of the menstrual cycle. *American Journal of Clinical Nutrition, 49*, 1164–1168.

Mac, K., & Chang, A. (1985). The premenstrual syndrome in Chinese. *Australian and New Zealand Journal of Obstetrics and Gynecology, 25*, 118–120.

Maddocks, S., Hahn, P., Moller, F., & Reid, R. L. (1986). A double-blind placebo-controlled trial of progesterone vaginal suppositories in the treatment of premenstrual syndrome. *American Journal of Obstetrics and Gynecology, 154*, 573–581.

Magos, A. L., Brincat, M., & Studd, J.W.W. (1986). Treatment of the premenstrual syndrome by subcutaneous oestradiol implants and cyclical oral norethisterone: Placebo controlled study. *British Medical Journal, 292*, 1629–1633.

Magos, A., & Studd, J. (1985). Effects of the menstrual cycle on medical disorders. *British Journal of Hospital Medicine, 33*, 68–77.

Magos, A. L., & Studd, J.W.W. (1986). Assessment of menstrual cycle symptoms by trend analysis. *American Journal of Obstetrics and Gynecology, 155*, 271–277.

Mansfield, P. K., Hood, K. E., & Henderson, J. (1989). Women and their husbands: Mood and arousal fluctuations across the menstrual cycle and days of the week. *Psychosomatic Medicine, 51*, 66–80.

Markum, R. A. (1976). Assessment of the reliability of and the effect of neutral instructions on the symptom ratings on the Moos Menstrual Distress Questionnaire. *Psychosomatic Medicine, 38*, 163–172.

Martin, E. (1987). *The woman in the body: A cultural analysis of reproduction.* Boston: Beacon.

Matria, C., & Mullen, P. (1978). Reclaiming menstruation: A study of alienation and repossession. *Women and Health, 3*(3), 23–30.

Matsumoto, S., Igarashi, M., & Nagaoka, Y. (1968). Environmental anovulatory cycles. *International Journal of Fertility, 13*, 15–23.

May, R. R. (1976). Mood shifts and the menstrual cycle. *Journal of Psychosomatic Research 20*, 125–130.

McCance, R. A., Luff, M. C., & Widdowson, E. E. (1937). Physical and emotional periodicity in women. *Journal of Hygiene, 37*, 571–605.

McClintock, M. (1971). Menstrual synchrony and suppression. *Nature, 229,* 244–245.

McClintock, M. K. (1981). Major gaps in menstrual cycle research: Behavioral and physiological controls in a biological context. In P. Komnenich, M. McSweeney, J. A. Noack, & S. N. Elder (Eds.), *The menstrual cycle, Vol. 2: Research and implications for women's health* (pp. 7–23). New York: Springer.

McEwen, B. S. (1980). Steroid hormones and the brain: Cellular mechanisms underlying neural and behavioral plasticity. *Psychoneuroendocrinology, 5,* 1–11.

McEwen, B. S. (1988). Basic research perspectives: Ovarian hormone influence on brain neurochemical functions. In L. H. Gise, N. G. Kase, & R. L. Berkowitz (Eds.), *The premenstrual syndromes* (pp. 21–33). New York: Churchill Livingstone.

McFarlane, J., Martin, C. L., & Williams, T. M. (1988). Mood fluctuations: Women versus men and menstrual versus other cycles. *Psychology of Women Quarterly, 12,* 201–223.

McNair, D. M., Lorr, M., & Droppleman, L. F. (1971). *Profile of Mood States.* San Diego, CA: Educational and Industrial Testing Service.

Metcalf, M. G. (1983). Incidence of ovulation from menarche to menopause: Observations of 622 New Zealand women. *New Zealand Medical Journal, 96,* 645–648.

Metcalf, M. G., & Hudson, S. M. (1985). The premenstrual syndrome: Selection of women for treatment trials. *Journal of Psychosomatic Research, 29,* 631–638.

Mishler, E. G. (1986). *Research interviewing: Context and narrative.* Cambridge, MA: Harvard University Press.

Mitchell, E. S., Lentz, M. J., Woods, N. F., Lee, K., & Taylor, D. (1992). Methodological issues in the definition of premenstrual syndrome. In A. J. Dan & L. L. Lewis (Eds.), *Menstrual health in women's lives* (pp. 7–14). Urbana: University of Illinois Press.

Monagle, L. A., Dan, A. J., Chatterton, R. T., DeLeon-Jones, F. A., & Hudgens, G. A. (1986). Toward delineating menstrual symptom groupings: Examination of factor analytic results of menstrual symptom instruments. *Health Care for Women International, 6,* 131–143.

Moos, R. H. (1968). The development of a menstrual distress questionnaire. *Psychosomatic Medicine, 30,* 853–867.

Moos, R. H. (1969). Typology of menstrual cycle symptoms. *Obstetrics and Gynecology, 103,* 390–402.

Moos, R. H. (1985). *Perimenstrual symptoms: A manual and overview of research with the Menstrual Distress Questionnaire.* Stanford, CA: Social Ecology Laboratory, Stanford University.

Moos, R. H., Kopell, B. S., Melges, F. T., Yalom, I. D., Lunde, D. T., Clayton, R. B., & Hamburg, D. A. (1969). Fluctuations in symptoms and moods during the menstrual cycle. *Journal of Psychosomatic Research, 13,* 37–44.

Morawski, J. G. (1990). Toward the unimagined: Feminism and epistemology in psychology. In R. T. Hare-Mustin & J. Marecek (Eds.), *Making a difference: Psychology and the construction of gender* (pp. 150–183). New Haven, CT: Yale University Press.

Mulligan, N. (1983). Recent developments: Premenstrual syndrome. *Harvard Women's Law Journal, 6,* 219–227.

Muse, K. N., Cetel, N. S., Futterman, L. A., & Yen, S.S.C. (1984). The premenstrual syndrome: Effects of "medical ovaiectomy." *New England Journal of Medicine, 311,* 1345–1349.

Nadelson, C. C., Notman, M., & Ellis, E. A. (1983). Psychosomatic aspects of obstetrics and gynecology. *Obstetrics and Gynecology, 24*, 871–884.

Nance, D. M. (1983). The development and neural determinants of the effects of estrogen on feeding behavior in the rat: A theoretical perspective. *Neuroscience and Biobehavioral Review, 7*, 189–211.

Notman, M. (1982). The psychiatrist's approach. In C. Debrovner (Ed.), *Premenstrual tension: A multidisciplinary approach* (pp. 51–69). New York: Human Sciences Press.

Notman, M. T., & Nadelson, D. (1983). Fertility and reproduction. *Journal of Psychiatric Education, 1*, 37–44.

Nowlis, V. (1965). Research with the Mood Adjective Check List. In S. Tompkins & C. Izard (Eds.), *Affect, cognition, and personality* (pp. 353–389). New York: Springer.

O'Brien, P.M.S. (1987a). Controversies in premenstrual syndrome: Etiology and treatment. In B. E. Ginsburg & B. F. Carter (Eds.), *Premenstrual syndrome: Ethical and legal implications in a biomedical perspective* (pp. 317–328). New York: Plenum.

O'Brien, P.M.S. (1987b). *Premenstrual syndrome*. Oxford: Blackwell Scientific.

Olasov, B., & Jackson, J. (1987). Effects of expectancies on women's reports of moods during the menstrual cycle. *Psychosomatic Medicine, 49*, 65–78.

O'Neil, M. K., Lancee, W. J., & Freeman, S. J. (1984). Fluctuation in mood and psychological distress during the menstrual cycle. *Canadian Journal of Psychiatry, 29*, 373–378.

Osofsky, H. J., & Blumenthal, S. J. (Eds.). (1985). *Premenstrual syndrome: Current findings and future directions*. Washington, DC: American Psychiatric Press.

Paige, K. E. (1971). Effects of oral contraceptives on affective fluctuations associated with the menstrual cycle. *Psychosomatic Medicine, 33*, 515–537.

Paige, K. E. (1973, April). Women learn to sing the menstrual blues. *Psychology Today*, pp. 41–46.

Paige, K. E. (1983). Virginity rituals and chastity control during puberty: Cross-cultural patterns. In S. Golub (Ed.), *Menarche: An interdisciplinary view* (pp. 155–174). Lexington, MA: D. C. Heath.

Paige, K. E. (1987). Menstrual symptoms and menstrual beliefs: National and cross-national patterns. In B. E. Ginsburg & B. F. Carter (Eds.), *Premenstrual syndrome: Ethical and legal implications in a biomedical perspective* (pp. 175–187). New York: Plenum.

Paige, K. E., Magnus, E., Hahn, S., & Carrie, C. (1983). *The female reproductive cycle: An annotated bibliography*. Boston: G. K. Hall.

Paige, K. E., & Paige, J. M. (1981). *Politics of reproduction ritual*. Berkeley: University of California Press.

Parlee, M. B. (1973). Premenstrual syndrome. *Psychological Bulletin, 80*, 454–465.

Parlee, M. B. (1974). Stereotypic beliefs about menstruation: A methodological note on the Moos Menstrual Distress Questionnaire and some new data. *Psychosomatic Medicine, 36*, 229–240.

Parlee, M. B. (1975a). Menstruation and voluntary participation in a psychological experiment. In W. McKenna (Ed.), *A new psychology of menstruation*. Symposium presented at the 83rd Annual Meeting of the APA, Chicago.

Parlee, M. B. (1975b). Psychology. *Signs: Journal of Women in Culture and Society*, *1*(1), 119–138.

Parlee, M. B. (1979). Psychology and women. *Signs: Journal of Women in Culture and Society*, *5*(1), 121–133.

Parlee, M. B. (1981). Appropriate control groups in feminist research. *Psychology of Women Quarterly*, *5*, 637–644.

Parlee, M. B. (1982a). Changes in moods and activation levels during the menstrual cycle in experimentally naive subjects. *Psychology of Women Quarterly*, *7*, 119–131.

Parlee, M. B. (1982b). The psychology of the menstrual cycle: Biological and psychological perspectives. In R. C. Friedman (Ed.), *Behavior and the menstrual cycle* (pp. 77–99). New York: Marcel Dekker.

Parlee, M. B. (1983). Menstrual rhythms in sensory processes: A review of fluctuations in vision, olfaction, audition, taste, and touch. *Psychological Bulletin*, *93*, 35–48.

Parlee, M. B. (1987). Media treatment of PMS. In B. E. Ginsburg & B. F. Carter (Eds.), *Premenstrual syndrome* (pp. 189–206). New York: Plenum.

Parlee, M. B. (1988). Menstrual cycle changes in moods and emotions: Causal and interpretive processes in the construction of emotions. In H. Wagner (Ed.), *Social psychophysiology and emotion: Theory and clinical applications* (pp. 151–174). Chichester: Wiley.

Parlee, M. B. (1989, March). *The science and politics of PMS research.* Invited paper presented at the Association for Women in Psychology Annual Research Conference, Newport, RI.

Parlee, M. B. (1990). Integrating biological and social scientific research on menopause. *Annals of the New York Academy of Sciences*, *592*, 379–389.

Parlee, M. B. (1991). Happy birthday to Feminism & Psychology. *Feminism & Psychology*, *1*, 39-48.

Parlee, M. B. (1992). Feminism and psychology. In S. R. Zalk & J. Gordon-Kelter (Eds.), *Revolutions in knowledge: Feminism in the social sciences* (pp. 33–56). Boulder, CO: Westview Press.

Parry, B. L., & Rausch, J. L. (1988). Evaluation of biologic research. In L. H. Geise, N. G. Kase, & R. L. Berkowitz (Eds.), *The premenstrual syndrome* (pp. 47–58). New York: Churchill Livingstone.

Parry, B. L., Rosenthal, N. E., Tamarkin, L., & Wehr, T. A. (1987). Treatment of a patient with seasonal premenstrual syndrome. *American Journal of Psychiatry*, *144*, 762–766.

Patel, S., Cliff, K. S., & Machin, D. (1985). The premenstrual syndrome and its relationship to accidents. *Public Health, 99*, 45–50.

Patkai, P., Johannson, G., & Post, B. (1974). Mood, alertness and sympathetic-adrenal medullary activity during the menstrual cycle. *Psychosomatic Medicine*, *36*, 503–512.

Patterson, E. T., & Hale, E. S. (1985). Making sure: Integrating menstrual care practices into activities of daily living. *Advances in Nursing Science*, *7*, 18–31.

Persky, H., Lief, H. I., Strauss D., Miller, W. R., & O'Brien, C. P. (1978). Plasma testosterone level and sexual behavior of couples. *Archives of Sexual Behavior*, *7*, 157–173.

Pierson, W. R., & Lockhart, A. (1963). Effect of menstruation on simple reaction time and movement time. *British Medical Journal, 1*, 796–797.

Plutchick, R. (1980). *Emotion, a psychoevolutionary synthesis*. New York: Harper & Row.

Postuma, B. W., Bass, M. J., Bull, S. B., & Nisker, J. A. (1987). Detecting changes in functional ability in women with premenstrual syndrome. *American Journal of Obstetrics and Gynecology, 156*, 275–278.

Presser, H. B. (1974). Temporal data relating to the human menstrual cycle. In M. Ferin, F. Halberg, R. M. Richart, & K. L. vande Wiele (Eds.), *Biorhythms and human reproduction* (pp. 277–285). New York: Wiley.

Prior, J. C. (1984). Is premenstrual syndrome exaggerated molimina? [letter]. *American Journal of Psychiatry, 141*, 1495–1496.

Prior, J., Vigna, Y., Sciaretta, D., Alojado, N., & Schulzer, M. (1987). Conditioning exercise decreases premenstrual symptoms: A prospective, controlled six-month trial. *Fertility and Sterility, 47*, 402–408.

Procacci, P., Zoppi, M., Maresca, M., & Romano, S. (1974). Studies on the pain threshold in man. *Advances in Neurology, 4*, 107–113.

Procacci, P., Buzzelli, G., Posseri, I., Sassi, R., Voegelin, M. R., & Zoppi, M. (1972). Studies on the cutaneous pricking pain threshold in man: Circadian and circatrigintan changes. *Research and Clinical Studies in Headache, 3*, 260–276.

Quigly, M. E., & Yen, S.S.C. (1980). The role of endogenous opiates on LH secretion during the menstrual cycle. *Journal of Clinical Endocrinology and Metabolism, 51*, 179–181.

Ramey, E. (1973). Sex hormones and executive ability. *Annals of the New York Academy of Sciences, 208*, 237–245.

Rapkin, A. J., Chang, L. C., & Reading, A. E. (1988). Comparison of retrospective and prospective assessment of premenstrual symptoms. *Psychological Reports, 62*, 55–60.

Redgrove, J. A. (1971). Menstrual cycles. In W. O. Colquhoun (Ed.), *Biological rhythms and human performance* (pp. 211–240). New York: Academic Press.

Reid, R. (1985). Premenstrual syndrome. *Current Problems in Obstetrics, Gynecology, and Fertility, 8*, 1–57.

Reid, R. L. (1986). Disturbances of mood and behavior during the menstrual cycle. In L. Dennerstein & I. Fraser (Eds.), *Hormones and behavior* (pp. 120–129). Amsterdam: Elsevier.

Reid, R. L.. & Yen, S.S.C. (1981). Premenstrual syndrome. *American Journal of Obstetrics and Gynecology, 139*, 85–104.

Renik, O. (1984). An example of disavowal involving the menstrual cycle. *Psychoanalytic Quarterly, 53*, 523–532.

Richardson, J.T.E. (1990). Questionnaire studies of paramenstrual symptoms. *Psychology of Women Quarterly, 14*, 15–42.

Richter, C. P. (1968). Periodic phenomena in man and animals: Their relation to neuroendocrine mechanisms (a monthly or near monthly cycle). In R. P. Michael (Ed.), *Endocrinology and Human Behavior*. London: Oxford University Press.

Rierdan, J. (1983). Variations in the experience of menarche as a function of preparedness. In S. Golub (Ed.), *Menarche* (pp. 119–125). Lexington, MA: D.C. Heath.

Rierdan, J., & Koff, E. (1985). Timing of menarche and initial menstrual experience. *Journal of Youth and Adolescence, 14*, 237–244.

Rierdan, J., Koff, E., & Flaherty, J. (1985–1986). Conceptions and misconceptions of menstruation. *Women and Health*, *10*, 33–45.

Rivera-Tovar, A. D., & Frank, E. (1990). Late luteal phase dysphoric disorder in young women. *American Journal of Psychiatry*, *147*, 634–636.

Rodin, J. (1976). Menstruation, reattribution and competence. *Journal of Personality and Social Psychology*, *33*, 345–353.

Rogers, M. L., & Harding, S. S. (1981). Retrospective and daily menstrual distress measures in men and women using Moos's instruments and modified versions of Moos's instruments. In P. Komnenich, M. McSweeney, J. A. Noack, & S. N. Elder (Eds.), *The menstrual cycle, Vol. 2: Research and implications for women's health* (pp. 71–81). New York: Springer.

Rorty, E. O. (Ed.). (1980). *Explaining emotions*. Berkeley: University of California Press.

Rossi, A. S. (1980). Mood cycles by menstrual month and social week. In A. J. Dan, E. A. Graham, & C. P. Beecher (Eds.), *The menstrual cycle, Vol. 1: A synthesis of interdisciplinary research* (pp. 56–75). New York: Springer.

Rossi, A. S., & Rossi, P. E. (1977). Body time and social time: Mood patterns by menstrual cycle phase and day of week. *Social Science Research*, *6*, 273–308.

Rubinow, D. R. (1987). Chair, Summary Session, Committee on Biomedical Issues. In B. E. Ginsburg & B. F. Carter (Eds.), *Premenstrual syndrome: Ethical and legal implications in a biomedical perspective* (pp. 411–412). New York: Plenum.

Rubinow, D. R., Hoban, M. C., Grover, G. N., Galloway, D. S., Roy-Byrne, P., Anderson, R., & Merriam, G. R. (1988). Changes in plasma hormones across the menstrual cycle in patients with menstrually related mood disorder and in control subjects. *American Journal of Obstetrics and Gynecology*, *158*, 5–11.

Rubinow, D. R., Hoban, M. C., Roy-Byrne, P. P., Grover, G. N., & Post, R. M. (1985). Menstrually related mood disorders. In H. J. Osofsky & S. J. Blumenthal (Eds.), *PMS: Current findings and future directions*. Washington, DC: American Psychiatric Press.

Rubinow, D. R., & Roy-Byrne, D. (1984). Premenstrual syndromes: Overview from a methodologic perspective. *American Journal of Psychiatry*, *141*, 163–172.

Rubinow, D. R., Roy-Byrne, P., Hoban, M. C., Grover, G. N., Stambler, N., & Post, R. M. (1986). Premenstrual mood changes: Patterns in women with and without premenstrual syndrome. *Journal of Affective Disorders*, *10*, 85–90.

Rubinow, D. R., & Schmidt, P. J. (1989). Menstrual and formal mood disorders. In L. M. Demers, J. L. McGuire, A. Phillips, & D. R. Rubinow (Eds.), *Premenstrual, postpartum, and menopausal mood disorders* (pp. 35–52). Baltimore: Urban & Schwarzenberg.

Ruble, D. N. (1977). Premenstrual symptoms: A reinterpretation. *Science*, *197*, 291–292.

Ruble, D. N., & Brooks-Gunn, J. (1979). Menstrual symptoms: A social cognition analysis. *Behavioral Medicine*, *2*, 171–194.

Ruble, D. N., & Brooks-Gunn, J. (1982). A developmental analysis of menstrual distress in adolescence. In R. C. Friedman (Ed.), *Behavior and the menstrual cycle* (pp. 177–198). New York: Marcel Dekker.

Ruble, D. N., & Brooks-Gunn, J. (1987). Perceptions of menstrual and premenstrual symptoms: Self-definitional processes at menarche. In B. E. Ginsburg & B. F.

Carter (Eds.), *Premenstrual syndrome: Ethical and legal implications in a biomedical perspective* (pp. 237–251). New York: Plenum.

Ruble, D. N., Brooks-Gunn, J., & Clarke, A. (1980). Research on menstrual-related psychological states: Alternative perspectives. In J. E. Parsons (Ed.), *The psychobiology of sex differences and sex roles* (pp. 227–243). New York: Hemisphere.

Russell, J. A. (1979). Affective space is bipolar. *Journal of Personality and Social Psychology, 37,* 273–294.

Russell, M. J., Switz, G. M., & Thompson, K. (1980). Olfactory influences on the human menstrual cylcle. *Pharmacology, Biochemistry, and Behavior, 13,* 737–738.

Sampson, G. A. (1987). Premenstrual syndrome: Characterization, therapies, and the law. In B. E. Ginsburg & B. F. Carter (Eds.), *Premenstrual syndrome: Ethical and legal implications in a biomedical perspective* (pp. 301–316). New York: Plenum.

Sanders, D., Warner, P., Backstrom, T., & Bancroft, J. (1983). Mood, sexuality, hormones and the menstrual cycles. I. Changes in mood and physical state: Description of subjects and method. *Psychosomatic Medicine, 45,* 487–501.

Sayers, J. (1982). *Biological politics: Feminist and anti-feminist perspectives.* New York: Tavistock.

Schact, T. E. (1985). DSM-III and the politics of truth. *American Psychologist, 40,* 513–526.

Schechter, D., Bachmann, G. A., Vaitukaitis, J., Phillips, D., & Saperstein, D. (1989). Perimenstrual symptoms: Time course of symptom intensity in relation to endocrinologically defined segments of the menstrual cycle. *Psychosomatic Medicine, 51,* 173–194.

Schilling, K. M. (1981). What is a *real* difference: Content or method in menstrual findings. In P. Komnenich, M. McSweeney, J. A. Noack, & S. N. Elder (Eds.), *The menstrual cycle, Vol. 2: Research and implications for women's health* (pp. 82–92). New York: Springer.

Schmidt, P. J., Grover, G. N., & Rubinow, D. R. (1990). State-dependent alterations in the perception of life events in menstrual-related mood disorders. *American Journal of Psychiatry, 147,* 230–234.

Schmidt, P. J., Nieman, L. K., Muller, K. L., Merriam, G. R., & Rubinow, D. R. (1991). Lack of effect of induced menses on symptoms with premenstrual syndrome. *New England Journal of Medicine, 324,* 1174–1179.

Schultz, K. J., & Koulack, D. (1980). Dream affect and the menstrual cycle. *Journal of Nervous and Mental Diseases, 168,* 436–438.

Severino, S. K. (1988). The psychoanalyst in a bio-medical world: New opportunities for understanding women. *Academy Forum, 32,* 10–12.

Severino, S. K., Bucci, W., & Creelman, M. L. (1989). Cyclical changes in emotional information processing in sleep and dreams. *Journal of the American Academy of Psychoanalysis, 17,* 555–577.

Severino, S. K., & Moline, M. L. (1989). *Premenstrual syndrome: A clinician's manual.* New York: Guilford Press.

Seward, G. H. (1934). The female sex rhythms. *Psychological Bulletin, 31,* 153–192.

Seward, G. H. (1944). Psychological effects of the menstrual cycle on women workers. *Psychological Bulletin, 41,* 90–102.

Shainess, N. (1961). A re-evaluation of some aspects of femininity through a study of menstruation: A preliminary report. *Comprehensive Psychiatry, 2*, 20–26.

Sherif, C. W. (1980). A social psychological perspective on the menstrual cycle. In J. E. Parsons (Ed.), *The psychobiology of sex differences and sex roles* (pp. 245–268). New York: Hemisphere.

Sherman, J. A. (1970). *On the psychology of women.* Springfield, IL: C.C. Thomas.

Shields, S. (1975). Functionalism, Darwinism, and the psychology of women. *American Psychologist, 30* 739–754.

Siegel, J. P., Myers, B. J., & Dineen, M. K. (1987). Premenstrual tension syndrome clusters. *Journal of Reproductive Medicine, 32*, 395–399.

Skinner, B. F. (1959). *Cumulative Record.* New York: Appleton-Century-Crofts.

Slade, P. (1984). Premenstrual emotional changes in normal women: Fact or fiction. *Journal of Psychosomatic Research, 28*, 1–7.

Smith, S. L. (1975). Mood and the menstrual cycle. In E. J. Sacher (Ed.), *Topics in psychoendocrinology* (pp. 19–57). New York: Grune & Stratton.

Snowden, R., & Christian, B. (1984). *Patterns and perceptions of menstruation.* New York: St. Martin's Press.

Sommer, B. (1972). Menstrual cycle changes and intellectual performance. *Psychosomatic Medicine, 34*, 263–269.

Sommer, B. (1973). The effect of menstruation on cognitive and perceptual-motor behavior: A review. *Psychosomatic Medicine, 35*, 515–534.

Sommer, B. (1982). Cognitive behavior and the menstrual cycle. In R. C. Friedman (Ed.), *Behavior and the menstrual cycle* (pp. 101–127). New York: Marcel Dekker.

Sommer, B. (1984, August). PMS in the courts: Are all women on trial? *Psychology Today*, pp. 36–38.

Sommer, B. (1985). How does menstruation affect cognitive competence and psychophysiological response? In S. Golub (Ed.), *Lifting the curse of menstruation* (pp. 53–90). New York: Harrington Park Press.

Sommer, B. (1987). The file drawer effect and publication rates in menstrual cycle research. *Psychology of Women Quarterly, 11*, 233–242.

Spencer, S. W., & Snyder, M. L. (1984). The menstrual cycle and punitiveness. *Health Psychology, 3*, 143–155.

Spitzer, R. L., Severino, S. K., Williams, J. B. W., & Parry, B. L. (1989). Late Luteal Dysphoric Disorder and DSM-IIIR. *American Journal of Psychiatry, 146*, 892–897.

Spitzer, R. L., Williams, J. B. W., & Skodol, A. E. (1980). DSM III: The major achievements and an overview. *American Journal of Psychiatry, 137*, 151–163.

Steege, J. F. (1989). Symptom measurement in premenstrual syndrome. In L. M. Demers, J. L. McGuire, A. Phillips, & D. R. Rubinow (Eds.), *Premenstrual, postpartum, and menopausal mood disorders* (pp. 53–64). Baltimore, MD: Urban & Schwarzenberg.

Steege, J. F., Stout, A. L., & Rupp, S. L. (1985). Relationships among premenstrual symptoms and menstrual cycle characteristics. *Obstetrics and Gynecology, 65*, 398–402.

Steiner, M., Haskett, R. F., & Carroll, B. J. (1980). Premenstrual tension syndrome:

The development of research diagnostic criteria and new rating scales. *Acta Psychiatrica Scandinavica*, *61*, 96–102.

Steiner, M., Haskett, R. F., Carroll, B. J., Hays, S. E., & Rubin, R. T. (1984). Circadian hormone secretory profiles in women with severe premenstrual tension syndrome. *British Journal of Obstetrics and Gynecology*, *91*, 466–471.

Stenn, P. G., & Klinge, V. (1972). Relationship between the menstrual cycle and bodily activity in humans. *Hormones and Behavior*, *3*, 297–305.

Stephens, W. (1961). A cross-cultural study of menstrual taboos. *Genetic Psychology Monographs*, *72*, No. 11.

Stephenson, L. A., Denney, D. R., & Aberger, E. W. (1983). Factor structure of the Menstrual Symptom Questionnaire: Relationship to oral contraceptives, neuroticism, and life stress. *Behavior Research and Therapy*, *21*, 129–135.

Stewart, D. E. (1989). Positive changes in the premenstrual period. *Acta Psychiatrica Scandinavica*, *79*, 400–405.

Stoltzman, S. M. (1986). Menstrual attitudes, beliefs, and symptom experiences of adolescent females, their peers, and their mothers. *Health Care for Women International*, *7*, 97–114.

Strickler, R. C. (1987). Endocrine hypotheses for the etiology of premenstrual syndrome. *Clinical Obstetrics and Gynecology*, *30*, 377–385.

Sutherland, H., & Stewart, I. (1965). A critical analysis of the premenstrual syndrome. *The Lancet*, *1*, 1180–1193.

Swandby, J. R. (1981). A longitudinal study of daily mood self-reports and their relationship to the menstrual cycle. In P. Komnenich et al. (Eds.), *The menstrual cycle, Vol. 2: Research and implications for women's health* (pp. 93–103). New York: Springer.

The Tampax Report. (1981). Rudder, Finn and Rotman, 110 E 59th Street, New York, New York 10022.

Taylor, J. W. (1979). The timing of menstruation-related symptoms assessed by a daily symptom rating scale. *Acta Psychiatrica Scandinavica*, *60*, 87–105.

Tennov, D. (1973). *Mode of control of reinforcement density as a function of the sex of the behaver.* Paper delivered at the 81st Annual Meeting of the American Psychological Association, Montreal.

Thayer, R. E. (1967). Measurement of activation through self-report. *Psychological Reports*, *22*, 663–678.

Thayer, R. E. (1970). Activation states as assessed by verbal report and four psychophysical variables. *Psychophysiology*, *7*, 86–94.

Treolar, A. E., Boynton, R. E., Behn, B. G., & Brown, B. W. (1967). Variation of the human menstrual cycle through reproductive life. *International Journal of Fertility*, *12*, 77–126.

Van den Akker, O., & Steptoe, A. (1985). The pattern and prevalence of symptoms during the menstrual cycle. *British Journal of Psychiatry*, *147*, 164–169.

Vellacott, I. D., Shroff, N. E., Pearce, M. Y., Stratford, M. E., & Akbar, F. A. (1987). A double-blind, placebo-controlled evaluation of spironolactone in the premenstrual syndrome. *Current Medical Research and Opinion*, *10*, 450–456.

Vingilis, E. (1980). Feeling states and the menstrual cycle. In C. Stark-Adamec (Ed.), *Sex roles: Origins, influences, and implications for women* (pp. 206–216). Montreal: Eden Press.

Wallach, A., & Rubin, L. (1971). The premenstrual syndrome and premenstrual responsibility. *UCLA Law Review*, *19*, 209–311.

Webster, S. K., Martin, H. J., Uchalik, D., & Gannon, L. (1979). The menstrual symptom questionnaire and spasmotic/congestive dysmenorrhea: Measurement of an invalid construct. *Journal of Behavioral Medicine*, *2*, 1–19.

Weideger, P. (1976). *Menstruation and menopause*. New York: Knopf.

Weizenbaum, F., Benson, B., Solomon, L., & Brehony, K. (1980). Relationships among reproductive variables, sucrose taste reactivity and feeding behavior in humans. *Physiology and Behavior*, *24*, 1053–1056.

Whalen, R. E. (1975). Cyclic changes in hormones and behavior. *Archives of Sexual Behavior*, *4*, 313–314.

Whelan, E. M. (1975). Attitudes toward menstruation. *Studies in Family Planning*, *6*, 106–108.

Whisnant, L., & Zegans, L. (1975). A study of attitudes toward menarche in white middle-class American adolescent girls. *American Journal of Psychiatry*, *132*, 809–814.

Widholm, O. (1979). Dysmenorrhea during adolescence. *Acta Obstetricia et Gynecologica Scandinavica*, *87*, 61–66.

Widholm, O. M., Frisk, T., & Hortling, H. (1967). Gynecological findings in adolescence: A study of 514 patients. *Acta Obstetricia et Gynecologica Scandinavica*, *46*, 1–27.

Widholm, O., & Kantero, R. L. (1971). Gynecological findings in adolescence. Part III. Menstrual pattern of adolescent girls according to chronological and gynecological ages. *Acta Obstetricia et Gynecologica Scandinavica*, *14*, 19–29.

Wilcoxon, L. A., Schrader, S. L., & Sherif, C. W. (1976). Daily self-reports on activities, life events, moods, and somatic changes during the menstrual cycle. *Psychosomatic Medicine*, *38*, 399–417.

Williams, G. D., & Williams, A. M. (1982). Sexual behavior and the menstrual cycle. In R. C. Friedman (Ed.), *Behavior and the menstrual cycle* (pp. 155–176). New York: Marcel Dekker.

Williams, M. J., Harris, R. I., & Dean, B. C. (1985). Controlled trial of pyridoxine in the premenstrual syndrome. *Journal of International Medical Research*, *13*, 174–179.

Woods, N. F., Most, C., Devy, G. (1982). Prevalence of perimenstrual symptoms. *American Journal of Public Health*, *72*, 1257–1264.

World Health Organization Task Force on Psychosocial Research in Family Planning. (1981). A cross-cultural study of menstruation. *Studies in Family Planning*, *12*, 3–16.

Wurtman, R. J., & Wurtman, J. J. (1989). Carbohydrates and depression. *Scientific American*, *260*, 68–75.

Wuttke, W., Arnold, P., Becker, D., Creutzfeldt, O., Langenstein, S., & Tirsch, W. (1986). Hormonal profiles and variations of the EEG and performances in psychological tests in women with spontaneous menstrual cycles and under oral contraceptives. In T. M. Itil (Ed.), *Psychotropic action of hormones* (pp. 169–182). New York: Spectrum.

Young, A. (1982). The anthropology of sickness and the anthropology of illness. *Annual Review of Anthropology*, *11*, 257–285.

Young, F., & Bacdayan, A. (1965). Menstrual taboos and social rigidity. *Ethnology*, *4*, 225–240.

Yuk, V. J., Jugdutt, A. V., Cumming, C. E., Fox, E. E., & Cumming, D. C. (1990). Towards a definition of PMS—a factor analytic evaluation of premenstrual change in noncomplaining owmen. *Journal of Psychosomatic Research*, *34*, 439–446.

Zimmerman, E., & Parlee, M. B. (1973). Behavioral changes associated with the menstrual cycle: An experimental investigation. *Journal of Applied Social Psychology*, *3*, 335–344.

Zola, I. K. (1966). Culture and symptoms: An analysis of patients' presenting symptoms. *American Sociological Review*, *31*, 615–630.

Zola, I. K. (1973). Pathways to the doctor: From person to patient. *Social Science and Medicine*, *7*, 677–689.

Zuckerman, M., & Lubin, B. (1965). *Manual for the Multiple Affect Adjective Check List*. San Diego, CA: Educational and Industrial Testing Service.

11

Women and Mental Health

Nancy Felipe Russo and Beth L. Green

Research on women's mental health has reflected the values and assumptions of the larger society and culture. This has meant gender bias in psychological theories and research methods, stereotypical conceptions of normality and mental illness, a lack of understanding of women's realities, a devaluation of women's activities, and a denial of women's contributions to the field. The need for feminist perspectives to ameliorate the distortions and gaps produced by such bias in mental health research, training, and practice has been underscored by a variety of authors (Alpert, 1986; Carmen, Russo & Miller, 1981; Dutton-Douglas & Walker, 1988; Rieker & Carmen, 1984; Russo, 1985, 1990; Rosewater & Walker, 1985).

A feminist perspective goes beyond critique and amelioration, however. Feminists have developed new theories, methods, and techniques and offered innovative perspectives on women's experiences, circumstances, and development over the life cycle. Women's mental health is viewed in its social/political context, and consumer issues are of importance (Liss-Levinson et al., 1985; American Psychological Association, 1987). Feminist theory has stimulated the development of a variety of feminist therapies that reflect integration of feminist principles into therapy theories. Feminists have also examined alternatives to therapy, including assertiveness training and consciousness raising (Brody, 1984; Dutton-Douglas & Walker, 1988; Rosewater & Walker, 1985).

An understanding of women's experiences is the foundation for effective therapeutic technique. As can be seen in the works cited in this chapter and in the other chapters of this book, feminist researchers have explored neglected areas in women's lives such as AIDS, anger, autonomy, body image, breast cancer, dependency, discrimination and stereotyping, eating disorders, elderly women's issues, ethnic minority women's issues, family and job stress, lesbian issues, menstruation and menopause, motherhood and other reproductive events, job stress, sexual harassment, and poverty (see also Travis, 1988a, 1988b). They have reexamined relationships and forced attention to effects of intimate violence, incest, and marital disruption.

In applying feminist principles, researchers and practitioners have emphasized the destructive effects of powerlessness and dependency for women and forged a shift of emphasis in therapy from adjustment to agency. In doing so, they have pointed to the importance of examining power inequities and social control mechanisms at home, at work, and in therapeutic relationships. Feminists have also sought to identify and celebrate women's strengths and to enhance visibility and valuing of women's contributions to their families and communities.

Feminists have articulated new roles for psychologists to promote feminist values (Sobel & Russo, 1981). They have formed coalitions to promote the value of cultural diversity, and among their successes is a cultural diversity section in the accreditation criteria of the American Psychological Association (1983) so that future generations of mental health researchers and practitioners will have a broader vision of psychological knowledge and its application. They have also sought coalitions across the disciplines to work for improvement in women's mental health research, service delivery, and public policy (Subpanel on the Mental Health of Women, 1978; Russo, 1985, 1990; Walker, 1984). As a result, numerous public policy reports have emphasized the importance of incorporating the new scholarship on women in mental health research, training, and service delivery (e.g., Eichler & Parron, 1987; Public Health Service, 1985; Subpanel on the Mental Health of Women, 1978).

It is impossible for one chapter to provide a detailed discussion of the issues, concerns, and contributions of feminist researchers, practitioners, and policy-makers to understanding women's mental health. Recent overviews and bibliographies can be found in Alpert (1986), Amaro and Russo (1987), Bernay and Cantor (1986), Brody (1984), Brody (1987), Brown and Root (1990), Coll and Mattei (1989), Dilling and Claster (1985), Dutton-Douglas and Walker (1988), Fine and Asch (1988), Fitzgerald and Nutt (1986), Franks and Rothblum (1983), Helms (1989), Lerman (1986), Lerner (1988), McGrath, Keita, Strickland, and Russo (1990), Notman and Nadelson (1990), Rieker and Carmen (1984), Robbins and Siegel (1985), Rosewater and Walker (1985), Russo (1985, 1990), Travis (1988a, 1988b), and Walker (1984).

Despite the burgeoning theory and research on women's issues, the existing scientific knowledge base continues to be inadequate for understanding the large and complex gender differences in patterns of mental disorder and its treatment. Advances in understanding gender differences in psychological distress and mental disorder will require a more sophisticated and in-depth examination of women's development, roles, and life circumstances. Such an examination is made more difficult by the continuing changes that are occurring in the roles, status, and life circumstances of women in the United States.

GENDER-RELATED SOCIAL ROLES: SOME DISTINCTIONS

The lack of precision in the concepts of gender, gender identity, gender-related traits, and gender-related social roles compounds the difficulty of reviewing the mental health literature. These concepts are muddled, and we suggest some distinctions to clarify the relationship of being a woman and mental health.

Sex versus Gender

We define sex as a biological category, based on biological characteristics used to define male and female. It is a variable used in empirical studies to define gender operationally. Gender is a social category, based on a social definition of the way males and females should differ physically, cognitively, emotionally, and behaviorally. *Gender identity* is the self-recognition that one belongs to a gender category.

These distinctions are congruent with existing definitions in the literature (cf. Matlin, 1993), except we add the recognition that biological characteristics are included in the social category of gender. Any dieter or body builder will affirm the fact that males and females have vast differences in their physical standards that are clearly related to gender ideals, and not biological sex!

We believe advancing conceptions of gender rests on (1) recognizing that the concepts of genetics and biology, although related, are not identical; (2) incorporating biological considerations in conceptions of gender; and (3) fully appreciating the implications of the fact that gender is a social category—that is, no trait or behavior intrinsically belongs to a specific gender. Research on reproductive events that is described below demonstrates the complex interplay among biology, the social context, gender, and social roles. Traits and behaviors, such as instrumentality or wearing skirts, are gender-related because they are defined as such and people are expected to act accordingly. Gender is thus a dynamic social construct that varies across cultures, classes, and ethnic groups (Amaro & Russo, 1987). It is also tied to the position of women in such groups.

Gender-related traits or other *personal attributes* are qualities that reflect differential gender-role socialization of males and females (formerly identified as masculine or feminine qualities) as well as current expectations for behavior. The term *gender-related* is used to emphasize that personal attributes and behaviors have no intrinsic link to gender. They reflect an average *group* difference, not a difference always found between male and female individuals. Concepts that assume the existence of masculine and feminine personal attributes (e.g., androgyny) are thus inappropriate or obsolete. Femininity is in the eye of the beholder and is not an intrinsic quality of a particular attribute, which could be part of a masculine or feminine gender role, depending on the situational or cultural context that defines it as part of such a role.

Gender difference is the term used in a gender comparison to describe group differences between women and men when no causal relationship is implied. Gender differences may reflect effects of gender-related attributes, women's social roles, life circumstances, or some other factor—they merely show that something is correlated with gender. Gender comparisons also involve gender similarities, which take on new meaning in this theoretical framework, which makes distinctions between a woman's feminine gender role and other sex roles.

Social roles are clusters of attitudes and behaviors associated with social positions. *Sex roles* are social roles assigned on the basis of biological sex. Women's *gender role* is thus one type of sex role. There are at least two kinds of gender roles in U.S. society: the masculine gender role and the feminine gender role (this is not the case for all societies; see, e.g., Williams, 1986). This conceptualization of gender puts "masculinity" and "femininity" in the eye of the beholder and not in the person. One's degree of masculinity or femininity thus depends on social definitions, not personal attributes.

The concepts of gender role and sex role have been muddled in the literature, sometimes used interchangeably. Historically, women's social roles have overlapped, and there has been no functional need for distinctions among types of sex roles. The expectation was that normal, "real" women became wives and mothers. Socialization to be a woman was socialization for wife and mother roles. Change in women's status and position in society, however, has resulted in the need for more complex conceptions of women's social roles.

Gender, as a social category, defines separate statuses and positions for men and women. Thus, we use *feminine gender role* to refer to the bundle of expectations and norms assigned to women by virtue of their female gender, whereby women are expected to possess feminine attributes and act in a feminine manner in keeping with the position of woman in society: "woman's role." Women must deal with the expectations of this feminine gender role, however those are defined.

Women's feminine gender role, as we view it, is a unique kind of sex role, for it is tied to the overall position of women in the larger society. Gender roles are thus different from other sex roles because they are not tied to the characteristics of a social institution within society, such as the family. Because gender roles are not setting-specific, they may be less likely to require reciprocity (i.e., change in the gender role of the opposite sex). Further, if other characteristics (e.g., race or ethnicity) interact in determining the position of subgroups of women in society, those characteristics are inseparably part of such women's feminine gender role (thus, e.g., the gender role of black women will conceptually differ from that of white women as long as racism in society makes for a different position for black women in society. We specifically use the term *black* in this case as racism against blacks in society has been based on exactly that: skin color).

In contrast, other sex roles are roles that reflect norms and expectations associated with positions that are assigned by sex in social organizations within society, such as the family, for example, wife, mother, aunt, sister. These norms and expectations also may or may not differ by ethnic group and may or may not parallel gender-role norms and expectations. Thus, for example, gender-role expectations may differ for black and white women (e.g., black women are seen as strong, white women as delicate), while mother role expectations may not (mothers are nurturant and caring, whatever their race). In this context, lesbian families, in particular, may provide some fascinating opportunities to study interrelationships among gender and motherhood roles for women.

Sex role stereotypes are stereotypes about the characteristics of individuals holding particular sex roles; for example, mothers are nurturant, daughters obedient. Women's sex-role stereotypes (e.g., wives make sure their husbands have clean shirts, mothers take care of babies that are sick) overlap feminine gender-role stereotypes, but are not necessarily identical (e.g., women are incompetent). *Gender role stereotypes* are a subset of sex-role stereotypes; they are the stereotypes that apply to gender role. Thus, the feminine gender-role stereotype is that women are nurturant whether or not they are engaged in other sex roles; that is, women should like and nurture babies even if they are not themselves mothers.

We thus differ from the prevailing literature in that we emphasize woman's feminine gender role as but one of a number of social roles assigned to the female sex, for example, wife and mother. Confusion in the literature has partially stemmed from the double use of the term *sex role* to refer both to the overarching category as well as to the subset of the social roles within the category. People appear to have difficulty maintaining distinctions among concepts without separate labels for them (witness the problems that have resulted from the double use of the word *man*). Thus, we will use the phrase *sex roles* to refer to the overarching category; *gender role* will refer to the feminine and masculine gender roles for women and men that are based on the position of their gender in society. Other sex roles that are social roles assigned by sex in social organizations within society, such as the family, will be designated by the name of the specific role (e.g., mother role) or by the organization to which they are tied (e.g., family sex roles). Family sex roles include marital roles (wife/husband), parental roles (mother/father), offspring roles (daughter/son), and kin roles (aunt/uncle). Differential sex-role expectations for offspring become increasingly salient in our aging society as daughters differentially assume the burden of caring for aged parents. The differential contributions of gender-role expectations (women are caretakers, not men) versus sex-role expectations (physically caring for parents is part of the daughter role, financially providing for them part of the son role) to the stress and strain of having elder parents have yet to be fully determined. In the United States, sex roles are largely confined to the family; assignment of most work roles by sex is now illegal. Nonetheless, it is still legal to assign some occupational roles on the basis of sex, for example, actress, dancer, model, and athlete in most (not all) sports. The persistence of occupational segregation attests to the existence of de facto sex roles in the workplace, however.

Women's social roles are interrelated. Gender-role socialization overlaps with socialization for other sex roles (particularly motherhood socialization). We suspect that socialization into women's multiple sex roles does not diverge at least until gender constancy is established, if not later. We also suspect that they diverge earlier for boys than girls; boys can be lots of things besides being fathers, but little girls go for a long time equating being a woman (gender role) with being a mother (family sex role). Some women have internalized a traditional "motherhood mandate" (Russo, 1976) for women's gender role, however, and if they are infertile, they report feeling "damaged" (Mazor, 1984; McGrath et al., 1990).

Distinguishing gender role from other sex roles is important here because it has implications for women's mental health and for intervention in the development of psychopathology. If characteristics and behaviors associated with work and family sex roles change (perhaps divergently) faster than gender-role socialization, coping skills may be undermined. Expectations among sex roles may conflict—for example, women's feminine gender role may be expected to be deferent and passive, while mothers are expected aggressively to defend their children—and such conflicts may undermine women's well-being and increase their risk for psychopathology. Further, women's family sex roles often rest on reciprocity and division of labor (particularly the marital roles of wife/husband and parental roles of mother/father). Thus, it is difficult to change one without disturbance in others. Change in the mother role is particularly complicated, as it is related to the roles of both father and child. Our review of the literature on the mental health risk factors associated with work and family roles suggests that stress associated with the sex role of mother is more important than the wife role in understanding symptoms of psychopathology that are found in married women (see chapter 18, this volume).

The remainder of this chapter summarizes selected recent research related to women's mental health. We first summarize epidemiological findings on gender differences in patterns of mental disorder, with particular attention to differences in patterns by race/ethnicity and marital roles. The next section provides additional information on high prevalence disorders for women: mood, anxiety, and eating disorders. Then, using a stress and coping perspective, we examine risk factors contributing to women's excess in psychopathology associated with reproductive events over women's life cycle. We only briefly touch on women's work and family roles in these discussions, as they are considered in another chapter in this book (see chapter 18). It is hoped that this selective summary of research findings will stimulate new research as well as facilitate the changes that are occurring in psychological education, training, and practice.

THE EPIDEMIOLOGICAL PICTURE

Large and complex gender differences in patterns of mental health disorder continue to be found in community surveys and in service delivery statistics.

Prevalence of Psychological Disorder

There are substantial gender differences in patterns of mental disorder; whether or not women are at higher risk for mental disorder than men is the subject of debate. In large part it depends on whether or not one believes that alcohol and drug abuse should be defined as mental disorders (Gove, 1980). Even then, to date there has been no comprehensive comparative assessment of the mental health of men and women.

The initial reports of the NIMH Epidemiological Catchment Area (ECA) Program presented data on prevalence of mental disorder in the noninstitutionalized population (18 years of age and older) in three ECA sites (Robins et al., 1984). This research does not present a full estimate of the prevalence of mental disorder. All adult disorders covered by the *Diagnostic and Statistical Manual, 3rd Edition* (DSM-III; American Psychiatric Association, 1987) were not covered in the Diagnostic Interview Schedule (DIS) used in the study. Further, only major categories were covered for some disorders. Multiple diagnosis was possible. Thus, totaling the rates of disorder for each gender to make conclusions about gender differences in overall prevalence rates is not appropriate, particularly when generalized anxiety disorder and posttraumatic stress disorder were not included in the original 15 DIS disorders studied. Unfortunately, the articles and press releases that accompanied the initial publication of this work (Myers et al., 1984; Robins et al., 1984) have led to the impression that there are no gender differences in mental disorder, and this impression has been perpetuated in the literature (e.g., Cleary, 1987). Whether or not this conclusion is accurate has yet to be appropriately documented.

The ECA research does provide information on prevalence of the major categories of disorder, however. Gender differences in lifetime prevalence were found for the majority of the 15 diagnoses that were assessed in samples from all three of the initial sites of the study: New Haven, Baltimore, and St. Louis.

The lifetime diagnoses with highest rates were alcohol abuse/dependence, phobia, drug abuse and dependence, major depressive episode, dysthymia, antisocial personality, and obsessive-compulsive disorder. Phobia was the most variable, ranging from 8 to 9% of individuals in New Haven and St. Louis to 23% in Baltimore. Alcohol abuse/dependence affected 11–16% of individuals; drug abuse, 5–7%; major depressive episode, 4–7%. Dysthymia, antisocial personality, and obsessive-compulsive disorder all affected from 2 to 4% of individuals.

Less frequent disorders, affecting from 1 to 2%, included schizophrenia, panic, and severe cognitive impairment. Manic episode affected .6–1.1% of individuals. Schizophreniform disorder, somatization, and anorexia did not exceed .3% of individuals at any site.

Gender Differences

Rates of major depressive disorder, simple phobia, and agoraphobia were significantly higher for women than men in all three sites. Women's rates ranged from 4.3 to 1.8 times those of men for these diagnoses.

Rates of dysthymia, obsessive-compulsive disorder, panic disorder, schizophrenia, and somatization disorder were significantly higher in women in at least one site. Rates ranged from 3.5 to 1.1 times those of men. In all sites, the rates for women were higher than the rates for men, even though the differences did not always attain statistical significance.

Insufficient proportions of individuals were diagnosed with anorexia to assess gender differences. However, evidence from other research has documented significant gender differences in eating disorders. Among hospitalized patients, the ratio of female to male anorexics is 8:1; for the population in general, the estimated ratio is 15:1 (Travis, 1988b, p. 140).

No gender differences in manic episode or cognitive impairment were apparent, and insufficient numbers prohibited assessment of gender differences in schizophreniform disorder.

Rates of alcohol abuse/dependence and antisocial personality were significantly higher for men than women in all three sites. For these diagnoses, men's rates ranged from 7.8 to 4.0 times those of women's. Drug abuse/dependence was significantly higher for men in two sites, men's rates ranging from 1.9 to 1.3 times those of women.

Thus, for the 15 diagnoses discussed above, there is evidence for gender differences in prevalence rates in 12 of them. Myers et al. (1984) reported that patterns of gender differences for six-month prevalence rates were similar to those of lifetime prevalence rates. Unfortunately, variation in gender differences by race were not reported in either study.

Although press releases from NIMH have emphasized the lack of gender differences in overall rates of disorder (Russo, 1985), the apparent equality in the disorders studied stems largely from men's high rate of diagnosis for substance abuse disorders, particularly alcohol abuse/dependence disorders. It may also reflect the lack of inclusion of other anxiety disorders in the research.

This chapter will focus on women's excess in mental disorder and thus will not discuss alcohol and drug disorders in detail. A recent review of the literature can be found in Travis (1988b). Two things should be remembered, however. First, simply because there is a gender difference in the rate of a disorder does not mean that the disorder does not have a significant impact on the mental health of the gender with the lower rate. For example, women have lower rates of alcohol and drug disorders than men. However, in the ECA rates for New Haven, for example, the percentages of women with alcohol and drug disorders (4.8% and 5.1%, respectively) were higher than the percentages of women with dysthymia (3.7%), obsessive-compulsive (3.1%), panic (2.1%), and somatization disorder (.3%). Second, important gender differences may be related to other aspects of a disorder than merely rate. For example, women heroin addicts have shorter addict careers, enter treatment earlier than men, and are more influenced by their partners. Women appear to seek treatment, comply with treatment regimens, and then fail to maintain abstinence (Hser, Anglin & Booth, 1987). This research suggests that treatment regimens for drug disorders should go beyond a focus on intrapsychic gender-related attributes and consider gender- and sex-role dynamics.

In any case, it is clear from the data that achieving significant advances in mental health research will require understanding the relationship among gender, gender- and sex-role dynamics, and mental health. Attempts to downplay the importance of gender by pointing to alleged equality of rates of mental disorder have been sadly misguided. Understanding the complex ways that gender and its correlates affect mental health is a fundamental challenge to mental health researchers and a necessary condition for improving the mental health of the U.S. population. Its significance cannot be understated.

Service Utilization

In 1980, females predominated in admissions to outpatient facilities (Russo & Sobel, 1981; Russo & Olmedo, 1983). They were also a greater proportion of admissions to inpatient facilities in nonfederal general hospitals and private mental hospitals. In contrast, men predominated in admission to state and county mental hospitals and Veterans Administration hospitals (Russo, Amaro, & Winter, 1987; Mowbray & Benedek, 1988).

Gender differences in service utilization statistics point to social and cultural variables as potent mental health influences. Use of facilities obviously does not solely reflect prevalence and incidence of mental disorder. Gender and ethnic differences in such things as help seeking, diagnostic practices, and treatment can also contribute to gender differences in utilization statistics. Gender differences in such data vary with type of facility and reveal the importance to diagnosis and service delivery of understanding the relationship between social and cultural factors associated with gender, marital roles and status, and ethnicity.

Gender, Marital Status, Ethnicity

Gender makes a difference depending on marital role and ethnicity. Service delivery data reveal never-married and separated/divorced men had higher overall admission rates to mental health facilities than women in the same marital status categories. In contrast, women with marital sex roles (i.e., married women) had higher admission rates than men with marital roles (Russo & Sobel, 1981; Russo et al., 1987). This finding is widely known and contrasts with findings from community surveys that report a gender difference in symptomatology, regardless of marital status, with women reporting more symptoms than men (Aneshensel, Frerichs & Clark, 1981; Cleary & Mechanic, 1983; Kessler & McRae, 1981, 1982).

When inpatient admission rates are examined more closely, however, the discrepancies become better understood: effects of gender and marital status vary with ethnicity and psychological disorder. Russo et al. (1987) found, for inpatients diagnosed with affective disorders in 1980 (now classified as mood disorders in the 1987 revision of the DSM-III (DSM-III-R), that women had a higher risk for such disorders, regardless of marital status. In contrast, men had higher rates of alcohol disorders, regardless of marital status (Russo et al., 1987).

Marital role was also important for inpatients diagnosed with schizophrenia, where there were higher admission rates for married women compared with married men. Gender had a reverse effect in other marital status categories, where men's rates were higher than women's.

When non-Hispanics and Hispanics were compared (note: members of both categories may be of any race), the above overall findings held for non-Hispanics, but Hispanics showed a different pattern. Hispanic men had higher admission rates in nearly every one of the three diagnostic groupings examined, regardless of marital status. There were two important exceptions: Hispanic women diagnosed with affective disorders had higher rates than Hispanic men in both married and never-married categories. Thus, for affective disorders, the gender differences among married and never-married are similar for Hispanics and non-Hispanics.

Parallel analyses are not available for African-American women at this time. However, for combined inpatient and outpatient 1975 admission data, men had higher admission rates than women in all marital status categories except for married, where women's rates were higher. This pattern held for both whites and blacks (Russo & Sobel, 1981). How these figures would vary with diagnosis is unknown. Because depressive disorders were the leading diagnosis for women of either racial grouping, it is likely that the overall pattern reflects the pattern for that diagnosis.

Unfortunately, such statistics do not identify parental status. Some authors have suggested that women's excess in affective disorder is due entirely to their childbearing rather than gender roles or gender-related attributes (Gater, Dean & Morris, 1989).

Three points are particularly important here. First, non-Hispanic whites are the largest patient subpopulation, and affective disorders are the most prevalent diagnostic category. Global summaries of epidemiological data can mask important interaction effects by gender, ethnicity, and diagnosis. Research that explores the effects of ethnicity may particularly profit from exploring the differential mental health effects of gender-related attributes and sex and gender roles across ethnic groups.

Second, measurement issues require investigation. The findings from community surveys, which often rely on measures sensitive to affective distress, parallel the global treatment statistics for affective disorders. Epidemiological analyses must become more detailed and sensitive to methodological limitations if they are not to be Eurocentric and misleading. Ultimately, understanding utilization of mental health services requires sophisticated research approaches that simultaneously consider effects of gender and race/ethnicity in a biopsychosocial context over the life cycle.

Finally, as Russo (1984) has pointed out, interactive effects of gender, race, and age on the most frequently diagnosed types of disorders may reflect the paradoxical effects of gender stereotyping: women are both overrepresented and underserved as a treatment population. Disorders that are congruent with society's view of "femininity" (e.g., anxiety, depression) show higher rates of treatment. In treatments for disorders that are incongruent with society's idealized view of "femininity" (e.g., alcoholism), women have been invisible and neglected. To what extent congruence between expectations about women's gender and sex roles and definition of mental disorder affects diagnosis and treatment judgments needs to be thoroughly explored. Among other things such congruence may reflect overpathologizing (inappropriately perceiving patients whose behavior violates norms as more disturbed), overdiagnosis (inappropriately applying a diagnosis as a function of group membership), and underdiagnosis (inappropriately avoiding application of a diagnosis as a function of group membership) (Lopez, 1989).

In a classic study, Rosenfield (1982) reported a greater probability of hospitalization for diagnoses inconsistent with gender-role stereotypes. More recent evidence for overpathologizing by psychologists has been found in the cases of men diagnosed with major depression and women diagnosed with antisocial personality or alcohol abuse disorders. Case history descriptions of such individuals were rated as more severely disturbed and more likely to elicit recommendations for drug treatment than individuals of the opposite sex receiving similar diagnoses (Waisberg & Page, 1988). Male psychiatrists' overdiagnosis of women as depressed was found in clinical judgments of a case description of undifferentiated schizophrenia with a dependent personality disorder. This bias was found whether or not the patient was described as black or white. Female psychiatrists did not exhibit this bias toward a diagnosis of depression for women patients of either race, although they did have a tendency to diagnose white female patients as having a brief reactive psychosis (Loring & Powell, 1988). Underdiagnosis has been a particular concern for women who abuse alcohol and drugs (Russo, 1985).

Women receive prescriptions for psychotropic drugs at a higher rate than men, for a variety of reasons, including gender differences in age, physical illnesses, psychiatric disorders, help seeking that leads to exposure to the medical system (which results in more prescriptions), and stressful life events (for a more complete discussion, see Travis, 1988b). Both excessive and inappropriate drug treatment continue to be major issues, particularly for older women (Russo, 1985). Waisberg and Page (1988) found that female patients were associated with stronger recommendations for drug treatment in all diagnostic categories except depression, where male patients were associated with stronger recommendations for drug treatment. A tendency to misdiagnose other disorders in women as depression may lead to inappropiate treatment; drugs that are appropriate to treat major depression are not necessarily effective in treating other disorders.

This brief epidemiological picture points to both the complexity and the psychosocial nature of the relationships among gender, ethnicity, marital status, and mental health. Gender differences in mental disorder are associated with age, race/ethnicity, marital roles, parental roles, and economic status, whether identified by community surveys or research on service utilization (Mowbray & Benedek, 1988). Narrow intrapsychic or biological approaches are not sufficient to achieve understanding of the etiology, diagnosis, treatment, and prevention of mental disorders in women. Further, the overlapping of symptoms of psychopathology with gender stereotypes makes misdiagnosis a substantial concern (Russo, 1984, 1985; McGrath et al., 1990).

HIGH PREVALENCE DISORDERS FOR WOMEN: MOOD AND ANXIETY DISORDERS

Mood and anxiety disorders are heterogeneous diagnostic categories in the DSM-III-R that often involve overlapping symptomatology. A variety of summary scales currently in use assess the presence of depressive symptoms such as crying, feelings of sadness and unhappiness, and eating and sleep disorders. High levels of depressive symptoms have been found in 20–25% of community samples (Kaplan, Roberts, Camacho & Coyne, 1987). Such symptoms of depression may reflect sadness, hopelessness, demoralization, and physical conditions as well as a variety of psychiatric disorders, including those classified as anxiety disorders (Weissman & Myers, 1980; Weissman, Leaf, & Bruce, 1987). Misdiagnosis of posttraumatic stress due to rape or battering as clinical depression is of particular concern (McGrath et al., 1990).

A number of researchers have suggested that the largest gender differences in such symptomatology are found for less severe symptoms (Clark, Aneshensel, Frerichs & Morgan, 1981; Craig & Van Natta, 1979). Thus, as Newmann (1984) has pointed out, gender differences found in research using summary scales may be misleading, since summary scales do not separate milder forms of distress, such as as sadness, from more severe psychiatric disorder. Issues related to definition and measurement of subtypes of depression that also apply to anxiety disorders can be found in McGrath et al. (1990).

Hamilton, Gallant, and Lloyd (1989) suggest that mood changes associated with the menstrual cycle may also contribute to elevations in women's symptom levels, particularly for research using the Center for Epidemiological Studies Depression scale (CES-D), which substantially overlaps with the Menstrual Distress Questionnaire (Moos, 1986).

Interestingly, research by Golding (1988) found that gender differences on the CES-D among a community sample of white women reflected an excess of extreme scorers among women rather than a difference in the distribution of depressive symptomatology between women and men. In examining the variables that contributed to the gender differences in score, she unfortunately did not distinguish between gender role, sex role, and gender-related attributes and life circumstances. She appeared to equate gender with unspecified gender-related attributes. The data appeared to rule out the effects of such attributes once gender-related life circumstances were controlled, which would suggest that menstrual cycle effects made a minimal contribution to elevations in women's depression scores. Unfortunately, by lumping marital status (married/not married), employment status, age, job status, education, and income under a concept of "demographic disadvantage," separating the effects of sex and gender roles and associated life circumstances is not possible.

Depression

The gender differences in rate of major depression and dysthymia identified above represent one of the most consistent findings in the literature: women are at higher risk for depression. Depression represents such a significant threat to women's mental health that the American Psychological Association (APA) established a President's Task Force to study risk factors and treatment issues in women's depression. The report of that task force summarizes research on risk factors and treatment related to depression in women (McGrath et al., 1990). Selected findings from the report are described below.

Women's higher risk for depression holds whether one looks at case records or community surveys (Ensel, 1982; Goldman & Ravid, 1980; Nolen-Hoeksema, 1987, 1990; Radloff, 1975; Weissman & Klerman, 1977, 1985; Weissman, Leaf, Holzer, Myers & Tischler, 1984), is found for white, black, and Hispanic women (Russo & Sobel, 1981; Russo et al., 1987), and is not explained by gender differences in willingness to report symptoms or help seeking (Nolen-Hoeksema, 1987, 1990; Weissman & Klerman, 1977, 1985).

Sets of symptoms that are persistent are defined as depressive syndromes (some of which have become defined as disorders). It should not be assumed that depression varies along a single continuum from common symptoms to major depression. Depressions differ in kind and severity. Different depressive syndromes may have different precursors (Hamilton, 1988). Psychological and/or pharmacological treatments that have been based on clinical trials for major depression may be totally inappropriate for treatment of depressive symptoms (Weissman & Myers, 1980; Weissman et al., 1987).

Although there is some evidence for continuity between depressive symptoms and the syndromes of clinical depression (Akiskal, 1987; Weissman, Myers, Thompson & Belanger, 1986), whether or not depressive symptoms signal higher risk for depression is not known. Depressive symptomatology correlates with other precursors to clinical depression. Indeed, Brown and colleagues (1986) reported that preclinical depressive symptoms had no increased risk for subsequent clinical depression after low self-esteem and stressful life events were controlled.

In reviewing these issues, APA's task force observed that interest in clinical major depression should not result in lack of research and therapeutic attention to less severe forms of depression. Approximately half of high scorers on self-report measures appear clinically impaired (Link & Dohrenwend, 1980). Further, depressive symptomatology does not necessarily reflect a minor or transitory state (Kaplan et al., 1987). Sadness, depressed mood, and other depressive symptoms themselves reflect suffering, whether or not they are risk factors for onset of a major depression.

Major depression and dysthymia are classified as depressive disorders, which are, in turn, classified along with "bipolar disorders" under the category "mood disorders" in the DSM-III-R (American Psychiatric Association, 1987). Descriptions of the most relevant diagnostic categories for women as they appear in DSM-III-R can be found in the APA task force report. Depressive-related subtypes recognized in the DSM-III-R include major (unipolar) depression, dysthymia, bipolar adjustment disorder with depressed mood, organic mood disorder, and the controversial schizoaffective disorder. In particular, the proposed category late luteal phase dysphoric disorder, which is found in the appendix of DSM-III-R, has been a focus of feminist opposition (for discussion of the controversy, see Gallant & Hamilton, 1988).

Gender differences have not been substantiated for all depressive subtypes (Nolen-Hoeksema, 1987, 1990). Women are at greater risk for major depression (Boyd & Weissman, 1981; Nolen-Hoeksema, 1987; O'Connell & Mayo, 1988; Robins et al., 1984; Weissman & Klerman, 1985) and for dysthymia (Weissman et al., 1984; Robins et al., 1984), but there is no evidence of greater risk for bipolar disorder. Thus, women's excess in affective disorder appears to be largely due to greater risk of unipolar depressions.

The DSM-III-R is a basic reference for diagnosing depression, and a substantial amount of research rests on DSM diagnostic definitions. But it should be recognized that diagnostic definitions change with time and, like most human concepts, reflect the values, visions, purposes, and limited wisdom of the individuals who create them. There is a lack of consensus about definitions of depression-related diagnostic categories, particularly the proposed category late luteal phase dysphoric disorder.

Hamilton and her colleagues (1984) have identified other categories of novel subtypes for which women appear to have higher risk: "atypical depression" (characterized by hypersomnia, hyperphagia, and increased libido; Klein, Gittelman, Quitkin & Rifken, 1980; Quitkin, Steward & McGrath, 1988); rapid-cycling bipolar illness (defined as having four or more affective episodes a year; Parry, 1989); and seasonal affective disorder (marked by changes in symptoms in response to seasonal changes such as decreased sunlight; Jacobsen et al., 1987).

No one theory or set of theories fully explains gender differences in depression. Current theories of women's depression span biological, psychological, social, and cultural variables (Herman, 1983; Klerman & Weissman, 1985a, 1985b; Nolen-Hoeksema, 1987, 1990). The task force report contains detailed discussion and lengthy bibliography on research relating to risk factors for women's depression, including psychological attributes as well as work and family roles, poverty, and violence. Both greater exposure to stressful life events and lack of access to coping resources (personal, social, and economic) appear to contribute to women's excess in depression (McGrath et al., 1990).

Anxiety Disorders

The ECA studies reported above identified women as having a higher risk for simple phobia, agoraphobia, obsessive-compulsive disorder, and panic disorder. These are classified as anxiety disorders by the DSM-III-R. The common features for this category are symptoms of anxiety and avoidance behavior. Although simple phobia is most frequently found in the general population, panic disorder is most commonly found among people seeking treatment (American Psychiatric Association, 1987). Perhaps as a consequence, individuals with panic disorder have been found to be the highest users of psychotropic drugs, particularly the minor tranquilizers (Weissman & Merikangas, 1986).

Having one anxiety disorder increases the probability of having others. In one study, over 30% of individuals with phobias also had experienced a panic disorder. Over 80% of individuals with a generalized anxiety disorder had at least one other anxiety disorder (Weissman & Merikangas, 1986). In addition to panic disorder (with and without agoraphobia), agoraphobia (without history of panic disorder), obsessive-compulsive disorder, and simple phobia, this category also includes social phobia, posttraumatic stress disorder, and generalized anxiety disorder. Related disorders include adjustment disorder with anxious mood, eating disorders, dream anxiety disorder, organic anxiety disorder, and avoidant personality disorder.

More needs to be learned about risk factors for anxiety disorders. It has been suggested that loss of social support and disruption of interpersonal relationships are risk factors for panic disorder (American Psychiatric Association, 1987). Similarly, Weissman et al. (1987) found that panic disorders were higher among single mothers than married mothers, for both black and white women. Interestingly, those researchers also reported that married mothers had higher risk for obsessive-compulsive disorder than single mothers. This was particularly true for black married mothers, whose rates exceeded those of black single mothers by nearly 7 to 1. The comparable figure for white mothers was nearly 3 to 1. These findings suggest that risk factors may differ for subtypes of anxiety disorders.

Agoraphobic women exhibit extreme forms of personal attributes associated with the feminine gender role, including helplessness, overdependency, and passivity (Chambless, 1982; Mathews, Gelder & Johnston, 1981). Haimo and Blitman (1985) point out, however, that a discussion solely focusing on an excess in feminine gender-related attributes is incomplete. Lack of instrumentality (an attribute associated with the masculine gender role) also characterizes agoraphobics. They document changes in the instrumentality of agoraphobic women as a result of assertiveness training.

Symptoms of anxiety disorders are correlated with other disorders, complicating diagnosis. For example, the symptoms of posttraumatic stress syndrome overlap with depression, including depressed mood, sleep and appetite disturbance, social withdrawal, lowered self-esteem, psychomotor retardation or agitation (American Psychiatric Association, 1987). Research that clarifies the relationships among symptoms of depression and anxiety disorders is clearly needed. Taken together, these symptoms constitute a large proportion of women's excess in psychopathology.

Both anxiety and depressive diagnoses are also correlated with personality disorders (for a more complete discussion of the implications of this overlap, see McGrath et al., 1990). Misdiagnosis may account for some of that overlap, and possible misdiagnosis of women who have experienced physical and sexual abuse is a particular concern. It has been estimated that, depending on the sample, up to 72% of psychiatric inpatients have histories of physical or sexual abuse (Carmen & Rieker, 1989). Bryer et al. (1987) found that childhood physical and sexual abuse and suicidal symptoms were associated with a high proportion of borderline personality diagnoses. Thus, a number of authors have argued for using posttraumatic stress syndrome as the initial diagnosis for abused patients rather than a personality disorder (Gelinas, 1983; Van der Kolk, 1988; Van der Kolk, Herman & Perry 1987).

Eating Disorders

Eating disorders are characterized by gross disturbances in eating behavior (American Psychiatric Association, 1987). Although anorexia and bulimia nervosa are distinct diagnoses, they can be related, and they typically begin in adolescence or early adulthood. Since 1980 bulimia has been distinguished from anorexia in the DSM-III.

The essential features of anorexia nervosa as defined by the DSM-III-R are distorted body image, refusal to maintain body weight at a normal level, intense fear of gaining weight or becoming fat, even though underweight, and, in females, amenorrhea (p. 65). Weight loss in excess of 15% of normal body weight has been an arbitrary guideline for alerting professionals to anorexia in their patients.

In contrast, bulimia nervosa is characterized by a "binge-purge" cycle, in which there are recurrent episodes of consuming large amounts of food and then "purging" them by extreme methods such as self-induced vomiting, laxative and diuretic abuse, excessive exercise, or fasting. Purging may or may not be a symptom of anorexia nervosa. The typical bulimic woman is of normal body weight, though she perceives herself as being overweight.

Both anorexia and bulimia are associated with other major psychological disorders, such as depression, anxiety, obsessive-compulsive disorder, and substance abuse disorder (Hinz & Williamson, 1987; Pyle et al., 1983; Wooley & Wooley, 1981). In particular, patients diagnosed with anorexia often have strong family histories of major depression and are themselves depressed (Cantwell et al., 1977; Winokur, March & Mendels, 1980). (For a description of behaviors associated with anorexia and bulimia, see Travis, 1988b.)

The gender difference in both of these disorders is clearly pronounced. Approximately 90% of all people suffering from either bulimia or anorexia nervosa are women (Halmi, Falk & Schwartz, 1981; Katzman, Wolchik, & Braver, 1984; Pope, Hudson, Yurgelun-Todd, & Hudson, 1984; Striegel-Moore, Silberstein, & Rodin, 1986). Although the estimated prevalence of eating disorders in the population is not high, ranging from 1 to 5% of all women (Pyle et al., 1983; Cooper & Fairburn, 1983; Hsu, 1983), the past two decades have witnessed a rapid increase in the number of reported cases of eating disorders.

Bulimia rates, in particular, appear to be rapidly increasing. Shisslak et al. (1987) reported that the incidence of bulimia in college women tripled between 1980 and 1983, suggesting gender roles in late adolescence/early adulthood need investigation. Dykens and Gerrard (1986) estimate that in college women the incidence of bulimia may be as high as 13%–20%. Further, work roles with a large gender-related component (some actually assigned by sex) may be a factor. Women in professions with sex roles such as modeling, dance, sports, and acting, in which thinness is also mandated, are also at higher risk for anorexia and bulimia (Garner & Garfinkel, 1980; Striegel-Moore et al., 1986). Treatment rates also vary by geography, with hospitalization rates in the north central states three times those in the South and West (Travis, 1988b). Travis (1988b) provides a more detailed discussion of eating disorders.

The accuracy of prevalence estimates for eating disorders has been subject to debate. Estimates vary considerably depending on the criteria used for diagnosis. Assessing bulimia is especially problematical, as researchers have not agreed on definitions for such central concepts as what constitutes a binge (e.g., number of calories versus duration of eating) or how to document frequency of binging and purging. Compounding these difficulties are the reluctance of many bulimic women to report their behaviors and the inaccuracy of self-report measures (Boskind-White & White, 1987; Dykens & Gerrard, 1986; Wilson, 1987). Again, distinctions between symptoms and disorders need to be made. In a discussion of methodological issues in bulimia treatment outcome research, Wilson (1987) argues that change in bulimic behavior alone is insufficient for evaluating improvement; changes in body image disturbance, feelings of self-efficacy, nutrition, and eating patterns must also be assessed. Research has provided some evidence that there are differences in pathology associated with increasing severity of the eating disorders (Mintz & Betz, 1988; Striegel-Moore et al., 1986). Research is needed that continues to address these definitional, diagnostic, and treatment issues, including the relationship of disordered eating to specific classes of stressful life events, such as sexual assault (Root, 1991).

There are class as well as gender differences in eating disorders, which typically involve women who are young, middle and upper class, and white. Some researchers have even gone so far as to call eating disorders a "culture-bound" syndrome, that is, a syndrome specific to a culture and one in which cultural factors play an important etiological role (Nasser, 1988). Many authors have pointed to Western culture's increasingly thin standards for female beauty and accompanying stigmatization of obesity as important factors explaining the rapid increase in rates of eating disorders (Boskind-White & White, 1987; Garner & Garfinkel, 1980; Striegel-Moore et al., 1986).

Rodin, Silberstein, and Striegel-Moore (1985) suggest that dieting and weight concerns have become so pervasive in Western society as to be considered normative for women (Polivy & Herman, 1985; Pyle et al., 1983; Wooley & Wooley, 1985). A study by Mintz and Betz (1988) found that in their sample of 682 college women, only one-third could be characterized as "normal eaters"; 82% reported one or more dieting behaviors daily, and another third reported using laxatives, vomiting, or fasting as a weight control measure one or more times a month. Dietary restraint is considered to be a central risk factor for the development and maintenance of eating disorders (Polivy & Herman, 1985; Davis, Freeman & Garner, 1988).

Even if dieting behaviors are the norm, which this evidence certainly suggests is true, the question remains as to why only a minority of U.S. women, mostly white women, develop clinical eating disorders in response to sociocultural pressures for thinness. In this regard, self-esteem and perceived control are once again implicated in the development of gender differences in psychological disorder (Travis, 1988b). It has even been suggested that the self-esteem of females with eating disorders rests on approval of others and adherence to social ideals, with a tenuous balance between self-regard and social confirmation that results in an other-directedness so extreme that bodily needs can be more readily ignored (Travis, 1988b, pp. 151–152). The fact that bulimia is more likely to be found in white women suggests that the social ideals are tied to the gender role of white women in society, one that differs from that of black women in ways that have etiological significance.

An other-directed sense of self-esteem and locus of control in the context of a diet-oriented culture may thus be the disastrous combination for women's mental health. Bulimic women are found to be more likely to endorse such statements as "Thin is beautiful" and to have internalized these standards to a greater extent than other women (Rodin, Silberstein & Striegel-Moore, 1985). Further, there is some evidence suggesting that bulimic women have overendorsed a stereotypical gender role in which physical beauty, defined in white women's terms, has been a central component (Brownmiller, 1984). Other theorists suggest that women with eating disorders, as perfectionists, view the feminine ideal as being a "superwoman," involving both traditionally masculine and feminine gender roles. Research utilizing measures such as the Bem's Sex Role Inventory has typically not found that bulimics are more likely to be feminine gender-typed, however (Dunn & Ondercin, 1981; Lewis & Johnson, 1985). This discrepancy suggests that research focusing on perceptions of gender roles rather than gender-related attributes or sex roles might be particularly illuminating.

In addition to examining the contribution of sociocultural factors to risk for eating disorders, a number of theories have attempted to explain eating disorders in terms of such factors as personality disturbance (Katzman & Wolchik, 1984), social impairment (Norman & Herzog, 1984; Johnson & Berndt, 1983; Herzog et al., 1987), family systems theory (Minuchin, 1974; Shisslak et al., 1987; Strober & Humphrey, 1987), and biological disturbances (Hinz & Williamson, 1987; Lee, Rush & Mitchell, 1985). Unfortunately, no one of these theories seems to address fully the complicated etiological questions that are central to understanding, treating, and preventing eating disorders. Further, explanations of eating disorders must not ignore the dynamics of gender roles that appear so central to the development of pathological eating behaviors.

UNDERSTANDING WOMEN'S EXCESS IN PSYCHOLOGICAL DISTRESS AND DISORDER

As the Subpanel on the Mental Health of Women of the President's Commission on Mental Health observed, "Circumstances and conditions that American society has come to accept as normal or ordinary lead to profound unhappiness, anguish, and mental illness in women. Marriage, family relationships, pregnancy, childrearing, divorce, work and aging all have a powerful impact on the well-being of women. . . . Compounding these ordinary events, women are also subject to some extraordinary experiences such as rape, marital violence, and incest, which leave them vulnerable to mental illness" (Subpanel, 1978, p. 1038). More than a decade later, these observations are confirmed in research that links mental health to sex and gender roles and gender-related life circumstances such as violence and poverty.

A Stress and Coping Perspective

Approaches to understanding women's excess in psychological distress and disorder can be placed in four categories: (1) person-centered (focuses on women's vulnerability or resistance to disorder due to biological or psychological characteristics that make women more or less responsive to stressful life events); (2) situation-centered (focuses on stressors or coping resources related to women's sex roles and life circumstances); (3) interactionist (examines interrelationships between the first two, including women's perceptions and cognitions of events and internal and external coping resources to deal with them); and (4) methodological (explains excess as artifact of such things as measurement, sampling, lack of appropriate controls, or bias in diagnosis).

Although an interactionist research perspective is the ideal, most research has traditionally fallen into either category 1 or 2. Hopefully, future research will aim for models that are interactionist in nature, controlling for methodological biases.

Genetic factors have been directly implicated in a variety of mental disorders. However, there is no evidence that such direct action operates differently for men and women, and thus seeking to explain women's excess in mental disorder by genetic factors does not appear promising (McGrath et al., 1990). Thus, they will not be discussed in this chapter.

A framework that includes both stress and coping provides a useful interactionist model for conceptualizing the conditions that contribute to increased risk for such mental disorders for women. A stress and coping framework considers events in context and examines the interaction of sources of stress, coping resources, coping strategies, and social support, all of which may involve physical, psychological, social, or environmental factors. This perspective reflects the broader shift in mental health research that has documented the mental health impact of daily hassles and chronic stress as well as major negative life events (Kessler, Price & Wortman, 1985; Thoits, 1987b, 1987c).

Life Events and Life Crises

As we have seen above, stress has been found to precipitate anxiety and mood disorders—disorders with a clear excess for women compared with men (see also Thoits, 1984, 1987a, 1987c; Brown & Harris, 1978). Negative life events and life crises are one reason for women's higher rates of distress and disorder. Evidence suggests that women experience stressful life events more often than men (Aneshensel et al., 1981; Cleary & Mechanic, 1983; Gore & Mangione, 1983). Women are more likely to experience social isolation, absence of a spouse, economic hardship, and chronic health problems (Newmann, 1986; Belle, 1990). Women report significantly more exposure to death than do men (Kessler & McLeod, 1984).

In 1988, nearly 100,000 women experienced forcible rape. Over 90% of rape victims are women. Child sexual abuse is a fact of life for both black and white women (Wyatt, 1985). Sexual assault and abuse have been experienced by 38–67% of adult women; approximately 31% of married women report violence in their recent relationships (Koss, 1990). Unwanted pregnancy continues to be common. In addition to the 1.5–1.6 million abortions that occur each year, an estimated 7% of all births are unwanted (i.e., born to women who did not want a(nother) child at that particular time or at any future time) (David, Dytrych, Matejcek, & Schüller (1988). Thus, reproductive-related life events and work and family roles all contribute to risk factors for mental health problems in women over the life cycle.

As Zautra, Reich, and Guarnaccia (1989) observe, different stressful life events pose different adaptive challenges, such that personal attributes that enhance coping in one scenario may be irrelevant to others. This may be particularly true for negative life events more likely to be experienced by women. For example, control-enhancing internal attributions may have negative effects on the mental health of rape victims through undermining their self-esteem (Koss & Burkhart, 1989; Wyatt, Notgrass, & Newcomb, 1990). The differential adaptive challenges posed by gender-related life events have yet to be articulated, but some evidence suggests that attitudes toward women's roles will moderate them (Kristiansen & Giulietti, 1990).

Women's Response to Stressful Life Events

Exposure to stressors is not sufficient to produce mental disorder, however (Kessler et al., 1985; Thoits, 1983, 1987c). Recent research has focused on identifying the variables, internal and external, that separate individuals who develop mental health problems in response to negative life events and life crises from those who do not.

To avoid stereotyping, we prefer the term *risk factors* rather than *vulnerability factors* to designate such variables. Given the congruence between the label *vulnerability* and women's stereotypical gender role, special care should be taken to avoid stereotyping and to explore causal dynamics. Congruence with stereotypes has all too often led to uncritical acceptance of theories and research results. Thus *vulnerable* is not a desirable label when discussing research findings related to gender.

In this vein, researchers have begun to examine the gender differences in responsiveness and resistance to stress (Kessler, 1979a, 1979b; Kessler et al., 1985). Some research has suggested that given equal exposure to stressors, women are more likely than men to report distress or seek help (Cronkite & Moos, 1985; Thoits, 1982, 1984). Such findings have been used to suggest a gender difference in women's responsiveness to negative life events compared with men's. However, Kessler, McLeod, and Wethington (1984) reported that women's greater level of responsiveness was not found in all types of events, but generally reflected those involving "network crises that have the capacity to provoke distress through the creation of empathic concern" (Kessler et al., 1985, p. 538).

Research has yet to fully explain gender differences in responsiveness to stress. Nonetheless, the stress of caring for others appears to be a crucial factor in the mental health gender gap found for married people (Belle, 1982b; Kessler & McLeod, 1984; Thoits, 1986, 1987a, 1987b, 1987c). It has been postulated that female sex-role socialization results in the development of maladaptive personal attributes and styles of coping that contribute to risk for psychopathology in response to stress (Abramson & Andrews, 1982; Kessler, 1979a; Kessler & McLeod, 1984; Kessler et al., 1984; Nolen-Hoeksema, 1987; Radloff & Rae, 1981). In some of these formulations, women are seen as having a psychic "cost of caring" due to their psychological orientation toward other people.

Expressiveness, Instrumentality, and the Cost of Caring

Does the gender-related personality trait of expressiveness (i.e., orientation toward, and concern for, others; Spence, Helmreich & Stapp, 1974) correlate with levels of psychopathology? Several reviews of research have reported that this is not the case. It is instrumentality—that is, a sense of agency or mastery— not concern with others, that significantly correlates with measures of well-being or symptomatology in the majority of research studies. Most measures of mental health used in this research have emphasized anxiety and affective and soma- toform disorders. It may be that by definition such disorders reflect a lack of mastery, autonomy, efficacy, or competence. Most of this research is conducted on college populations and deals with symptomatology rather than psychiatric disorder, however.

It may be that gender role—which for women means lack of power and the normative expectation that women should always respond to the needs of others— is more important than the gender-related psychological trait of expressiveness in the development of psychopathology. Snodgrass (1985) reports that interper- sonal sensitivity is an interactive process, more related to the status than the gender of individuals (although gender has also been conceptualized as a status variable). It may also be that the trait of expressiveness will not correlate with psychopathology unless a provoking agent, such as relationship loss, occurs (Brown & Harris, 1978).

Another possibility is that women's orientation toward others puts them at higher risk for psychopathology due to effects of shame (Lewis, 1976). Wright, O'Leary, and Balkin (1989) found shame to be more strongly related to depressive symptomatology than guilt, for both women and men. Although they did not find a gender difference in levels of shame in their sample, their research was based on a college student population. The concept of shame may be very different in college women compared with women in the general population. The effects of social support on the contribution of shame to women's psycho- pathology are a promising area of study. The role of shame is particularly important to understand because of its possible implications for treatment. If guilt is contributing to the problem, sharing the information with a therapist would be expected to have cathartic effects, and an active therapeutic stance is not necessarily needed. If shame is the underlying factor, exposure of shame experiences may make the client "only feel worse" unless the therapist takes an active stance and communicates "positive regard" to the client (Wright et al., 1989, p. 229).

Instrumentality, Mastery, and Perceived Control

Instrumentality, mastery, and perceived control—the obverse of powerlessness—have been positively associated with health and well-being and negatively associated with psychopathology (see Bassoff & Glass, 1982; Thomas & Reznikoff, 1984; Whitely, 1985, for reviews; also see Horwitz & White, 1987; Marsh & Weary, 1989; Seaman & Seaman, 1983; Warren & McEachren, 1983; Weary, Elbin & Hill, 1987; Weary, Jordan & Hill, 1985).

Women who are lower in instrumentality, mastery, and/or perceived control may also be more likely to have both helplessness expectancies (i.e., the expectation that outcomes are not controllable) and negative outcome expectancies (i.e., not being able to attain highly valued outcomes or to avoid aversive outcomes). These are postulated to combine to create hopelessness, which leads to depression in response to negative life events (Abramson, Metalsky & Alloy, 1989). The interrelationships between gender and sex roles, and expectancies of helplessless and hopelessness have yet to be explored systematically.

Instrumentality and its related concepts are predictive of self-esteem, which is clearly an important factor in psychopathology, particularly depression. Brown and Harris (1978) suggested a model that includes both risk factors and provoking agents, arguing that the presence of a risk factor does not in itself increase the risk for depression in the absence of a provoking agent. In their model, low self-esteem establishes a predisposition for depression (Brown, Bifulco, Harris & Bridge, 1986), with life events interacting to increase risk (e.g., lack of an intimate relationship with husband, the presence of three or more children aged 14 or under at home, lack of paid employment) (Brown & Prudo, 1981; Campbell, Cope & Teasdale, 1983). Unfortunately, the research does not include male participants so that contributors to excess in women's psychopathology cannot be identified. Assessment of the mental health outcomes of interaction of gender-related attributes with sex and gender-role provoking agents is a promising research area.

Attributes such as instrumentality, mastery, and perceived control may be most effectively conceptualized as moderating variables in an interactionist framework. As Reich and Zautra (1990) point out, however, the concept of perceived control is multidimensional, and perceived control beliefs are themselves influenced by life events, positive and negative. Although overall beliefs about personal control are predictive of behaviors in response to stress, assessment of control beliefs about specific classes of outcomes, such as health, increases prediction (Wallston & Wallston, 1978; Wallston, Wallston, & DeVellis, 1978). A lowered sense of personal control has been found to be associated with poorer self-health ratings, less self-initiated health care, less optimism regarding the efficacy of early treatment, and greater use of the health care system, including more dependence on the physician. Further, these associations were stronger for women compared with men (Seaman & Seaman, 1983). Exploration of how control beliefs that specifically pertain to sex- and gender-role domains relate to coping with stress and expression of psychopathology would be an important extension of this research.

For example, Reich and Zautra (1990) suggest that social support is differentially related to symptomatology in individuals low in internal control compared with individuals high in internal control. This finding comes from longitudinal research on older subjects (the majority of them female), in which research participants received a control-enhancement intervention, a placebo manipulation that involved social contact with a friendly investigator, or no contact. The mental health of high internals improved in the control-enhancement condition; the mental health of low internals improved in the social contact condition.

These findings support the work of Hobfoll (1986a, 1986b), who has proposed a model of ecological congruence to predict the effectiveness of specific resources to buffer the effects of stressful life events. In Hobfoll's model, resource effectiveness is situation-dependent and is related to personal and cultural values, time since the event, and stage in the individual's development, among other things. Lazarus and Folkman (1984) also consider the fit between coping resources and situational demands, but their work has a greater focus on cognitive resources than Hobfoll's model does. Because stress and coping are thus situation-specific, study of specific types of events is needed to assess matching stressful event, resource, and situation. This model suggests that lack of congruence among gender-related attributes, attitudes, and values of the person, the meanings of the coping responses (to the person as well as the person's reference groups), and the expected consequences and meaning of coping processes may contribute to increased risk of psychopathology in women (see Hobfoll, 1986a, for reviews of literature related to women's stress and social support).

In studying gender-related differences in social support, however, it will be important to separate the contribution of gender-related attributes (e.g., expressiveness, nurturance) and the qualities of women's feminine gender, wife, and mother roles. The fact that women's roles are characterized by lack of access to instrumental resources and sex segregation of activities at home and at work continues to be a hallmark of U.S. society (irrespective of women's personal attributes related to instrumentality or related qualities) and should be incorporated in models that seek to understand gender differences in social support.

Coping Processes

More research is needed on the mechanisms by which instrumentality may mediate or moderate women's responses to stressful life events (McGrath et al., 1990). One possibility is that it interacts with a tendency to make internal, stable, and global explanations for negative events (i.e., with a pessimistic explanatory style), which in turn affects coping mechanisms (Brewin, 1985; Sweeney, Anderson & Bailey, 1986; Seligman et al., 1988). One study (Baucom & Danker-Brown, 1984) reported that high-instrumental women were more likely than low-instrumental women to use self-protective attributional patterns to enhance their egos—they attributed success to ability and effort, and failure to task difficulty. Indeed, for low-instrumental women, failure impaired subsequent task performance, while success did not affect it. For high-instrumental women, success facilitated performance on subsequent tasks; failure did not.

Similarly, Wortman and Brehm (1975) have pointed out that learned helplessness does not always lead to depression in response to negative life events, suggesting that whether or not a person responds with helplessness or reactance (i.e., desire to regain control) to such events depends on control expectations. In a recent study using a college sample, Marsh and Weary (1989) explored the relationship between depression and attributional complexity (i.e., motivation to make attributions, preference for complex explanations over simple ones, and higher awareness of the power of situational influences in determining behavior). Attributional complexity was considered to indicate a desire to regain control through seeking of social information. Marsh and Weary found that mildly and moderately depressed individuals (i.e., those with higher expectations for control) had higher attributional complexity scores compared with severely depressed (i.e., those with lower expectations for control) or nondepressed individuals, regardless of sex. Further, women were both more attributionally complex and more depressed than their male peers. This work is interesting because it suggests that perceived control and orientation toward others (via attributional complexity) may work together to moderate depression. More research is needed before causal dynamics are understood, however. The finding of women's higher attributional complexity is not surprising given that women have a feminine gender role of lower status and power. Attributional complexity in women thus reflects both a situation-specific need to regain control as well as the need for lower-status individuals to monitor situations more closely. It may be that the lower status of women's feminine gender role contributes to other factors that contribute to risk for depression (e.g., lowered self-esteem). Marsh and Weary (1989) used a sample of college students, and their approach would appear to be likely to tap into gender roles in this population. How attributional complexity and perceived control relate to depression in the context of wife and mother roles should also be studied. Unfortunately, unless age and marital status are controlled in studies using college populations, they may be comparing depression scores of reentry mothers with those of young adult males, so that gender- and sex-role expectations for the two groups are not parallel.

Depressed men and women have been found to be more likely to use emotion-focused responses and less likely to use problem-solving coping responses in response to stressful life events (Billings, Cronkite, & Moos, 1983). Nolen-Hoeksema (1987) further argued that gender differences in depression may be due to women's ruminative response styles, which amplify and prolong depressive episodes, in contrast to men's active response styles, which dampen depressive episodes. Women's ruminative response set may interfere with instrumental behavior, increasing failure and feelings of helplessness. It may also increase the likelihood that an individual will develop depressive explanations for his or her depression and increase the accessibility of negative memories. Males do appear less likely than females to recall depressive symptomatology (Angst & Dobler-Mikola, 1983).

Self-Disclosure as Protection from Psychopathology

Newmann (1986) reviewed evidence to assess the relative contributions of psychological attributes versus greater exposure to stressful life events to women's higher risk for depression. She found that, indeed, women had greater exposure to stressful life events, but women were no more vulnerable to developing depressive syndrome than were men after exposure to stress was controlled. There was a gender difference in reporting depressive symptoms that were unrelated to depressive syndrome, but that was related to age and marital role. Young married women reported higher levels of sadness than men or never-married women. It is not clear how this expression of sadness relates to risk for the development of depression. A gender difference in the normal expression of feelings may reflect sex- or gender-role expectations or simply be a gender-related attribute that is not related to clinical depression.

Further, as Newmann (1984) observed, "The capacity to experience and express feelings of sadness in the face of loss or disappointment is generally viewed as a mark of mental health and may be an effective deterrent to the development of more severe symptomatology" (p. 137). Self-disclosure may directly provide catharsis or indirectly elicit more effective social support.

Before a causal attribution for the excess in women's mental health problems is made to gender-related psychological characteristics, however, it must be recognized that "responsivity" and "vulnerability" are labels that are used to describe unexplained variance in differences in symptom levels for women and men (Thoits, 1987c). They are not explanations for those differences. Further, caring and nurturing are central aspects of women's gender, gender role, and the sex roles of wife and mother. Are women more responsive because of a gender-related psychological trait, such as nurturance? Or are they more responsive because they are fulfilling gender-role expectations about women held by themselves or by others, for example, that women should be nurturant, warm, and caring? Or are they responding to sex-role expectations held by themselves or others related to their roles as wife, mother, daughter, sister, or aunt? Or perhaps all of the above? Systematic research from a stress and coping perspective has potential for answering these questions.

Again, we use the term *responsive* rather than *vulnerable* for a reason. The use of the label *responsive* recognizes the fact that women have shown greater responsivity than men to both positive and negative life events (Cronkite & Moos, 1985; Thoits, 1987c). It also avoids the gender stereotypes of women as weak, delicate, and helpless (Cronkite & Moos, 1985).

The female excess in psychopathology begins to appear in adolescence (Horwitz & White, 1987; Kandel & Davies, 1982; Nolen-Hoeksema, 1990) and changes developmentally in complex ways (Abrahams, Feldman & Nash, 1978; Cunningham & Antill, 1984; Feldman, Biringen, & Nash, 1981; Horwitz & White, 1987; Puglisi, 1983; Flett, Vredenburg & Pliner, 1985). Given that adolescence and young adulthood are major formative periods in the development of adult gender- and sex-role identities, adolescence is a particularly interesting developmental period for research on the origins of women's excess in psychopathology.

In conceptualizing causal dynamics in the development of gender differences in psychopathology, it is important to recognize that personal attributes such as instrumentality, perceived control, and self-esteem may be both a cause and a consequence of stressful life events (Hamilton & Abramson, 1983). Kessler et al. (1985) summarize methodological and conceptual issues in research on life events, life stress, and life crises. Both longitudinal and experimental research designs that are based on transactional models will be needed for causal dynamics to be more fully understood. Even then, mental health problems themselves can also be both a cause and a consequence of stressful life events such as unwanted pregnancy, marital disruption, and job loss. It is not possible to explore all of the stress-related life events associated with women's work and family roles (see chapter 18, this volume, for further discussion). However, in the remainder of this chapter we do focus on two classes of life events related to women's bodies: physical and sexual abuse and reproductive-related events.

PHYSICAL AND SEXUAL ABUSE

Issues related to physical and sexual abuse are discussed elsewhere in this book, and a number of reviews of the empirical literature are available (Koss, 1990; Browne & Finkelhor, 1986). Nonetheless, a chapter discussing women's mental health would be incomplete without drawing attention to the pervasive mental health impact of such experiences (McGrath et al., 1990). A recent analysis of ECA data from Los Angeles compared risk for selected mental disorder for individuals reporting an experience of sexual assault (includes childhood sexual abuse) in their lifetime and for individuals who did not. Sexual assault experiences contributed to increased risk for major depressive episode, substance use disorders, and the three anxiety disorders studied: phobia, panic, and obsessive-compulsive disorder. Nearly 18% of sexually assaulted individuals were found to meet criteria for major depressive episode, compared with 5% of nonassaulted individuals. For drug abuse, the figures were 20% versus 6% for assaulted versus nonassaulted individuals; for phobia, 22% versus 10%; for panic disorder, 6% versus 1%; for obsessive-compulsive disorder, 5% versus 1%.

With variables associated with onset before assault controlled, it was found that the risk ratio for assaulted versus nonassaulted individuals ranged from 4 to 1 for phobia, panic disorder, and obsessive-compulsive disorder and from 2.3–2.5 to 1 for drug abuse/dependence, major depression, and alcohol abuse/ dependence. Gender, Hispanic background, and education were not related to the overall probability of developing a disorder after abuse experiences. Thus, although sexual assault contributes to women's higher rates of mental disorder, it appears it is because women are more likely to have assault experiences, not because they are more "vulnerable" to mental disorder than assaulted men after such experiences.

There was a gender difference in risk for only one specific disorder studied: sexually assaulted men were more likely subsequently to develop alcohol abuse/ dependence disorder than women. No relationship was found between onset after sexual assault and the other disorders studied (mania, schizophreniform disorder, and antisocial personality) (Burnam et al., 1988).

In that study, assault in childhood was associated with higher risk for subsequent disorder than assault in adulthood. It is clear that child sexual abuse has widespread and long-lasting mental health effects for both women and men. Reactions of victims of sexual abuse include aggression, anxiety, depression, fear, hostility, and sexually inappropriate behavior. Long-term effects have been empirically documented and include anxiety, depression, feelings of isolation and stigma, low self-esteem, impairment of ability to trust others, self-destructive behavior, substance abuse, and sexual maladjustment. Browne and Finkelhor (1986) provide a review of the empirical literature on the impact of child sexual abuse.

Although a history of sexual abuse in childhood increased risk for psychopathology in adulthood, not all victims of sexual abuse exhibit severe mental health problems. Abuse by fathers or stepfathers, genital contact, and use of force have been associated with more severe impairment of the victim (Browne & Finkelhor, 1986). Carmen and Rieker (1989) provide an insightful model of the victim-to-patient process in which the damage to the self caused by sexual abuse begins a variety of psychological and social processes that may result in a variety of forms of mental illness. They point to the overlapping symptoms of posttraumatic stress disorder with borderline and multiple personality diagnoses as well, diagnoses not included in the ECA study. They also report knowledge of cases of anorexia with histories of sexual abuse. They creatively link the damaged self of sexual abuse victims to AIDS risk in adolescent runaway, homeless, and mentally ill populations, providing recommendations for clinical interventions. Their model is particularly interesting because it relates the psychopathology generated by the abuse experience to elements of the social context, including ongoing family relationships, that disconfirm and transform the abuse in destructive ways.

Their work is a rich source of hypotheses for future research. It also provides insights into the processes that might underlie Gold's (1986) finding that sexually abused women had more pessimistic attributional styles than nonvictims. More specifically, they were more likely to attribute negative events to internal, stable, global factors, blame themselves for negative events and attribute positive events to external factors. They were also less likely to blame other people for negative events. Although causal relationships could not be determined, attributional style was related to low self-esteem, psychological distress, and depression in these victims.

REPRODUCTIVE-RELATED EVENTS

Reproductive life events are a normal part of women's lives and relate uniquely to women's biology. They are critical to a feminist perspective, as women's biology is so often used to justify women's disadvantaged social, economic, and political status. They also offer superb examples of the need for biopsychosocial models of stress and coping, point to the importance of distinguishing between acute and chronic sources of stress, and underscore the importance of viewing women as active agents in the stress and coping process.

Reproductive-related events—including menstruation, pregnancy and child-birth, and menopause—are stressful life events for women, and fluctuations in women's hormones do not explain responses to them. Mood and behavior changes correlated with reproductive events occur for both women and men, and neuroendocrine response is altered by social roles, status, and other socio-cultural variables (Hamilton, 1984).

There has yet to be widespread, systematic application of a stress and coping model that incorporates a combination of gender-related biological, psycholog-ical, and social factors in examining the implications of these events for women's risk for psychopathology. Such a model would recognize that meanings and outcomes of reproductive-related events are socially constructed and that the link between the biological variables and mental health outcomes depends on the psychosocial context. It would also seek to account for the fact that moods and behaviors often remain stable despite substantial changes in hormones and neu-rotransmitters (McGrath et al., 1990).

Most research has focused on the relationship of reproductive-related events to psychological distress and affective disorders. The report of the APA Task Force on Women's Depression of the American Psychological Association (McGrath et al., 1990) provides a recent review of the literature on reproductive-related events and women's depression.

Responses to reproductive events are intercorrelated, suggesting that risk fac-tors and personal and social coping resources for such events are interrelated. Premenstrual changes have been correlated with symptoms of depression post-partum (Brockington & Kumar, 1982; Hamilton, 1984; Stout, Steege, Blazer & George, 1986). Prenatal depression is correlated with postpartum depression (Buesching, Glasser & Frate, 1986). Reactions to reproductive-related events over the life cycle may reflect a lifetime history of major affective disorder (Hamilton, Parry & Blumenthal, 1988a).

Menstruation

In the framework of the APA Task Force on Women's Depression that is used here, menstruation is classified under the rubric *reproductive-related events* (McGrath et al., 1990). The use of *related* in this label is in keeping with the concerns of the Society for Menstrual Cycle Research, which has maintained "that reproduction is but one aspect of this pervasive female experience" and has resisted the definition of menstrual phenomena as "reproductive" (Dan & Leppa, 1988, p. 143).

Significant mood and behavior changes are associated with the menstrual cycle for some, although not all, women. Common symptoms include anxiety, depression, hostility, irritability, somatic symptoms, and changes in sleep, appetite, energy, and libido. Hamilton, Parry, and Blumenthal (1988a, 1988b) and Travis (1988a) provide excellent reviews of this literature. An estimated 1 in 20 women experience severe premenstrual symptoms, and from 20 to 80% of women report mild to minimal premenstrual mood or somatic changes. Premenstrual symptoms appear in adolescence, but have their highest prevalence in the late twenties and early thirties and may continue to occur even after ovaries have ceased to function (Hamilton et al., 1988a).

Greene and Dalton (1953) proposed the term *premenstrual syndrome* (PMS) to describe the somatic, affective, and behavior changes experienced during the latter part of the menstrual cycle. However, there is heterogeneity in the set of symptoms that women report under the label PMS, and there is substantial controversy over whether PMS is a unitary concept. Richardson (1990) discusses the current status of research on PMS and conceptual and methodological controversies associated with it.

Clarification of the definition and diagnosis of premenstrual syndrome continues to be needed (Logue & Moos, 1986; Gallant & Hamilton, 1988; Richardson, 1990; Schnurr, 1988). Schnurr (1988) suggested that up to 50% of women reporting premenstrual syndrome may not meet diagnostic criteria. Further, women with "false" premenstrual syndrome were twice as likely to have a history of psychiatric disorder (DeJong et al., 1985).

A cyclic mood disorder may operate independently from the menstrual cycle in which cycles of affective symptoms and menstruation overlap and then disassociate (Hamilton et al., 1988a). Premenstrual mood changes have been associated with history of affective disorder (Endicott et al., 1981; Hamilton et al., 1985; Logue & Moos, 1986). Many of the symptoms that lead women to seek help from a PMS clinic mirror presenting symptoms for major psychological disorder, suggesting misdiagnosis of psychiatric disorder as PMS as an important concern. Stout et al. (1986) compared a sample of women from a premenstrual syndrome (PMS) clinic with a community sample, finding that the clinic group was significantly more likely to meet DSM-III-R criteria for lifetime psychiatric disorder for several major disorders, including phobia, dysthymia, and alcohol and drug dependence.

Risk factors for PMS have not been clearly identified. Friedman and Jaffe (1985) found that housewives reported more symptoms than employed women and that level of education was negatively correlated with number of symptoms reported. In contrast, Schnurr (1988) found employed women were more likely to report PMS. Some researchers have found that menstrual symptoms increase with age (Logue & Moos, 1986), while others report the opposite effect (Schnurr, 1988). This may reflect reporting differences by age: one study reported that older women appeared to experience more symptoms (but not report them), while younger women did tend to report them (Timonen & Procope, 1973). It may also reflect methodological differences among the studies.

More research is needed on the relationship between menstrual symptoms and sex and gender roles. Slade and Jenner (1980) found that the extremes of both positive and negative attitude toward traditional gender roles were associated with higher levels of menstrual symptoms. They suggest that higher rates of menstrual symptoms among traditional women may reflect their comfort with a sick role while higher rates of such symptoms among egalitarian women may reflect stress from role conflict. Their results could also reflect a general response bias on the part of depressed individuals, however. Clarification of risk factors as they are associated with gender-related attributes and women's social roles is clearly needed.

Although biological explanations of the causes of PMS are common, few researchers have attempted to test biopsychosocial models of PMS in which the interaction of biological and psychosocial variables is taken into account (Brooks-Gunn, 1986). Gallant and Hamilton (1988) suggest that to better understand PMS and its effects, researchers must utilize more complex biopsychosocial models that take into account such variables as individual beliefs and expectancies, demographic factors, and possible positive effects.

Menstrual cycle research is difficult and complex. It has been influenced by cultural attitudes and beliefs, confounded occasional and recurrent symptoms, focused on negative symptomatology, relied on retrospective reports, failed to disguise the purpose of the research, neglected to include male control groups, and used instruments of questionable reliability and validity (for a more complete discussion of methodological limitations and issues, see Travis, 1988a). Richardson (1990) provides a recent review and critique of questionnaires used to study paramenstrual symptomatology that contains a lengthy bibliography. Among his conclusions is reassurance that women's retrospective reports of their experienced premenstrual symptoms are reliable and accurate. However, his review did not include an important study that found that only 20–50% of women who retrospectively report premenstrual complaints were actually observed to have such complaints when daily reports are kept (Hamilton et al., 1985). Similarly, McFarlane, Martin, and Williams (1988), who compared concurrent and retrospective measures of mood fluctuation in a sample of women and men, found a retrospective reporting bias. They discovered that although women did not exhibit the stereotypic "menstrual mood pattern" in daily reports, it did appear when the data for the same days were gathered retrospectively. Moods fluctuated more during the week than over the menstrual cycle, and women's moods were not less stable than those of men, either within a day or day-to-day.

Another problem in menstrual cycle research is that typical measures of menstrual symptoms often fail to distinguish between number and severity of symptoms. Busch, Costa, Whitehead, and Heller (1988) note that many measures obscure possible effects of severity by relying only on reports of the number of symptoms. They found that severity of symptoms was a reliable measure of the level of distress experienced and was a significant predictor of absenteeism among working women.

Pregnancy and Childbirth

Pregnancy is associated with a low incidence of psychiatric disorders, which may reflect selection (mentally healthy women may be more likely to have partners and become pregnant), coping resources (partners may be more supportive during pregnancy), or differential diagnosis (practitioners may be less likely to label a pregnant women as having a psychiatric disorder).

Hamilton et al. (1988a) point out that the relative lack of psychiatric disorder during pregnancy, despite elevated levels of steroid hormones, contrasts with the changes in symptoms that sometimes occur with cyclic hormonal elevations. They suggest that these differences may reflect adaptations in gonadal steroid receptor functioning. A focus on gonadal steroids, such as androgen, which are found in both men and women, is needed to counterbalance a research bias in the literature toward steroids of primarily ovarian origin, particularly estrogen (Hamilton, 1984). Gender-comparative research is required to ascertain if there are, indeed, specific clinical correlates of biological changes at childbirth.

Pregnancy, whether it is resolved by childbirth or abortion, can be viewed as a stressful life event and thus can lead to an exacerbation of problems for women with histories of mental health problems (Adler & Dolcini, 1986). Problems in pregnancy most often occur in women who have a history of such disorders (Hamilton et al., 1988a). The appropriateness of a biopsychosocial stress and coping model, rather than one that focuses solely on biological changes in pregnancy, is indicated in the findings that pregnancy and delivery are associated with bipolar and psychotic illness in women's partners (Hamilton, 1984; Freeman, 1951; Towne & Afterman, 1955).

Hobfoll and Leiberman (1987) tested Hobfoll's stress and coping model to compare women's emotional response to normal delivery, miscarriage (spontaneous abortion), and delivery by cesarean section and preterm delivery, at the time of the event and three months later. Although all of these events involve acute stress, preterm delivery was also seen as involving the chronic stress of coping with a preterm infant and was thus predicted to have longer-term effects than the other three groups. Indeed, although there was no significant difference in depression among the groups at time one, the group-by-time interaction effect was significant. The spontaneous abortion and cesarean-section acute-stress groups decreased more on depression than the preterm chronic stress or the normal delivery (considered baseline stress) groups. This points to the importance of separating acute from chronic sources of stress involved with reproductive-related events.

High self-esteem was found to be a personal resource associated with lower depressive symptomatology at both times of measurement for all groups. Intimacy with spouse was associated with lowered symptomatology at the time of the event, but not later. Hobfoll and Leiberman suggest that high self-esteem is a transituational personal resource always available for women having it, while spouse support was viewed as dependent on situational demands and constraints.

Intimate violence is a common experience for women and recognized as destructive to women's physical and mental health. Recent reviews of this literature are available (Koss, 1990; McGrath et al., 1990; see also chapter 13, this volume). Although the issue of intimate violence in pregnancy has been recognized for more than a decade (Gelles, 1975), the contribution of such violence to low self-esteem and other symptoms of psychopathology before, during, and after pregnancy has yet to be adequately investigated. Hilliard (1985) reported that 11% of the pregnant women in a sample obtained from an obstetric clinic had a history of physical abuse. Stark et al. (1979, 1981) reported that pregnant battered women were more likely to have a history of psychosocial problems; a substantial proportion of these battered women (29%) reported escalation of violence during pregnancy. These researchers also suggest that battering during pregnancy is associated with a higher risk for spontaneous abortion, which is also a source of acute stress for women. Stacey and Shupe (1983) reported that 42% of their sample of women entering shelters for battered women said they had been battered during pregnancy, with reported injuries being slaps, kicks, and punches to genitals and abdomen. They suggest that the violence was directed at the fetus as well as the woman.

Abuse must be studied in context and may be correlated with different high-risk behaviors in different samples. For example, in a study of adolescent mothers, Amaro and her colleagues (1989) found that adolescents who used illicit drugs during pregnancy were more than twice as likely to be exposed to physical abuse than were pregnant adolescents who did not use drugs (24% compared with 9%). This difference was significant when maternal race and age were controlled as well. Pregnant adolescent drug users were also more likely to be North American black (as opposed to foreign-born), have a history of venereal disease and of elective abortion, and report more negative life events (violent and nonviolent) (Amaro, Zuckerman & Cabral, 1989). The link between violence and reproductive-related events is clearly an underresearched area of critical importance.

The rising prevalence of AIDS among women is also a critical mental health issue, particularly for ethnic minority women. Women are 7% of individuals diagnosed with AIDS; 70% of those women are ethnic minority (black, white, and Hispanic women comprise 49%, 30%, and 20% of women with AIDS, respectively). A larger percentage of women diagnosed with AIDS have died of the disease compared with men, regardless of ethnic group (Fullilove, 1988).

The link between pregnancy and intravenous (IV) drug abuse is a new and insidious source of chronic reproductive-related stress. In 1988, 80%, 74%, and 52% of AIDS cases among Hispanic, black, and white women, respectively, were IV drug-related. That year black and Hispanic children accounted for 55% and 20% of pediatric AIDS cases, respectively (Selik, Castro & Pappaioanou, 1988). Meanwhile, their proportions in the U.S. population that year were only 15% and 11% (U.S. Bureau of the Census, 1989). Intravenous drug use by pregnant women was implicated in 72%, 62%, and 31% of pediatric AIDS cases among Hispanic, black, and white children, respectively (Selik et al., 1988). The mental health implications of AIDS in pregnant women have yet to be fully assessed, but must be included in the efforts of researchers, service providers, and policymakers as they attempt to deal with the staggering psychological, social, and societal consequences of AIDS and its related diseases.

Postpartum illness may resemble several major categories of psychiatric disorder, including depression, mania, delirium, organic syndromes, and schizophrenia. "Baby blues" (i.e., mild postpartum dysphoria) is distinguished from severe postpartum depression by the severity and frequency of symptoms, timing of the course of the disorder, and epidemiology. The illness, which is reported in between 39–85% of women, occurs about the third or fourth day after delivery, and lasts from one to two days to one to two weeks. Severe postpartum depression occurs in about 10% of women, may occur from six weeks to three to four months after delivery, and can last from six months to a year (Hamilton et al., 1988a; O'Hara, Zekowski, Phillips & Wright, 1990).

Stern and Kruckman (1983) conducted a cross-cultural study of postpartum depression that supports the conception of postpartum depression as socially constructed. They suggest that postpartum depression in the United States may reflect a lack of social support for the women's transition to her motherhood role and a lack of social structuring during the postpartum period.

Although there has been substantial research devoted to examination of biological contributors to postpartum depression, little research has investigated gender- and sex-role variables that contribute to a positive or negative postpartum experience. Three psychosocial variables have been consistently associated with postpartum depression: cognitive vulnerability (Cutrona, 1983; O'Hara, Rehm & Campbell, 1982), marital role dissatisfaction (Cox, Connor & Kendell, 1982; Paykel, Emms, Fletcher & Rassaby, 1980), and stressful life events during pregnancy and immediately postpartum (O'Hara, Neunaber & Zekoski, 1984; Paykel et al., 1980). Whiffen (1988b) assessed the impact of these variables on postpartum depression in a prospective study. Prepartum marital tension and depressive symptomatology significantly predicted postpartum depressive symptomatology. Negative life events also significantly predicted postpartum depressive symptomatology.

Whiffen (1988a) also reported that mothers' perceptions of their infants as "difficult" were positively correlated with depression. Such perceptions may be a result of depressed mood. However, research is needed to assess whether mothers who are prone to depression are more likely to have infants who cry more and are more temperamental, thus creating a source of stress that results in depressive symptomatology. Perceiving the infant as difficult was most strongly related to depression if the mother had expressed optimistic expectations about the child's behavior before birth. Lack of congruence between expectancies and outcomes may be particularly stressful for new mothers. Researchers have linked postpartum depression to stress related to transition to motherhood role (Cutrona, 1983; O'Hara et al., 1984).

Abortion

In 1988, 1.6 million abortions were performed in the United States (Henshaw & Van Vort, 1990). Emotional responses after abortion have been the subject of investigation by countless researchers. As Schwartz (1986) observed, a 1981 review of the literature identified more than 1,000 articles, in the English language alone, on psychological and social consequences of abortion. Unfortunately, much of the research on emotional consequences of abortion has been based on clinical samples, conducted with inadequate methodology, and has focused on negative consequences. Although there is a myth that severe guilt and depression often result from abortion, this is not substantiated in the scientific literature (Adler et al., 1990; Schwartz, 1986).

Schwartz (1986) identified 32 systematic and scientifically sound studies on the psychological consequences of abortion. Psychiatric problems were rare, 1–2% in most studies where preexisting history was controlled. Previous psychiatric history and pressure to have an abortion (against own judgment or religious beliefs) were found to be risk factors for serious psychiatric responses that did occur.

A recent in-depth review of the well-controlled empirical studies conducted in the United States documents the relatively minor risks of abortion to women's psychological well-being (Adler et al., 1990). That review found that the predominant response to an abortion experience is relief. Feelings of guilt, depression, and regret may also be experienced after the procedure, but they are typically mild and transitory and do not affect general functioning (Adler, 1975a, 1975b; Adler & Dolcini, 1986; Belsey et al., 1977; David, Rasmussen & Holst,

1981; Ewing & Rouse, 1973; E. W. Freeman, 1977; Marecek, 1986; Shusterman, 1979).

Adler (1975) identified three clusters of emotions after abortion. One cluster was based on positive emotions such as relief and happiness. The other two were based on negative emotions. One of them was internally based, including anxiety, depression, regret, doubt, and anger; the other was socially based, including shame, guilt, and fear of disapproval. The positive emotions were experienced much more strongly than the negative emotions (3.96 on a 4-point scale for positive emotions, compared with 2.26 and 1.81 for internally based and socially based emotions, respectively).

Abortion's relative risk of mental disorder compared with other reproductive-related events has yet to be fully ascertained. Wilmoth and Adelstein (1988) attempted to review the pertinent literature to develop a portrait of the relative risks of abortion, childbirth (with and without adoption), miscarriage, single motherhood, and other medical procedures. They found a deplorable paucity of research on women's reproductive lives, but concluded from their examination of the existing literature that abortion held no more risks for depression than other significant life events, including childbirth.

One U.S. study did compare women who experienced early abortion, late abortion, or term delivery (Athanasiou, Oppel, Michelson, Unger, & Yager, 1973). Those authors concluded that compared with term births, abortion was a "benign procedure . . . psychologically and physically" (p. 231). A comparison of risk of postabortion psychosis and postpartum psychosis in England yielded an estimate of 0.3 psychoses per 1,000 legal abortions compared with 1.7 psychoses per 1,000 deliveries (Brewer, 1977). David et al. (1981) examined first admissions to psychiatric hospitals three months postpartum or postabortion for all women under 50 years of age in Denmark. First-admission risk was low and similar for abortions and deliveries, 12 per 10,000 compared with 7 per 10,000 women, respectively, for all women of reproductive age. The importance of the situational context is seen in the elevated risk for admission for separated, divorced, and widowed women having abortions or carrying to term (64 versus 17 per 10,000 women, respectively). The authors suggest that the higher risk for such women may reflect original intendedness of the pregnancy. The low first-admission rate found, despite the stressful conditions of marital disruption, suggests that in a social context accepting of sexuality and contraceptive use and tolerant of reproductive choices, neither abortion nor delivery poses substantial risk for severe psychopathology.

Adler and her colleagues suggest that women's emotional responses after abortion can best be understood in a stress and coping framework. Although the abortion experience per se does not appear to be a significant risk factor for psychopathology, some women are at higher risk for emotional responses after an unwanted pregnancy that is terminated by abortion. Risk factors include a history of emotional disturbance, not expecting to cope well with the abortion, feeling coerced to have the abortion, difficulty in deciding to have an abortion, termination of a pregnancy that was originally wanted, abortion in the second trimester of pregnancy, self-blame for the unwanted pregnancy, and limited or no social support (Adler et al., 1990).

Major and her colleagues (Major et al., 1990) used a stress and coping model to examine the relationships among self-efficacy for coping, perceived social support, and women's adjustment after first-trimester abortion. Source of support made a difference. Women who told their families and received support were less depressed and anticipated fewer negative responses than other women. However, women who told supportive partners were not different from those women who did not tell them; these two groups, however, were significantly less depressed than women who told partners who were not supportive. It may be that women were more selective in telling their families, doing so only when they anticipated support. In contrast, they may have felt obligated to tell their partner, whether or not his support was anticipated. The authors suggest that the presence of negative supportive transactions might be more important than the absence of positive support transactions in determining adjustment for stressful life events. If so, policies that mandate a woman's informing others about her abortion decisions without regard to their reaction to her may undermine women's mental health. This work also suggests that stress and coping models must conceptualize individuals as active agents, who seek to manage stress by selecting alternatives that are perceived as less stressful and that more closely match their coping resources.

Major and her colleagues also found that the effect of social support was indirect: it enhanced adjustment through its impact on women's self-efficacy for coping. In a follow-up study, Mueller and Major (1989) used an experimental design to evaluate a counseling intervention aimed at enhancing self-efficacy for coping and lowering self-blame for the pregnancy. Women who received the self-efficacy intervention were less depressed after the abortion than women who received the attribution intervention, and both groups were less depressed than the control group, which received the standard abortion counseling session. This study causally links perceived self-efficacy to mental health outcome of abortion and suggests that interventions oriented to promote self-efficacy may have preventative effects.

This pattern of findings supports an ecological congruence model of stress and coping such as that of Hobfoll (1986a, 1986b) and suggests that emotional response to abortion (as well as other reproductive-related life events) may differ across groups (e.g., ethnic or religious groups) that hold differential attitudes toward abortion and whose members vary in access to economic and psychosocial coping resources. Researchers who examine such responses cross-culturally should be wary of cultural stereotyping. For example, even among low-income and relatively unacculturated Mexican American women, Amaro (1988) found great heterogeneity in attitudes toward reproductive-related events, including abortion. Her findings contrast with the stereotype found in the literature of Mexican American women as passive and "content in having many babies and in not undertaking an extended education or participating in the labor force" (Andrade, 1982, p. 225).

Research has typically sought to identify negative abortion outcomes. Positive psychological outcomes have not been fully assessed, although they might have implications for understanding women's lack of psychopathology after abortion despite experiencing the stress of an unwanted pregnancy. E. W. Freeman (1977) found that after an abortion, women reported feeling more self-directed and instrumental, suggesting that the experience may enhance women's personal coping resources. Abortion may also have indirect effects on women's mental health by reducing family size. Morris and Sison (1974) found that high parity was associated with feelings of powerlessness among women, feelings that were not explained by a link between powerlessness and contraceptive use. They reported that the correlation between female powerlessness and parity persisted after controlling for age, education, husband's occupation, family income, and use of contraception. They did not assess the mental health of women in their study, however, so they did not investigate the link between powerlessness and psychopathology among mothers that is found in other research (see chapter 18, this volume, for a review of this literature).

The relationship between abortion and childbearing is complex, however, and must be considered in the context of coping resources. Russo and Zierk (1992) examined the relationship of abortion to women's well-being in the context of childbearing experiences and coping resources in a national sample of 5,295 U.S. women followed over a span of eight years. Family size was negatively correlated with well-being, even when controlling for presence of spouse, education, income, employment, and number of births not wanted at the time or any future time. Abortion and motherhood overlapped: two out of three women having abortions were mothers, and mothers with unwanted births were more likely to have had an abortion than mothers with wanted births. Women having repeat abortions had a significantly higher number of children than other women. Women having one abortion had higher global self-esteem, particularly with regard to feelings of self-worth, capableness, and not feeling one is a failure. Repeated unwanted pregnancy, whether resolved by birth or abortion, was correlated with fewer coping resources as indexed by lower income and education. Interestingly, preexisting low levels of self-esteem were predictive of both wanted and unwanted births. Multiple regression analyses revealed that when income, education, employment, childbearing variables (number and wantedness of children), and preexisting levels of well-being were controlled, having either one abortion or repeat abortions was not independently related to women's subsequent well-being. When women who had abortions seven years previously were compared with women who had more recent abortions, no differences in well-being were identified. These results were considered to be incompatible with assertion of the existence of "postabortion syndrome."

Antiabortion activists have engaged in efforts to define women's response to abortion as a clinical disease, postabortion syndrome (Speckhard, 1987). Emotional response after abortion is conceptualized as a type of posttraumatic stress disorder (PTSD). There is no scientific basis for such a category. While unwanted pregnancy and its resolution are a potential source of stress, under what conditions an abortion might compound, relieve, or otherwise affect such stress has yet to be determined. However, since the psychological impact of abortion is affected by social support for the women's decision (Adler et al., 1990), such things as attacks on abortion clinics and harassment of women seeking abortions may produce negative effects that will be correlated with the abortion experience. Research on the relationship of such activities to the production of both guilt and shame may be useful.

Adoption is sometimes proposed as an alternative to abortion for resolution of unwanted pregnancy, but little research has been conducted on the psychological consequences of adoption. As in the case of abortion, clinical and case studies do suggest that some women may be at risk for psychological and interpersonal difficulties after giving up a child for adoption, and for some people such risks persist over long periods of time (Pannor, Baron & Sorosky, 1978). Studies of the postadoption experience suffer many of the same limitations of those of postabortion experience, however, including reliance on clinical samples and a focus on negative experiences.

Research on postabortion emotional responses would suggest that some postadoption women would be at higher risk than others. Individual coping resources, characteristics of the adoption experience, and social support would be expected to affect postadoption emotional responses. One study of the members of Concerned United Birthparents, a national organization that emerged from an initial support group for people dealing with postadoption emotional responses, found such individuals to perceive adoption as having a long-lasting negative impact in the areas of marriage, childbearing, and parenting (Deykin, Campbell & Patti, 1984). Most of these individuals reported lack of social support in the form of family opposition to their decision, a decision made under pressure by physicians or social workers, and a lack of financial resources. This is not a random sample of parents who surrender children for adoption, so rates and level of risk cannot be ascertained. However, it is noteworthy that these risk factors are similar to those that put women at higher risk of emotional responses after abortion. Giving up a child clearly was an emotionally charged decision for these individuals; 65% of the sample had initiated a search for the surrendered child. Predictors of search activity, which suggests a higher level of distress, were more likely to reflect external pressure on the decision and time lapsed since surrender than personal reasons such as lack of preparation for parenthood or age. Interestingly, childlessness was not a predictor of search activity, and the majority of searching parents had other children.

Individuals who hold negative attitudes toward adoption and perceive themselves as unable to cope with the experience may be at higher risk for negative mental health outcomes. Thus, studies of surrendering parents before abortion became legal may not be comparable with those after access to legal abortion, given that it could be that individuals who perceive themselves with the fewest coping resources may choose the abortion alternative. Indeed, Deykin et al., (1984), who found length of time since adoption to be significantly associated with search activity, gathered their data in 1980, seven years after *Roe v. Wade* (although *Roe v. Wade* was decided in 1973, a number of states had begun to make abortion more accessible in the late 1960s). Percentages of searchers among individuals who surrendered children were 37%, 43%, 69%, and 81% for intervals of less than 7, 8–12, 13–17, and 18 or more years since adoption, respectively. These findings may reflect the fact that adoption, like the birth of a premature infant, involves chronic stress that does not dissipate over time (as opposed, e. g., to the acute stress involved in abortion). Alternatively, it may be that under conditions of choice, individuals are able to self-select the alternative that is least stressful. Thus, the correlation of length of time since adoption and search activity might reflect the difference between adoption when no alternative to abortion is available and adoption under conditions of legal abortion. Although the researchers did not relate their findings to abortion availability, their work suggests the need for research that separates cohort effects from length of time since adoption. Ironically, if efforts to encourage women to use adoption as an alternative to abortion become coercive, the risk for psychopathology after adoption may increase.

Once again, the importance of viewing women as active agents and providing them with choices so they can manage stress through selection of alternatives that match coping resources must be emphasized. Women's access to abortion since 1973 has enabled them to self-select abortion versus childbirth based on a host of psychological, social, and economic factors, including their perception of whether or not they could cope with that alternative. Thus, both the population of women who give birth and keep their babies and the population of such women who give their babies up for adoption have changed since 1973. For example, there has been an increasing proportion of teenage mothers who keep their babies rather than give them up for adoption. This is a reflection of the loss of women in the childbirth population who did not wish to keep a child yet also did not wish to give it up for adoption. The removal of such women from the childbirth population can explain the increased well-being and reduction of psychopathology seen in teenage mothers in studies after 1973 (Barth, Schinke & Maxwell, 1983) and would suggest that the well-being of women who place children for adoption after 1973 would be enhanced as well.

In considering the full mental health impact of reproductive choices, it will be important to examine risk for psychopathology for other family members as well as for the woman. Deykin et al. (1984) reported that 80% of their sample stated that surrendering a child had potent effects on their parenting practices, including overprotectiveness and difficulty in dealing with children's independence. Research has documented risk for long-lasting and negative effects of being unwanted during pregnancy for children who are subsequently born and raised with their natural parents (see David et al., 1988, for a review). Little is known, however, about the risks associated with adoption for the mental health of the child adopted away or to other children in the family of the woman surrendering a child.

In reviewing the literature on pregnancy and its resolution, its most remarkable feature is the relative lack of it. It is rather incredible that there is such little scientific knowledge about pregnancy-related decisions, behaviors, and outcomes given their momentous consequences for the lives of so many individuals.

Menopause

Women are defined as postmenopausal if they have not had menstrual bleeding for one year. Menopause occurs at approximately age 50, and symptoms include "hot flashes," "night sweats," sleep disturbance, fatigue, irritability, and other mood changes (Hamilton et al., 1988b; Travis, 1988a).

The contribution of hormonal changes in menopause is not clear. Depression may be a precursor, rather than a consequence, of emotional responses associated with menopause. Longitudinal research has found that depressed women were twice as likely to report menopausal symptoms, such as hot flashes, and were more likely to seek medical help for menopausal symptoms compared with other women (McKinlay, McKinlay & Brambilla, 1987a, 1987b). There is an increase in consultations for emotional problems in perimenopausal (one to two years before cessation of menstruation) and early postmenopausal (one to two years after such cessation) women. Women of this age group historically have received more prescriptions for psychotropic drugs than women of other ages and men of similar ages (Skegg, Doll & Parry, 1977). Interestingly, some research suggests that physicians are more likely to perceive menopausal symptoms as more severe and of psychological origin than women themselves (Cowan, Warren & Young, 1985).

Longitudinal research using a community sample suggests that a stress and coping perspective focused on gender- and sex-role issues can illuminate the relationship between menopause and psychopathology (McKinlay et al., 1987b). That research found that the most marked increases in depression with menopause were associated with multiple social sources of stress, much of it having to do with role obligations (e.g., adolescent children, ailing husbands, and aging parents) rather than biological factors. Menopause was not associated with either physical or mental health problems. Most of the variance in health status of menopausal women was explained by previous health status and help-seeking behavior (McKinlay et al., 1987a). This contrasts with the stereotype of the menopausal women, which has reflected research based on women in treatment populations.

Gender differences at age 50 are found in some symptoms related to depression, but not others, and they may be related to sex or gender roles. Bungay and colleagues (1980) found no gender differences in difficulty sleeping, loss of interest in sexual relations, or loss of appetite. However, in addition to night sweats, gender differences were found in anxiety, loss of confidence, difficulty in making decisions, difficulty in concentration, forgetfulness, tiredness, and feelings of worthlessness (after controlling for some age-related life events, such as children's leaving home).

By age 50, nearly 30% of U.S. women have undergone surgical menopause instead of experiencing the natural cessation of ovarian function. The cessation of menstruation following surgical hysterectomy with oophorectomy is a more stressful life event than normal menopause and carries a higher mental health risk for women. Depression is correlated with surgical menopause, although the effects appear to be short-lived (McKinlay et al., 1987b). The proportion of women who have surgical menopause varies with age, and studies by age grouping alone are inadequate (Hamilton et al., 1988b). McKinlay et al. (1987b) reported that most of women's self-perceptions of health status and concomitant use of health services in menopause were related to the experience of surgical menopause (McKinlay et al., 1987a).

The importance of investigating gender- and sex-role variables across social classes is found in the work of Nadelson, Notman, and Ellis (1983). They concluded from their review of the literature that psychosocial variables at menopause were more clearly associated with depression than were endocrine changes. Women experiencing the most distress at menopause were women who had relied on their childbearing and childbearing roles for status and self-esteem. Middle- and upper-class women were more likely than lower-class women to report menopause as liberating because of increased opportunities resulting from cessation of childbearing.

In summary, although research suggests that gender-related attributes and sex- and gender-role issues are related to women's risk for psychopathology after stressful reproductive-related life events, there has been little systematic research to explore them. Women's responses to reproductive-related events can be understood in a stress and coping framework, whereby risk factors and coping resources interact to influence the relationship between stressful events and the development of psychopathology. Women's mental health is a broad topic, impossible to cover in one brief chapter. We have focused here on reproductive-related life events to demonstrate the importance of examining the interrelationships among biological, psychological, and social variables over the life cycle if women's higher risk for psychopathology is to be understood.

WOMEN'S MENTAL HEALTH: CURRENT STATUS, FUTURE PROSPECTS

This review has documented substantial gender differences in psychopathology, identifying such differences in current expressions of symptoms, syndromes, and mental disorders. The implications of gender as a social category are complex and vary across class, race, and ethnic group. We argue that future advances in understanding gender differences in mental health require recognizing that women's feminine gender role is but one of women's many sex roles and appreciating the violence, powerlessness, and lack of access to resources that pervade women's lives. Advances will also require the recognition that definitions of categories of psychopathology—from symptom to syndrome to mental disorder—are social constructions that reflect the values and vision of fallible human beings. Symptoms of mental disorders that have high prevalence for women overlap with each other, as well as with women's gender stereotypes. Misdiagnosis—of one disorder for another or of normal role behavior for psychopathology—continues to be a critical issue in women's mental health. Gender-related attributes (particularly those of instrumentality and perceived control), gender- and sex-role expectations and obligations (particularly with regard to caring, nurturance, and actual control and access to resources), and gender-related stressful life events (particularly with regard to physical and sexual abuse, reproduction, and poverty) all contribute to women's risk for psychopathology. Examination of reproductive-related events in women's lives, events that are most clearly tied to women's unique biology, underscores the contribution of psychosocial variables in constructing the adaptive challenges of such events. A stress and coping framework that includes biological, psychological, social, and cultural variables related to gender and considers the behaviors of women in their larger context appears to hold exceptional promise for mental health research and theory. The paucity of mental health research on outcomes of reproductive-related events, however, reminds us of the importance of the larger social context to the setting of research priorities. We must remember that, despite pervasive gender differences in mental health, they were identified as a priority of the National Institute of Mental Health only when forced to do so by Congress (Russo, 1990). Continued monitoring of mental health funding and service delivery bodies will be needed as long as women's position in society is devalued.

NOTE

We would like to thank Laurie Chassen, Nancy Eisenberg, Ria Hermann, Jody Horn, and Teresa Levitan for feedback on the manuscript. Jan Lameroux, Carolyn Powers, Irina Feier, and Sharu Kakar provided invaluable assistance in assembling materials and typing references.

REFERENCES

Abrahams, B., Feldman, S. S., & Nash, S. C. (1978). Sex role self-concept and sex role attitudes: Enduring personality characteristics or adaptations to changing life situations? *Developmental Psychology, 14*, 393–400.

Abramson, L. Y., & Andrews, D. E. (1982). Cognitive models of depression: Implications for sex differences in vulnerability to depression. *International Journal of Mental Health, 11*, 77–94.

Abramson, L. Y., Metalsky, G. I., & Alloy, L. B. (1989). Hopelessness depression: A theory-based subtype of depression. *Psychological Review, 96*, 358–372.

Adler, N. (1975a). Abortion: A social psychological perspective. *Journal of Social Issues*, *35*, 100–119.

Adler, N. (1975b). Emotional responses of women following therapeutic abortion. *American Journal of Orthopsychiatry*, *45*, 446–456.

Adler, N., David, H. P., Major, B. N., Roth, S. H., Russo, N. F., & Wyatt, G. E. (1990). Psychological responses after abortion. *Science*, *248* (April 6), 41–44.

Adler, N., & Dolcini, P. (1986). Psychological issues in abortion for adolescents. In G. B. Melton (Ed.), *Adolescent abortion: Psychological and legal issues* (pp. 74–95). Lincoln: University of Nebraska Press.

Akiskal, H. S. (1987). The milder spectrum of bipolar disorders: Diagnostic, characteristic, and pharmacologic. *Psychiatry Annals*, *17*, 32–37.

Alpert, J. (Ed.). (1986). *Psychoanalysis in women*. Hillsdale, NJ: Analytic Press.

Amaro, H. (1988). Women in the Mexican American community: Religion, culture, and reproductive attitudes and experiences. *Journal of Community Psychology*, *16*, 6–20.

Amaro, H., & Russo, N. F. (Eds.). (1987). *Hispanic women and mental health*. New York: Cambridge University Press. [Special Issue, *Psychology of Women Quarterly*, *11* (4)].

Amaro, H., Russo, N. F., & Johnson, J. (1987). Family and work predictors of psychological well-being among Hispanic women professionals. *Psychology of Women Quarterly*, *11*, 505–521.

Amaro, H., Zuckerman, B., & Cabral, H. (1989). Drug use among adolescent mothers: Profile of risk. *Pediatrics*, *84*(1), 144–151.

American Psychiatric Association. (1987). *Diagnostic and statistical manual of mental disorders* (3rd ed., rev.). Washington, DC: Author.

American Psychological Association, Committee on Accreditation. (1983). *Accreditation handbook* (rev. ed.). Washington, DC: American Psychological Association.

American Psychological Association, Committee on Women in Psychology. (1987). *If sex enters into the psychotherapy relationship*. Washington, DC: American Psychological Association.

Andrade, S. J. (1982). Social science stereotypes of the Mexican American woman: Policy implications for research. *Hispanic Journal of Behavioral Sciences*, *4*, 223–244.

Aneshensel, C., Frerichs, S. R., & Clark, V. (1981). Family roles and sex differences in depression. *Journal of Health and Social Behavior*, *22*, 379–393.

Angst, J., & Dobler-Mikola, A. (1983, December). *Do the diagnostic criteria determine the sex ratio in depression?* Presented at the 22nd Annual Meeting of the American College of Neuropsychopharmacology, San Juan, Puerto Rico.

Athanasiou, R., Oppel, W., Michelson, L., Unger, I., & Yager, M. (1973). Psychiatric sequelae to term birth and induced early and later abortion: A longitudinal study. *Family Planning Perspectives*, *5*, 227–231.

Barth, R. P., Schinke, S. P., & Maxwell, J. S. (1983). Psychological correlates of teenage motherhood. *Journal of Youth and Adolescence*, *12*(6), 471–487.

Bassoff, E. S., & Glass, G. V. (1982). The relationship between sex roles and mental health: A meta-analysis of twenty-six studies. *Counseling Psychologist*, *10*, 105–112.

Baucom, D. H., & Danker-Brown, P. (1984). Sex role identity and sex-stereotyped tasks in the development of learned helplessness in women. *Journal of Personality and Social Psychology, 46*, 422–430.

Belle, D. (Ed.). (1982a). *Lives in stress: Women and depression*. Beverly Hills: Sage.

Belle, D. (1982b). Social ties and social support. In D. Belle (Ed.), *Lives in stress: Women and depression*. Beverly Hills: Sage.

Belle, D. (1982c). The stress of caring: Women as providers of social support. In L. Goldberger & S. Breznitz (Eds.), *Handbook of stress: Theoretical and clinical aspects*. New York: Free Press.

Belle, D. (1990). Poverty and women's mental health. *American Psychologist, 45*(3), 385–389.

Belsey, E. M., Greer, H. S., Lai, S., Lewis, S. C., & Beard, R. W. (1977). Predictive factors in emotional response to abortion: Kings termination study—IV. *Social Science and Medicine, 11*, 71–82.

Bernay, T., & Cantor, D. W. (Eds.). (1986). *The psychology of today's woman: New psychoanalytic visions*. Hillsdale, NJ: Erlbaum.

Billings, A. G., Cronkite, R. C., & Moos, R. H. (1983). Social-environmental factors in unipolar depression: Comparisons of depressed patients and nondepressed controls. *Journal of Abnormal Psychology, 92*(2), 119–133.

Boskind-White, M., & White, W. C. (Eds.). (1987). *Bulimarexia: The binge/purge cycle* (2nd ed.). New York: Norton.

Boyd, J. H., & Weissman, M. M. (1981). Epidemiology of affective disorders: A reexamination and future directions. *Archives of General Psychiatry, 38*, 1039–1046.

Brewer, J. C. (1977). Incidence of post-abortion psychosis: A prospective study. *British Medical Journal, 1*, 476.

Brewin, C. R. (1985). Depression and causal attributions: What is their relation? *Psychological Bulletin, 98*, 297–309.

Brockington, I. F., & Kumar, R. (1982). *Motherhood and mental illness*. New York: Grune & Stratton.

Brody, C. M. (1984). *Women therapists working with women: New theory and process of feminist therapy*. New York: Springer.

Brody, C. M. (Ed.). (1987). *Women's therapy groups: Paradigms for feminist treatment*. New York: Springer.

Brooks-Gunn, J. (1986). The relationship of maternal beliefs about sex typing to maternal and young children's behavior. *Sex Roles, 14*, 21–35.

Brown, G. W., Bifulco, A., Harris, T., & Bridge, L. (1986). Life stress, chronic subclinical symptoms and vulnerability to clinical depression. *Journal of Affective Disorders, 11*, 1–19.

Brown, G. W., & Harris, T. (1978). *Social origins of depression: A study of psychiatric disorder in women*. New York: Free Press.

Brown, G. W., & Prudo, R. (1981). Psychiatric disorder in a rural and urban population: 1. Aetiology of depression. *Psychological Medicine, 11*, 581–599.

Brown, L. S., & Root, M. P. (Eds.). (1990). *Diversity and complexity in feminist therapy*. New York: Haworth Press.

Browne, A., & Finkelhor, D. (1986). Impact of child sexual abuse: A review of research. *Psychological Bulletin, 99*(1), 66–77.

Brownmiller, S. (1984). *Femininity*. New York: Simon & Schuster.

Bryer, J. B., Nelson, B. A., Miller, J. B., & Krol, P. A. (1987). Childhood sexual and physical abuse as factors in adult psychiatric illness. *American Journal of Psychiatry, 114*, 1426–1430.

Buesching, D. P., Glasser, M. L., & Frate, D. A. (1986). Progression of depression in the prenatal and postpartum periods. *Women and Health, 11*, 61–78.

Bungay, G. T., Vessey, M. P., & McPherson, C. K. (1980). Study of symptoms in middle life with special reference to the menopause. *British Medical Journal, 281*, 181–183.

Burnam, M. A., Stein, J. A., Golding, J. M., Siegel, J. M., Sorenson, S. B., Forsythe, A. B., & Telles, C. A. (1988). Sexual assault and mental disorders in a community population. *Journal of Consulting and Clinical Psychology, 56*(6), 843–850.

Busch, C. M., Costa, P. T., Whitehead, W. E., & Heller, B. R. (1988). Severe perimenstrual symptoms: Prevalence and effects on absenteeism and health care seeking in a nonclinical sample. *Women and Health, 14*, 59–74.

Campbell, E. A., Cope, S. J., & Teasdale, J. D. (1983). Social factors and affective disorders: An investigation of Brown and Harris's model. *British Journal of Psychiatry, 143*, 548–553.

Cantwell, D. P., Sturzenberger, S., Burroughs, J., Salkin, B., & Green, J. K. (1977). Anorexia nervosa: An affective disorder? *Archives of General Psychiatry, 34*, 1087–1093.

Carmen, E. H., & Rieker, P. P. (1989). A psychosocial model of the victim-to-patient process. *Psychiatric Clinics of North America, 12*(2), 431–443.

Carmen, E. H., Russo, N. F., & Miller, J. B. (1981). Inequality and women's mental health: An overview. *American Journal of Psychiatry, 138*(10), 1319–1330.

Chambless, D. (1982). Characteristics of agoraphobics. In D. Chambless & A. J. Goldstein (Eds.), *Agoraphobia: Multiple perspectives on theory and treatment* (pp. 215–219). New York: Wiley.

Clark, V. A., Aneshensel, C. S., Frerichs, R. R., & Morgan, T. M. (1981). Analysis of effects of sex and age on response to items on the CES-D Scale. *Psychiatry Research, 5*, 171–181.

Cleary, P. D. (1987). Gender differences in stress-related disorders. In R. C. Barnett, L. Biener, & G. K. Baruch (Eds.), *Gender and stress* (pp. 39–73). New York: Free Press.

Cleary, P. D., & Mechanic, D. (1983). Sex differences in psychological distress among married people. *Journal of Health and Social Behavior, 24*, 111–121.

Coleman, L., Antonucci, T., & Adelmann, P. (1987). Role involvement, gender, and well-being. In F. Crosby (Ed.), *Spouse, parent, worker: On gender and multiple roles* (pp. 138–154). New Haven, CT: Yale University Press.

Coll, C. G., & Mattei, M. (Eds.). (1989). *The Puerto Rican woman: A psychosocial approach to lifespan developmental issues.* New York: Praeger.

Cooper, P.J., & Fairburn, C. G. (1983). Binge-eating and self-induced vomiting in the community: A preliminary study. *British Journal of Psychiatry, 142*, 139–144.

Cowan, G., Warren, L. W., & Young, J. L. (1985). Medical perceptions of menopausal symptoms. *Psychology of Women Quarterly, 9*(1), 3–14.

Cox, J. L., Connor, Y., & Kendell, R. E. (1982). Prospective study of the psychiatric disorders of childbirth. *British Journal of Psychiatry, 140*, 111–117.

Craig, T. J., & Van Natta, P. A. (1979). Influence of demographic characteristics on two measures of depressive symptoms. *Archives of General Psychiatry, 36*, 149–154.

Cronkite, R. C., & Moos, R. H. (1985). The role of predisposing and moderating factors in the stress-illness relationship. *Journal of Health and Social Behavior*, *25*, 372–393.

Cunningham, J. D., & Antill, J. K. (1984). Changes in masculinity and femininity across the family life cycle: A reexamination. *Developmental Psychology*, *20*, 1135–1141.

Cutrona, C. E. (1983). Causal attributions and perinatal depression. *Journal of Abnormal Psychology*, *92*, 161–172.

Dan, A. J., & Leppa, C. (1988). The menstrual cycle. *Women's Health Perspective: Annual Review*, 143–160.

David, H. P., Dytrych, Z., Matejcek, Z., & Schüller, V. (1988). *Born unwanted: Developmental effects of denied abortion*. New York: Springer.

David, H. P., Rasmussen, N., & Holst, E. (1981). Postpartum and postabortion psychotic reactions. *Family Planning Perspectives*, *13*(2), 88–93.

Davis, R., Freeman, R. J., & Garner, D. M. (1988). A naturalistic investigation of eating behavior in bulimia nervosa. *Journal of Consulting and Clinical Psychology*, *56*(2), 273–279.

DeJong, R., Rubinow, D. R., Roy-Byrne, P., Hobran, M. C., Grover, G. N., & Post, R. M. (1985). Premenstrual mood disorder and psychiatric illness. *American Journal of Psychiatry*, *142*, 1359–1361.

Deykin, E. Y., Campbell, L., & Patti, P. (1984). The postadoption experience of surrendering parents. *American Journal of Orthopsychiatry*, *54*(2), 271–280.

Dilling, C., & Claster, B. (Eds.). (1985). *Female psychology: A partially annotated bibliography*. New York: Coalition for Women's Mental Health.

Dunn, P. K., & Ondercin, P. (1981). Personality variables related to compulsive eating in college women. *Journal of Clinical Psychology*, *37*, 43–49.

Dutton-Douglas, M. A., & Walker, L. (Eds.). (1988). *Feminist psychotherapies: Interaction of therapeutic and feminist systems*. Norwood, NJ: Ablex.

Dykens, E. M., & Gerrard, M. (1986). Psychological profiles of purging bulimics, repeat dieters, and controls. *Journal of Consulting and Clinical Psychology*, *54*, 283–288.

Eichler, A., & Parron, D. L. (1987). *Women's mental health agenda for research*. Rockville, MD: National Institute of Mental Health.

Endicott, J., Halbreich, U., Schact, S., & Nee, J. (1981). Premenstrual changes and affective disorders. *Psychosomatic Medicine*, *43*, 519–530.

Ensel, W. M. (1982). The role of age and the relationship of gender and marital status to depression. *Journal of Nervous and Mental Disease*, *170*, 536–543.

Ewing, J. A., & Rouse, B. A. (1973). Therapeutic abortion and a prior psychiatric history. *American Journal of Psychiatry*, *130*, 37–40.

Feldman, S. S., Biringen, Z. C., & Nash, S. C. (1981). Fluctuations of sex-related self-attributions as a function of stage of family life cycle. *Developmental Psychology*, *17*, 24–35.

Fine, M., & Asch, A. (1988). *Women with disabilities: Essays in women, culture, and politics*. Philadelphia: Temple University Press.

Fitzgerald, L., & Nutt, R. (1986). The Division 17 principles concerning the counseling/psychotherapy of women: Rationale and implementation. *Counseling Psychologist*, *14*, 180–216.

Flett, G. L., Vredenburg, K., & Pliner, P. (1985). Sex roles and depression: A preliminary investigation of the direction of causality. *Journal of Research in Personality,* *19,* 429–435.

Franks, V., & Rothblum, E. D. (Eds.). (1983). *The stereotyping of women: Its effects on mental health.* New York: Springer.

Freeman, E. W. (1977). Abortion: Subjective attitudes and feelings. *Family Planning Perspectives, 10,* 150–155.

Freeman, T. (1951). Pregnancy as a precipitant of mental illness in men. *British Journal of Medical Psychology, 24,* 49–54.

Friedman, D., & Jaffe, A. (1985). Influence of lifestyle on the premenstrual syndrome. *Journal of Reproductive Medicine, 30,* 715–719.

Fullilove, M. (1988). Ethnic minority women and AIDS. *Multicultural Inquiry and Research on AIDS, 2*(2), 4–5.

Gallant, S. J., & Hamilton, J. A. (1988). On a premenstrual psychiatric diagnosis: What's in a name? *Professional Psychology: Research and Practice, 19,* 271–278.

Garner, D. M., & Garfinkel, P. E. (1980). Sociocultural factors in the development of anorexia nervosa. *Psychological Medicine, 10,* 647–656.

Garner, D. M., Garfinkel, P. E., Schwartz, D., & Thompson, M. (1980). Cultural expectations of thinness in women. *Psychological Reports, 47,* 483–491.

Gater, R. A., Dean, C., & Morris, J. (1989). The contribution of childbearing to the sex difference in first admission rates for affective psychosis. *Psychological Medicine, 19*(3), 719.

Gelinas, D. J. (1983). The persisting negative effects of incest. *Psychiatry, 46,* 312–332.

Gelles, R. (1975). Violence and pregnancy: A note on the extent of the problem and needed services. *Family Coordinator, 24,* 81–86.

Gold, E. R. (1986). Long-term effects of sexual victimization in childhood: An attributional approach. *Journal of Consulting and Clinical Psychology, 54,* 471–475.

Golding, J. M. (1988). Gender differences in depressive symptoms. *Psychology of Women Quarterly, 12,* 61–74.

Goldman, N., & Ravid, R. (1980). Community surveys: Sex differences in mental illness. In M. Guttentag, S. Salasin, & D. Belle (Eds.), *The mental health of women* (pp. 31–35). New York: Academic Press.

Gore, S., & Mangione, T. W. (1983). Social roles, sex roles, and psychological distress: Additive and interactive models of sex differences. *Journal of Health and Social Behavior, 24,* 300–312.

Gove, W. R. (1980). Mental illness and psychiatric treatment among women. *Psychology of Women Quarterly, 4,* 345–362.

Greene, R., & Dalton, K. (1953). The premenstrual syndrome. *British Medical Journal, 1,* 1007–1014.

Haimo, S., & Blitman, F. (1985). The effects of assertive training on sex role concept in female agoraphobics. *Women and Therapy, 4*(2), 53–61.

Halmi, K. A., Falk, J. R., & Schwartz, E. (1981). Binge-eating and vomiting: A survey of a college population. *Psychological Medicine, 11,* 697–706.

Hamilton, E. W., & Abramson, L. Y. (1983). Cognitive patterns and major depressive disorder: A longitudinal study in a hospital setting. *Journal of Abnormal Psychology, 92*(2), 173–184.

Hamilton, J. A. (1984). Psychobiology in context: Reproductive-related events in men's and women's lives. [Review of *Motherhood and mental illness*]. *Contemporary Psychiatry*, *3*(1), 12–16.

Hamilton, J. A. (Ed.). (1988). *Risk factors for depression in women and diagnostic subtypes.* Report from the Committee on Etiology and Diagnosis, Task Force on Women and Depression, American Psychological Association.

Hamilton, J. A., Alagna, S. W., Parry, B., Herz, E. K., Blumenthal, S., & Conrad, C. (1985). An update on premenstrual depression: Evaluation and treatment. In J. H. Gold (Ed.), *The psychiatric implications of menstruation* (pp. 3–19). Washington, DC: American Psychiatric Press.

Hamilton, J. A., Gallant, S., & Lloyd, C. (1989). Evidence for a menstrual-linked artifact in determining rates of depression. *Journal of Nervous and Mental Disease*, *177*, 359–365.

Hamilton, J. A., Parry, B. L., & Blumenthal, S. J. (1988a). The menstrual cycle in context I: Affective syndromes associated with reproductive hormonal changes. *Journal of Clinical Psychiatry*, *49*, 474–480.

Hamilton, J. A., Parry, B. L., & Blumenthal, S. J. (1988b). The menstrual cycle in context II: Human gonadal steroid hormone variation. *Journal of Clinical Psychiatry*, *49*, 481.

Hamilton, J. A., Parry, B., & Herz, E. K. (1984). Premenstrual mood changes: A guide to evaluation and treatment. *Psychiatric Annals*, *14*, 426–435.

Helms, J. E. (1989). Considering some methodological issues in racial identity counseling research. *Counseling Psychologist*, *17*, 227–252.

Henshaw, S. K., & Van Vort, J. (1990). Abortion services in the United States, 1987 and 1988. *Family Planning Perspectives*, *22*(3), 102–142.

Herman, M. F. (1983). Depression and women: Theories and research. *Journal of the American Academy of Psychoanalysis*, *11*(4), 493–512.

Herzog, D. B., Heller, M. B., Lavori, P. W., & Off, I. L. (1987). Social impairment in bulimia. *International Journal of Eating Disorders*, *6*, 741–747.

Hilliard, P. (1985). Physical abuse in pregnancy. *Ob-Gyn*, *66*(2), 185–190.

Hinz, L. D., & Williamson, D. A. (1987). Bulimia and depression: A review of the affective variant hypothesis. *Psychological Bulletin*, *102*, 150–158.

Hobfoll, S. E. (1986a). The ecology of stress and social support among women. In S. E. Hobfoll (Ed.), *Stress, social support and women* (pp. 3–14). Washington, DC: Hemisphere.

Hobfoll, S. E. (1986b). The limitations of social support in the stress process. In G. Sarason & B. R. Sarason (Eds.), *Social support: Theory, research, and applications* (pp. 391–414). The Hague: Martinus Nijhof.

Hobfoll, S. E., & Leiberman, J. R. (1987). Personality and social resources in immediate and continued stress resistance among women. *Journal of Personality and Social Psychology*, *52*(1), 18–26.

Horwitz, A. V., & White, H. R. (1987). Gender role orientations and types of pathology among adolescents. *Journal of Health and Social Behavior*, *28*, 158–170.

Hser, Y. I., Anglin, M.D., & Booth, M. W. (1987). Sex differences in addict careers, Part 3: Addiction. *American Journal of Drug and Alcohol Abuse*, *13*(3), 231–251.

Hsu, L. K. (1983). The aetiology of anorexia nervosa. *Psychological Medicine*, *13*, 231–238.

Jacobsen, F. M., Wehr, T. A., Sack, D. A., James, S. P., & Rosenthal, N. E. (1987).

Seasonal affective disorder: A review of the syndrome and its public health implications. *American Journal of Public Health, 77*(1), 57–60.

Johnson, C. L., & Berndt, D. J. (1983). Preliminary investigation of bulimia and life adjustment. *American Journal of Psychiatry, 140*, 774–777.

Kandel, D. B., & Davies, M. (1982). Epidemiology of depressive mood in adolescents. *Archives of General Psychiatry, 39*, 1205–1212.

Kaplan, A. G., Roberts, R., Camacho, T., & Coyne, J. (1987). Psychosocial predictors of depression: Prospective evidence from the Human Population Laboratory Studies. *American Journal of Epidemiology, 125*, 206–220.

Katzman, M. A., & Wolchik, S. A. (1984). Bulimia and binge eating in college women: A comparison of personality and behavioral characteristics. *Journal of Consulting and Clinical Psychology, 52*(3), 423–428.

Katzman, M., Wolchik, S., & Braver, S. (1984). The prevalence of frequent binge eating and bulimia in a nonclinical college sample. *International Journal of Eating Disorders, 3*, 53–61.

Kessler, R. C. (1979a). A strategy for studying differential vulnerability to the psychological consequences of stress. *Journal of Health and Social Behavior, 20*, 100–108.

Kessler, R. C. (1979b). Stress, social status, and psychological distress. *Journal of Health and Social Behavior, 20*, 259–272.

Kessler, R. C., & McLeod, J. D. (1984). Sex differences in vulnerability to undesirable life events. *American Sociological Review, 49*, 620–631.

Kessler, R. C., McLeod, J. D., & Wethington, E. (1984). The cost of caring: A perspective on the relationship between sex and psychological distress. In I. G. Sarason & B. R. Sarason (Eds.), *Social support: Theory, research and applications* (pp. 491–506). The Hague: Martinus Nijhof.

Kessler, R., & McRae, J. A., Jr. (1981). Trends in the relationship between sex and psychological distress. *American Sociological Review, 46*, 443–452.

Kessler, R., & McRae, J. A., Jr. (1982). The effect of wives' employment on the mental health of married men and women. *American Sociological Review, 47*, 216–227.

Kessler, R. C., Price, R. H., & Wortman, C. B. (1985). Social factors in psychopathology: Stress, social support, and coping processes. *Annual Review of Psychology, 36*, 531–572.

Klein, D. F., Gittelman, R., Quitkin, F., & Rifkin, A. (1980). *Diagnosis and drug treatment of psychiatric disorders*. Baltimore, MD: Williams & Wilkins.

Klerman, G. L., & Weissman, M. M. (1985a). Depressions among women. In J. H. Williams (Ed.), *Psychology of women: Selected readings*. New York: W. W. Norton.

Klerman, G. L., & Weissman, M. M. (1985b). Gender and depression. *Trends in Neurosciences, 8*(9), 416–420.

Koss, M. P. (1990). The women's mental health research agenda: Violence against women. *American Psychologist, 45*(3), 374–380.

Koss, M. P., & Burkhart, B. (1989). A conceptual analysis of rape victimization. *Psychology of Women Quarterly, 13*, 27–40.

Kristiansen, C. M., & Giulietti, R. (1990). Perceptions of wife abuse. *Psychology of Women Quarterly, 14*, 177–189.

Lazarus, R. S., & Folkman, S. (1984). *Stress, appraisal, and coping*. New York: Springer.

Lee, N. F., Rush, A. J., & Mitchell, J. E. (1985). Bulimia and depression. *Journal of Affective Disorders, 9*, 231–238.

Lerman, H. (1986). *A note in Freud's eye: From psychoanalysis to the psychology of women*. New York: Springer.

Lerner, H. G. (1988). *Women in the therapy*. Northdale, NJ: Aronson.

Lewis, H. (1976). *Psychic war in men and women*. New York: New York University Press.

Lewis, L., & Johnson, C. (1985). A comparison of sex role orientation between women with bulimia and normal controls. *International Journal of Eating Disorders, 4*, 247–257.

Link, B., & Dohrenwend, B. P. (1980). Formulation of hypotheses about the true prevalence of demoralization in the United States. In B. P. Dohrenwend, M. Schwartz-Gould, R. Neugebauer, & R. Wunsch-Hitzig (Eds.), *Mental illness in the United States: Epidemiological estimates* (pp. 114–132). New York: Praeger.

Liss-Levinson, N., Clamar, A., Ehrenberg, M., Ehrenberg, O., Fidell, L., Maffeo, P., Redstone, J., Russo, N. F., Solomons, D., & Tennov, D. (1985). *Women and psychotherapy: A consumer handbook*. Washington, DC: National Coalition for Women's Mental Health.

Logue, C. M., & Moos, R. H. (1986). Perimenstrual symptoms: Prevalence and risk factors. *Psychosomatic Medicine, 48*, 388–414.

Lopez, S. (1989). Patient variable biases in clinical judgment: Conceptual overview and methodological considerations. *Psychological Bulletin, 106*, 184–203.

Loring, M., & Powell, B. (1988). Gender, race and DSM-III: A study of the objectivity of psychiatric diagnostic behavior. *Journal of Health and Social Behavior, 29*, 1–22.

Major, B., Cozzarelli, C., Sciacchitano, A. M., Cooper, M. L., Testa, M., & Mueller, P. M. (1990). Perceived social support, self-efficacy, and adjustment to abortion. *Journal of Personality and Social Psychology, 59*, 452–463.

Marecek, J. (1986). Legal and ethical issues in counseling pregnant adolescents. In G. B. Melton (Ed.), *Adolescent abortion: Psychological and legal issues* (96–115). Lincoln: University of Nebraska Press.

Marsh, K. L., & Weary, G. (1989). Depression and attributional complexity. *Personality and Social Psychology Bulletin, 15*(3), 325–336.

Mathews, A. M., Gelder, M. G., & Johnston, D. W. (1981). *Agoraphobia, nature and treatment*. New York: Guilford Press.

Matlin, M. W. (1993). *The psychology of women*. Orlando, FL: Harcourt, Brace, & Jovanovich.

Mazor, M. D. (1984). Emotional reactions to infertility. In M. D. Mazor & H. P. Simons (Eds.), *Infertility: Medical emotional and social considerations* (pp. 23–36). New York: Human Sciences Press.

McFarlane, J., Martin, C. L., & Williams, T. M. (1988). Mood Fluctuations: Women versus men and menstrual versus other cycles. *Psychology of Women Quarterly, 12*(2), 201–224.

McGrath, E. Keita, G. P., Strickland, B. R., & Russo, N. F. (Eds.). (1990). *Women and depression: Research, risk factors and treatment*. Final report of the American Psychological Association Task Force on Women and Depression. Washington, DC: American Psychological Association.

McKinlay, J. B., McKinlay, S. M., & Brambilla, D. J. (1987a). Health status and utilization behavior associated with menopause. *American Journal of Epidemiology, 125*(1), 110–121.

McKinlay, J. B., McKinlay, S. M., & Brambilla, D. J. (1987b). The relative contributions of endocrine changes and social circumstances to depression in mid-aged women. *Journal of Health and Social Behavior, 28,* 345–363.

Melton, G. B. (Ed.). (1986). *Adolescent abortion: Psychological and legal issues.* Lincoln: University of Nebraska Press.

Mintz, L. B., & Betz, N. E. (1988). Prevalence and correlates of eating disordered behaviors among undergraduate women. *Journal of Counseling Psychology, 35*(4), 463–471.

Minuchin, S. (1974). *Families and family therapy.* Cambridge: Harvard University Press.

Moos, R. H. (1986). *Perimenstrual symptoms: A manual and overview of research with the Menstrual Distress Questionnaire.* Palo Alto, CA: Stanford University, Social Ecology Laboratory.

Morris, N. M., & Sison, B. S. (1974). Correlates of female powerlessness: Parity, methods of birth control, pregnancy. *Journal of Marriage and the Family, 36,* 708–712.

Mowbray, C. T., & Benedek, E. P. (1988). *Women's mental health research agenda: Services and treatment of mental disorders in women* (Women's Mental Health Occasional Paper Series). Rockville, MD: National Institute of Mental Health.

Mueller, P., & Major, B. (1989). Self-blame, self-efficacy, and adjustment to abortion. *Journal of Personality and Social Psychology, 57*(6), 1059–1068.

Myers, J. K., Weissman, M. M., Tischler, G. L., Holzer, C. E., Leaf, P. J., Orvaschel, H., Anthony, J. C., Boyd, J. H., Burke, J. D., Kramer, M., & Stoltzman, R. (1984). Six-month prevalence of psychiatric disorders in three communities. *Archives of General Psychiatry, 41,* 959–967.

Nadelson, C. C., Notman, M. T., & Ellis, E. A. (1983). Psychosomatic aspects of obstetrics and gynecology. [Special Issue]. *Psychosomatics, 24*(10), 871–884.

Nasser, M. (1988). Culture and weight consciousness. *Journal of Psychosomatic Research, 32*(6), 573–577.

Newmann, J. P. (1984). Sex differences in symptoms of depression: Clinical disorder or normal distress? *Journal of Health and Social Behavior, 25,* 136–160.

Newmann, J. P. (1986). Gender, life strains, and depression. *Journal of Health and Social Behavior, 27,* 161–178.

Nolen-Hoeksema, S. (1987). Sex differences in unipolar depression: Evidence and theory. *Psychological Bulletin, 101*(2), 259–282.

Nolen-Hoeksema, S. (1990). *Sex differences in depression.* Stanford, CA: Stanford University Press.

Norman, D. K., & Herzog, D. B. (1984). Persistent social maladjustment in bulimia: A one-year follow up. *American Journal of Psychiatry, 141,* 444–446.

Norman, D. K., Herzog, D. B., & Chauncey, S. (1986). A one-year outcome study of bulimia: Psychological and eating symptom changes in a treatment and nontreatment group. *International Journal of Eating Disorders, 5,* 47–58.

Notman, M. T., & Nadelson, C. (1990). *Women and men: New perspectives on gender.* Washington, DC: American Psychiatric Press.

O'Connell, R. A., & Mayo, J. A. (1988). The role of social factors in affective disorders: A review. *Hospital and Community Psychiatry, 39*(8), 842–851.

O'Hara, M. W., Neunaber, D. J., & Zekoski, E. M. (1984). Prospective study of postpartum depression: Prevalence, course, and predictive factors. *Journal of Abnormal Psychology, 93*(2), 158–171.

O'Hara, M. W., Rehm, L. P., & Campbell, S. B. (1982). Predicting depressive symptomatology: Cognitive-behavioral models and postpartum depression. *Journal of Abnormal Psychology, 91*, 457–461.

O'Hara, M. W., Zekoski, E. M., Phillipps, L. H., & Wright, E. J. (1990). Controlled prospective study of postpartum mood disorders: Comparison of childbearing and nonchildbearing women. *Journal of Abnormal Psychology, 99*, 3–15.

Pannor, R., Baron, P., & Sorosky, A. (1978). Birthparents who relinquished babies for adoption revisited. *Family Child Placement Practice, 17*, 329–337.

Parry, B. L. (1989). Reproductive factors affecting the course of affective illness in women. *Psychiatric Clinics of North America, 12*, 207–220.

Paykel, E. S., Emms, E. M., Fletcher, J., & Rassaby, E. S. (1980). Life events and social support in puerperal depression. *British Journal of Psychiatry, 136*, 339–346.

Polivy, J., & Herman, C. P. (1985). Dieting and binging. *American Psychologist, 40*, 193–201.

Pope, H. G., Hudson, J. I., Yurgelun-Todd, D., & Hudson, M. S. (1984). Prevalence of anorexia nervosa and bulimia in three student populations. *International Journal of Eating Disorders, 3*, 45–51.

Public Health Service. (1985). *Women's health (Vol. 1)*, Report of the Public Health Service Task Force on Women's Health Issues (DHHS Publication No. PHS 85-50206). Washington, DC: U.S. Department of Health and Human Services.

Puglisi, J. T. (1983). Self-perceived age changes in sex role self concept. *International Journal of Aging and Human Development, 16*, 183–191.

Pyle, R. L., Mitchell, J. E., Eckert, E. D., Halvorson, P. A., Neuman, P. A., & Goff, G. M. (1983). The incidence of bulimia in freshman college students. *International Journal of Eating Disorders, 2*, 75–85.

Quitkin, F. M., Steward, J. W., & McGrath, P. J. (1988). Phenelzine versus imipramine in the treatment of probable atypical depression: Defining syndrome boundaries of selective MAOI responses. *American Journal of Psychiatry, 45*, 306–311.

Radloff, L. S. (1975). Sex difference in depression: The effects of occupation and marital status. *Sex Roles, 1*, 249–265.

Radloff, L. S., & Rae, D. S. (1981). Components of the sex difference in depression. In R. G. Simmons (Ed.), *Research in community and mental health* (pp. 76–95). Greenwich, CT: JAI Press.

Reich, J. W., & Zautra, A. J. (1990). Dispositional control beliefs and the consequences of a control-enhancing intervention. *Journal of Gerontology, 45*, 46–51.

Richardson, J. (1990). Questionnaire studies of paramenstrual symptoms. *Psychology of Women Quarterly, 14*(1), 15–42.

Rieker, P., & Carmen, E. (Eds.). (1984). *The gender gap in psychotherapy: Social realities and psychological processes*. New York: Plenum Press.

Robbins, J. H., & Siegel, R. J. (Eds.). (1985). *Women changing therapy: New assessments, values, and strategies in feminist therapy*. New York: Harrington Park Press.

Robins, L. N., Helzer, J. E., Weissman, M. M., Orvaschel, H., Gruenberg, E., Burke, J. D., & Regier, D. A. (1984). Lifetime prevalence of specific psychiatric disorders in three sites. *Archives of General Psychiatry, 41*, 949–958.

Rodin, J., Silberstein, L. R., & Striegel-Moore, R. H. (1985). Women and weight: A normative discontent. In T. B. Sonderegger (Ed.), *Psychology and gender: Ne-*

braska symposium on motivation (pp. 267–307). Lincoln: University of Nebraska Press.

Root, M. P. (1991). Persistent disordered eating as a gender-specific, post-traumatic stress response to sexual assault. Special Issue: Psychotherapy with victims. *Psychotherapy: Theory, Research, and Practice, 28,* 96–102.

Rosenfield, S. (1982). Sex roles and societal reactions to mental illness: The labeling of "deviant" deviance. *Journal of Health and Social Behavior, 23,* 18–24.

Rosewater, L., & Walker, L. (Eds.). (1985). *The handbook of feminist therapy: Women's issues in psychotherapy.* New York: Springer.

Russo, N. F. (1976). The motherhood mandate. *Journal of Social Issues, 32,* 143–154.

Russo, N. F. (1984). Sex role stereotyping, socialization, and sexism. In A. Sargent (Ed.), *Beyond sex roles* (2nd ed., pp. 150–167). St. Paul, MN: West.

Russo, N. F. (Ed.). (1985). *A woman's mental health agenda.* Washington, DC: American Psychological Association.

Russo, N. F. (1990). Reconstructing the psychology of women. In M. T. Notman & C. Nadelsen, *Women and men: New perspectives on gender* (pp. 43–62). Washington, DC: American Psychiatric Press.

Russo, N. F., Amaro, H., & Winter, M. (1987). The use of inpatient mental health services by Hispanic women. *Psychology of Women Quarterly, 11*(4), 427–442.

Russo, N. F., & Olmedo, E. L. (1983). Women's utilization of outpatient psychiatric services: Some emerging priorities for rehabilitation psychologists. *Rehabilitation Psychology, 28*(3), 141–155.

Russo, N. F., & Sobel, S. B. (1981). Sex differences in the utilization of mental health facilities. *Professional Psychology, 12*(1), 7–19.

Russo, N. F., & Zierk, K. L. (1992). Abortion, childbearing, and women's well-being. *Professional Psychology, 23,* 269–280.

Schnur, R. E., & MacDonald, M. L. (1988). Stages of identity development and problem drinking in college women. *Journal of Youth and Adolescence, 17,* 349–369.

Schnurr, P. P. (1988). Some correlates of prospectively defined premenstrual syndrome. *American Journal of Psychiatry, 145,* 491–494.

Schwartz, R. A. (1986). Abortion on request: The psychiatric implications. In J. D. Butler & D. F. Walbert (Eds.), *Abortion medicine and the law* (3rd ed., pp. 323–337). New York: Facts on File.

Seaman, M., & Seaman, T. E. (1983). Health behavior and personal autonomy: A longitudinal study of the sense of control in illness. *Journal of Health and Social Behavior, 24,* 144–160.

Seligman, M., Castellon, C., Cacciola, J., Schulman, P., Luborsky, L., Ollove, M., & Downing, R. (1988). Explanatory style change during cognitive therapy for unipolar depression. *Journal of Abnormal Psychology, 97*(1), 13–18.

Selik, R. M., Castro, K. G., & Pappaioanou, M. (1988). Distribution of AIDS cases, by racial/ethnic group and exposure category, United States, June 1, 1981–July 4, 1988. *MMWR CDC Surveillance Summary,* July, 1–10.

Shisslak, C. M., Crago, M., Neal, M. E., & Swain, B. (1987). Primary prevention of eating disorders. *Journal of Consulting and Clinical Psychology, 55*(5), 660–667.

Shusterman, L. R. (1979). Predicting the psychological consequences of abortion. *Social Science and Medicine, 13*(A), 683–689.

Skegg, D. C., Doll, R., & Parry, J. (1977). Use of medicines in general practice. *British Medical Journal, 1,* 1561–1563.

Slade, P., & Jenner, F. A. (1980). Attitudes toward female roles, aspects of menstruation and complaining of menstrual symptoms. *British Journal of Social and Clinical Psychology, 19*, 109–113.

Snodgrass, S. E. (1985). Women's intuition: The effect of subordinate role on interpersonal sensitivity. *Journal of Personality and Social Psychology, 49*(1), 146–155.

Sobel, S. B., & Russo, N. F. (Eds.). (1981). *Sex roles, equality, and mental health.* Washington, DC: American Psychological Association. (Special Issue of *Professional Psychology, 22* [Whole No. 1].)

Speckhard, A. (1987). *Post abortion counseling: A manual for Christian counselors.* Falls Church, VA: PACE.

Spence, J. T., Helmreich, R. L., & Stapp, J. (1974). The Personal Attributes Questionnaire: A measure of sex role stereotypes and masculinity-femininity. *JSAS Catalog of Selected Documents in Psychology, 43*, (Ms. No. 617).

Stacey, W., & Shupe, A. (1983). *The family secret.* Boston: Beacon Press.

Stark, E., Flitcraft, A., & Frazier, W. (1979). Medicine and patriarchal violence: The social construction of a private event. *International Journal of Health Service, 9*, 461–493.

Stark, E., Flitcraft, A., Zuckerman, D., Grey, A., Robinson, J., & Frazier, W. (1981). Wife abuse in the medical setting. *Domestic Violence, 7*, 7–41.

Stern, G., & Kruckman, L. (1983). Multi-disciplinary perspectives on post-partum depression: An anthropological critique. *Social Science & Medicine, 17*(5), 1027–1041.

Stout, A. L., Steege, J. F., Blazer, D. G., & George, L. K. (1986). Comparison of lifetime psychiatric diagnoses in premenstrual syndrome clinic and community samples. *Journal of Nervous and Mental Disease, 174*, 517–522.

Striegel-Moore, R. H., Silberstein, L. R., & Rodin, J. (1986). Toward an understanding of risk factors for bulimia. *American Psychologist, 41*(3), 246–263.

Strober, M., & Humphrey, L. L. (1987). Familial contributions to the etiology and course of anorexia nervosa and bulimia. *Journal of Consulting and Clinical Psychology, 55*, 654–659.

Subpanel on the Mental Health of Women, President's Commission on Mental Health. (1978). Report of the Special Population Subpanel on Mental Health of Women. *Task Panel Report submitted to the President's Commission on Mental Health* (Vol. 3). Washington, DC: U.S. Government Printing Office.

Sweeney, P. D., Anderson, K., & Bailey, S. (1986). Attributional style in depression: A meta-analytic review. *Journal of Personality and Social Psychology, 50*, 974–991.

Thoits, P. A. (1982). Life stress, social support, and psychological vulnerability: Epidemiological considerations. *Journal of Community Psychology, 10*, 341–362.

Thoits, P. A. (1984). Explaining distributions of psychological vulnerability: Lack of social support in face of life stress. *Social Forces, 63*, 463–481.

Thoits, P. A. (1986). Multiple identities: Examining gender and marital status differences in distress. *American Sociological Review, 51*, 259–272.

Thoits, P. A. (1987a). Gender and marital status differences in control and distress: Common stress versus unique stress explanations. *Journal of Health and Social Behavior, 28*, 7–22.

Thoits, P. A. (1987b). Negotiating roles. In F. J. Crosby (Ed.), *Spouse-parent worker: On gender and multiple roles* (pp. 11–22). New Haven, CT: Yale University Press.

Thoits, P. A. (1987c). Position paper. In A. Eichler, & D. L., Parron, *Women's mental health: Agenda for research* (pp. 80–102). Washington, DC: NIMH.

Thomas, D. A., & Reznikoff, M. (1984). Sex role orientation, personality structure, and adjustment in women. *Journal of Personality Assessment, 48*(1), 28–36.

Timonen, S., & Procope, B. J. (1973). The premenstrual syndrome: Frequency and association of symptoms. *Annual Chir Gyn Fenniae, 62*, 108–116.

Towne, R. D., & Afterman, J. (1955). Psychosis in males related to parenthood. *Bulletin of the Menninger Clinic, 19*(1), 19–26.

Travis, C. B. (1988a). *Women and health psychology: Biomedical issues.* Hillsdale, NJ: Erlbaum.

Travis, C. B. (1988b). *Women and health psychology: Mental health issues.* Hillsdale, NJ: Erlbaum.

U.S. Bureau of the Census. (1989). *Studies in marriage and the family* (Current Population Reports, Series P-23, No. 162). Washington, DC: U.S. Government Printing Office.

Van der Kolk, B. A. (1988). The trauma spectrum: The interaction of biological and social events in the genesis of the trauma response. *Journal of Traumatic Stress, 1*, 273–290.

Van der Kolk, B. A., Herman, J. L., & Perry, C. (1987, October). *Traumatic antecedents of borderline personality disorder.* Paper presented at the Fourth Annual Meeting of the Society for Traumatic Stress Studies, Baltimore, MD.

Waisberg, J., & Page, S. (1988). Gender role nonconformity and perception of mental illness. *Women and Health, 14*(1), 3–16.

Walker, L. E. (Ed.). (1984). *Women in mental health policy.* Beverly Hills: Sage.

Walker, L. E. (1985a). Feminist therapy with victims/survivors of interpersonal violence. In L. B. Rosewater & L. E. Walker (Eds.), *Handbook of feminist therapy* (pp. 203–214). New York: Springer.

Walker, L. E. (1985b). *Statement on proposed diagnosis of masochistic personality disorder.* Paper presented to the American Psychiatric Association's Work Group to Revise *DSM-III*, New York.

Wallston, B. S., & Wallston, K. A. (1978). Locus of control and health. A review of the literature. *Health Education Monographs, 6*, 197–217.

Wallston, K. A., Wallston, B. S., & De Vellis, R. (1978). Development of the Multidimensional Health Locus of Control (MHLC) Scales. *Health Education Monographs, 6*, 160–170.

Warren, L. W., & McEachren, L. (1983). Psychosocial correlates of depressive symptomatology in adult women. *Journal of Abnormal Psychology, 92*(2), 151–160.

Weary, G., Elbin, S., & Hill, M. G. (1987). Attributional and social comparison processes in depression. *Journal of Personality and Social Psychology, 52*, 605–610.

Weary, G., Jordan, J. S., & Hill, M. G. (1985). The attributional norm of internality and depression in sensitivity to social information. *Journal of Personality and Social Psychology, 3*, 2–8.

Weissman, M. M., John, K., Merikangas, K., Prusoff, B., Wickramaratne, P., Gammon, G., Angold, A., & Warner, V. (1986). Depressed parents and their children: General health, social and psychiatric problems. *American Journal of Diseases of Children, 140*, 801–805.

Weissman, M. M., & Klerman, G. L. (1977). Sex differences and epidemiology of depression. *Archives of General Psychiatry, 34*, 98–111.

Weissman, M. M., & Klerman, G. L. (1985). Gender and depression. *Trends in NeuroSciences, 8*(9), 416–420.

Weissman, M. M., Leaf, F. J., & Bruce, M. L. (1987). Single-parent women: A community study. *Social Psychiatry, 22*, 29–36.

Weissman, M. M., Leaf, P. J., Holzer, C. E., Myers, J. K., & Tischler, G. T. (1984). The epidemiology of depression: An update on sex differences in rates. *Journal of Affective Disorders, 7*, 179–188.

Weissman, M. M., & Merikangas, K. R. (1986). The epidemiology of anxiety and panic disorders: An update. *Journal of Clinical Psychiatry, 47* (6-Supplement), 11–17.

Weissman, M. M., & Myers, J. K. (1980). The New Haven Community Survey 1967–75: Depressive symptoms and diagnosis. In S. B. Sells & R. Crandall (Eds.), *Human functioning in longitudinal perspective* (pp. 74–88). Baltimore: Williams & Wilkins.

Weissman, M. M., Myers, J., Thompson, W., & Belanger, A. (1986). Depressive symptoms as a risk factor for mortality and for major depression. In L. Erlenmeyer-Kimling & N. Miller (Eds.), *Life span research on the prediction of psychopathology* (pp. 251–260). Hillsdale, NJ: Erlbaum.

Whiffen, V. E. (1988a). Screening for postpartum depression: A methodological note. *Journal of Clinical Psychology, 44*, 367–371.

Whiffen, V. E. (1988b). Vulnerability to postpartum depression: A prospective multivariate study. *Journal of Abnormal Psychology, 97*, 467–474.

Whitely, B. E., Jr. (1985). Sex role orientation and psychological well-being: Two meta-analyses. *Sex Roles, 12*, 207–225.

Williams, W. L. (1986). *The spirit and the flesh: Sexual diversity in American Indian culture.* Boston: Beacon Press.

Wilmoth, G., & Adelstein, D. (1988). *Psychological sequelae of abortion and public policy.* Paper presented at the 96th American Psychological Association Convention, Atlanta, GA.

Wilson, G. (1987). Assessing treatment outcome in bulimia nervosa: A methodological note. *International Journal of Eating Disorders, 6*(3), 339–348.

Winokur, A., March, V., & Mendels, J. (1980). Primary affective disorder in relatives of patients with anorexia nervosa. *American Journal of Psychiatry, 137*, 695–698.

Wooley, S. C., & Wooley, O. W. (1981). Overeating as substance abuse. *Advances in Substance Abuse, 2*, 41–67.

Wooley, S. C., & Wooley, O. W. (1985). Intensive outpatient and residential treatment for bulimia. In D. M. Garner & P. E. Garfinkel (Eds.), *Handbook of psychotherapy for anorexia nervosa and bulimia.* New York: Guilford Press.

Wortman, C. B., & Brehm, J. W. (1975). Responses to uncontrollable outcomes: An integration of reactance theory and the learned helplessness model. In L. Berkowitz (Ed.), *Advances in experimental social psychology* (Vol. 8). Orlando, FL: Academic Press.

Wright, F., O'Leary, J., & Balkin, J. (1989). Shame, guilt, narcissism and depression: Correlates and sex differences. *Psychoanalytic Psychology, 6*, 217–230.

Wyatt, G. E. (1985). The sexual abuse of Afro-American and white-American women in childhood. *Child Abuse and Neglect*, *9*, 507–519.

Wyatt, G. E., Notgrass, C. M., & Newcomb, M. (1990). Internal and external mediators of women's rape experiences. *Psychology of Women Quarterly*, *14*, 153–176.

Zautra, A. J., Reich, J. W., & Guarnaccia, C. A. (1989). The effects of daily life events on negative affective states. *Journal of Personality*. In P. Kendal & D. Watson (Eds.), *Anxiety and depression* (pp. 225–251). New York: Academic Press.

12

Pregnancy

Bonnie Seegmiller

Motherhood is an extremely important issue to all women. In all societies throughout the world, women are expected to marry and bear children. This expectation is termed the "motherhood mandate" (Russo, 1976). Most women, in fact, do meet these expectations; they marry and bear children through biological pregnancy achieved through sexual intercourse. Others have traditionally become mothers through adoption, stepparenting, or foster care. More recently, reproductive technologies such as donor insemination, invitro fertilization, embryo transfer, and surrogacy have been developed that provide women with other possible means of becoming mothers. Women who were previously unable to have children are now able to do so. In contrast, however, other women are making choices that fail to conform to some or all of societal expectations. Thus, an increasing number of unmarried heterosexual and lesbian women are choosing motherhood, while other women are choosing to remain child-free.

This chapter deals with pregnancy: how cultures shape and maintain individuals' attitudes toward pregnancy, what the experience of pregnancy is like, how women change and adapt during pregnancy, and how they interact with the medical establishment during this period.

Although the purpose of this book is to enhance sociocultural awareness and understanding of women, a review of the literature on the above topics has shown that women of color and ethnicity have been sorely neglected with regard to most issues surrounding pregnancy. The scarcity of such data clearly indicates that there are major gaps in our knowledge and that further research is needed.

THE PREGNANCY EXPERIENCE

Introduction: Folktales, Prescriptions, and Taboos

Most women who want to become mothers do so as a result of a biological pregnancy. All cultures mark pregnancy as a special event and shape attitudes and behaviors associated with it. Many unfounded beliefs (frequently referred to as "old wives' tales") about pregnancy exist. Just as there is a "society of children," there is a "society of women" through which this folklore of pregnancy is passed, from woman to woman, intergenerationally and between peers. This folklore touches on many aspects of pregnancy. A number of stories, for example, suggest ways that one can predict the fetus's sex: if the fetus is carried in the hips ("low") or has a slow heart rate, it is thought to be a girl, while if it is carried out in front ("high"), has a fast heart rate, or kicks early, a boy. Some of the folklore relates to the symptoms of pregnancy, such as the notion that heartburn means the baby will be hairy. Women also pass on advice about how to induce labor, such as by using large doses of castor oil or laxatives (they don't work) (Brown, 1981).

Some view pregnancy as akin to spirit possession, with the following being true for both: the individual's body has been invaded by an alien; its presence supplies explanations of the person's behavior; the person is exempt from responsibilities; society attempts to tame the spirit; specialists are required for diagnosis and prognosis; both serve as a way of gaining status; and both are more frequent in women (Graham, 1976). Realistically, pregnancy and childbirth are uncertain events over which individuals have only limited control. In most cultures, pregnancy is surrounded by magical belief systems and prescriptions of things to do or avoid that most likely represent attempts to increase subjective feelings of control (Brown, 1981). Some actions are recommended to increase the chances of an easy or successful pregnancy and birth. For example, some pregnant Spanish-speaking women in the southwestern United States wear a cord, or *muñeco* beneath the breasts and knotted over the umbilicus to prevent morning sickness and ensure a safe delivery. Some Puerto Rican and Mexican women ingest particular kinds of teas to prevent morning sickness, while in the United States, saltines and benedictine are used for the same purpose. Puerto Rican culture instructs the pregnant woman to eat oatmeal and cornstarch pudding to decrease the amount of wrinkling in the child (Brown, 1981).

In contrast to these prescriptive activities, other things are taboo. These taboos derive from fears of causing harm to the woman, fetus, or others, as well as from beliefs that the pregnant woman has supernatural powers (Graham, 1976). Breaking the taboo is believed to result in immediate punishment. Stephens (1963) names three classes of taboos: food, action, and sex. Food taboos are the most ubiquitous. Many involve prohibiting food with physical characteristics considered undesirable for the child. Thus, pregnant Polynesian women avoid eating any eggs with double yolks or fruit partially joined with another, believing that twins would result, and some women in the United States avoid eating strawberries, which are thought by some to produce strawberry birthmarks (Brown, 1981). Puerto Rican taboos include not drinking strong tea (thought to lead to miscarriage), avoiding Carnation milk (thought to cause nausea), not eating fruit with milk (it will poison you), not eating extremely hot or cold foods (they'll hurt the baby), and avoiding sour foods (they aren't good for the baby and will make you skinny in pregnancy) (Lazarus, 1984). Vietnamese women avoid salty food, fish, and rice for similar reasons. Some women in the United States believe eating potatoes during pregnancy will cause the child to be deformed. (Finger, 1984, has pointed out that this belief may have arisen from the relatively higher incidence of spina bifida—an open lesion anywhere along the spinal cord—in people of Irish descent.)

In many cultures, fetuses are thought to take on characteristics of things seen by the mother; consequently, activity taboos include not looking at certain things, like snakes, other animals, or the full moon, to avoid crippling or deforming the fetus. Looking at fire is thought to cause birthmarks in some cultures (Hilliard, 1986), and riding horseback is often avoided because it is thought to lead to a difficult delivery (Joesting, 1973). Pregnant Vietnamese woman are forbidden to attend weddings or funerals (Brown, 1981). Many Puerto Rican women believe that sleeping with a chain on will result in the baby's having a line around its neck when it is born and, also, that disliking an individual may result in the baby's resembling that person. Thinking evil thoughts is thought to harm the baby (Lazarus, 1984). According to Kitzinger (1978), in some places it is believed that if a pregnant woman is frightened by a mouse, the fetus will develop a mouse-shaped birthmark. Some blacks in Louisiana believe that lifting the arms above the head will result in the umbilical cord's twisting around the child's neck (Scott & Stern, 1986). Based on her fieldwork, Kitzinger (1978) describes some of the many rules for the pregnant Jamaican woman:

She is not to step over a donkey's tethering rope lest the birth be overdue, or put corks in bottles in case she has a difficult, prolonged labor and does not "open up." She must not see a corpse lest her blood become chilled and the baby turn cold inside her and die . . . she must drink with discretion because too much water drowns the child. [They] must not make too many preparations ahead of time or the baby will be stillborn, a belief which corresponds to the English [and American] superstition that if an expectant mother buys the pram [or baby furniture or a layette] before the baby's birth, her baby may not survive. . . . If she sees anything shocking or ugly, or becomes upset about something, the baby may be marked. If she notices a person without a leg, for example, her baby may be born like that, or if she wrings a chicken's neck and feels sorry for the bird, the baby can be born resembling a chicken. (p. 70)

In many industrialized societies, many restrictions placed on the pregnant woman's physical and social activities may also be classified as activity taboos since they are totally unnecessary. For example, until relatively recently in the United States, pregnancy was not a public event. Pregnant teachers were banned from their classrooms, and other pregnant women were not permitted to work. These taboos were enforced through both formal and informal sanctioning. In addition to the ''negative moral influence'' that such exposure to sexuality was thought to have on children and other adults, there was the supposed threat of harm to the fetus from too much activity!

Sex taboos usually take the form of prohibitions against engaging in intercourse so as to avoid alleged harm to the fetus and pollution of one's body. Such beliefs are not unusual in the United States (Brown, 1981). Masters and Johnson (1966) reported 77% of the women they interviewed had been told by their physicians to avoid sex during the third trimester (only 21% complied, by the way). Pregnant Mbuti women (in Zaire) are prohibited from accompanying men on the hunt, and intercourse is banned during pregnancy as well as before the hunt (Turnbull, cited in Kitzinger, 1978). As will be discussed later in the chapter, in most cases there is no medical reason to avoid intercourse during pregnancy. Paige and Paige (1981) suggest that sex taboos may reflect psychological conflicts aroused by the birth event: having to avoid something removes the cause of conflict. Others (e.g., Young, 1965) view sex and other taboos (as well as instructions for positive activities) as part of the transitional rites of passage marking and culminating in the child's birth.

In some cultures, men also are subject to certain prescriptions and taboos during their wife's pregnancy, labor, or birth. Most notable among these, in some (e.g., South American) cultures, men are expected to engage in couvade, in which they either pretend to experience (couvade ritual) or actually experience (couvade syndrome) some of the symptoms of pregnancy, labor, or birth, including nausea, vomiting, toothache, loss of appetite, and/or pain (Trethowan & Conlon, 1965). That there are rituals and taboos surrounding pregnancy that apply to men may seem curious at first given the exclusively female nature of pregnancy. This very exclusivity, however, may provide one of the major explanations for the occurrence of couvade. Rituals such as couvade and other actions either required of, or prohibited for, the fathers serve as public attempts to establish social recognition of the man's rights, paternity, and control of the process and the child. They may be ways for the men to emphasize their contributions, to draw attention away from the women (Bettelheim, 1962; Paige & Paige, 1981). Reproductive rituals that involve males, in their varied forms from couvade to the medicalization of childbearing by physicians who are usually men, may serve political functions. (Medicalization involves procedures such as general anesthesia, delivery in the supine position, use of drugs to time labor, episiotomies, and immediate clamping of the umbilical cord.) Such rituals have the effect of increasing the woman's powerlessness while the male is given more control (Paige & Paige, 1981).

Other explanations of these rituals and taboos have also been proposed. Some view them as ways for the male to establish for himself an identity as a father. They may also reflect the male image of the laboring woman as in pain and need of protection (Slochower, personal communication, 1989). Some view them as forms of sympathetic magic, through which any evil spirits that may be around are tricked into pursuing the father instead of the mother or fetus (Colman & Colman, 1971). From a psychoanalytic perspective, the rituals may represent attempts to get the child to attend to the father instead of the mother in order to prevent incestuous desires for the mother (Reik, 1931). They may be reaction formations in males who are extremely ambivalent about the pregnancy, serving to repress any unconscious aggression the man feels toward the mother and the fetus or child (Brown, 1981; Reik, 1931). Paige and Paige (1981) have also stated that in some cases, paternal fasting expresses the urge to devour the child and is the atonement for guilt from this urge. In addition, male rituals may be expressions of male identification with the female role ("womb envy"), serving to reduce envy of this role and enabling the man to share in the experience (Bettelheim, 1962; Burton & Whiting, 1961; Kitzinger, 1972, 1978). The rituals may also represent socially acceptable outlets for cross-sex identifications (Bettelheim, 1962; Colman & Colman, 1971).

Attitudes Toward Pregnancy and How They Are Shaped

In most industrialized societies, the medical model is applied to pregnancy, turning it into a pathological event, rather than a normal physiological process or stage of development. Pregnancy is considered to be a time of illness; the pregnant woman is thought of as sick, and this view is reinforced by the fact that pregnant women visit physicians, that is, people who care for the ill, not the well. The effect for some women is a self-fulfilling prophecy: the inclination to treat women "as if" they are ill may in some cases actually encourage the adoption of the sick role (McKinlay, 1972).

Many view pregnancy as a period of increased psychological and physiological vulnerability, often accompanied by severe psychological or psychogenic problems. Some believe that these problems result directly from actual physiological changes that occur during pregnancy, such as increases in progesterone and estrogen (possibly directly resulting in emotional lability), increases in adrenal cortical hormones (which are related to stress), and reduced norepinephrine levels (which relate to depression) (see Treadway, Kane, Jarrahi-Zadeh & Lipton, 1969; Unger, 1979). On the other hand, others argue cogently that identical physiological changes interact with the woman's individual psychological makeup as well as with social and cultural influences to produce different reactions in each woman (Unger, 1979). A good example of the need to consider the interaction between these factors is provided by Unger's discussion of the high desirability of slimness as a cultural norm in the United States. Of biological necessity, pregnancy involves the loss of this valued state, causing many women to feel depressed. So not only are the physiological changes of pregnancy important, but perhaps even more important is how the physiological changes affect the woman's level of body comfort, her self-image, and/or her actual appearance through psychological channels. Thus, in order to understand how women view pregnancy and themselves while pregnant, psychological, social, and cultural influences must be considered along with the physiological processes.

Women receive information throughout their entire lives that shapes their views of pregnancy. A partial list of the sources of such information includes the woman's own mother, her early socialization experiences, the woman's peers, other pregnant women, responses from medical personnel, how other people respond to her, and messages transmitted through the broader culture, such as the media. In regard to early socialization experiences, imagine the effect one would expect from being exposed to a mother, grandmother, aunts, and other adult women who viewed pregnancy positively, remained active during their pregnancy, actually spoke about the pregnancy, and in general conveyed the positive message that pregnancy was a normal physiological process. Imagine further that the men involved also responded positively. Contrast this with an environment in which the women, if they spoke of it at all, viewed pregnancy negatively, dwelt on their being sick and on the pain and difficulties experienced, and assumed the martyr role, and the men involved also viewed pregnancy as an illness. Theories of personality development such as psychoanalytic theory, identification theory, social learning theory, and cognitive theory would all predict these differential attitudes would be internalized by children (both girls and boys) exposed to them. Women whose mothers and other significant female figures displayed positive attitudes and reactions to pregnancy would be expected to feel more positively about pregnancy than those who had been exposed to models with more negative attitudes. Early experiences with openness about the process would be expected to result in more openness, less secretiveness, and less shame and embarrassment in adulthood.

Adult peers would be expected to exert similar types of influence, especially given the importance of social acceptance and support. Imagine the difference between peers who share factual information and positive experiences as opposed to those who shock you with horror stories. (A personal communication from Rabinowitz, 1988, tells of one woman who, when pregnant, was cautioned to wipe herself carefully after urinating, since the woman telling her the story reported feeling her own fetus's hand on one such occasion.) Medical personnel also shape attitudes toward pregnancy. Despite the fact that enormous physiological changes occur during pregnancy, many physicians continue to view such symptoms are purely psychogenic. This frequently results in women's receiving inadequate treatment and derisive responses from medical personnel who view symptoms as reflecting the woman's maladjustment or her rejection of the fetus (Lennane & Lennane, 1973). Other medical personnel may take the opposite attitude, by interpreting psychological symptoms as physical (Slochower, personal communication, 1989).

The media also depict pregnant women in ways that convey information about, and attitudes toward, pregnancy. Until the 1960s, one might have concluded from watching television that there were no pregnant females since they were never shown (and were rarely alluded or referred to). Beginning with "I Love

Lucy," however, the situation began to change, although many restrictions applied. In the late 1970s, for example, a local newscaster in New York City wore a shirt during a broadcast with the word *baby* and a downward pointing arrow aimed at her pregnant midsection, which was discretely hidden behind the news desk. Most women who are currently portrayed on TV as being pregnant are slim except for a slight bulge in the abdominal area. Although things have changed since "Little Ricky" Arnaz was gestated on "I Love Lucy," and soap operas frequently depend on babies born out of wedlock and on miscarriages for their plots, few, if any, television serials foster the view that pregnancy is a normal event. On the contrary, pregnancy is portrayed as either a condition requiring urgent medical attention or the butt of jokes.

The print media also send messages through their portrayal of pregnant women. Graham (1976) summarized the message sent by a number of magazines aimed at pregnant women:

Pregnancy, as socially portrayed, epitomizes femininity: it offers woman her ultimate social and psychic fulfillment. But it is also a time of emotional and physical vulnerability; the expectant mother is in need of protection. Dormant emotions are awakened through the hormonal or psychotic imbalances resulting from the baby *in utero*. Nonetheless, perhaps as a compensation, pregnancy is an occasion to enjoy activities and objects normally denied; the expectant mother can and should be spoiled. (pp. 295–296)

People's attitudes toward events and themselves are also in part shaped by interpersonal relationships, that is, by how others respond to them. Pregnancy brings about a change in these responses. Pregnancy has been described as "the most stereotyped stage of a woman's life, with attitudes toward pregnancy serving as one of the most prevalent sources of discrimination against women" (Leifer, 1980, p. 754). Although discrimination against pregnant workers in regard to hiring and fringe benefits was outlawed by the U.S. Civil Rights Law of 1964, discrimination, both in the form of conveying the idea that pregnancy means inferiority and in more economic terms such as pregnant women's being denied jobs or raises, still exists.

Other changes occur in how other people react to the pregnant woman. Foremost among these is the fact that pregnant women are responded to on the basis of an identification that is biologically based rather than personal, in terms of their being pregnant rather than on the basis of individual characteristics (Colman & Colman, 1971). One notices that other individuals or groups are more accepting or, at the very least, act differently toward the pregnant woman: she is no longer ignored. At social gatherings, pregnant women, especially those who are most noticeably pregnant and close to term, become the biologically based dominant focus of attention (Colman & Colman, 1971). The presence of pregnant women frequently makes others anxious. On game shows, for instance, it seems inevitable that the hosts make some comment or joke about how the woman should remain calm if she wins so as not to induce labor.

Another oft-noted change occurs in regard to personal boundaries (Colman & Colman, 1971). People infantilize pregnant women and in many ways become intrusive. Individuals who would never under ''ordinary circumstances'' do so, feel at liberty to touch the pregnant woman and her swollen abdomen. Distal intrusions also increase as people, both known and unknown, smile (knowingly? approvingly?) and stare. Anecdotal evidence shows that unsolicited advice is given freely to pregnant women by complete strangers. Others with whom one is not on close terms discuss intimate details of their own pregnancies and childbearing experiences (and so the transmission of more folklore continues).

The above findings suggest that pregnancy elicits rather complex responses from others, possibly including envy, anxiety, identification, and hope, to name a few (Slochower, personal communication, 1989). Most of these reactions have not yet been studied. Studies have, however, shown quite clearly that pregnancy is reacted to as if it were a social stigma akin to mental and physical disability or obesity and that people hold expectations about how pregnant women should behave, that is, passively. Taylor and Langer (1977), in a study of interpersonal interaction, showed that although individuals liked a passive pregnant woman more than an assertive one, they preferred to interact with a nonpregnant woman rather than a pregnant one. In other studies, people were overly solicitous of pregnant women while simultaneously preferring to stand farther away from them (Davis & Lennon, 1983; Langer, Fiske, Taylor & Chanowitz, 1976; Taylor & Langer, 1977). In these studies, many furtive glances were directed at the pregnant women, which parallels behavior shown toward the handicapped (although, to be sure, the reactions to the two groups may result from different reasons). Pregnancy may be a statistically novel sight since the pregnant woman's discomfort in social situations may lead her to engage in social interaction less often. Because individuals frequently respond socially to novelty with both unwarranted attention to novel characteristics and avoidance of the unusual person, the pregnant woman's sense of social deviance may be increased along with her social isolation, thus reinforcing her view of pregnancy as a deviant condition (Unger, 1979). This response to social novelty also explains the simultaneous increase in both stares and furtive glances, as well as the increased touching and standing farther away mentioned earlier.

Some evidence suggests social class differences in how women view pregnancy, but the findings have been conflicting. The view of pregnancy as illness and the assumption of the sick role was found to be more common in women of lower socioeconomic status in some studies (Rosengren, 1961, 1962) but less common in other studies (McKinlay, 1972). Horgan (1983), using another approach to study social class differences, demonstrated that stores catering to women of different social classes handled maternity clothing differently. Most of the high-status stores did not even carry maternity clothes. Those that did had very few, and these were located by the lingerie or loungewear. In contrast to this, maternity clothes in lower-status stores were usually placed with uniforms or large sizes. These differential placements were seen as reflecting different attitudes toward pregnancy and women. The higher-status stores conveyed the message that pregnancy is "feminine, delicate, luxurious, joyous, personal, and private. In lower status stores, pregnancy is viewed as a job, a period when one is fat" (Horgan, 1983, p. 337). A questionnaire administered to pregnant women at the stores confirmed that women from the different socioeconomic classes viewed themselves differently: pregnant women from the higher social classes were more likely to feel sexy and less likely to report being treated differently by others, while lower social status women felt fat. Anecdotal evidence suggests that higher-status stores may be moving toward a more integrated attitude toward pregnancy: in some of these stores, maternity wear may now be found next to infant wear.

There has been some movement in the United States toward viewing pregnancy as a normal developmental stage (Rapoport, Rapoport & Streilitz, 1972). However, as has been shown throughout this chapter, many still hold the view that pregnancy is a sickness, and many still attribute failure to become pregnant and a mother as due to immaturity and psychological conflicts. In addition, most studies of pregnancy continue to examine the individual and do not put enough (if any) emphasis on the wider context in which pregnancy occurs (Bronfenbrenner, 1979). It should be clear from the above discussion that many social and cultural factors influence a woman's attitudes to pregnancy, yet only minimal attention has been paid to such factors. Notably, only a few studies have dealt with how factors related to race or ethnicity influence attitudes toward pregnancy. The evidence that does exist is conflicting. Lazarus (1984), for instance, had expected, but failed to find, that the health-related beliefs in Puerto Rican culture, such as the hot-cold therapeutic theory, extreme modesty, different ways of classifying illness, and the strong family support system, would result in Puerto Rican women's differing from non–Puerto Rican women with regard to their beliefs about, and experiences of, their pregnancies. In contrast, Harris, Linn, Good, and Hunter (1981) found that Cuban and other Hispanic women were more positive in their attitudes toward pregnancy than were black or white women. To the extent that women of color and ethnicity are exposed to different social and cultural influences, one would expect differences in their attitudes and reactions to pregnancy. Yet such studies of the psychological experiences of pregnancy as influenced by social and cultural factors have not been conducted.

REACTIONS TO PREGNANCY

Pregnancy is a period of enormous change. The woman who is pregnant experiences physiological, psychological, interpersonal, and social status changes simultaneously with the more obvious changes in appearance (Leifer, 1980). To some, pregnancy is inherently a crisis, necessarily a time of enormous stress and emotional upheaval when old conflicts surrounding issues such as dependency, nurturance, and separation are resurrected, thus creating psychological disequilibrium. The woman attempts to resolve these old conflicts by renegotiating her relations—with herself, her parents, her partner, and society in general. Thus, although emotional changes occurring during pregnancy constitute a significant crisis, the woman's reactions to the crisis can potentially (though not necessarily) lead to psychological growth (Benedek, 1949, 1952, 1959, 1970; Bibring, 1959; Bibring, Dwyer, Huntington & Valenstein, 1961; Chertok, 1966; Deutsch, 1945). Others have suggested that emotional upheaval is not inherent to pregnancy, and some have even described pregnancy as a period of bliss, of "vegetative calm," or of particular well-being (Cohen, 1966; Hooke & Marks, 1962). The view that is most compelling, however, is that pregnancy is neither a crisis nor a time of absolute bliss, but a developmental transition in which the accompanying emotional upheavals are intrinsically neither positive nor negative; they can be either (Leifer, 1977; Osofsky & Osofsky, 1984). Whether one believes pregnancy to be a crisis or a transition, all would agree that pregnancy is a time of change during which previous ways of reacting are no longer adequate, and new responses become necessary.

The major topics covered in this section include the tasks of pregnancy that women must deal with (attachment, separation-individuation, and identity formation); how women react to pregnancy in general; how they adjust to pregnancy; how changes in one's body are responded to; the affective changes that occur in mood, anxieties and fears, and self-preoccupation; and the changes in fantasies and dreams and in sexuality that occur during pregnancy.

The Tasks of Pregnancy

Pregnant women tackle extremely important tasks. Although different investigators use varying labels, most agree that the major tasks of pregnancy are attachment, separation-individuation, and identity formation. These involve adjusting to being pregnant, incorporating (feeling the fetus to be a part of you) and accepting the fetus, forming an attachment to it, differentiating and separating from the fetus, reconciling with one's own mother by forming a new relationship with her through separation and individuation, and internalizing the identity of "mother." These tasks result in the woman's developing a new sense of self, of the child, of one's own mother, and of one's partner (Ballou, 1978; Bibring et al., 1961; Colman & Colman, 1971; Doering, Entwisle & Quinlan, 1980; Leifer, 1977; Sherwin, 1987).

During the first trimester, the fetus is experienced as part of the self rather than as a separate entity, and there is little sense of attachment to it as a separate being. The woman's awareness of these changes results in her viewing the fetus as a foreign object that she attempts to cope with by incorporating it into her body image (Bibring et al., 1961). Thus, during this stage, the fetus is viewed as an extension of herself, not as separate. During this early part of pregnancy, the woman begins to become preoccupied with herself (or narcissistic) as she becomes more aware of, and focused on, the subtle changes that are occurring in her body. Not being visibly pregnant causes some women to question the existence of the child. Fear of miscarriage (Leifer, 1977) or of the possibility of an elective abortion depending upon the results of amniocentesis also results in a hesitancy to become attached to the fetus. Katz Rothman (1987), in fact, has written of ''the tentative pregnancy,'' which refers to the delay in attachment feelings engendered by prenatal screening procedures such as amniocentesis. (On the other hand, procedures such as ultrasound, conducted even earlier in the pregnancy than amniocentesis, may accelerate the development of attachment.) During this early part of pregnancy, the woman may hold long conversations with others about the child, especially her partner, thus beginning the incorporation of the child into their relationship. She may also try out different names on the fetus in a further attempt to make the fetus feel real (Leifer, 1977; Sherwin, 1987).

Quickening in the second trimester has traditionally been viewed as a turning point in the process of accepting the fetus as an individual, as separate and apart, and as an object of attachment. Its movements help to make the fetus real, as do the noticeable changes in the woman's body that necessitate the purchase of maternity clothes. During the second trimester, the woman may respond to fetal movements by talking, offering reassurance, affection, or reprimands for moving too quickly or forcefully, or, if she is eating, she may offer the fetus food. Frequently, at this point, the woman's language also reflects the growing sense of attachment, with many references to ''we'' (Sherwin, 1987). Many women encourage their partner's participation in the conversations, in feeling the movements, and attending prenatal classes (Leifer, 1977). The woman usually becomes concerned with her relationship with her own mother during this time as the identification of herself as a mother begins to develop (Bibring et al., 1961).

The attachment and separation processes continue during the third trimester as the woman becomes particularly aware of the fetus's body parts, activity level, and temperament (Sherwin, 1987) and as she ascribes personal characteristics to the fetus. The woman's increasing self-preoccupation may in part result from her attempts to deal with the problems of separation and identity diffusion between the fetus and herself (Colman & Colman, 1971). During the third trimester, the reality of the fetus is further increased by changes in her body; also, it is often during this time that she names the child. Some have also described what have been called ''nesting behaviors'' (e.g., buying things for the child, decorating its room or area, cleaning) at this time and have found them to be related to the degree of emotional attachment the woman has to her fetus (Leifer, 1977). Furthermore, one's body size is a constant reminder that the baby will soon separate (Slochower, personal communication, 1989). Women frequently experience their large bodies as discontinuous from (i.e., not) their real selves (Schuzman, cited in Sherwin, 1987).

Clearly, the development of attachment to the fetus varies widely from woman to woman. Leifer (1977), for example, described three patterns of attachment formation over the course of pregnancy. For some women, there was minimal attachment throughout; these women perceived the fetus as an intrusion and an annoyance. A second pattern was shown by women who did not experience closeness early in the pregnancy, but whose feelings of attachment were evident after the quickening. The third pattern was evidenced by women who showed early attachment that continued throughout the pregnancy. The dynamics of the attachment process are extremely important as researchers have shown that the degree of emotional attachment achieved during pregnancy relates strongly to postpartum maternal feelings and adjustment (Leifer, 1977; Lester & Notman, 1986).

Working out the relationship with her fetus can be difficult for a woman and is certainly an individual process. The kind of attachment that one develops is influenced by the woman's relationships with other people, in both the past and the present. These relations determine what she expects of others and what she believes people are like (Ballou, 1978). One set of relations that are particularly relevant to pregnancy concern those involving the woman's own mother, particularly her own early experience of having been mothered. Investigators such as Ballou (1978), Benedek (1970), Lester and Notman (1986), Pines (1972), and Shereshefsky and Yarrow (1973) have noted that a positive sense of having been mothered facilitates the ability to mother someone else well. Women who themselves had good experiences being mothered—who saw their mothers as empathic, satisfied with their maternal role, supportive, and close—showed greater ego strength during pregnancy and less anxiety. Those who had difficulty adjusting to pregnancy were less likely to have perceived their mothers as good mothers (Ballou, 1978; Leifer, 1980).

Some have described pregnancy as regressive in the sense of its being a time when the woman becomes more concerned with earlier issues of dependency and autonomy vis-à-vis her own mother (Benedek, 1970; Bibring et al., 1961). During pregnancy, the woman attempts to psychologically reconcile conflicts with her mother and consequently to renegotiate their dependency relationship. Ballou (1978) found that during pregnancy, a more positive view of one's own mother often develops, along with a more positive view of one's own childhood. This is especially true if the woman was able to tolerate her own dependency. Ballou points out, "If she is going to accept the dependency of her child, she must accept her own dependency" (Ballou, 1978, p. 46). Such dependency should be viewed as healthy.

This process of reconciliation can vary in its difficulty. For some, the problems that the pregnant woman's mother may herself have may make things more difficult. Some common situations in which this occurs include when the woman's mother attempts to prove she's a better mother, when she finds her internal conflicts about aging exacerbated by her daughter's pregnancy, and when she is confronted with the unwanted necessity of finally accepting her daughter as an adult. (To some women, adulthood requires pregnancy and motherhood.) Some women find it difficult to separate from their mothers as their mother continues to attempt to control them. In contrast, for some women, this may become a time of increased sharing with their mothers. For the first time, the older woman may share her own experiences and feelings about pregnancy and motherhood with her daughter. Some researchers have found that during this period, the pregnant woman may permit her mother to be more openly affectionate to her than ever before. Given the daughter's conflicts about autonomy and dependency and the difficulties involved in establishing oneself as an adult rather than a child to one's parents, the daughter may previously have had to mistrust and reject any such expressions of affection as possessive or overprotective (Leifer, 1977). The daughter's new status of imminent motherhood may automatically confer adult status. Colman and Colman (1971) have noted that pregnancy involves establishing a new identity, that of "mother," which is separate from that of one's own mother and which involves feelings of adult competence and effectiveness.

General Reactions to Pregnancy

Earlier in the chapter, some of the factors influencing the formation of attitudes toward pregnancy in general were discussed. How a woman actually reacts to her pregnancy is shaped by a host of factors in addition to her attitudes. Some of these include background and life history factors, such as her relationship with her own parents, her own experiences of being mothered, early influences on her personality such as identification with her parent(s), and her experiences with children. Some are personality factors, including the woman's predominant defenses, characteristic ways of expressing feelings, her sense of her own identity, achievement of an adult role, qualities of feminine identification and gender-role attitudes in general, adaptive behaviors, and emotional stability. Others relate to her current life situation, such as her adaptation to her marriage or relationship, compatibility with her partner, their relationship as a couple, her mate's reactions and supportiveness, his capacity for empathy and affection, the anticipated relation of her partner to the expected child, her emotional responses to the pregnancy, her employment status, and socioeconomic influences. Additional factors concern the pregnancy experience itself, such as whether the pregnancy is wanted and planned, whether the pregnancy is an easy or difficult one physically, her reactions to the physical changes of pregnancy, and her expectations about the sex of the child. The fears and anxieties she experiences about the child and about her own body may also influence her reactions to her pregnancy, as might her responses to labor and delivery. Her dependency relations with others, her narcissism, her feelings of competency regarding child-rearing and her capacity to see herself in the mothering role, and her movement toward identifying as a larger family unit may also affect how she experiences her pregnancy. Other influences relate to the physical, psychological, economic, and social support available to her and to the role conflicts that she may feel. Similarly, her experiences in school, with peers, and at work all may influence a woman's reactions toward pregnancy, as may her interpretation of all of the factors (Hunter College Women's Studies Collective, 1983; Shereshefsky & Yarrow, 1973).

Given these many influences, it is not surprising to find that reactions to pregnancy are individual, that is, that there is no one way of reacting to pregnancy. One of the most consistent findings regarding pregnancy is that how a woman adjusts is consistent with how she adapted to situations before the pregnancy. A study by Leifer (1977), for example, found that women who showed positive adjustments early in pregnancy and whose positive adjustments continued throughout pregnancy tended to have had stable, well-integrated prepregnancy personalities that included feelings of satisfaction with themselves (in regard to both self-concept and body image), stable and positive need, satisfaction with sexual relations, absence of menstrual stress, and high levels of growth motivation. In addition, they had planned their pregnancies. These women reacted positively to most aspects of pregnancy. They evidenced little symptomatology (physical problems) and took pride in their pregnant appearance. These women also felt increased self-esteem and a sense of growth as pregnancy progressed. Women who adapted more gradually to pregnancy were less satisfied with themselves before the pregnancy and showed moderate rankings on the personality variables referred to above. They experienced more ambivalent feelings about their pregnancy and their appearance and showed moderate to high levels of symptomatology. They felt less confident about themselves as mothers. However, despite these difficulties, many of these women experienced increases in self-esteem during pregnancy. The third group in Leifer's study was comprised of women who adjusted poorly to pregnancy. They were found to have poor personality integration, they were dissatisfied with their sexual relations, they experienced more negative affect, they felt very negatively about their appearance, and they had very low self-esteem both before and during pregnancy, as well as high symptomatology during pregnancy. Similarly, Shereshefsky and Yarrow (1973) found that overall adjustment to pregnancy was related to prior ego strength, to nurturance, and to the ability to visualize oneself as a mother. The woman's personality before pregnancy was found to relate to her reactions during pregnancy: women who were passive, dependent, emotional, and excitable, all traits associated with stereotyped femininity, experienced the greatest difficulties during pregnancy, perhaps because they lacked the strength, assertiveness, and independence necessary for childbearing. In sum, "each woman entered upon, confronted, and dealt with the pregnancy experience according to the strengths and weaknesses she possessed prior to the pregnancy experience" (Shereshefsky & Yarrow, 1973, p. 47). Another consistent finding has been that over the course of pregnancy, ambivalent and moderately positive attitudes usually become more prevalent, regardless of how negative or positive the women were at the beginning of pregnancy. This occurs as she attempts to deal with all of the tasks and changes discussed above. Most women focus on the delivery date during the third trimester and, as it approaches, become impatient to get the birth over with. Simultaneously, however, they may experience a feeling of loss for this unique relationship with the fetus (Jessner, Weigert, & Foy, 1970).

Adjustment to Pregnancy

Factors related to the social context such as the amount and quality of support provided by one's social network—one's mate, friends, family, and coworkers— all affect whether pregnancy is experienced and adapted to negatively or positively (Cohen, 1966; Gladieux, 1978; Leifer, 1980; Nadelson, 1978; Shereshefsky & Yarrow, 1973). Strong social support has the effect of mediating the adverse effects of stress during pregnancy (Brown, 1986; Gladieux, 1978; Nuckolls, Cassel & Kaplan, 1972; Reading, 1983; Tilden, 1983). Jurich (1987), for example, found anxiety at three, six, and eight months of pregnancy was highly related to the woman's need for emotional support and her satisfaction with her relationship with her partner. Mead and Newton (1967) have stressed how little support the structure of American society provides to the pregnant woman (and mother) in comparison with other societies (see also Leifer, 1980; Nadelson, 1978).

The finding that the first pregnancy is frequently a more positive experience than later pregnancies may in part be due to the higher level of support generally available for pregnancy when it is a new experience. For later pregnancies, one's family and friends may no longer respond to the uniqueness of the situation. The differing amounts of support available based on parity need to be studied cross-culturally, for in cultures that prize high fertility, the amount of support might, in fact, increase with each additional pregnancy.

Other important social context variables are associated with socioeconomic status. To the degree that women are subject to greater stress as a result of the conditions that accompany poverty, one would expect less adjustment to pregnancy. However, although many studies (Richardson & Guttmacher, 1967) consistently confirm that physical problems in pregnancy, birth, and the neonatal period are related to socioeconomic status, women of low socioeconomic status do not show poorer psychological adjustment to pregnancy than those who are more affluent. This finding may reflect the fact that women of color and ethnicity, who comprise a disproportionate part of the lower socioeconomic groups, have been shown to have more reliable and extensive support networks than other women (Stack, 1974). Support has been shown to mediate the negative effects of stress (Nuckolls et al., 1972).

Little or no information is available regarding the effects of the partner's supportiveness in nonmarital heterosexual relationships or those of shorter duration or in lesbian relationships of any duration. Most studies of the psychological aspects of pregnancy, such as adjustment and adaptation, have been conducted on couples who have been legally married. Those studies generally show that pregnancy is accompanied by decreased marital satisfaction, although more so for the husband (Leifer, 1977). Pregnancy may cause considerable disequilibrium for the couple, since it necessarily results in a major change in the couple's identity and communication pattern, and a shift toward more traditional roles (Leifer, 1980). On the other hand, Shereshefsky and Yarrow (1973) found a positive relationship between the woman's adaptation to pregnancy and her husband's response to the pregnancy: when the couple experienced an emerging sense of a common goal, their relationship deepened. Kazama (1988), too, found that marital intimacy had a significant buffering effect on stress. Although Tietjen and Bradley (1985) found no relationship between the husband's support and the woman's overall attitude to pregnancy, they did find that support from the husband related to the woman's adjusting positively with regard to her attitudes toward the child, perceived stress, and postpartum marital adjustment. Cohen (cited in Leifer, 1977) found that the woman's sense of her husband, as well as her relationship with her mother, influenced her satisfaction with pregnancy. Women who adjusted well early in the pregnancy had good relationships with their husbands. Those who had problems early in the pregnancy but who did well later also had positive relations with their husbands, but poor relations with their mothers. Those with problems throughout the pregnancy had poor relations with both their husbands and their mothers.

Although there is some evidence that pregnancy changes one's relationships with friends (Thrasher & Falicov, cited in Leifer, 1980), this phenomenon has received little direct attention, despite the important part friendships play in many women's lives. As the number of voluntarily and involuntarily single mothers continues to increase, this factor would be expected to gain in importance. Social networks and support systems that involve both family and friends are an integral part of the cultures of many women of color and ethnicity. There is evidence to indicate that Puerto Rican (Lazarus, 1984) and black (Stack, 1974) women with good family support respond more positively to pregnancy than those lacking such support. The practice of "passing-on" children, that is, either temporarily or permanently giving them to a family member or close friend, deserves more study (Boyd-Franklin, 1983; Stack, 1974). Knowing that there will be a familiar, trusted person to care for the child when it is born may alleviate some of the problems related to adjustment to pregnancy.

In sum, the most consistent finding regarding support is that it acts to mediate the negative effects of stress (Leifer, 1977; Nuckolls et al., 1972; Reading, 1983). Different sources of support are differentially effective (partner, friends, peers, family, siblings) in buffering different types of stress. Whatever its sources, support is extremely important and is a subject that needs further study.

CHANGES DURING PREGNANCY

Physical Changes

Symptomatology

Generally, the less satisfied one is with one's body before pregnancy, the greater the symptomatology (physical problems) and the more negative or ambivalent one's feelings during pregnancy (Leifer, 1977; Shereshefsky & Yarrow, 1973). One common symptom is morning sickness. There is conflicting evidence as to whether nausea and vomiting have purely biochemical causes as opposed to being psychogenic. It is clear, however, that these symptoms do not indicate a rejection of the fetus. Symptomatology is also unrelated to marital status, race, number of pregnancies, and age (Newton, 1955). The types of symptomatology and the degree to which they are expressed have been shown to be culturally influenced (Carrie, 1981; Leifer, 1980; Mead, 1949).

Body Changes

The conflicting evidence describing how pregnant women feel about their changing bodies may reflect the great individuality of women (Leifer, 1980; Tolor & DiGrazia, 1977). Many investigators report that the emotional reactions to one's pregnant appearance usually become at least somewhat more negative throughout pregnancy (Schuzman, cited in Sherwin, 1987). However, another consistent finding (e.g., Leifer, 1977; Schuzman, cited in Sherwin, 1987) is that attitudes toward one's appearance during pregnancy relate closely to how the woman felt about her body before the pregnancy started as well as to her more general attitudes about the pregnancy. Leifer, for example, found that women who were highly satisfied with their bodies before the pregnancy began and who held positive attitudes about pregnancy were the only women who were unqualifiedly positive about their pregnant appearances. Leifer further describes the women in her study who responded to pregnancy early with positive feelings as taking more pride in their pregnant appearance, enjoying the attention of others, being very involved in their body changes, and experiencing an enhanced sense of womanliness. The women who at first were ambivalent or held negative attitudes toward their pregnancies were more apprehensive about their body changes and the possible loss of attractiveness. Their anxieties increased throughout the pregnancy.

In addition to reactions to one's changing appearance, there is also an increased awareness throughout pregnancy of one's body and body parts. Furthermore, Schuzman (cited in Sherwin, 1987) describes how all pregnant women experience some degree (usually not a great deal) of body image distortion (their sense of what their bodies look like). Harris (1979), in one of the few studies specifically conducted to compare such distortions in black and white women, found that black and white women perceive their bodies differently. The white women were more aware of their stomachs during their pregnancies than were black women. For white women, this awareness related directly to the actual physical state of their stomachs and therefore indicated less body image distortion. For black women, stomach awareness related to emotional and financial factors rather than to the realistic physical states of their stomachs. In addition, the black woman experienced more body distortion throughout pregnancy. Her attitude toward herself was the best predictor of the degree of distortion: the more positively she felt about herself, the less body distortion she experienced. Black women of low socioeconomic status also reported higher levels of body distortion. For the white women, the degree of distortion was more closely related to their physical state: the less active they perceived pregnancy to be, the more distortion they felt. Although Harris attributes these differences to cultural factors, the explanation of how such factors might operate remains unclear.

One's sense of one's body boundary in relation to the environment also changes during pregnancy. Various studies have shown that throughout pregnancy women increasingly experience their bodies as providing protection and acting as a barrier for the fetus. Body space, the distance from another person at which one feels comfortable, also increases throughout pregnancy (Schuzman, cited in Sherwin, 1987; Fawcett, Bliss-Holtz, Haas & Leventhal, 1986).

Women also commonly experience an increased feeling of a loss of control throughout their pregnancies. In addition to reflecting the actual loss of control over body changes, increased clumsiness, and a loss of balance, the feelings may also reflect reactions to the intrusive medical procedures used throughout the prenatal period and to labor and delivery (Leifer, 1977, 1980; Schuzman, cited in Sherwin, 1987; Slochower, personal communication, 1989).

Affective Changes

Mood

Although many studies have attributed the emotional changes of pregnancy entirely to hormones, the impact of social beliefs about hormonal changes has largely been ignored (Parlee, 1978). Whatever the cause, the physiological and physical changes that occur during pregnancy are often seen to evoke negative mood change. There is increasing evidence, however, that the kind and degree of mood change during pregnancy reflect more pervasive personality factors: in general, the more positive the prepregnancy mood, the less the disruption during pregnancy (Leifer, 1977).

Some degree of emotional lability and feelings of psychological disequilibrium are common during pregnancy. By the third trimester, many women experience their emotions as closer to the surface and less easily defended against, and many experience marked mood swings. Many women also feel less able to cope with stress and react with more irritability to minor frustrations (Leifer, 1977).

Reliable and valid statistics on depression during pregnancy are lacking. As part of normal gestation, women often experience the same symptoms as those present in depressive disorders, including fatigue, weight gain, psychomotor retardation, increased somatic concern, and mood fluctuation. However, not all pregnant women with these symptoms are depressed. Therefore, these symptoms seem best attributable to physiological, rather than psychological, causes. Kaplan (1986) emphasizes that physiological functioning and psychological functioning interact in pregnancy and both must be considered. She suggests that, along with physiological causes, for some women depression in pregnancy may be due in part to learned helplessness, given the inevitable feeling of loss of control, and in part to the internalization of cultural ideas that portray pregnancy as a time of dependency and inability to function.

Finally, the mood changes that may occur during pregnancy are expected in most cultures. So, for example, it is expected that pregnant Dakota Indian women may show such great personality changes that they may hit their children, which is an extremely rare act in Dakota society (Kitzinger, 1978). As was the case with women's reactions to changes in their bodies, there is a positive relationship between the woman's mood and depression before pregnancy and her reactions during pregnancy and the postpartum period (Buesching, Glaser & Frate, 1986).

Anxiety and Fears During Pregnancy

Studies of fear and anxiety during pregnancy have examined how positive and negative attitudes toward pregnancy relate to differing anxiety levels, the kinds and intensity of anxieties felt, how fears and anxieties change throughout the course of pregnancy, and the functions served by anxiety and fears.

Various kinds of fears and anxieties are extremely common during pregnancy (Leifer, 1977). They relate to the woman's attitude toward the pregnancy, with the focus and intensity of the anxiety changing over time (Leifer, 1977). Women who are most attached to the fetus direct most of their fears and anxiety toward the fetus. Those who are moderately invested experience anxiety toward both the fetus and themselves, whereas those who are minimally invested either focus their anxieties on themselves or show no or very low anxiety levels. Anxiety also changes throughout the duration of the pregnancy, with most of the anxieties and fears becoming increasingly realistic. Early in pregnancy common fears reflect a sense of protectiveness, including fear of miscarriage, fear that the child might be deformed, anxiety about being responsible for the child, and concern about proper diet and avoiding drugs. After the quickening, during the second trimester, there is decreased concern about miscarriage and increased concern about the child's normalcy. During the third trimester, especially as delivery nears, women become more concerned about themselves, particularly experiencing anxiety and fear about the delivery, about death, and about future roles, responsibilities, sex, attractiveness, marriage, and career plans. Many women fear losing their husbands, either through the husband's accidental death or to another woman (Leifer, 1977).

Stressful life events are also associated with anxiety and fear (Telles, 1987). As mentioned earlier, the effects of anxiety produced by life events may be mediated by how adequate a support system the woman has available to her (Leifer, 1977; Nuckolls et al., 1972).

Increased Self-Preoccupation

Pregnancy is frequently accompanied by an increased preoccupation with self and a corresponding decline of emotional investment in the external world (Caplan, 1960; Leifer, 1977). In the first trimester, as the signs of pregnancy increase, the woman may feel some need to be alone for physical and emotional replenishment. During the second trimester, stimulated by the quickening, there is an increase in the interaction between the woman and her fetus, with a concomitant feeling of "us" as a unit. The woman may withdraw from things that are not related to the pregnancy. During the third trimester, this withdrawal continues and is most intense as the woman prepares for the birth and motherhood. This withdrawal is not a passive withdrawal but rather entails an active focus on the fetus. Thus the self-preoccupation serves an adaptive function (Leifer, 1977).

For many, pregnancy is a time of increased vulnerability, accompanied by an increased need for succorance (Caplan, 1960; Gerson, Alpert, & Richardson, 1984; Leifer, 1977), which is most commonly experienced in relation to one's partner, family, and friends. This need serves an adaptive role. It may also permit the expectant mother to satisfy some of her own dependency needs that were not satisfied in her own infancy and childhood (Leifer, 1977).

For many, pregnancy is a period during which, along with the increased stress, there is an intensified feeling of well-being (Leifer, 1977). For most, however, well-being is not the prevailing mood. Rather, such feelings alternate with feelings of emotional upheaval.

To sum up, pregnancy is not a time period characterized by a single affect. Increased self-preoccupation, anxiety, and emotional lability are all potentially normal, not pathological, responses. They seem to channel the expectant mother's energy toward herself and the fetus and thus may facilitate the formation of a mother-child bond. Thus some of the emotional changes in pregnancy that have traditionally been considered as negative may actually play adaptive roles.

In the first trimester, depression and fatigue are common. During the second trimester, many experience the quickening as the beginning of a time of particular well-being. This may result from the visibility of the pregnancy and the acceptance of its reality, relief that the fetus is alive, and relief from the symptoms of the first trimester. During the second trimester, also, there may be an increase in dependency and the desire to be alone, which peaks during the third trimester. Toward the end of the pregnancy, some women experience increased anxiety and stress resulting from the imminent changes in their roles and relationships and from the anticipated process of childbearing. Kaij and Nilsson's (1972) conclusion that "there is a substantial neurotic response during pregnancy" (p. 368) may reflect their failure to see the potentially positive aspects of some of the symptoms shown. The evidence is conflicting, but the most plausible conclusion is that the way a woman adapts to pregnancy is a reflection of the interaction among biological, psychological, and societal factors and is related to what her personality was like before pregnancy.

Fantasies and Dreams

Waking fantasies and sleeping fantasies (i.e., dreams) during pregnancy, both representing the same underlying processes, contain unmistakable references to the pregnancy. A number of researchers have found both quantitative and qualitative differences in the dreams of pregnant and nonpregnant women. Pregnant women report a greater number of dreams than nonpregnant women, as well as more dreams containing references to babies (e.g., Gillman, 1968; Van De Castle & Kindler, cited in Sherwin, 1987). Their dreams contain more references to architectural features, concerns related to pregnancy, more instances of their husbands' finding other women more attractive, and more references relating to dependency. Pregnant women also report more anxiety dreams than nonpregnant women (Gillman, 1968). More of the dreams of pregnant women deal with misfortune, harm, or environmental threats. There are many dreams of the woman's being trapped, assaulted, or in danger, and many dreams that her fetus or baby is deformed, crippled, or threatened. On the other hand, there are also many dreams with positive themes in which emotions such as ecstatic joy and anticipation are expressed (Colman & Colman, 1971; Deutsch, 1945; Gillman, 1968; Sherwin, 1987; Winget & Kapp, cited in Sherwin, 1987).

These fantasies may serve a number of different purposes, such as providing opportunities for expressing and working through anxieties and fears (e.g., about pregnancy, delivery, being hurt and hurting the baby, loss of control), attempting to deal with anticipated stresses, and solving problems (e.g., Benedek, 1970; Colman & Colman, 1971; Gillman, 1968; Lederman, 1984; Leifer, 1977; Sherwin, 1987). Many researchers (Lederman, 1984; Sherwin, 1987; Rubin, 1984) interpret such fantasies as indicating the beginning of the internalization of the maternal role. The fantasies enable the woman to relate to the idea of her own child and to the idea of herself as mother. Simultaneously, they permit her to resolve her grief for the loss of her past life and lost roles (Rubin, 1984). Fantasies, according to Benedek (1970), are influenced by the general course of pregnancy and relate to the woman's attitude toward her pregnancy.

The content of fantasies about the fetus also changes during the course of pregnancy. During the first trimester, the fetus is felt as a diffuse presence (Leifer, 1977; Rubin, 1984). Fantasies may be symbolically linked to the pregnancy, for instance, by an egg (Rubin, 1984), and there are many dreams involving injury to the self (Gillman, 1968). During the second trimester, particularly after the quickening, these dreams are gradually replaced by views of the fetus as a person with the fetus and baby seen in very warm, vivid, detailed images and as much larger than a newborn child (Gillman, 1968; Leifer, 1977). Dreams of injury to the self generally decrease while dreams about harm to and from strangers increase. During the third trimester, particularly as the time for delivery nears, anxieties and fears about self-injury again surface in fantasies. In some dreams, labor and delivery are totally bypassed; in others, horrible, mutilating accidents occur in which the woman or the baby is mutilated or dies (Colman & Colman, 1971; Gillman, 1968; Leifer, 1977; Rubin, 1984; Sherwin, 1987). Of course, dreams may also be extremely pleasant: for example, one woman dreamed that she gave birth to a baby that crawled up her and hugged her. In all of these fantasies, the newborn child is usually depicted as mature, with its image very differentiated (Leifer, 1977; Rubin, 1984).

Sexuality

Many individuals believe in the asexuality of motherhood; that is, they hold the belief that mothers are not and should not be sexual. This culturally transmitted belief prescribes behaviors and feelings that individuals hold about mothers. As Weiskopf (1980) has pointed out, "For some, being a mother-to-be and being sexual are internally conflictual" (p. 775). Some pregnant women view themselves as "sacred vessels of new life and thus should not be contaminated by sex" (Kitzinger, cited in Weiskopf, 1980, p. 777). The often expressed fear of injuring the child during sex may, indeed, reflect fear of harm from their partner's activity. However, such fears may also reflect the idea that their own sexuality might harm the child; in other words, since mothers are not supposed to be sexual beings, they believe that if they are at all sexual, the child may be harmed in retaliation (Weiskopf, 1980).

In any case, sexuality during pregnancy is affected by both psychological and physical factors and may show just about any pattern of change (Osofsky & Osofsky, 1980; Sherwin, 1987; White & Reamy, 1982). However, many studies have reported a decrease, followed by an increase, and then another decrease in sexual interest and activity throughout the three trimesters of pregnancy, respectively (Battachi, cited in Sherwin, 1987; Falicov, 1973; Kumar, Brant, & Robson, 1981; Masters & Johnson, 1966; Reading, 1983; Robson, Brant, & Kumar, 1981; Sherwin, 1987; Solberg, Dultler, & Wagner, 1973; Tolor & DiGrazia, 1976). During the first trimester, common reasons cited for decreased sexual interest and/or activity include physiological changes, such as fatigue and nausea, that cause discomfort, fear of injuring the fetus, general loss of interest in sex, awkwardness, compliance with a physician's instructions or the recommendation of a friend, not feeling attractive, beliefs in the asexuality of motherhood, and the belief that the only purpose of sex is procreation (Tolor & DiGrazia, 1976).

During the second trimester, many women report increased eroticism with a desire for more frequent sexual intercourse and a greater number of sexual fantasies. This may in part result from a lessening of the discomforts felt during the first trimester. During the third trimester, many women report decreased sexual interest and activity. For some, sex may become more physically difficult or uncomfortable at this time. For others, the physician may prohibit it. Some women become increasingly fearful that the baby will be hurt or that intercourse will bring on labor (Colman & Colman, 1971). Sherwin (1987) concluded that if the pregnancy is normal (i.e., if there are no problems such as bleeding, a tendency to abort spontaneously, cervical incompetence or weakness, or a history of premature labor), then intercourse per se probably will not induce labor. As the woman approaches term, however, orgasm might induce labor because of hormonal changes that accompany it.

HEALTH CARE DURING PREGNANCY

As part of the pregnancy experience, most women must interact with the health care delivery system. In the United States, this system is fraught with difficulties ranging from inadequate prenatal care to the unnecessary medicalization of pregnancy and childbirth.

The Prenatal Care Delivery System

Although the importance of early and quality prenatal care is well established, in the United States, racial and ethnic differences in ease of access to care are readily apparent. White women start prenatal care earliest, and fewer have no prenatal care at all. Black women and Hispanic women (except for Cubans) start prenatal care much later than any other group, and a greater number of these women have no prenatal care. Native American women also start their care later than women in the other groups or have no care. Chinese and Japanese women surpass white women, although other Asian women are less likely than white women to start care in the first trimester and are more likely to delay care or have no care. However, Asian women also start earlier and receive more prenatal care than do black women. Low birth weight (less than 2,500 grams), a major risk factor for the neonate, is much more common among women who have had less frequent, late, or inadequate prenatal care (Reading, 1983). Strikingly, in 1985, 12.4% of black babies were of low birth weight, while the percentages for other racial and ethnic groups ranged from 4.9 for Chinese babies to 8.9 for Puerto Rican babies (Taffel, 1987).

The 1985 Natality Report for the United States (National Center for Health Statistics, 1987) indicated a slight increase over previous years in prenatal care for all groups of women combined, to a median of 11.8 visits. However, the racial and ethnic differential is still strongly observable: the median number of visits was 12.0 for white mothers, but only 10.3 for black mothers. In addition, the percentage of premature babies has increased recently to 9.8% (from 8.9% in 1980). This increase was found for both black and white babies, but the racial differential is considerable: the percentage rose from 16.8% to 17.5% for black babies, as compared with 7.9% to 8.2% for white babies. Infant mortality, associated with low birth weight and lack of early and comprehensive prenatal care, is twice as high for blacks as for whites in the United States.

There are many reasons for these differentials. Reading (1983) and others have noted that more appropriate use of prenatal care was made by women who were married, had higher levels of education, and believed in the usefulness of preventive care, all more likely for white women. Gaviría, Stern, and Schensul (1982), studying Mexican-Americans, found that in addition to economic and educational variables, prenatal care also varied with time since immigration to the United States: more recent immigrants delayed use of prenatal care much longer than long-term migrants. For many Mexican-American women, preventive health care has a low priority given the many difficulties they have to deal with (Chavez, Cornelius, & Jones, 1985; Marin, Marin, Padilla & De la Rocha, 1983), and immigrant Mexican-American women report feelings of less responsibility and control over their health (Castro, Furth, & Karlow, 1984), which become manifest in their failure to obtain early prenatal care.

There are many problems surrounding health care in the United States, especially prenatal care. There are many barriers to quality prenatal care, particularly for women who are poor. A few of these are costs, how clinics are organized, women's lack of familiarity with the system, inaccessibility of care, and language barriers (Ehrenreich & English, 1979). Often, individuals in control try to impose white, middle-class models indiscriminately, ignoring interpersonal interactions and sociocultural differences in beliefs and attitudes toward pregnancy. Ehrenreich and English state that "ethnics and minorities, coming from different health care backgrounds, often feel they lose control over their bodies while their cultural knowledge is not tolerated" (quoted in Lazarus, 1984, p. 15). Physicians want passive patients. The providers of medical care often hold attitudes toward women (and particularly toward women of color and ethnicity) that are degrading and that reflect their belief that women are incompetent. Health care personnel also often try to reduce the anxiety that women feel by joking with them, instead of by providing them with information, and the personnel frequently disregard what the woman tells them (Graham & Oakley, 1981). Note the following quotation from Graham and Oakley, in which the physician actually contradicts the patient with regard to how many children she has:

Doctor (reading case notes): Ah, I see you've got a boy and a girl.
Patient: No, two girls.
Doctor: Really. *Are you sure* [italics added]? I thought it said . . . [checks in notes]. Oh no, you're quite right, two girls. (p. 66)

The quality of the first prenatal visit affects compliance with the medical advice offered. The oft-cited negative experiences of most women who attend clinics do not encourage their use. Clinic care can be extremely depersonalized and humiliating. Clinics (as well as private physicians) tend to show their devaluation of patients' time by imposing long waiting periods, which, in addition, can be quite physically uncomfortable. Clinics generally offer no continuity in terms of the medical personnel that a particular woman deals with. This might increase the anxiety that some women feel about gynecological exams. Clinics are frequently not located in the communities where the women live, causing difficulties involving transportation and child care. Indeed, child care may be problematic even if the clinic is located within one's community. The fact that some women are in the United States illegally may also interfere with their access to prenatal care (Alvarez, 1985).

A number of major problems result in the clinic visits being particularly negative for women of color and ethnicity. Not only are most clinics understaffed, but whatever staff does exist is usually not of backgrounds similar to the women who are attending the clinic. The staff frequently are not sufficiently empathic due to a lack of understanding of how social and cultural factors shape attitudes toward, and behavior during, pregnancy (Alvarez, 1985; Lazarus, 1984). Staff members frequently stereotype minority women and consequently may fail to deal with the real problems they experience as individuals (Jorgensen & Adams, 1987). Researchers such as Fuentes (1972), Medina (1980), and Reading (1983) stress that when dealing with patients, it is extremely important to take into account such factors as disease etiology, attitudes toward illness, decision making in illness situations, the importance of elders, religion, and respect in the culture, the degree to which hospitalization is considered to be a family affair, and attitudes toward impersonality and specialization. The importance of medical personnel's responses to pregnant Philippino immigrant women in the United States probably also applies equally well to other groups (Stern, Tilden, & Maxwell, 1986). These researchers found that the Philippino women were subjected to three major and unnecessary sources of stress. First, there were major conflicts relating to customs, beliefs, and cultural practices associated with childbearing. For example, medical personnel recommended a diet that contained foods that were not readily accessible to these women. Also, the women did not want to eat extra food since they believed that not eating would keep the baby small for an easier delivery. In addition, in the Philippines, obstetric personnel are always women, while in the United States, pregnant women most often encounter men in these roles. Espín (1986) found similar results with Hispanic women, who usually discuss pregnancy-related issues with other women as they find it too distressing and embarrassing to discuss such topics with males. This results in their failing to bring problems to the attention of male physicians. Similarly, Scott and Stern (1986) stressed the difficulties black women in Louisiana experience in their attempts to resolve contradictory information from their two most important sources of health information: their elders (especially grandmothers), who pass on traditional taboos and traditions, and the dominant culture, which provides them with new health prescriptions and information from education, the media, and resources such as prenatal classes and social networks. Scott and Stern concluded that from the very first visit (as noted above, shown to strongly influence later use of prenatal resources), health care clinics must consider the woman's views and beliefs about childbearing, must provide culturally sensitive care (including styles of approach, customs, and language), and need to give advice (such as what to eat) that fits in with the woman's life-style and diet, while simultaneously providing information about pregnancy and childbirth (see also Powers, 1982; Snow, 1974).

Stern, Tilden, and Maxwell (1986) also note that conflicts between interpersonal styles and social approach produced difficulties for pregnant Philippino women. In that culture, women feel shame when told something directly; they prefer indirect chitchat. The direct approach of the health care providers in the United States thus subjected these women to unintentional shaming. Their third point was that the language barrier made communication more difficult. If the personnel do not speak one's language, it is even more difficult to ask any questions. Lazarus (1984) found similar results for Puerto Rican and other low-income women. To remedy some of these problems and to attempt to increase clinic attendance and acceptance of services, Lee (1976) and Medina (1980) have recommended that aides who are indigenous to the community in which the clinics are located be employed to staff the clinics. The hiring of female aides may also make a significant difference.

Health care in the United States is based on a profit motive. High costs, failure to meet eligibility requirements for assistance, and inadequate insurance also present problems for women that may lead to either delayed care or no care at all. The federal government has three major programs through which funding is provided for prenatal care: Medicaid, Title V funds, and the Special Supplemental Food Program for Women, Infants, and Children (WIC). However, because of cuts in these programs at the federal level, every state has reduced its Medicaid programs (through tightened eligibility requirements or service cutbacks), 47 states have cut back their Title V funds, and other federal cuts have resulted in 725,000 people, 64% of whom are women and children, losing services. In addition, these programs are aimed at high-risk pregnancies and provide little or no support for normal pregnancies (Collins & Natapoff, 1984).

Prenatal Screening

Prenatal screening reflects the medicalization of childbearing, because these procedures depend on increasingly complex technology. Various procedures are used during pregnancy for prenatal screening. These techniques provide information about, and diagnose problems in, the fetus. Their ostensible purpose is to improve the health and genetic characteristics of fetuses and newborns. The following discussion of these techniques relies heavily on information from Reading (1983) and *The New Our Bodies, Ourselves* (Boston Women's Health Book Collective, 1985).

Methods

The methods used in prenatal screening vary widely in terms of timing, use, intrusiveness, and risk factors. A fetoscopy involves direct visualization of external defects in the fetus. Compared with other techniques, the spontaneous abortion rate of 3–6% is high (Rodbeck & Campbell, 1979).

Used more frequently is ultrasound, in which high-frequency, low-intensity sound waves are passed through the woman's abdomen, and immediate images are created of the echoes that result. Ultrasound is used to enhance the safety and the effectiveness of amniocentesis, establish fetal age, detect abnormal growth rates, diagnose multiple pregnancies, detect changes in the volume of the amniotic fluid, and detect abnormalities of fetal structures and of the placenta. It may be carried out any time during pregnancy. Ultrasound is a noninvasive procedure, and therefore no risk of miscarriage accompanies it. Although its long-term effects on the woman and fetus are unknown, they are presently presumed to be negligible.

Amniocentesis provides information about chromosome disorders, neural tube defects, metabolic disorders, and the sex of the fetus. Usually conducted between 14 and 16 weeks, amniocentesis is most often performed on women who are over 35, those who have previously given birth to a child with a neural tube defect (e.g., spina bifida), with Down's syndrome, or with some other defect caused by a chromosomal abnormality, those who have had spontaneous abortions repeatedly or who have histories of certain diseases, and those who are carriers of certain sex-linked (e.g., hemophilia) or other characteristics (e.g., Tay-Sachs disease or sickle-cell anemia) (Boston Women's Health Book Collective, 1985; Reading, 1983). Amniocentesis may also be conducted shortly before delivery when its purpose is to assess the condition of the fetal lungs. To perform amniocentesis, the physician inserts a long, thin needle into the uterus through the abdominal wall and removes about four teaspoons of fluid, containing some of the fetus's cells. Amniocentesis is always immediately preceded by an ultrasound picture that ensures proper placement of the needle. The cells are cultured, and the chromosomes in the cells are photographed. The sex of the fetus is readily discernible through the analysis and the photograph of the chromosomes. Results of the procedure are available two to three weeks after the amniocentesis is carried out. Amniocentesis, which is done on an outpatient basis, is usually not painful; the insertion of the needle may cause a mild sting (some physician's use local anesthetic), and a sensation of pressure is usually felt as the fluid is withdrawn. Sometimes mild cramps or spotting may follow the procedure. More serious, however, are the risks of maternal bleeding, injury to the fetus, and miscarriage (slightly less than 1%).

A Chorionic Villus Sampling Test is a procedure currently being perfected to provide information earlier (at 8–10 weeks) than is possible through amniocentesis, thus permitting a first trimester abortion if chosen. In this test, small amounts of tissue from the chorion, one of the membranes surrounding the fetus, are removed and analyzed. The danger of miscarriage is currently around 1%. This technique offers advantages over amniocentesis because of the possibility of early diagnosis.

Alpha-Fetoprotein (AFP) Tests are blood tests conducted between 14 and 19 weeks that detect the level of AFP proteins. These proteins are elevated for women whose fetuses are affected by neural tube defects. AFP analyses are also carried out routinely on fluid withdrawn during amniocentesis. About 2 in 1,000 babies are born each year in the United States with neural tube defects. These are defects in which the neural tube, which forms the brain, spinal cord, and spinal column, has not completely closed. Neural tube defects may result in an opening at the top (anencephaly, which is fatal) or along the backbone (spina bifida, which varies in degree of severity). The risks accompanying AFP Tests when done along with an amniocentesis are the same as those associated with amniocentesis alone. There are no risks associated with blood withdrawn for an AFP Test through an ordinary blood test. AFP Tests have an 85% accuracy in detecting neural tube defects; there is a small risk of getting a "false positive" result.

Other tests may also be performed to determine if the fetus is healthy enough to remain in the uterus. These include Estriol Tests, usually taking the form of a blood test to measure the level of estriol, which indicates how well the placenta is functioning. A Non-Stress Test involves attaching a fetal monitor and measuring whether the fetus's heart rate accelerates, to indicate movement. The purpose of the Contraction Stress Test is to measure how well the placenta responds to a contraction. The test involves nipple stimulation, which results in the production of oxytocin, a hormone that causes contractions; thus the test measures the body's ability to produce contractions. The fetal monitor is an instrument to which the fetus is attached (usually during labor) to measure fetal heart rate changes as contractions occur. The Oxytocin Challenge Test (OCT) administers pitocin (a synthetic oxytocin hormone) intravenously, in order to test further the body's ability to produce contractions. It is used when nipple stimulation fails to bring on contractions in the Contraction Stress Test. At times, the OCT may result in early labor, which may necessitate a consequent cesarian section and immature birth.

Psychological Reactions

The few researchers who have studied the psychological impact of these screening procedures have found that women show a great deal of variation in how they respond to them (Dixson, Richards & Reinsch, 1981). Most women expressed very positive feelings about counseling they had received before a medical procedure was performed. More than 50% reported insignificant, while 7% reported severe, pain or discomfort. Although all reported high levels of anxiety while waiting for the results of the test, they were almost unanimous in saying they would do it again (Chervin, cited in Reading, 1983). On the other hand, Wilson (cited in Reading, 1983) reported the following reasons for women's declining amniocentesis: concerns about the safety of the procedure, alleviation of their anxieties by counseling alone, fear of spontaneous abortion, deciding not to have an abortion whatever the results of the test, pregnancies too advanced for simple abortions, and a preference for not knowing about the condition of the fetus. Dixson et al. (1981) compared women who had gone ahead with an amniocentesis with those who had declined to have the procedure performed, based on their fears of injuring the fetus or of miscarriage or because of religious beliefs. More of the women who had the amniocentesis felt that having an abnormal baby would have a greater impact on their lives, most reported less pain than they had expected, and over half felt increased attachment to the fetus after the procedure because they had been able to see a picture (from ultrasound) of the fetus. The picture may have served to increase the reality and individuality of the fetus for the woman. Of the women who had opted not to undergo the procedure, 63% felt they could not have terminated the pregnancy if an abnormality had been found, whereas only 7% of the amniocentesis group felt this way. Other studies have found that fewer women of color and ethnicity have amniocentesis, while more women with higher educations and incomes undergo the procedure (Reading, 1983).

Responses to ultrasound have generally been positive, with increased attachment to the fetus and more positive attitudes toward the pregnancy frequently being reported. Many women feel that ultrasound scanning is both informative and emotionally rewarding. They feel more confident, informed, involved, reassured, relieved, and less uncertain. Many describe their emotional state after ultrasound as "wonderful" (Campbell, Townes & Beach, 1982; Petchesky, 1987).

Issues Regarding Prenatal Screening

There is much debate as to whether prenatal screening is desirable or overused. On the one hand, these procedures can detect many conditions prenatally that are handicapping (e.g., spina bifida, Down's syndrome) or incompatible with life (such as anencephaly). They may enable therapeutic abortions to be performed early. The procedures can also detect some conditions that are amenable to correction in utero (e.g., Rh incompatibility, some heart defects). They thus have the potential to provide women with the opportunity to make choices about the children they will bear and therefore may increase her sense of control.

On the other hand, there are many unknowns as well as potential and actual abuses surrounding the use of these procedures. For example, although amniocentesis does induce miscarriage about 1% of the time and the long-term effects of procedures such as ultrasound on mother or child are unknown, they are touted as completely safe. The effects of the anxiety felt while waiting for the results of tests are largely also undocumented. Katz Rothman (1987) labeled this period before learning the results of the tests the "tentative pregnancy." How such procedures affect attachment to the fetus and later interactions is also unknown. Fletcher and Evans (1983) caution about the potential misuse of the procedures as a weapon against abortions, having found that some women spontaneously commented that once they had seen the ultrasound picture, they considered the fetus to be alive and never could have considered an abortion thereafter. Thus some fear the possibility that such viewing might be required before all requested abortions or that such techniques might be used to obtain court-ordered intervention for fetal therapy. In addition, as noted previously, all of these procedures represent an example of increased obstetrical management of pregnancy, in which the woman must depend upon physicians.

Little is known about the psychological effects and impact of the detection of fetal abnormalities on the woman and her family (Zuskar, 1987). On the one hand, such detection might have quite negative effects. The decision to have, or necessity of having, an abortion can be quite difficult and depressing under such circumstances (Blumberg, Golbus, & Hanson, 1975). Reactions similar to those shown to the birth of a handicapped child—mourning for the fantasized, perfect child (Solnit & Stark, cited in Zuskar, 1987), searching for the cause (Mercer, cited in Zuskar, 1987), and placing of blame (Helmrath & Steinitz, 1978)—might all be expected. When an abnormality is detected, in many cases the severity of the abnormality and prognosis might not be known, resulting in decisions being made on the basis of incomplete information (Horger & Pai, cited in Zuskar, 1987). Some of the salutary processes usually in evidence after a child with defects is born cannot be called upon prenatally. Parents who have given birth to a handicapped child have described the time spent waiting to see the child as particularly difficult (D'Arcy, cited in Zuskar, 1987). The greater waiting time for a child who has been prenatally diagnosed as having a defect would be expected to be at least as, if not more, difficult since it is longer.

On the other hand, prenatal diagnosis of an abnormality provides the woman with the opportunity to make a choice as to whether she wants to terminate the pregnancy through abortion or continue the pregnancy. If she decides to continue the pregnancy, the prenatal diagnosis probably permits her to prepare better for the child and its special needs. Prenatal diagnosis may permit the parents the mourning for the perfect child mentioned above at a time when they have more energy to deal with this. By the time the baby is born, they may be further along in the adjustment process than those who have not availed themselves of these technologies (Solnit & Stark, cited in Zuskar, 1987).

The absolute incidence of defects is small for women in most age groups. However, for any particular woman, if it is her child who is disabled, the small incidence in general is meaningless, as she (and her family) are the ones who will be responsible for dealing with the disability. Society generally fails to provide adequate support for children (and later adults) born with special needs. Given this situation, some feel that if a defect is discovered through prenatal screening, those women who might otherwise elect to continue their pregnancies are under direct and indirect pressure to abort the fetus (Snitow, 1986). On the other hand, however, many women feel that they could not or do not want to cope with a disabled child. Prenatal screening allows them the choice of increasing the probability that they will not have to do so.

There are strong, implicit social values based on eugenic assumptions underlying the use of these prenatal screening methods (Hubbard, 1982). The procedures are described as solving the "problems" of severely physically and mentally disabled babies, but many disabled individuals consider the procedures as a means of devaluing them. They consider the problems to result from the lack of societal supports rather than from the disabilities per se (Parlee, 1986).

The issues of choice, control, and consent are raised in relation to how the procedures and their results are used. Physicians who are concerned about mal-practice suits and lawsuits claiming wrongful birth (e.g., in which the parents of an unwanted child conceived after sterilization or of a child whose disabilities could have been detected prenatally but weren't, sue the physician) and wrongful life (in which the child sues after birth) may place unwarranted reliance upon these tests. The increased use of fetal monitoring is frequently cited as a major explanation of the astounding increase in the number of cesarian sections in the United States over the past 20 years, from 5% in 1968 to almost 20% in 1981 (Boston Women's Health Book Collective, 1985). Interestingly, despite the increased use of fetal monitoring and cesarian sections, the number of neonatal deaths has not decreased (Friedman, 1986).

Another issue that is relevant in this context is that of sex preselection. Throughout the world, parents have preferences about the number and sex of children they desire, with most preferring males and a male child first if two children are desired (Rowland, 1985; Williamson, 1976). A number of the prescreening techniques provide information about the sex of the fetus. Of concern are demographic and social effects resulting from using the information provided by the prenatal screening techniques to choose the sex of their child(ren) through selective abortion. For example, a study conducted in China found 29 of 46 women whose fetuses were female elected abortions, while only 1 of 53 who were carrying male fetuses did so (Boston Women's Health Book Collective, 1985). The ramifications of preselecting sex require careful consideration. Based on the expressed preference for males, some have suggested that sex preselection will result in a surplus of male firstborns. One can only speculate on the consequences of this occurrence, given the personality characteristics such as achievement orientation and achievement more frequently associated with first-borns as opposed to later-borns.

In brief, prenatal diagnostic tests may be used in ways to make them assets or liabilities. In either case, they raise complicated questions about their desirability, necessity, safety, and accessibility that are not easily answerable. One must ask why society fails to deal with the underlying social and economic problems that cause many of the disorders identifiable through the tests. Society creates certain avoidable problems and then develops tests to detect these problems rather than dealing with the basic source of the problems.

Importantly, however, these prenatal screening procedures have the potential to permit women to continue their pregnancies to term with less anxiety than would otherwise be the case. It may thus be even more important that these procedures be equally available to all women. Low-income women, who have the greatest incidence of pregnancy complications, may have less access to these prenatal screening procedures than women with higher incomes (Snitow, 1986). These procedures have the potential to increase women's control through increasing her choice. All women need to become better informed about these tests and the options they provide.

SOME CONCLUDING COMMENTS ABOUT PREGNANCY

Pregnancy is a normal stage in development (Leifer, 1980; Rapoport et al., 1972). Many continue to view pregnancy in a sexist fashion as a necessity for women: the optimal outcome of pregnancy is considered to be "adjustment or adaptation to a traditionally defined feminine role" (Leifer, 1980, p. 764). Failure to fulfill this ideal continues to be perceived as equivalent to immaturity, or due to unresolved conflicts (Leifer, 1980).

Most studies have failed to consider pregnancy within the social context. Nevertheless, to understand such a complex phenomenon, one must understand the multitude of influences upon it (Bronfenbrenner, 1979). Leifer's (1980) call for more studies of other than middle-class women has not been answered. It has been clearly established that varying attitudes toward pregnancy shape the pregnancy experience differently even within the white middle class. Common sense alone would lead one to expect that women from different backgrounds, growing up in cultures with different views of pregnancy, would hold different beliefs and attitudes about pregnancy. Yet almost nothing is known about the psychological experience of pregnancy for women of color and ethnicity. Studies conducted within the United States as well as cross-culturally have devoted more attention to fertility and natality statistics and to rituals concerned with childbearing than to the psychological dynamics present throughout pregnancy. Furthermore, extremely current information applicable to any group of women is rare, despite the distinct possibility that attitudes and experiences have changed as a result of changes resulting from the women's movement. In addition, research that deals with the complex issues surrounding prenatal screening procedures and their safety is urgently needed.

Most women either continue to choose to become pregnant (through either intercourse or the employment of reproductive technologies such as donor insemination) or do so unintentionally. They consider their pregnancies to be among the most significant events in their lives. It should be obvious, therefore, that much additional research remains to be conducted on these topics.

NOTE

I would like to express my appreciation to my husband, Steve, for his extremely helpful, critical reading of, and comments regarding, this manuscript, as well as for his support. I am also grateful to Joyce Slochower for her generous help. Her knowledgeable comments and suggestions added much to this chapter. In addition, I would like to thank Myron Gershberg for his support and encouragement. Thanks, too, to Michele Paludi for her comments on an earlier version of this chapter.

REFERENCES

Alvarez, M. (1985). Health conditions of Mexican immigrants—A review of the literature. *Salud Frontera (Border Health)*, *1*, 48–52.

Ballou, J. W. (1978). *The psychology of pregnancy: Reconciliation and resolution.* Lexington, MA: Lexington Books.

Benedek, T. (1949). *The emotional structure of the family.* In R. N. Anshen (Ed.), *Science and culture series: Vol. 5. The family: Its function and destiny* (pp. 202–225). New York: Harper.

Benedek, T. (1952). *Psychosexual functioning in women.* New York: Ronald Press.

Benedek, T. (1959). Parenthood as a developmental phase. *Journal of the American Psychoanalytic Association, 7,* 339–417.

Benedek, T. (1970). The psychobiology of pregnancy. In E. J. Anthony & T. Benedek (Eds.), *Parenthood: Its psychology and psychopathology* (pp. 137–152). New York: Little, Brown.

Bettelheim, B. (1962). *Symbolic wounds: Puberty and the envious male.* New York: Collier Books.

Bibring, G. L. (1959). Some considerations of the psychological processes of pregnancy. *Psychoanalytic Study of the Child, 14,* 113–121.

Bibring, G. L., Dwyer, T., Huntington, D. S., & Valenstein, A. F. (1961). Study of the psychological processes in pregnancy and of the earliest mother-child relationship. I: Some propositions and comments. *Pychoanalytic Study of the Child, 16,* 9–24.

Blumberg, B. D., Globus, M. S., & Hanson, K. H. (1975). The psychological sequelae of abortion performed for a genetic indication. *American Journal of Obstetrics and Gynecology, 122,* 799–808.

The Boston Women's Health Book Collective. (1985). *The new our bodies, ourselves.* New York: Simon & Schuster.

Boyd-Franklin, N. (1983). Black family life-styles: A lesson in survival. In A. Swerdlow & H. Lessinger (Eds.), *Class, race, and sex: Dynamics of control* (pp. 52–83). Boston: G. K. Hall.

Bronfenbrenner, U. (1979). *The ecology of human development.* Cambridge: Harvard University Press.

Brown, M. S. (1981). Culture and childrearing. In A. N. Clark (Ed.), *Culture and childrearing* (pp. 3–35). Philadelphia: F. A. Davis.

Brown, M. (1986). Social support during pregnancy: A unidimensional or multidimensional construct? *Nursing Research, 35,* 4–9.

Buesching, D. P., Glaser, M. L., & Frate, D. A. (1986). Progression of depression in the prenatal and postpartum periods. *Women and Health, 11,* 61–78.

Burton, R., & Whiting, V. (1961). The absent father and cross-sex identity. *Merrill Palmer Quarterly of Behavior and Development, 7,* 85–95.

Campbell, F. L., Townes, B. D., & Beach, L. R. (1982). Motivational bases of child-bearing decisions. In G. L. Fox (Ed.), *The childbearing decision* (pp. 145–160). Beverly Hills: Sage.

Caplan, G. (1960). Emotional implications of pregnancy and influences on family relationships. In H. C. Stuart & D. G. Prugh (Eds.), *The healthy child.* Cambridge: Harvard University Press.

Carrie, C. M. (1981). Reproductive symptoms: Interrelations and determinants. *Psychology of Women Quarterly, 6,* 174–186.

Castro, F., Furth, P., & Karlow, H. (1984). The health beliefs of Mexican-American and Anglo-American women. *Hispanic Journal of Behavioral Science, 6,* 365–383.

Chavez, L. R., Cornelius, W., & Jones, O. W. (1985). Perinatal care among Mexican women in the United States. *Salud Frontera (Border Health)*, *1*, 2–6.

Chertok, L. (1966). *Motherhood and personality: Psychoanalytic aspects of childbirth.* New York: Lippincott.

Cohen, M. B. (1966). Personal identity and sexual identity. *Psychiatry*, *29*, 1–14.

Collins, M., & Natapoff, J. (1984). *A descriptive analysis of maternal and infant health care in New York State*. Report to the Mid-Atlantic Regional Nurses Association and New York State Nurses Association.

Colman, A. D., & Colman, L. L. (1971). *Pregnancy: The psychological experience.* New York: Herder & Herder.

Davis, L. L., & Lennon, S. J. (1983). Social stigma of pregnancy: Further evidence. *Psychological Reports*, *53*, 997–998.

Deutsch, H. (1945). *The psychology of women: Vol. 2. Motherhood.* New York: Grune & Stratton.

Dixson, B., Richards, T. L., & Reinsch, S. (1981). Midtrimester amniocentesis: Subjective maternal responses. *Journal of Reproductive Medicine*, *26*, 10–16.

Doering, S. G., Entwisle, D. R., & Quinlan, D. (1980). Modeling the quality of women's birth experience. *Journal of Health and Social Behavior*, *21*, 12–21.

Ehrenreich, B., & English, D. (1979). *For her own good: 150 years of the experts' advice to women.* London: Pluto Press.

Espín, O. M. (1986). *Hispanic female healers in urban centers in the United States.* Unpublished manuscript.

Falicov, C. J. (1973). Sexual adjustment during the first pregnancy and postpartum. *American Journal of Obstetrics and Gynecology*, *7*, 991–1000.

Fawcett, J., Bliss-Holtz, V. J., Haas, M. B., & Leventhal, M. (1986). Spouses' body image changes during and after pregnancy: A replication and extension. *Nursing Research*, *35*, 220–223.

Finger, A. M. (1984). Claiming our bodies: Reproductive rights and disability. In R. Arditti, R. Duelli Klein, & S. Minden (Eds.), *Test-tube women: What future for motherhood?* (pp. 281–297). London: Pandora Press.

Fletcher, J. C., & Evans, M. I. (1983). Maternal bonding examinations. *New England Journal of Medicine*, *308*, 392–393.

Friedman, E. (1986). The obstetrician's dilemma. *New England Journal of Medicine*, *315*, 615–619.

Fuentes, J. A. (1972). *Please doctor, listen to me!* Unpublished master's thesis, Loma Linda University, Loma Linda, CA.

Gaviría, M., Stern, G., & Schensul, S. L. (1982). Sociocultural factors and perinatal health in a Mexican-American community. *Journal of the National Medical Association*, *74*, 983–989.

Gerson, M. J., Alpert, J., & Richardson, M. S. (1984). Psychology of mothering: Review essay. *Signs*, *9*, 434–453.

Gillman, R. D. (1968). The dreams of pregnant women and maternal adaptation. *American Journal of Orthopsychiatry*, *38*, 688–692.

Gladieux, J. D. (1978). Pregnancy—The transition to parenthood—Satisfaction with the pregnancy experience as a function of sex role conceptions, marital relationship, and social network. In W. B. Miller & L. F. Newman (Eds.), *The first child and family formation* (pp. 275–295). Chapel Hill, NC: Carolina Population Center.

Gordon, R. E., & Gordon, K. K. (1959). Social factors in the prediction and treatment of emotional disorders of pregnancy. *American Journal of Obstetrics and Gynecology, 77,* 1074–1083.

Graham, H. (1976). The social image of pregnancy: Pregnancy as spirit possession. *Sociological Review, 24,* 291–308.

Graham, H., & Oakley, A. (1981). Competing ideologies of reproduction: Medical and maternal perspectives on pregnancy. In H. Roberts (Ed.), *Women, health, and reproduction* (pp. 50–74). London: Routledge & Kegan Paul.

Harris, R. (1979). Cultural differences in body perception during pregnancy. *British Journal of Medical Psychology, 52,* 347–352.

Harris, R., Linn, M. W., Good, R., & Hunter, K. (1981). Attitudes and perceptions of perinatal concepts during pregnancy in women of three cultures. *Journal of Clinical Psychology, 37,* 477–483.

Helmrath, T. A., & Steinitz, E. M. (1978). Death of an infant: Parental grieving and the failure of social support. *Journal of Family Practice, 6,* 785–790.

Hilliard, P. A. (1986, September). Old wives' tales. *Parents,* pp. 144–145.

Hooke, J. F., & Marks, P. A. (1962). MMPI characteristics of pregnant women. *Journal of Clinical Psychology, 18,* 316–317.

Horgan, D. (1983). The pregnant woman's place and where to find it. *Sex Roles, 9,* 333–340.

Hubbard, R. (1982). Legal and policy implications of recent advances in prenatal diagnosis and fetal therapy. *Women's Rights Law Reporter, 7,* 201–218.

Hunter College Women's Studies Collective. (1983). *Women's Realities, Women's Choices.* New York: Oxford University Press.

Jessner, L., Weigert, E., & Foy, J. L. (1970). The development of parental attitudes during pregnancy. In E. J. Anthony & T. Benedek (Eds.), *Parenthood: Its psychology and psychopathology* (pp. 209–244). Boston: Little, Brown.

Joesting, J. (1973). Texas folklore about childbirth. In D. Tennov & L. Hirsch (Eds.), *Proceedings of the first international childbirth conference* (pp.16–21). Stamford, CT: New Moon Publishers.

Jorgensen, S. R., & Adams, R. P. (1987). Family planning needs and behavior of health care professionals and their clientele. *Hispanic Journal of Behavioral Science, 9,* 265–286.

Jurich, J. A. (1987). The relationship of social support and social networks to anxiety during pregnancy. *Dissertation Abstracts International, 48,* 224-A.

Kaij, L. & Nilsson, A. (1972). Emotional and psychiatric illness following childbirth. In J. G. Howells (Ed.), *Modern perspectives in psycho-obstetrics* (pp. 364–384). New York: Brunner/Mazel.

Kaplan, B. J. (1986). A psychobiological review of depression during pregnancy. *Psychology of Women Quarterly, 10,* 35–48.

Katz Rothman, B. (1987). *The tentative pregnancy.* New York: Viking.

Kazama, S. W. (1988). The effects of stress and marital intimacy on pregnancy and birth complications. *Dissertation Abstracts International, 48* (9), 2244-A.

Kitzinger, S. (1972). *The experience of childbirth.* London: Pelican.

Kitzinger, S. (1978). *Women as mothers: How they see themselves in different cultures.* New York: Random House.

Kumar, R., Brant, H. A., & Robson, K. M. (1981). Childbearing and maternal sexuality: A prospective study. *Journal of Psychosomatic Research, 25,* 375–383.

Langer, E. J., Fiske, S., Taylor, S. E., & Chanowitz, B. (1976). Stigma, staring, and discomfort: A novel stimulus hypothesis. *Journal of Experimental Social Psychology, 12*, 451–463.

Lazarus, E. S. (1984). *Pregnancy and clinical care: An ethnographic investigation of perinatal management for Puerto Rican and low-income women in the U.S.* Unpublished doctoral dissertation, Case Western Reserve.

Lederman, R. P. (1984). *Psychosocial adaptation in pregnancy.* Englewood Cliffs, NJ: Prentice-Hall.

Lee, I. C. (1976). *Medical care in a Mexican-American community.* Los Alamitos, CA: Hwong.

Leifer, M. (1977). Psychological changes accompanying pregnancy and motherhood. *Genetic Psychology Monographs, 95*, 55–96.

Leifer, M. (1980). *Psychological effects of motherhood: A study of first pregnancy.* New York: Praeger.

Lennane, M. B., & Lennane, R. J. (1973). Alleged psychogenic disorders in women: A possible manifestation of sexual prejudice. *New England Journal of Medicine, 288*, 288–292.

Lester, E. P., & Notman, M. T. (1986). Pregnancy, developmental crisis, and object relations: Psychoanalytic considerations. *International Journal of Psychoanalysis, 67*, 357–366.

Marin, B. V., Marin, G., Padilla, A. M., & De la Rocha, C. (1983). Utilization of traditional and nontraditional sources of health care among Hispanics. *Hispanic Journal of Behavioral Science, 5*, 65–80.

Masters, W. H., & Johnson, V. E. (1966). *Human sexual response.* Boston: Little, Brown.

McKinlay, J. B. (1972). The sick-role: Illness and pregnancy. *Social Sciences and Medicine, 6*, 561–572.

Mead, M. (1949). *Male and female.* New York: Morrow.

Mead, M., & Newton, N. (1967). Cultural patterning of perinatal behavior. In S. A. Richardson & A. F. Guttmacher (Eds.), *Childbearing: Its social and psychological aspect* (pp. 142–244). Baltimore: Williams & Wilkins.

Medina, A. S. (1980). Hispanic maternity care: A study of deficiencies and recommended policies. *Public Affairs Report, 21*, 1–7.

Nadelson, C. C. (1978). "Normal" and "special" aspects of pregnancy: A psychological approach. In C. C. Nadelson & M. T. Notman (Eds.), *Women in context series: Vol. 6. The woman patient: Medical and psychological interfaces.* New York: Plenum.

National Center for Health Statistics: Advance report of final natality statistics, 1985. (1987, July 17). *Monthly Vital Statistics Report, 36*(4) Supplement (DHHS Pub. No. PHS 87-1120). Hyattsville, MD: Public Health Service.

Newton, N. (1955). *Maternal emotions: A study of women's feelings toward menstruation, pregnancy, childbirth, breast feeding, infant care and other aspects of their femininity.* New York: Hoeber.

Nuckolls, K. B., Cassel, J., & Kaplan, B. A. (1972). Psychosocial assets, life crises, and the prognosis of pregnancy. *American Journal of Epidemiology, 95*, 431–441.

Osofsky, H. J., & Osofsky, J. D. (1980). Normal adaptation to pregnancy and parenthood. In P. Taylor (Ed.), *Parent-infant relationships* (pp. 112–130). New York: Grune & Stratton.

Osofsky, J. D., & Osofsky, H. J. (1984). Psychological and developmental perspectives on expectant and new parenthood. In R. Parke (Ed.), *Review of child development research. Vol. 7* (pp. 372–397). Chicago: University of Chicago Press.

Paige, K. E., & Paige, J. M. (1981). *The politics of reproductive ritual.* Berkeley: University of California Press.

Parlee, M. B. (1978). Psychological aspects of menstruation, childbirth, and menopause: An overview with suggestions for further research. In J. Sherman & F. L. Denmark (Eds.), *Psychology of women: Future directions of research* (pp. 179–238). New York: Psychological Dimensions.

Parlee, M. B. (1986). Women and reproductive technologies. *Frontiers, 9,* 32–35.

Petchesky, R. P. (1987). Fetal images: The power of visual culture in the politics of reproduction. In M. Stanworth (Ed.), *Reproductive technologies: Gender, motherhood, and medicine* (pp. 57–80). Beverly Hills: Sage.

Pines, D. (1972). Pregnancy and motherhood: Interaction between fantasy and reality. *British Journal of Medical Psychology, 45,* 333–343.

Powers, B. (1982). The use of orthodox and black American folk medicine. *Advances in Nursing Science, 4,* 31–33.

Rapoport, R., Rapoport, R., & Streilitz, Z. (1972). *Fathers, mothers, and society.* New York: Basic Books.

Reading, A. (1983). *Psychological aspects of pregnancy.* New York: Longman.

Reik, T. (1931). *Ritual: Psychoanalytic studies.* New York: Hogarth.

Richardson, S. R., & Guttmacher, A. F. (1967). *Childbearing: Its social and psychological aspect.* Baltimore: Williams & Wilkins.

Robson, K. M., Brant, H. A., & Kumar, R. (1981). Maternal sexuality during first pregnancy and after childbirth. *British Journal of Obstetrics and Gynecology, 88,* 882–889.

Rodbeck, C. H., & Campbell, S. (1979). The early prenatal diagnosis of neural tube defects. *Trends in Neuroscience, 5,* 1–4.

Rosengren, W. R. (1961). Social sources of pregnancy as illness or normality. *Social Forces, 39,* 260–267.

Rosengren, W. R. (1962). Social instability and attitudes toward pregnancy and child-rearing attitudes. *Social Forces, 41,* 127–134.

Rowland, R. (1985). A child at any price? An overview of issues in the use of the new reproductive technologies, and the threat to women. *Women's Studies International Forum, 8,* 539–546.

Rubin, R. (1984). *Maternity identity and the maternal experience.* New York: Springer.

Russo, N. (1976). The motherhood mandate. *Journal of Social Issues, 32,* 143–154.

Scott, M.D.S., & Stern, P. N. (1986). The ethno-market theory: Factors influencing childbearing health practices of Northern Louisiana black women. In P. N. Stern (Ed.), *Women, health, and culture.* New York: Hemisphere.

Shereshefsky, M., & Yarrow, L. J. (1973). *Psychological aspects of a first pregnancy and early postnatal adaptation.* New York: Raven.

Sherwin, L. N. (1987). *Psychosocial dimensions of the pregnant family.* New York: Springer.

Snitow, A. (1986, December). The paradox of birth technology: Exploring the good, bad, and scary. *Ms. Magazine,* pp. 42–46.

Snow, L. (1974). Folk medicine beliefs and their implications for care of patients. *Annals of Internal Medicine, 81,* 82–96.

Solberg, D., Dultler, J., & Wagner, W. (1973). Sexual behavior in pregnancy. *New England Journal of Medicine, 288*, 1098–1103.

Stack, C. (1974). *All our kin*. New York: Harper & Row.

Stephens, W. N. (1963). *The family in cross-cultural perspective*. New York: Holt, Rinehart, & Winston.

Stern, P. N., Tilden, V. P., & Maxwell, E. K. (1986). Culturally induced stress during childbearing: The Philippino-American experience. In P. N. Stern (Ed.), *Women, health, and culture* (pp. 105–121). New York: Hemisphere.

Taffel, S. (1987, February 10). Characteristics of Asian births, United States, 1980. *Monthly Vital Statistics Report, 32*(10) (DHHS Pub. No. PHS 84-1120). Hyattsville, MD: Public Health Service.

Taylor, S., & Langer, E. (1977). Pregnancy: A social stigma? *Sex Roles, 3*, 27–35.

Telles, C. (1987). Psychological and physiological adaptation to pregnancy and childbirth in low-income Hispanic women. *Hispanic Journal of Behavioral Science, 9*, 34–38.

Tietjen, A. M., & Bradley, C. F. (1985). Social support and maternal psychosocial adjustment during the transition to parenthood. *Canadian Journal of Behavioral Sciences, 17*, 109–121.

Tilden, V. P. (1983). The relation of life stress and social support to emotional disequilibrium during pregnancy. *Research in Nursing and Health, 6*, 167–174.

Tolor, A., & DiGrazia, P. (1976). Sexual attitudes and behavior problems during and following pregnancy. *Archives of Sexual Behavior, 6*, 539–551.

Tolor, A., & DiGrazia, P. (1977). The body image of pregnant women as reflected in their human figure drawings. *Journal of Clinical Psychology, 33*, 566–571.

Treadway, C. R., Kane, F. J., Jarrahi-Zadeh, A., & Lipton, M. A. (1969). The psychoendocrine study of pregnancy and puerperium. *American Journal of Psychiatry, 125*, 1380–1386.

Trethowan, W. E., & Conlon, M. F. (1965). The Couvade syndrome. *British Journal of Psychiatry, 111*, 57–66.

Unger, R. K. (1979). *Female and male psychological perspectives*. New York: Harper & Row.

Weiskopf, S. C. (1980). Maternal sexuality and asexual mothering. *Signs, 5*, 766–782.

White, S., & Reamy, K. (1982). Sexuality and pregnancy: A review. *Archives of Sexual Behavior, 11*, 429–444.

Williamson, N. (1976). Sex preference, sex control, and the status of women. *Signs, 1*, 847–862.

Wood, C. H., & Bean, F. D. (1977). Offspring gender and family size: Implications for a comparison of Mexican Americans and Anglo-Americans. *Journal of Marriage and the Family, 39*, 129–139.

Young, F. W. (1965). *Initiation ceremonies: A cross-cultural study of status dramatization*. Indianapolis: Bobbs-Merrill.

Zuskar, D. M. (1987). The psychological impact of prenatal diagnosis of fetal abnormality. *Women and Health, 12*, 91–103.

Part V
Victimization of Women

13

Recovering Ourselves: The Frequency, Effects, and Resolution of Rape

Mary P. Koss and Takayo Mukai

There are many ways for women to be victimized. Within their relationships lie the risks of courtship violence and acquaintance rape. Walking on the streets risks victimization by crimes such as purse snatching, mugging, stalking, frottage, shootings, and rape by a stranger. Ethnic and poor women are disproportionately exposed to street crime (Bureau of Justice Statistics [BJS], 1992). Lesbian women are additionally vulnerable to hate crimes that can include verbal epithets, physical assault, and even rape (Berrill, 1990; Garnets, Herek, & Levy, 1990). But it is the fear of rape that unites all women (Gordon & Riger, 1989; Riger & Gordon, 1988). For urban women younger than 35, rape is feared even more than murder (Warr, 1985). In response to their fear, over half of women react with self-isolation, forgoing some activities such as evening entertainment. In contrast, most men (90%) deny taking steps to reduce their vulnerability to crime, even though statistics suggest that they are more likely to be victims of every violent crime except rape (Gordon & Riger, 1989). Thus, contemporary women in the United States live their lives under the threat of sexual violation and this fear constitutes a special burden not shared by men.

Rape is a crime of violence that uses sex as a weapon. Virtually all women and men are potential victims of rape. Its impact is multidimensional (physical, psychological, and social) and everlasting. Yet, rape is a crime that is and has been most underreported. This fact inevitably uncovers the sociocultural context against which rape must be examined. The purpose of this chapter is to review recent attempts to capture the multifaceted nature of rape in order to identify gaps and problems in existing research. We will examine the following aspects of rape: (1) representation of rape in surveys and statistical reports, (2) rape victims' experiences, (3) representative treatment methods, and (4) strategies for preventing rape.

DEFINITION OF RAPE

Criminal Definition of Rape

The traditional common law definition of rape was "carnal knowledge of a female forcibly and against her will" (Bienen, 1981, p. 174). Carnal knowledge was defined as penetration of the vagina by the penis, which restricted rape only to female victims and limited application of the term only to cases of penile-vaginal penetration. The current FBI definition of rape is very similar to the common law definition and differs only by substituting "her will" for "her consent."

As a consequence of pressure for legislative reform of rape statutes, the legal definition of rape has been broadened in most states to include fellatio, cunnilingus, and anal intercourse, and the sex of the victim or offender is no longer specified. However, the spouse of the victim is still excluded from the definition of an offender in some states. In addition often there is an age limit before forced intercourse is classified as child abuse. Most often, victims younger than 14–16 years old are excluded from the crime of rape.

Rape in Clinical Context

The criminal definition of rape has serious limitations because some cases of sexual assault, which may be conceptualized and experienced as rape by the victim, will be disqualified by legal definition. From a clinical point of view, rape is the extreme form of sexual victimization (Koss & Harvey, 1987), and in terms of the impact to the victim's mental and physical health, other forms of sexual assault are related to rape. For example, attempted rape differs from rape only by the absence of penetration. However, its traumatic aftereffect to the victim is often comparable to that of completed rape.

THE SCOPE OF RAPE

Empirical Data

Reported Crime Statistics

The Uniform Crime Reports (UCR) have been compiled by the Federal Bureau of Investigation (FBI) for the past five decades. They are the compiled numbers of crimes reported to local police authorities for several violent index offenses that include criminal homicide, forcible rape, aggravated assault, and robbery (e.g., Federal Bureau of Investigation [FBI], 1991). The Uniform Crime Reporting definitions limit the victims of forcible rape to women and further limit rape only to instances of penile-vaginal penetration. Included in the forcible rape rate are attempts to rape where no penetration took place. Excluded are statutory rapes without force and rapes where the offender was the legal or common law spouse of the victim.

With these limitations, 102,555 reported crimes qualified as rapes in 1990 (FBI, 1991). This figure translated into a victimization rape of 80 out of every 100,000 female Americans (FBI, 1991). Approximately 84% of the incidents were completed rapes. In 1986, rape comprised 7% of the violent crime volume and 1% of the crime index total. In the 40-year period from 1933 to 1973, the reported rape rate increased 557% (Hindelang & Davis, 1977); and since 1977, it has risen 21% (FBI, 1991).

Criminal Victimization Surveys

Surveys of the general public about crime victimizations they might have experienced, even when the incidents were not reported to the police, are the major avenue by which the true rate of crime has been estimated. In 1966, the President's Commission on Law Enforcement and Administration of Justice issued a contract to conduct the first nationwide victimization survey, the forerunner of what is today called the National Crime Victimization Survey (NCVS) (e.g., Bureau of Justice Statistics [BJS], 1992). To facilitate comparison with the UCR, the NCVS has been restricted to those crimes indexed by the FBI and consequently has adopted Uniform Crime Reporting definitions with the exception of the case of forcible rape, in which the NCVS includes male as well as female victims.

The results of the NCVS are reported annually. Once selected as a NCVS household, a given housing unit remains in the sample for three years, with interviews occurring every six months. During each contact, respondents are asked to indicate only those criminal victimizations that have occurred since the last interview. The initial interview is for bounding, and these data are not included in the annual crime victimization estimates. The first contact is in person; thereafter both telephone contacts and in-person interviews are used. The eighteenth NCVS report was based on findings from a survey of a representative sample of approximately 62,000 housing units across the United States, including about 127,000 inhabitants over age 12 (BJS, 1992).

Early versions of the survey reported only 15 rapes among 10,000 households (Hindelang & Davis, 1977). In successive versions of the NCVS, the methodology for questioning about rape experiences has changed little. Unlike earlier versions where respondents were asked about victimizations that happened to anyone in their household, respondents are currently asked only about victimizations that they have personally experienced. The crime screening question is designed to alert the interviewer to a possible rape: "Did someone try to attack you in *some other way*?" (BJS, 1992 p. 108; emphasis added). Even in their most recent version, the questions do not inquire directly about rape. Participants are not told that unwanted sexual behavior is considered a form of attack for NCVS purposes. It has been noted that this approach is "not straightforward" (Block & Block, 1984, p. 146). The NCVS approach to measurement of rape has been severely criticized (Koss, 1992).

On the basis of responses to this single item, rape was determined to be the rarest of all the NCVS-measured violent crimes, representing less than 1% of incidents. The victimization rate for rape among women and girls over age 12 was 1.0 per 1,000 during a six-month period. The rate for men and boys was statistically unreliable because only 10 or fewer cases were reported. Of the rapes, 97% involved a single victim and 88% involved a single perpetrator, all of whom were male. The perpetrator was a stranger in 42% of the instances; 17% of the incidents involved weapons; and 52.8% of the episodes were reported to police (BJS, 1992).

Epidemiologic Surveys

Crime victimization data are limited in mental health applications primarily because they are incidence figures; that is, they include rapes that occurred only during the preceding six-month period. If a woman has been raped more than six months ago, she is no longer considered to be victimized. This time period is too short to capture the full impact of rape. The posttraumatic stress disorder that victims of rape may experience is characterized as follows: "Reexperiencing symptoms may develop after a latency period of months or years following the trauma" (*DSM-III-R*, American Psychiatric Association, 1987, p. 249). Thus, prevalence data on rape that are based on a longer reference period may be more appropriate than incidence data for mental health applications.

Over the past several years, the methods of epidemiology have been utilized to assess the frequency of rape. Included in this group are studies that have focused on adolescents (Ageton, 1983a, 1983b; Hall & Flannery, 1984; Moore, Nord, & Peterson, 1989); college students (Koss, Gidycz, & Wisniewski, 1987); adult women (Essock-Vitale & McGuire, 1985; George, Winfield, & Blazer, 1992; Kilpatrick, Best, Veronen, Amick, Villeponteaux, & Ruff, 1985; Kilpatrick, Saunders, Veronen, Best, & Von, 1987; Koss, Koss, & Dinero, 1987; National Victims Center [NVC], 1992; Russell, 1982, 1990; Sorenson, Stein, Siegel, Golding, & Burnam, 1987; Wyatt, 1992); adult men (George & Winfield-Laird, 1986; Sorenson et al., 1987); special populations, including the elderly, nursing home residents, psychiatric patients, the homeless, and prisoners (D'Ercole & Struening, 1990; George & Winfield-Laird, 1986; Goodman, 1991; Jacobson & Richardson, 1987); and ethnic groups, including Hispanics (Sorenson & Siegel, 1992) and African-Americans (Wyatt, 1992).

The prevalence of completed rape has been estimated at approximately 20% of adult women in several sources (Goodman, 1991; Kilpatrick, Saunders, Veronen, Best, & Von, 1987; Koss, Woodruff, & Koss, 1991; Russell, 1982; Wyatt, 1992). However, a group of studies have reported lower rape prevalences of approximately 6 to 14% (Essock-Vitale & McGuire, 1985; Kilpatrick, Best,

Veronen, Amick, Villeponteaux, & Ruff, 1985; Gordon & Riger, 1989; NVC, 1992). Of course, developing a single prevalence number is artificial because the frequency of rape varies with age and sociodemographic characteristics (Sorenson & Siegel, 1992; George, Winfield, & Blazer, 1992).

Assessment of the Quality of the Database

Sources of Method Variance

A review of the extant studies on criminal victimization reveals not only differences in the prevalence rates obtained, but also considerable variation in the definitions of rape, samples, methods of data collection, participation rates, number and content of screening questions, and the contexts in which rape questioning appeared. This leads to the conclusion that rape prevalence rates are very sensitive to the methods used to measure them.

Although it may seem inconceivable, it is not difficult to find epidemiological studies characterized by the absence of a definition for the concept of sexual assault (George & Winfield-Laird, 1986; Hall & Flannery, 1984) or by global and vague definitions. Typical of a nonspecific definition is the following, "Sexual assault was defined as being pressured or forced to have sexual contact" (Sorenson et al., 1987, p. 1156). Such terminology not only is imprecise, but may result in confusion and miscommunication if used without specification of the connotation of the term.

Generally speaking, the UCR practice of including attempts to rape in the definition of rape has been adopted in victimization surveys. Because typically fewer than half of the "rapes" are completed rapes, separate reporting of attempted and completed rapes would be more precise (Block & Block, 1984). The sex neutrality of reform statutes has also been ignored in many cases. From a practical point of view, restricting the focus to female victims is sensible since the bulk of rapes reported in the NCVS involves female victims and male offenders. However, consideration of male victims is within the scope of the legal definition of rape. Two studies (George & Winfield-Laird, 1986; Sorenson et al., 1987) have reported prevalence rates for men, including situations in which men or boys were forced to participate involuntarily in undesired sexual activities with women who had psychologically coerced them. Inclusion of such incidents violates both legal usage and the psychological meaning of the term *rape*, which connotes "invasion" of a victim's body (Masters, 1986).

The term *screening questions* refers to the items used to identify respondents as sexually victimized so that they may be administered more detailed questions regarding their incidents. The function of screening questions is to jog the respondent's memory of incidents. The quality of data on victimization has been reported to depend upon how the task of remembering and reporting is structured and the way in which the interviewer uses the screening questions (Biederman & Reiss, 1987). An examination of the questions and structures of interview used in surveys revealed two major approaches to screening: gate questions and behaviorally specific scenarios.

Gate questions aim to identify the maximum number of sexually abused people from whom rape victims can be culled on the basis of subsequent detailed inquiry. A gate question is generally a global item such as, "In your lifetime, has anyone ever tried to pressure or force you to have sexual contact?" (Sorenson et al., 1987). This approach has been widely used in prevalence studies because of its perceived advantages of all-inclusiveness and inoffensiveness. Yet, there are reasons to question its efficacy. The usage of euphemistic language such as "sex" and "sexual relations" may miss some eligible repondents because the typical woman might not consider oral or anal sex or penetration with objects when she is asked to think of "sex" or "sexual relations." Such terms may also imply completion while only slight penetration is sufficient for rape. The incorporation of the word *rape* (e.g., Ageton, 1983a, 1983b) may fail to identify all eligible cases because many victims with an experience that legally qualifies as rape do not use this term to conceptualize their incident (Koss, 1988).

Behavioral scenarios are often used in an attempt to put before the respondent detailed examples of the types of experiences the interviewer seeks to identify. An example of such a specific scenario is the following: "Has a man made you have sex by using force or threatening to harm you? When we use the word *sex*, we mean a man putting his penis in your vagina, even if he didn't ejaculate (come)" (Koss et al., 1987).

It has been suggested that personal memories are stored in categories with similar content (e.g., Rubin, 1986). Certain memories are recalled simply because they differ from the typical experiences in that category. According to research on the NCVS data collection, presentation of additional items about crime and the seriousness of victimization before the main questionnaire stimulated the recall of more criminal incidents (Skogan, 1981). Therefore, the use of behavioral scenarios that begin with lesser degrees of victimization and build up to sexual assault may be more effective than gate questions in allowing the interviewer to cue the respondent to the specific types of behavior to be recalled. In return, this process may allow greater time for the respondent to think carefully about past experiences.

It is possible that the context in which the rape questions are presented impacts on the repondent's ability to delineate the appropriate set of experiences. However, in all of the large-scale epidemiological studies on criminal victimization or mental health, rape was but one variable, and the primary focus of the project dictated the context in which questioning about rape would occur. For example, a survey focused on crime may stimulate recall only of those sexual experiences the respondent viewed as police matters, which would fail to include the group of respondents who did not conceptualize their experience as any sort of crime.

Interviewer effects are reported to be most substantial for sensitive topics, particularly rape (Bailey, Moore, & Bailar, 1978). In rape prevalence studies that focused exclusively on women, female interviewers were uniformly used.

However, when both sexes were interviewed, sex-matching was either not discussed (Sorenson et al., 1987) or the sexes were not matched for the screening phase (George & Winfield-Laird, 1986). Because respondents will not be followed up if they are not identified as rape victims at the screening stage, this procedure is problematic. Confidential setting is another important, but often neglected, issue. Because of the intimate nature of sexual violence and the lack of confidentiality, such as the presence of other family members during the interview, the prevalence of sexual assault may be significantly underestimated (e.g., Skogan, 1981).

All major survey methods have been utilized to collect data on rape incidence and prevalence, including in-person interviews (Ageton, 1983a; Koss et al., 1987; George & Winfield-Laird, 1986; Russell, 1982; Sorenson et al., 1987; Wyatt, 1992), random digit telephone surveys (Hall & Flannery, 1984; Kilpatrick et al., 1985; NVC, 1992), mailed self-report surveys (Koss, Koss, & Woodruff, 1991), and group-administered self-report surveys (Koss et al., 1987a). Although all methods of data collection are thought to be essentially equivalent, one study reported prevalence rates twice as high when obtained in person compared to telephone administration (Gordon & Riger, 1989).

Studies have utilized sophisticated sampling plans that resulted in groups of respondents who well represented the population from which they were selected. These populations include adolescents, nationally, age 11–17 (Ageton, 1983a, 1983b); college students, nationally (Koss et al., 1987); adult women, nationally (NVC, 1992); urban working women (Koss et al., 1990); adult residents of rural and urban areas of North Carolina, including the elderly, nursing home residents, psychiatric patients, and prisoners (George & Winfield-Laird, 1986); Hispanic and white adult residents of Los Angeles (Sorenson et al., 1987); and African-American and white female adults aged 16–36 years residing in Los Angeles (Wyatt, 1992). Unfortunately, due to methodological differences, it is impossible to cumulate findings from these specialized samples.

The rates of participation in the studies typically ranged from 50 to 70%. Prevalence rates tended to be higher in studies with lower participation rates, and the rates of participation seem to be confounded by the context of questioning and the type of screening questions used. When nonoffensive, euphemistic language was used to prevent premature termination of participation, the participation rates were higher. It is quite possible that there is a direct trade-off between explicitness of questions and self-selection of participants. Since participants, compared with nonparticipants, were found to be more often single, young, and educated (Wyatt, 1992), this may inflate prevalence rates as rape is thought to increase with education and decrease with age, according to NCVS data (Skogan, 1981).

Threats to Validity

Fabrication refers to a respondents' tendency, for whatever reason, to make up a completely false report of victimization. The studies of self-reported burglary, robbery, and assault revealed fabrication not to be a serious problem (Sparks, 1982). Although fabrication of self-reported sexual victimization has received limited empirical attention, several studies have reported that credulity of self-reports was substantiated by the material shared with the interviewer (Ageton, 1983b; Koss et al., 1987; Koss & Gidycz, 1985).

Nonreporting is considered to be a much more serious threat to the validity of sexual victimization data than fabrication. There are two types of nonreporting: purposive nonreporting (withholding) and unintentional nonreporting (lack of recall due to memory decay, repression, or failure of screening questions to stimulate recall of relevant experiences). Some proportion of nonreporting can be due to differential productivity (Sudman & Bradburn, 1974), which refers to differences among subjects in willingness to adopt a productive role during an interview. Educated and test-wise respondents are reported to exhibit greater productivity in interviews (Skogan, 1981), which is suspected of masking hypothesized negative associations between social position and victimization.

Other factors that influence the number of victimizations reported to an interviewer are the placement of the detailed incident questions relative to the screening questions and the length of the recall period. If respondents are given detailed follow-up questions after they have given an affirmative reply, the total number of victimizations they report on the survey will be lower than if they were given all the screening items first (Sparks, 1982). In addition, since rape is clearly a salient event, longer recall periods may be feasible due to the formation of indelible, flashbulb-type memories (Brown & Kulik, 1977). Although the maximum interval over which recall can be expected has not been studied, it is possibile that older respondents have forgotten more relevant events than younger respondents simply because the recall period for the former group is much longer. This phenomenon could partially account for apparent increases in the rape rate in recent years (Russell, 1984).

Telescoping refers to a tendency for respondents incorrectly to place a victimization experience in time. Thus, experiences may be recalled as having happened closer to the present than they actually did (forward telescoping) or further from the present than they actually did (backward telescoping). Telescoping poses serious threats to the validity of incidence figures, which aim to stipulate that a given number of victimizations occurred within a fixed, relatively short time frame.

Some of the lower prevalence rates in the literature clearly stemmed from a relative lack of success in overcoming the forces that foster nondisclosure of rape. The higher prevalence rates raise concerns about differential participation by those who were younger, more educated, members of the majority culture, and more likely to have experienced sexual assault. The 14% prevalence released by the National Victims Center (1992) has the advantage of a national sample, and techniques for questioning about rape were state of the art. But there are reasons to consider this figure a conservative estimate. First, the sample excluded some high risk groups including young girls under age 18, women too poor to own a telephone, women living in college residences, institutions, and prisons, and women serving in the military. Second, data collection was by telephone, and reporting of rape has been found to be higher when obtained in person (Gordon & Riger, 1989). If the face-to-face interview is the gold standard in epidemiology, it must be concluded that an exemplary study of rape prevalence with a nationally generalizable database does not yet exist.

Public Policy Needs for Sound Data on Rape Prevalence

As discussed earlier, neither UCR or NCVS is designed to capture the full scope of rape. Various epidemiologic surveys have methodological problems, which make their direct comparison invalid. Under these circumstances, the following recommendations were formulated so that future research findings would be more cumulative.

1. A clear conceptualization of rape must be established as the foundation of the study. Separate categories of rape must be studied based on specific behavioral characteristics. An operational definition of rape in the screening questions or incident report must include the following elements: force, nonconsent, penetration, and statutory age.
2. Nationally representative samples must be attempted. "High-risk" groups or populations must be studied separately.
3. Children and adolescents should be studied directly rather than relying on retrospective reporting by adults.
4. More attention needs to be paid to the context of data collection, such as the match of sex between the respondent and the interviewer, to obtain more accurate information.

THE IMPACT OF RAPE ON MENTAL AND PHYSICAL HEALTH

Cognitive Responses to Rape

To understand psychological and behavioral postvictimization symptoms, it is crucial to examine the victim's perceptions and cognitive appraisals of her experience (e.g., Koss & Harvey, 1991). Cognitive appraisal refers to the process by which an individual evaluates a particular stressor (e.g., Folkman, 1984; Lazarus & Folkman, 1984). However, the amount of psychological distress experienced by an individual is determined not by the stressor alone but by the relationship between the person and the environment. The person factors that could influence the process of cognitive appraisal are commitments, beliefs, and existential beliefs (Lazarus & Folkman, 1984). The situation factors include predictability, duration, and ambiguity of the stressor (Lazarus & Folkman, 1984). The characteristic symptoms of posttraumatic stress disorder (PTSD) such as obsessions, nightmares, and phobias are considered to be the consequence of an inadequate emotional processing of the trauma (Rachman, 1980).

Behavioral models of PTSD suggest that experiencing a sudden, terrifying event creates a memory schema that consists of (1) information about the characteristics of the feared situation, (2) information about the verbal, physiological, and overt behavioral responses that occurred in that situation and that reoccur whenever the schema is activated, and (3) cognitions about the meaning of the feared situation and the responses that occurred in it (Foa, Steketee, & Olasov, 1989). People untouched by victimization often maintain beliefs, such as thoughts about personal invulnerability, that are incompatible with the experience of rape. The cognitive processing of rape involves changing the interpretation of the experience to fit inner models (assimilation) or altering beliefs to fit the experience (accommodation). An extensive array of beliefs are potentially challenged by rape including safety, power or efficacy, trust, esteem, and intimacy (McCann & Pearlman, 1990). Because these beliefs (or schemas) are the eyeglasses through which humans interpret and make sense of ongoing perceptions, rape-induced changes have the potential for far-reaching and long-lasting consequences. The cognitive activity typical of stress response is ignored in the criteria for the diagnosis of PTSD, which focuses on memory intrusions, emotional arousal, and avoidance behavior.

Among cognitive responses to rape, the victim's causal attribution has received the most empirical study. How a victim attempts to answer the question ''Why me?'' affects her later adjustment. Janoff-Bulman (1979) defines two types of self-blame as a form of causal attribution. Behavioral self-blame occurs when a victim assigns responsibility for her rape to her own modifiable behaviors. In contrast, characterological self-blame occurs when a victim attributes responsibility to stable aspects of her personality. According to Janoff-Bulman (1979), behavioral self-blame is associated with more positive adjustment because it would enhance the victim's sense of control, while characterological self-blame suggests the inevitability of the assault and, therefore, poor adjustment. More immediate cognitive reactions to rape include confusion, shock, and difficulty in remembering, concentrating, and making decisions (Ruch, Gartrell, Amedeo, & Coyne, 1991).

Most of the work on cognitive responses to victimization has been theoretical in nature, except for the empirical studies on people who experienced natural traumas. Due to the lack of adequate methodologies to assess the foregoing cognitive changes, the progress of the research on victims of human-induced violent crimes has been hampered.

Symptomatic Reactions to Rape

A large empirical literature documents the psychological symptoms experienced in the aftermath of rape (for reviews see Hanson, 1990; Lurigio & Resick, 1990; Resick, 1987, 1990; Roth & Lebowitz, 1988). Given the nature of the rape, it is understandable that immediate distress results, but what is surprising is the longevity of the effects. Rape victims typically show very high distress levels within the first week that peaks in severity by approximately 3 weeks postassault, continues at a high level for the next month, and then begins to improve by 2 to 3 months postassault. Many differences between victimized and nonvictimized women disappear after 3 months except for elevations in fear, anxiety, self-esteem, and sexual dysfunction that persist for up to 18 months (Resick, 1987). Approximately one-quarter of women who are several years beyond rape experience continuing negative effects (Hanson, 1990). Even when evaluated many years after sexual assault, data from the epidemiologic catchment area studies revealed that victims were more likely to receive several psychiatric diagnoses including major depression, alcohol abuse/dependence, drug abuse/ dependence, generalized anxiety, obsessive-compulsive disorder, and posttraumatic stress disorder (PTSD) (Burnam et al., 1988; Winfield et al., 1990).

Most rape victims qualify for the posttraumatic stress disorder (PTSD) diagnosis when evaluated in a trauma center. For example, an average of 12 days following assault, 94% of rape victims met PTSD criteria; 46% still met the criteria 3 months later (Rothbaum et al., 1992). Rape is more likely to induce PTSD than a range of traumatic events affecting civilians including robbery, physical assault, tragic death of a close friend or family member, combat service, or natural disaster (Norris, 1992).

Fear and Anxiety

The most frequently observed symptoms following rape are fear and anxiety. Ruch et al. (1991) administered the Sexual Assault Symptoms Assessment (SASA) to rape victims who reported to the sexual assault center within 72 hours of the assault. Immediately following the assault, 86% of victims reported intense fear of the assailant and fear for their personal safety and expressed heightened concern about others' reaction (what the authors call disclosure anxiety). Further, since 23% of the victims failed to complete SASA, the Clinical Trauma Assessment (CTA; Ruch, Gartrell, Ramelli, & Coyne, 1991) was developed. CTA supplements SASA with clinical assessment by the crisis intervention worker. The crisis workers rated the victim's symptoms of fear and concern about others' reactions as especially severe (Ruch et al., 1990). In all items except one, disorientation, all trauma symptoms correlated positively and significantly with the crisis workers' assessment.

Using the Modified Fear Survey (MFS; Veronen & Kilpatrick, 1980), an instrument specifically designed to assess fear in rape victims, or SCL-90 (Derogatis, 1977), which has a phobic anxiety subscale, several studies have found differences in fear levels between victims and nonvictims. In their longitudinal study, Kilpatrick and Veronen (1984) found that rape victims received elevated scores on seven of the eight MFS subscales and phobic anxiety at the 6–21-day, one-month, three-month, six-month, and one-year assessments. Fear decreased at 18 months, but reemerged at two and three years postcrime. Calhoun, Atkeson, and Resick (1982) found similar results. The victims exhibited improvement between two weeks and two months postcrime but continued to score significantly higher than nonvictimized women through one year postcrime.

Several studies have examined the development of general anxiety reactions in response to rape. The SCL-90 Anxiety Subscale and the State-Trait Anxiety Scale (Spielberger, Gorsuch, & Luchene, 1970) have both been used to assess these reactions. The weekly assessments of Peterson, Olasov, and Foa (1987) indicated that state anxiety is higher than trait anxiety for the first five weeks following rape, that both state and trait anxiety have a peak in the third week, and that trait anxiety is slightly higher at week five than at week one. Kilpatrick and Veronen (1984) found a somewhat different pattern. They found trait anxiety scores to be higher than state anxiety scores at all sessions. They also found rape victims to score higher than nonvictims at all sessions through one year postcrime.

Depression

There are three ways in which a rape victim may experience depression: short-term, long-term, and chronic or severe depression, which includes suicidal thoughts or attempts.

Immediately following the assault, the victims often expressed sad feelings about the assault, apathetic feelings about her life, or suicide thoughts (Ruch et al., in press). According to the Beck Depression Inventory (BDI) (Beck, Ward, Mendelsohn, Mock, & Erbaugh, 1961), administered within one month postcrime, nearly half of the victims fell into the moderately or severely depressed range (Frank & Stewart, 1984; Frank, Turner, & Duffy, 1979). The depression diminished by three months postcrime. Other studies have found similar initial levels of depression (Atkeson, Calhoun, Resick, & Ellis, 1982; Kilpatrick & Veronen, 1984; Peterson et al., 1987; Resick, 1987) using the BDI, the Hamilton Psychiatric Rating Scale for Depression (HPRS; Hamilton, 1960), the depression-dejection scale from the Profile of Mood States Scale (POMS; McNair, Lorr, & Droppleman, 1971), or the depression subscale from SCL-90 or BSI. However, when compared with nonvictims at one year after the assault, rape victims were found to be still significantly different in the depression scales of the SCL-90 and the POMS (Kilpatrick & Veronen, 1984).

According to cross-sectional studies of long-term effects of rape, victims 1–16 years postrape were found to be significantly more depressed than nonvictims as measured by the BDI (Ellis et al., 1981), and victims who were an average of 21.9 years postrape scored higher than nonvictims on the SCL-90 and the Mental Health Problem Interview (Kilpatrick et al., 1987). Kilpatrick et al. (1987) also found a stronger impact of series victimization (defined as repeated incidents) on the degree of victim's depression; 80% of two-incident victims met the lifetime diagnosis of major depressive disorder as compared with 45.7% of single-incident victims. Finally, the level of suicidal ideation and attempts among rape victims is notable, and studies report it to increase over time (Ellis, Atkeson, & Calhoun, 1981; Frank et al., 1979; Frank & Stewart, 1984).

Low Self-Esteem

Given that self-blame has been frequently noted in rape victims (Janoff-Bul-man, 1979; Libow & Doty, 1979; Meyer & Taylor, 1985; Ruch et al., 1991), it might be expected that self-esteem would be affected. However, few studies have addressed self-esteem, and none has examined the relationship between self-blame and self-esteem. In their longitudinal study using the Self-Report Inventory (SRI; Bown, 1961), Kilpatrick and Veronen (1984) found that victims reported significantly lower self-esteem than nonvictims on most of eight sub-scales. At one year after the crime, self, others, and parents were still sources of lower esteem for the victims.

Resick (1987) used the Tennessee Self-Concept Scale (TSCS; Fitts, 1965) in longitudinal comparison of rape, robbery, and rape-robbery victims. The TSCS consists of an overall self-esteem score and eight subscales that are different from those assessed by the SRI. Overall, rape-robbery victims had lower esteem regarding physical self, social self, and identity than either rape victims or robbery victims at least up to six months postassault.

Changes in Social Adjustment

Considering that the victims often express loss of trust in people (e.g., the assailant, men, social network) immediately following rape and that they are highly concerned about others' reactions to the assault, it is expected that the victim's social adjustment will be affected.

In their longitudinal study, Resick, Calhoun, Atkeson, and Ellis (1981) reported that the victims had poorer overall economic, social, and leisure adjustment for two months postcrime than nonvictims. Work adjustment was impaired for eight months. Marital, parental, and family unit adjustment were not affected at all, whereas extended family adjustment was affected for one month. The possible explanation of this finding was that participation in a longitudinal research lent credibility to the reactions of victims such that significant others provided more social support.

Studies of the long-term effects found that completed rape was particularly associated with problems in areas of social life and leisure, family unit, and marital adjustment (Kilpatrick et al., 1987). They also found that risk of developing social phobia is 4.5 times higher in rape victims than nonrape crime victims.

Although work adjustment appeared to be a particular problem following crime, no significant difference on this subscale was found between the rape and robbery victims at three and six months postcrime (Resick, 1986). On the other hand, the interpersonal sensitivity scale from the SCL-90 was more elevated in rape than robbery victims at three and six months postcrime (Resick, 1986) and than nonvictims at 18 months and two years postcrime (Kilpatrick & Veronen, 1984).

Impacts on Sexual Functioning

A number of researchers have reported problems in long-term sexual functioning. Sexual functions are among the most long-lasting problems experienced by rape victims. The most immediate reaction is probably avoidance of sex. However, according to Ellis, Calhoun, and Atkeson (1980), by one year postcrime, the frequency of sexual activity had returned to normal levels for those women who were sexually active before the crime.

Rape survivors are consistently found to have less sexual satisfaction (Feldman-Summers, Gordon, & Meager, 1979; Orlando & Koss, 1983; Resick, 1986) and more sexual dysfunctions (Becker, Skinner, Abel, & Cichon, 1986; Becker, Skinner, Abel, & Treacy, 1982; Kilpatrick et al., 1987; Resick, 1986), even when the assault was not conceptualized as a rape by the victim (Orlando & Koss, 1983). According to a large study of sexual functioning in sexual assault survivors by Becker et al. (1986), the majority of the sexual dysfunctions suffered by the assaulted victims were early-response-cycle-inhibiting problems. In particular, compared with the dysfunctional nonassaulted women, the sexual assault survivors were more likely to experience fear of sex and arousal dysfunction.

Victimization-Induced Somatic Changes

Between half and two-thirds of victims sustain no physical trauma (Beebe, 1991; NVC, 1992; Koss, Woodruff, & Koss, 1991). Of those who are injured about half receive formal medical care (Beebe, 1991; Koss et al., 1991). Sexually transmitted diseases (STDs) occur as a result of rape in 3.6% to 30% of victims (e.g., Murphy, 1990). AIDS is spontaneously mentioned as a concern by 26% of rape victims interviewed within three months of rape (Baker, Burgess, Brickman, & Davis, 1990). Pregnancy results from rape in approximately 5 percent of the cases (Beebe, 1991; Koss, Woodruff, & Koss, 1991). However, victimized women who seek medical intervention may not be receiving the emergency care that rape protocols recommend. In a recent national sample, no pregnancy testing or prophylaxis was received by 60% of rape victims, and no information or testing for exposure to HIV was reported by 73% of victims (NVC, 1992).

In primary care practice, women with a history of victimization by rape (and other crimes) report more symptoms of illness across virtually all body systems except the skin and eyes and perceive their health less favorably than nonvictimized women (Koss, Koss, & Woodruff, 1991). In addition, victimized women are more likely to report negative health behaviors including smoking, alcohol use, and failure to use seatbelts (Koss, Koss, et al., 1991). Given their greater perception of symptoms and exposure to more health risks, it is understandable that victimized women receive significantly more medical care than nonvictimized women (Golding, Stein, Siegel, Burnam, & Sorenson, 1988; Koss, Koss, et al., 1991). Adult women who had been raped or assaulted visited their physician twice as often, an average of 6.9 visits per year, compared to 3.5 visits for nonvictimized women (Koss, Koss, et al., 1991). Utilization data across five years preceding and following victimization ruled out the possibility that victims had been high utilizers of services from some earlier point preceding their crime.

A number of chronic conditions are diagnosed disproportionately among rape victims including chronic pelvic pain, gastrointestinal disorders, headaches, chronic pain, psychogenic seizures, and premenstrual symptoms (Koss & Heslet, in press). In many instances elevated prevalence of victimization is found both among those patients with and those patients lacking medical explanations for their symptoms. In response to these findings the American Medical Association (1992) has recently adopted a policy that urges physicians to undertake routine screening for victimization at the entry points to the health care system, validate disclosures of victimization, and develop the ability to link patients to trauma-specific resources in the community.

Variables Affecting Recovery

Preassault Variables

There are several reliable predictors of the victim most likely to adjust successfully in the aftermath of rape (Hanson, 1990; Lurigio & Resick, 1990). Demographic variables have been reported to have little effect on victims' responses to crime (Kilpatrick & Veronen, 1984; Kilpatrick, Best, et al., 1985) or subsequent recovery (Becker et al., 1982; Ruch & Leon, 1983). However, elderly women, Asian, and Mexican-American women are all thought to have more difficult recoveries than other women (Atkeson et al., 1982; Ruch & Leon, 1983; Ruch, Gartrell, Amedeo, & Coyne, 1991; Williams & Holmes, 1981). Women with previous victimization have greater assault impact and longer recoveries.

Prior psychological functioning or life stressors are reported to influence recovery. Preexisting mental health problems were found to be one of the most significant predictors of the initial level of trauma (Ruch & Leon, 1983). Although a history of psychotherapy or hospitalization was not associated with elevations in depression, fear, or anxiety, a history of psychotropic medication, alcohol abuse, or suicidal ideation or attempts was related to stronger distress in the first month postcrime (Frank, Turner, Stewart, Jacob, & West, 1981). A prior diagnosis of a psychiatric disorder is also identified as a predictor for victim's short-term response and recovery (Frank & Anderson, 1987). As for long-term effect, depression, suicidal history, and sexual adjustment prior to the rape were significantly related to depression scores at four months postassault (Atkeson et al., 1982).

The research on the effect of prior victimization has been very inconsistent. Ruch and Leon (1983) reported that trauma scores for women with prior victimization increased during two weeks after the crime while the scores for women without prior victimization decreased. In contrast, Frank, Turner, and Stewart

(1980) and Frank and Anderson (1987) did not find a significant difference between single-incident victims and multiple-incident victims on measures of depression, anxiety, or fear from one to four months postcrime. However, the multiple-incident victims did report poorer overall social adjustment and greater disruption in social functioning in their immediate household. With regard to longer-term reactions, multiple-incident victims were not found to be different from single-incident victims at one year postcrime, but they reported more intense nightmares and a greater fear of being home alone (McCahill, Meyer, & Fishman, 1979).

A history of domestic violence, child abuse, incest, or observing parental violence was found to be predictive of problems in both reaction and recovery (Glenn & Resick, 1986). Moreover, Resick (1986) found that severity of prior criminal victimization was predictive of problems with symptoms such as flashbacks, nightmares, anxiety attacks, avoidance, and intrusion of memories. With regard to other life stressors, Ruch, Chandler, and Harter (1980) found a curvilinear relationship between women's reported degree of trauma and the number of changes in life during the year prior to rape. It seems that experience with some life stress may have an inoculating effect, but too high a level of stress interferes with the development of coping methods after the assault.

The effect of preassault cognitive appraisals on postassault functioning has not been studied extensively. However, a perception of unique invulnerability may exacerbate reactions to traumatic events (Perloff, 1983). It is understandable that those who believe they control their lives and environments make the poorest adjustments to events that are out of their control. Further, victims who appraised the situation as "safe" prior to the assault had greater fear and depressive reactions than women who perceived themselves in a dangerous situation prior to the assault (Frank & Stewart, 1984; Scheppele & Bart, 1983). The role of preassault cognitive appraisals and attributions warrants further study.

Assault Variables

There has been a common assumption in the public arena that some rapes are worse than others. Rapes by strangers and those that are more violent are assumed to be more traumatic for the victim. However, this may not be the case. The fear that one will be injured or killed is equally common among women who are raped by husbands and dates as it is among those raped by total strangers (NVC, 1992). Acquaintance rapes are as equally devastating to the victim as stranger rapes, as measured by standard measures of psychopathology (Katz, 1991). The prevalence of psychiatric diagnoses among women sexually assaulted by acquaintances is approximately equal (anxiety, depression, and sexual adjustment) or even higher (obsessive-compulsive disorder, phobias, and panic disorders) compared to women victimized by strangers (Burnam et al., 1988). Acquaintanceship with the assailant may affect the victim in other ways, however. For example, it was reported that women who delayed treatment were more likely to have known their assailants and less likely to have physically defended themselves (Stewart et al., 1987).

Brutality scores or indices were developed to examine the effect of brutality upon the victim's reactions. Research findings have been mixed. Perceived severity of rape did not predict later reactions (Atkeson et al., 1982). Neither the presence nor extent of violence per se was strongly associated with victim reactions (Sales, Baum, & Shore, 1984), but a combination of assault variables was found to predict greater distress on some measures. For example, the "threat index" was significantly and positively correlated with self-esteem at an initial assessment but not at the 6- or 12-month follow-up (Cluss, Boughton, Frank, Stewart, & West, 1983). In Norris and Feldman-Summers's study (1981), assault variables predicted psychosomatic symptoms but not sexual satisfaction or frequency or the level of reclusiveness.

Examination of individual assault variables has yielded mixed results. Threats against the victim's life were found to predict symptomatology within the first three months but not at the six-month follow-up (Sales et al., 1984). The assault variables that predicted follow-up symptomatology were the number of assailants, physical threat, and injury requiring medical care and causing medical complications (Sales et al., 1984). The display of a weapon did predict life-style changes and avoidance at one month postassault, while restraint, threat, and length of the crime predicted avoidance and intrusion at six months postcrime (Resick, 1986).

The possibility that "the actual violence of an attack is less crucial to victim reaction than the felt threat" was proposed by Sales et al. (1984). Subsequent studies found that subjective distress was predictive of later fear reactions (Girelli, Resnick, Marhoefer-Dvorak, & Hutter, 1986), that cognitive appraisal of life threat predicted later PTSD (Kilpatrick et al., 1987), and that the perception of imminent death or injury of others predicted fear symptoms and avoidance at one month and six months, respectively (Resick, 1986).

Postassault Variables

Of the variables that may affect recovery, postassault factors are the least studied. Among the variables that have not been paid enough attention are the effect of participating in the criminal justice system, the effectiveness of the type of counseling, social support, coping methods by the victim, attributions, and the effect of initial reactions.

In general, the level of distress experienced within the first few weeks after rape is highly correlated with subsequent distress (Kilpatrick, Veronen, & Best, 1985). In most of the longitudinal studies, victim reactions have stabilized at three months and then continued at the same level until the end of the assessment. A variable that has received some empirical consideration is participation in the criminal justice system. Although no difference was found at one year postrape in the level of depression or social adjustment between those who wished to prosecute and those who did not (Cluss et al., 1983), women who wished to prosecute reported greater self-esteem. Further, women who wished to prosecute, but were not able to, showed better work adjustment and more rapid improvement in self-esteem compared with those who did not wish to prosecute. Among those who prosecuted, Sales et al. (1984) reported a tendency of increasing numbers of symptoms as the processes progressed toward trial. The authors suggested that extended court proceedings may inflict additional demands on these women and keep them in a victim role. In a partial support for this argument, two studies have found that participating in court may be quite stressful and fear provoking for victims (Calhoun et al., 1982; Kilpatrick, Veronen, & Resick, 1979).

The role of postrape social support on adjustment has also been examined. Sales et al. (1984) discussed the difficulty of measuring and interpreting the effects of social support on victims' reactions and recovery. Postassault support is inevitably confounded by the quality and quantity of prerape relationships. Support may vary depending on the nature of the assault. For example, family closeness and the violence of an assault were found to be correlated, victims with greater family closeness reporting fewer symptoms (Sales et al., 1984) and experiencing lower levels of trauma fairly soon after the assault (Ruch & Chandler, 1980). Overall, social support (e.g., the presence of understanding men and women in the victim's life) predicted lower level of depression (Atkeson et al., 1982) and less reclusiveness over the long term (Norris & Feldman-Summers, 1981). Unsupportive behavior in particular predicts poorer social adjustment (Davis, Brickman, & Baker, 1991). Proceeding with prosecution appears to prolong recovery (Sales et al., 1984). Finally, positive and negative social network responses were found to be unrelated to whether women wished to prosecute the assault (Cluss et al., 1983).

Postrape cognitive appraisals and attributions can be viewed as reactions to the assault and as attempts to cope with the event and reactions. People have a strong need to search for the meaning of negative events (Janoff-Bulman, 1979; Taylor, 1983). Any kind of criminal victimization destroys the illusion that we live in a predictable, controllable, meaningful world. In a study of incest victims, Silver, Boon, and Stones (1983) found that women who had reported that they were able to make some sense out of their experience reported less psychological distress, better social adjustment, greater self-esteem, and greater resolution of the experience than women who were not able to find any meaning but were still searching.

Meyer and Taylor (1986) empirically tested Janoff-Bulman's (1979) hypotheses on the types of self-blame employed by a victim and her level of adjustment. Contrary to the prediction, both behavioral and characterological self-blame were found to be associated with poor adjustment. The only form of causal attribution that was unassociated with the level of adjustment was societal blame, in which a victim assigns responsibility to the society, which allows sexual assault to happen (Meyer & Taylor, 1986).

As an alternative to Janoff-Bulman's behavioral-characterological distinction, Abbey (1987) provides alterable-unalterable distinction as a more important predictor for the impact of self-attribution on postrape adjustment level. Based on the standardized interview with 24 rape victims, Abbey (1987) found consistently high attributions of responsibility to the rapist, while attributions to the victims themselves were rare. Therefore, Abbey (1987) argues that victims may be making subtle distinctions between avoidability and responsibility. Further, according to Abbey (1987), by focusing on alterable-unalterable aspects of the assault, the victims may feel that they can avoid recurrent attack while still attributing the responsibility of the previous attack to the rapist.

The Process of Resolution

Health-Promoting Reappraisals

The resolution of a traumatic experience such as rape requires several components. According to Taylor (1983), in order for a successful adjustment to happen, a victim must (1) search for meaning of her experience, (2) attempt to gain control of her own life, and (3) attempt to promote self-enhancement. A victim must (re)discover her own ability to cope, adapt, learn, grow, and become self-reliant and self-confident (Finkel, 1975). No study has examined whether the specific content of cognitive reappraisal makes any difference in the victim's level of adjustment. However, some kinds of reappraisals, especially the ones that do not affirm the validity of the victim's sense of victimization, seem more likely to be harmful to the victim's emotional adjustment in the long term.

In addition to the stress caused by the act of violence, women victims of violence must deal with a culture that often attributes the assault to women's provocation (Burt, 1980). Victims are often ignored (Reiff, 1979), seen as losers (Bard & Sangrey, 1979), or avoided because they are depressed (Coates, Wortman, & Abbey, 1979). Rape victims are not exceptional to this societal treatment. Under these circumstances, one of the ways that victims approach the cognitive reappraisals is through "devictimization," which includes trying to "pass" as nonvictims. In fact, the desire to avoid identification as a victim is frequently very high among rape victims (e.g., Curtis, 1976). Selective evaluation is another often-employed strategy by victims. It allows victims to limit the extent to which they see themselves as victims, thereby assisting them to maintain their level of functioning.

Illness Promoting Encapsulation and Assimilation

The devictimization strategies may be adaptive in that they will help victims to survive through the most stressful situation following the violent assault. On the other hand, they may be maladaptive because by using them, victims will not face the significant reality of their experiences or seek adequate assistance from available resources.

The expression "victim-to-patient process" describes women's attempts to adjust to the judgments made by others about their experiences and the subsequent detrimental impact on mental health of these adjustments. According to Reicker and Carmen (1986), victims often become psychologically impaired as a consequence of trying to accommodate to others' judgments on their assault. Victims may (1) deny the assault, (2) alter or minimize their affective responses to the assault, and (3) change the meaning of the assault often by assigning the responsibility to themselves. These types of accommodations are more common among younger victims whose sense of self has yet to be established (Hymer, 1984). These accommodations, while seen as immediate survival strategies, have been reported to hinder emotional development of victims and ultimately form the basis of the damaged sense of self (Carmen et al., 1984; Reiker & Carmen, 1986; Summit, 1983).

TREATMENT AND SERVICES

Recovery is a process during which there are multiple points when victims may require services including the period surrounding the immediate crisis, whenever judicial procedures reactivate the incident, and after many months of trying to cope alone have failed to resolve persistent somatic and psychological distress.

Community Services

The adequacy of community response to rape is reflected by the availability, accessibility, quantity, quality, and legitimacy of services (Koss & Harvey, 1991). Prior to 1970 there existed no service agency or advocacy group giving attention to rape victims. Grass-roots rape crisis centers opened across the United States during the 1970s and grew during the 1980s into influential settings for community action, legal advocacy, and reform of victim services. However, limited funding in recent years has forced many agencies to prioritize services, which has usually resulted in the maintenance of crisis intervention services while other components shrink or disappear. Focus groups with victims of rape within New York State revealed limited or nonexistent services available to survivors of rape and their families, especially in rural areas, and wide variation in the quality of programs (Avner, 1990).

Crisis Intervention

Based on crisis theory (Burgess & Holmstrom, 1976), crisis intervention incorporates dissemination of information, active listening, and emotional support (e.g., Forman, 1980). Although this is one of the most common procedures used in rape crisis centers (Koss & Harvey, 1991), empirical investigations of their efficacy are scarce. Treatment by dynamic psychotherapy has often been advocated as a supplement to crisis intervention, but formal evaluation of effectiveness is absent (e.g., Burgess & Holmstrom, 1974; Evans, 1978; Fox & Scheri, 1972).

The brief behavioral intervention (BBIP) was designed for use immediately after the rape has occurred (Kilpatrick & Veronen, 1983). This four- to six-hour treatment package was viewed as a prophylactic treatment to prevent the development of phobic reactions and other PTSD symptoms. First, the victim was encouraged to reexperience the rape events in imagery and to permit herself to express feelings associated with the rape. She was then educated in learning theory models of the development and maintenance of fear as in the three systems' model of fear responses (behavioral, cognitive, physiological). In the third phase, attempts were made to reduce feelings of guilt and responsibility for the rape via discussion of societal expectations and myths about rape. Finally, coping skills such as self-assertion, relaxation, thought stopping, and methods for resuming normal activities were taught. The outcome of a study in which 15 recent victims were randomly assigned to one of three treatment conditions, repeated assessment, delayed assessment, or BBIP, indicated that repeated assessment, not true treatment condition, had the greatest therapeutic effect.

Clinical Treatment

Relatively few victims seek formal mental health treatment immediately after rape (Golding, Stein, Siegel, Burnam, & Sorenson, 1988). Even those who receive emergency medical care hesitate to commit to an ongoing therapeutic relationship (Kilpatrick & Veronen, 1983). Rape victims strongly resist the identity of "psychiatric patient" (Foa, Rothbaum, Riggs, & Murdock, 1991). Often they hope that the rape will resolve itself if they go back to their normal routine and don't think or talk about it. However, resolution of rape on one's own is difficult because victims face a culture that challenges their credibility and holds them at least partially culpable for their own rape. Given the expected recovery environment and the persistent impacts of rape, it is understandable that as many as 48% of one sample of victims reported that they had eventually sought psychotherapy (Ellis, Atkeson, & Calhoun, 1981). Among the reasons given for finally seeking aid were impending trial, persistent symptoms that did not diminish with time, first sexual encounter after the assault, breakup or argument with significant other, and withdrawal of support by family or friends (Stewart et al., 1987).

Research on treatment outcome for rape victims has focused almost exclusively on cognitive-behavioral methods. The treatments employed have concentrated primarily on rape-related symptoms as targets for the treatment intervention. Such targets included fear or anxiety and accompanying avoidance patterns, depression, and social and sexual dysfunctioning.

Psychotherapeutic interventions with empirical documentation of effectiveness with rape victims include: systematic desensitization (Frank, Stewart, Dancu, Hughes, & West, 1988), prolonged exposure (Foa et al., 1991), cognitive therapy (Frank & Stewart, 1984), stress inoculation therapy (Foa et al., 1991; Resick et al., 1989; Resick & Schnicke, 1992), cognitive processing therapy (Resick

& Schnicke, in press), and treatment for sexual dysfunction (Becker & Skinner, 1984). Eye movement desensitization and reprocessing therapy also has been proposed as an effective treatment for rape victims, but empirical evidence of effectiveness is not yet available (e.g., Shapiro, 1991).

Systematic Desensitization

The aim of systematic desensitization is to decrease the anxiety associated with situations or objects that are not realistically dangerous by the use of imaginal exposure with relaxation. Frank, Stewart, Dancu, Hughes, and West (1988) and Frank and Stewart (1983, 1984) described the procedure as follows. Subjects were first taught progressive relaxation training (Jacobson, 1938, 1970). Usually by the fourth visit, the three main target complaints were discussed and divided into specific scenes. All scenes were rated by the clients on a 1-to-10 scale, and a hierarchy was constructed arranging scenes from the least fearful to the most fearful. Clients were asked to imagine each scene while relaxing, starting with the least fearful one. The client signaled when she experienced anxiety, and the scene was then discontinued. Treatment continued until the client imagined each scene in the hierarchy without anxiety. Clients with several hierarchies were presented with one scene from each hierarchy per session.

Fourteen sessions of systematic desensitization as described above resulted in a decrease in the targeted fear, as well as an increase in social adjustment. However, in the absence of a comparison group, the effects are difficult to interpret. Since the criteria for inclusion in the study allowed the clients to receive treatment immediately following the rape, some of this improvement may have reflected the natural reduction of symptoms over the first several months following assault.

Cognitive Therapy

Cognitive techniques attempt to help clients identify distorted beliefs and test their reality. Frank and Stewart (1984) reported the effects of cognitive therapy targeted at depression and anxiety in rape victims who entered treatment an average of two weeks after their assault. This treatment, based on Beck's (1972) procedure, included self-monitoring of activities, for example, mastery and pleasure responses, as well as graded task assignments and identification and modification of maladaptive cognition. The treatment consisted of three phases. The first phase focused on challenging maladaptive thinking and encouraging novel thinking. During the second phase, cognitive distortions were identified, and rational, adaptive responses were constructed. During the final phase, basic assumptions about the world were explored.

According to the reported studies (Frank, 1979; Frank & Stewart, 1984; Turner & Frank, 1981), the outcome of cognitive therapy was similar to that of systematic desensitization: ratings of fear, anxiety, depression, and social maladjustment showed significant decrements. However, the absence of a comparison group and the failure to exclude clients who were raped recently limited the conclusion on the efficacy of cognitive therapy.

Flooding

Flooding (prolonged imaginal or in vivo exposure to moderately disturbing fear cues) has been markedly successful in treating anxiety disorders (Fairbank & Keane, 1982; Keane & Kalopek, 1982; Minisek, 1984). Although there is evidence for the effectiveness of imaginal flooding on sexual assault victims (Foa et al., 1991), serious concerns have been expressed concerning the use of flooding with sexual assault victims. They include (1) flooding focuses excessively on anxiety as a target for change to the exclusion of irrational cognitions, (2) flooding may result in an inappropriate reduction of anxiety to nonconsensual forced sex, (3) flooding may result in higher treatment dropout rates due to its aversive procedure, and (4) flooding fails to enhance the development of coping strategies (Kilpatrick, Veronen, & Resick, 1982).

In a rebuttal to these criticisms, Rychtarik et al. (1984) noted that irrational thoughts, feelings of anxiety, and avoidance are not independent of each other. Therefore, reduction of anxiety to rape-related cues may result in the amelioration of associated, negative, irrational cognitions. Moreover, cognitive mechanisms underlie some of the changes produced by exposure (flooding) and therefore are expected to influence fear, avoidance, and associated thoughts (Foa & Kozak, 1986). In addition, since flooding has often been directed at unduly intense fears of realistic concerns, decreasing such fears does not lead to carelessness about one's safety. Similarly, decreasing a woman's emotional distress to the memory of her rape need not lead to disregard for her well-being. Overall, the evaluation of flooding with rape victims awaits further investigation.

Packaged Treatments

Two treatment packages that aim at providing such coping strategies were developed by Kilpatrick, Veronen, and other colleagues. In addition to BBIP, which is designed to be used immediately after the assault, stress inculation training (SIT) was developed for victims who remained highly fearful three months after the assault (Kilpatrick et al., 1982). The program consisted of two phases: an educational phase and the training of coping skills. In the first phase, the program was described as a cognitive-behavioral approach to the management of rape-related fear and anxiety. Rape-related fear was explained as a classical conditioning phenomenon. Anxiety was described according to Lang's (1977) multichannel systems, which included behavioral/motoric, cognitive, and physiological responses. In addition, anxiety was presented as occurring in stages as opposed to being an all-or-none phenomenon.

The second phase started with deep muscle relaxation (Jacobson, 1938) and breathing control, followed by the training of communication skills through role playing. Covert modeling was also incorporated. This technique was similar to role playing but used imagery rather than in vivo practice. To control obsessive thinking, thought stopping (Wolpe, 1958) was also taught until the client became able to produce the troublesome thought and then silently verbalize the word "Stop!" The last technique, guided self-dialogue, was considered the most important. The therapist taught the client to focus on her internal dialogue and to identify irrational, faulty, or negative self-statements. Rational and positive statements were generated and substituted for the negative ones following Meichenbaum's (1974) stress-inoculation training.

Although a clear treatment effect was indicated with improvements on rape-related fear, anxiety, phobic anxiety, tension, and depression, the interpretation of the data is limited without a control group.

A study comparing SIT, exposure treatment, supportive counseling, and a no-treatment control was conducted by Foa and colleagues (1991). All clients are at least three months postassault and meet diagnostic criteria for posttraumatic stress disorder. SIT treatment is conducted in a similar manner described by Kilpatrick et al. (1982) except that instructions for in vivo exposure to feared situations are not included. Exposure treatment consists of nine biweekly, 90-minute sessions. The first two sessions are devoted to information gathering, explanations of treatment rationale, and treatment planning. A hierarchy is constructed of avoided situations for in vivo exposure homework. Exposure begins with situations that evoke relatively low levels of anxiety and moves up the hierarchy to more feared situations. The next seven sessions are devoted to reliving the rape scene in imagination. Clients are instructed to try to imagine as vividly as possible the assault scene and describe it aloud. At first, the clients are instructed not to verbalize details that are extremely upsetting. Later, they are encouraged to describe the rape in its entirety in order to facilitate habituation. At the last session, clients are reminded that avoiding safe situations and rape-related thoughts may increase PTSD symptoms and are asked to practice this approach in their everyday life. Supportive counseling follows the same nine-session format. Treatment focuses on assisting clients in solving daily problems that may or may not be rape-related and thus aims at promoting perception of self-control. The therapist plays an indirect and unconditionally supportive role.

The results indicated improvement on measures of PTSD, Beck Depression Inventory, State-Trait Anxiety Inventory, and self- and assessor-rated measures of target complaints. This improvement was maintained at three-month follow-up. Interestingly, improvement on core PTSD symptoms was evident only after the full course of treatment, whereas improvement of other symptoms was noted by midtreatment.

These treatments are predominately practiced in the individual psychotherapy format. However, many clinicians believe that group settings are the intervention of choice for rape victims (Koss & Harvey, 1991). The rationale is that groups of survivors are in a unique position to counter rape-induced isolation, provide support, validate feelings, confirm the experience, counteract self-blame and promote self-esteem, share grief, provide opportunities for safe attachment, and empower survivors within an egalitarian structure (Koss & Harvey, 1991).

Resick, Jordan, Girelli, Hutter, and Marhoefer-Dvorak (1989) compared three types of group therapy: stress inoculation, assertion training, and supportive psychotherapy plus information with a naturally occurring wait-list control group. SIT was similar to that described by Kilpatrick et al. (1982) with two exceptions: (1) cognitive restructuring, assertiveness training, and role play were excluded since they were used in the comparative treatment, and (2) exposure in vivo was added to the application phase. Assertion training treatment began with an educational phase that included an explanation of how assertion can be used to counter fear and avoidance. The specific techniques were adopted from Lange and Jakubowski (1976) and from Rational Emotive Therapy (RET; Ellis & Grieger, 1977). Training included behavioral rehearsal via role play with feedback regarding performance. Supportive psychotherapy plus information consisted of an educational phase, after which participants selected topics for discussion. Topics included the reactions of others to their assault and the degree of support they encountered, as well as assault-induced anxiety. The group was designed to validate the members' reactions to sexual assault as well as to offer general support. Results indicated that all three treatments were highly effective in reducing symptoms, with no group differences evident. Improvement was maintained at six-month follow-up on rape-related fear measures, but not on depression, self-esteem, and social fears. No improvements were found in the wait-list control group.

Peer Group Treatment

Cryer and Beutler (1980) reported a significant reduction in fear and hostility as a result of short-term supportive group therapy. However, three of the seven victims who completed the study reported only slight change in their overall condition. In addition, without a specific report on the content of the therapy, the results of the study remain inconclusive.

The effect of time-limited group therapy was reported by Peal, Westin, and Peterson (1985). The treatment focused on helping clients reach realistic solutions for specific problems emphasizing here-and-now issues, rather than psychodynamic processes. Although the authors report striking improvements on all symptoms following therapy, total reliance on clients' subjective evaluations limits interpretability of the data.

An Assessment of the Quality of the Treatment Database

No one therapy has demonstrated superiority for rape-related symptoms nor has any therapy proved effective for every client (Resick & Markaway, 1991). All therapies have common features including the avoidance of victim-blame, a supportive, nonstigmatizing view of rape as a criminal victimization, an environment to overcome cognitive and behavioral avoidance, and information about trauma reactions as well as the expectation that symptoms will improve (Resick & Markaway, 1991). Therapies differ in whether processing of traumatic memories is explicitly undertaken and if so, whether it is accomplished by low or high arousal methods, and in the degree of attention to cognitive reformulation. Although measures of outcome have improved considerably since early studies, no single scale assesses the full range of rape-induced symptoms. Nor have investigators begun to assess the effectiveness of treatments in fostering adaptive accommodation and altering maladaptive schema changes. Interventions do not currently acknowledge specific concerns about rape among various ethnic groups in the United States, even though recovery is known to be more different within certain cultures. Nor do treatment programs address the developmental implications of rape for adolescents—the group who experiences the highest rate of assault. Finally, most of the treatment studies have been relatively brief and have involved uncomplicated cases. Clearly, rape is one of the most serious human traumas and resolving it may take considerable time, particularly when a recent rape has compounded effects with past victimizations. In short, the empirical database is insufficient to guide a prescriptive approach to treatment wherein interventions are matched to the types and severity of symptoms and victim characteristics.

PREVENTING SEXUAL ASSAULT

Deficit-Oriented Approaches

Based on the reasoning that murder and mutilation are always possible outcomes of rape, Storaska (1975) recommended women not to offend or upset her assailant. Although this view was once well supported by law enforcement agencies and officers, recently, it has been heavily criticized. Storaska's recommendation implies that since a woman is usually more powerless than her assailant, she should remain passive and cooperative rather than attempting to fight back. It implies that a woman may have to accept rape when her life seems to be at risk. Such a view not only supports women's sense of powerlessness but discourages women's ability to defend themselves.

Moreover, findings from empirical studies (e.g., Bart, 1981; Bart & O'Brien, 1985; Sanders, 1980) contradict Storaska's reasoning in that those women who have successfully avoided rape were more likely to have actively resisted their assailants. For example, using the data from the Los Angeles Epidemiologic Catchment Area study (consisting of 3,132 adult victims), Siegel, Sorenson, Golding, Burnam, and Stein (1989) report that overall, those who experienced no physical contact were more likely to have resisted than those with contact. More specifically, those who successfully avoided contact reported a greater use of verbal strategies. Although there are women who were raped due to uncontrollable situational factors, what must be emphasized is that cooperation with the assailant does not guarantee the woman's safety while resistance does not increase her risk (Koss & Harvey, 1987).

Competence-Oriented Approaches

In 1983, Storaska's recommendation was formally condemned by the National Coalition Against Sexual Assault (NCASA). Out of the criticisms against Storaska's deficit-oriented approach to rape prevention, the need for an approach that enhances women's sense of power and control has emerged. As described by Brodyaga, Gates, Singer, Tucker, and White (1975), this approach emphasizes a woman's (1) active resistance through physical self-defense, screaming, and fleeing; (2) passive resistance by talking to persuade a rapist to forgo his attempt, and (3) submission if her life is in serious danger. As discussed elsewhere (Koss & Harvey, 1987), submission is not cooperation with the assailant but should be seen as an act of survival for women faced with the danger of violent assault. In order for this competence-oriented approach to be widely adopted, the societal condition needs to be reexamined and challenged. Recent development of such rape prevention strategies is called primary prevention.

Primary Prevention

Recent activities initiated by rape crisis centers and other community programs have been analogous to those of a public health care system. Some activities have aimed at global social change by establishing new resources and networks to prevent rape. Other activities have aimed at more specific changes in community by inoculating knowledge, attitudes, and skills and by offering self-defense courses. In addition to these similarities, there are limitations in public health analogy. Unlike in public health activities, it is extremely difficult to determine the incidence of rape, let alone estimate its decrease as a measure of effectiveness of a given activity. Moreover, at risk populations in cases of rape include virtually all women and girls and many men and boys. Under these circumstances, it is essential to develop specific prevention programs for groups at particularly high risk: children, adolescent and young adult women, elderly women, minority women, handicapped people, and gay men. It is equally important to note frequency of different types of sexual assault reported across different groups. For example, adolescent and young adult women are at the particular risk of acquaintance and date rape, while children are more likely to be sexually abused by adult family members or relatives. Thus, primary prevention efforts are directly targeted toward societal conditions that foster and tolerate rape while increasing vulnerability of women and children.

CONCLUSIONS—A RESEARCH AGENDA

Considering that the history of scientific studies on rape dates back only to the late 1970s, tremendous progress has been achieved. As reviewed in this chapter, the survey techniques have been examined and the efforts have been made to capture the multifaceted trauma of rape and to examine the assault experiences in terms of the victim's development. Despite these accomplishments, there are still gaps in existing empirical research, which often lacks an adequate comparison group or relies on victims' retrospective accounts. More attention must be paid to overcome these limitations. An increase in quality of research will enhance the quality of the treatment methods. Finally, in order to combat prolonged, multifaceted trauma of rape, prevention strategies also must be multidimensional and based on in-depth understanding of this significant social problem.

REFERENCES

Abbey, A. (1987). Perceptions of personal avoidability versus responsibility: How do they differ? *Basic and Applied Social Psychology, 8(1&2),* 3–19.

Ageton, S. S. (1983a). *Sexual assault among adolescents.* Lexington, MA: Lexington Books.

Ageton, S. S. (1983b). *Sexual assault among adolescents: A national study.* Final report, submitted to the National Institute of Mental Health.

American Psychiatric Association. (1987). *Diagnostic and statistical manual of mental disorders* (4th ed.). Washington, DC: Author.

Atkeson, B. M., Calhoun, K. S., Resick, P. A., & Ellis, E. M. (1982). Victims of rape: Repeated assessment of depressive symptoms. *Journal of Consulting and Clinical Psychology, 50,* 96–102.

Avner, J. I. (1990). *Rape, sexual assault, and child sexual abuse: Working towards a more responsive society.* Final report of the governor's Task Force on Rape and Sexual Assault. Albany, NY: New York State Division for Women.

Bailey, L., Moore, T. F., & Bailar, B. A. (1978). An interviewer variance study for the eight impact cities of the National Crime Survey cities sample. *Journal of the American Statistical Association, 73,* 23–30.

Baker, T. C., Burgess, A. W., Brickman, E., & Davis, R.C. (1990). Rape victims' concerns about possible exposure to HIV infection. *Journal of Interpersonal Violence, 5,* 49–60.

Bard, M., & Sangrey, D. (1979). *The crime victim's book.* New York: Basic Books.

Bart, P. B. (1981). A study of women who both were raped and avoided rape. *Journal of Social Issues, 37,* 123–136.

Bart, P., & O'Brien, P. (1985). *Stopping rape: Successful survival strategies.* New York: Pergamon Press.

Beck, A. T. (1972). *Depression: Causes and treatment.* Philadelphia: University of Pennsylvania Press.

Beck, A. T., Ward, C. H., Mendelsohn, M., Mock, J., & Erbaugh, J. (1961). An inventory for measuring depression. *Archives of General Psychiatry, 41,* 561–571.

Becker, J. V., & Skinner, L. J. (1984). Behavioral treatment of sexual dysfunctions in sexual assault survivors. In I. Stuart & J. Greer (Eds.), *Victims of sexual aggression,* (pp. 211–234). New York: Van Nostrand Reinhold.

Becker, J. V., Skinner, L. J., Abel, G. G., & Cichon, J. (1986). Level of postassault sexual functioning in rape and incest victims. *Archives of Sexual Behavior, 15,* 37–49.

Becker, J. V., Skinner, L. J., Abel, G. G., & Treacy, E. C. (1982). Incidence and types of sexual dysfunctions in rape and incest victims. *Journal of Sex and Marital Therapy, 8*, 65–74.

Beebe, D. K. (1991). Emergency management of the adult female rape victim. *American Family Physician, 43*, 2041–2046.

Berrill, K. T. (1990). Anti-gay violence and victimization in the United States: An overview. *Journal of Interpersonal Violence, 5*, 274–294.

Bienen, L. B. (1981). Rape III—National developments in rape reform legislation. *Women's Rights Law Reporter*, 171–213.

Block, C. R., & Block, R. L. (1984). Crime victimization, crime measurement, and victim surveys. *Journal of Social Issues, 40*, 137–160.

Bown, O. (1961). The development of a self-report inventory and its function in a mental health assessment battery. *American Psychologist, 16*, 402.

Brodyaga, L., Gates, M., Singer, S., Tucker, M., and White, R. (1975). *Rape and its victims: A report for citizens, health facilities and criminal justice agencies.* Washington, DC: National Institute of Law Enforcement and Criminal Justice.

Brown, R., & Kulik, J. (1977). Flashbulb memories. *Cognition, 5*, 73–79.

Bureau of Justice Statistics (BJS). (1992). *Criminal Victimization in the United States. 1991.* Washington, DC: U.S. Department of Justice.

Burgess, A. W., & Holmstrom, L. L. (1974). *Rape: Victims of crisis* (chaps. 3, 15). Bowie, MD: R. J. Brady.

Burgess, A. W., & Holmstrom, L. L. (1976). Coping behavior of the rape victim. *American Journal of Psychiatry, 131*, 981–986.

Burnam, M. A., Stein, J. A., Golding, J. M., Siegel, J. M., Sorenson, S. B., Forsythe, A. B., & Telles, C. A. (1988). Sexual assault and mental disorders in a community population. *Journal of Consulting and Clinical Psychology, 56*, 843–850.

Burt, M. R. (1980). Cultural myths and supports for rape. *Journal of Personality and Social Psychology, 38*, 217–230.

Calhoun, K. S., Atkeson, B. M., & Resick, P. A. (1982). A longitudinal examination of fear reactions in victims of rape. *Journal of Counseling Psychology, 29*, 655–661.

Cluss, P. A., Boughton, J., Frank, L. E., Stewart, B. D., & West, D. (1983). The rape victims: Psychological correlates of participation in the legal process. *Criminal Justice and Behavior, 10*, 342–357.

Coates, D., Wortman, C. B., & Abbey, A. (1979). Reactions to victims. In I. H. Frieze, D. Bar-Tal, & J. S. Carroll (Eds.), *New approaches to social problems: Applications to attribution theory* (pp. 21-52). San Francisco, CA: Jossey-Bass.

Council on Scientific Affairs. (1992). Violence against women: Relevance for medical practitioners. *Journal of the American Medical Association, 267*, (23), 3184–3189.

Cryer, L., & Beutler, L. (1980). Group therapy: An alternative treatment approach for rape victims. *Journal of Sex and Marital Therapy, 6*, 40–46.

Curtis, L. A. (1976). Present and future measures of victimization in forcible rape. In M. J. Walker & S. L. Brodsky (Eds.), *Sexual assault* (pp. 61–68). Lexington, MA: D.C. Heath.

Davis, R. C., Brickman, E., & Baker, T. (1991). Supportive and unsupportive responses of others to rape victims: Effects on concurrent victim adjustment. *American Journal of Community Psychology, 19*, 443–451.

D'Ercole, A., & Struening, E. (1990). Victimization among homeless women: Implications for service delivery. *Journal of Community Psychology, 18*, 141–152.

Derogatis, L. R. (1977). *SCL-90-R manual.* Baltimore: Johns Hopkins University Press.

Ellis, A., & Grieger, R., (Eds.). (1977) *Handbook of rational-emotive therapy.* New York: Springer.

Ellis, E. M., Atkeson, B. M., & Calhoun, K. S. (1981). An assessment of long-term reaction to rape. *Journal of Abnormal Psychology, 90*, 263–266.

Ellis, E. M., Calhoun, K. S., & Atkeson, B. M. (1980). Sexual dysfunctions in victims of rape: Victims may experience a loss of sexual arousal and frightening flashbacks even one year after the assault. *Women and Health, 5*, 39–47.

Essock-Vitale, S. M., & McGuire, M. T. (1985). Women's lives viewed from an evolutionary perspective. I. Sexual histories, reproductive success, and demographic characteristics of a random sample of American women. *Ethology and Sociobiology, 6*, 137–154.

Evans, H. I. (1978). Psychotherapy for the rape victim: Some treatment models. *Hospital and Community Psychiatry, 29*, 309–312.

Fairbank, J. A., & Keane, T. M. (1982). Flooding for combat-related stress disorders: Assessment of anxiety reduction across traumatic memories. *Behavior Therapy, 13*, 499–510.

Federal Bureau of Investigation. (1991). *Uniform Crime Reports.* Washington, DC: U.S. Department of Justice.

Feldman-Summers, S., Gordon, P. E., & Meager, J. R. (1979). The impact of rape on sexual satisfaction. *Journal of Abnormal Psychology, 88*, 101–105.

Finkel, N. J. (1975). Stress, traumas, and trauma resolution. *American Journal of Communty Psychology, 3*, 173–178.

Fitts, W. H. (1965). *Manual: Tennessee self-concept scale.* Nashville, TN: Counselor Recordings and Tests.

Foa, E. B., & Kozak, M. J. (1986). Emotional processing of fear: Exposure to corrective information. *Psychological Bulletin, 99*, 20–35.

Foa, E. B., Rothbaum, B. O., Riggs, D. S., & Murdock, T. B. (1991). Treatment of posttraumatic stress disorder in rape victims: A comparison between cognitive-behavioral procedures and counseling. *Journal of Consulting and Clinical Psychology, 59*, 715–723.

Foa, E. B., Steketee, G., & Olasov, B. (1989). Behavioral/cognitive conceptualization of post-traumatic stress order. *Behavior Therapy, 20*, 155–176.

Folkman, S. (1984). Personal control and stress and coping processes: A theoretical analysis. *Journal of Personality and Social Psychology, 46*, 839–852.

Forman, B. D. (1980). Cognitive modification of obsessive-thinking in a rape victim: A preliminary study. *Psychological Reports 47*, 819–822.

Fox, S. S., & Scherl, D. J. (1972). Crisis intervention with victims of rape. *Social Work, 17*, 37–42.

Frank, E. (1979). Psychological response to rape: An analysis of response patterns. Unpublished doctoral dissertation, University of Pittsburgh.

Frank, E., & Anderson, B. P. (1987). Psychiatric disorders in rape victims: Past history and current symptomatology. *Comprehensive Psychiatry, 28*, 77–82.

Frank, E., & Stewart, B. D. (1983). Treating depression in victims of rape. *The Clinical Psychologist, 36*, 95–98.

Frank, E., & Stewart, B. D. (1984). Depressive symptoms in rape victims: A revisit. *Journal of Affective Disorders, 7*, 77–85.

Frank, E., Stewart, B. D,., Dancu, C., Hughes, C., & West, D. (1988). Efficacy of cognitive behavior therapy and systematic desensitization in the treatment of rape trauma. *Behavior Therapy, 19*, 403–420.

Frank, E., Turner, S. M., & Duffy, B. (1979). Depressive symptoms in rape victims. *Journal of Affective Disorders, 1*, 269–277.

Frank, E., Turner, S. M., & Stewart, B. D. (1980). Initial response to rape: The impact of factors within the rape situation. *Journal of Behavioral Assessment, 2*, 39–53.

Frank, E., Turner, S. M., Stewart, B. D., Jacob, J., & West, D. (1981). Past psychiatric symptoms and the response to sexual assault. *Comprehensive Psychiatry, 22*, 479–487.

Garnets, L., Herek, G. M., & Levy, B. (1990). Violence and victimization of lesbians and gay men: Mental health consequences. *Journal of Interpersonal Violence, 5*, 366–383.

George, L. K., Winfield, I., & Blazer, D. G. (1992). Sociocultural factors in sexual assault: Comparison of two representative samples of women. *Journal of Social Issues, 48*, 105–126.

Girelli, S. A., Resick, P. A., Marhoefer-Dvorak, S., & Hutter, C. K. (1986). Subjective distress and violence during rape: Their effects on long-term fear. *Victims and Violence, 1*, 35–45.

Glenn, F., & Resick, P. A. (1986). *The effects of family violence on coping ability to a later victimization*. Unpublished manuscript, University of Missouri-St. Louis.

Golding, J. M., Stein, J. A., Siegel, J. M., Burnam, M. A., & Sorenson, S. B. (1988). Sexual assault history and use of health and mental health services. *American Journal of Community Psychology, 16*, 625–644.

Goodman, L. (1991). The prevalence of abuse among homeless and housed poor mothers: A comparison study. *American Journal of Orthopsychiatry, 61*, 163–169.

Gordon, M. T., & Riger, S. (1989). *The female fear*. New York: Free Press.

Hall, E. R., & Flannery, P. J. (1984). Prevalence and correlates of sexual assault experiences in adolescents. *Victimology 9*, 398–408.

Hamilton, M. (1960). A rating scale for depression. *Journal of Neurology, Neurosurgery, and Psychiatry, 23*, 56–62.

Hanson, R. K. (1990). The psychological impact of sexual assault on women and children: A review. *Annals of Sex Research, 3*, 187–232.

Hassell, R. A. (1981, March). *The impact of stranger vs. nonstranger rape: A longitudinal study*. Paper presented at the Eighth Annual Conference of the Association for Women in Psychology, Boston.

Haynes, S. N., & Mooney, D. K. (1975). Nightmares: Etiological, theoretical and behavioral treatment considerations. *Psychological Record, 25*, 225–236.

Hindelang, M. J., & Davis, B. J. (1977). Forcible rape in the United States: A statistical profile. In D. Chappel, R. Geis, & G. Geis (Eds.), *Forcible rape: The crime, the victim, and the offender* (pp. 87–114). New York: Columbia University Press.

Holmes, M. R., & St. Lawrence, J. S. (1983). Treatment of rape-induced trauma: Proposed behavioral conceptualization and review of the literature. *Clinical Psychology Review, 3*, 417–433.

Horowits, M. J., Wilner, N., Marmar, C., & Krupnick, J. (1980). Pathological grief and the activation of latent self-images. *American Journal of Psychiatry, 137,* 1137–1162.

Hymer, S. (1984). The self in victimization: Conflict and developmental perspectives. *Victimology: An International Journal, 9,* 142–150.

Jacobson, A., & Richardson, B. (1987). Assault experiences of 100 psychiatric inpatients: Evidence of the need for routine inquiry. *American Journal of Psychiatry, 144,* 908–913.

Jacobson, E. (1938). *Progressive relaxation.* Chicago: University of Chicago Press.

Jacobson, E. (1970). *Modern treatment of tense patients.* Springfield, IL: Thomas.

Janoff-Bulman, R. (1979). Characterological versus behavioral self-blame: Inquiries into depression and rape. *Journal of Personality and Social Psychology, 37,* 1798–1809.

Janoff-Bulman, R. (1985). Criminal vs. non-criminal victimization: Victim's reactions. *Victimology, 10,* 498–511.

Katz, B. L. (1991). The effects of acquaintance rape on the female victimm. In A. Parrot & L. Bechhofer (Eds.), *Acquaintance rape: The hidden crime* (pp. 251–269). New York: John Wiley.

Keane, T. M., & Kalopek, D. G. (1982). Imaginal flooding in the treatment of a post-traumatic stress disorder. *Journal of Consulting and Clinical Psychology, 50,* 138–140.

Kilpatrick, D. G., Best, C. L., Veronen, L. J., Amick, A. E., Villeponteaux, L. A., & Ruff, G. A. (1985). Mental health correlates of criminal victimization: A random community survey. *Journal of Consulting and Clinical Psychology, 53,* 866–873.

Kilpatrick, D. G., Saunders, B. E., Veronen, L. J., Best, C. L. & Von, J. M. (1987). Criminal victimization: Lifetime prevalence, reporting to police, and psychological impact. *Crime and Delinquency, 33,* 479–489.

Kilpatrick, D. G., & Veronen, L. J. (1983). Treatment for rape-related problems: Crisis intervention is not enough. In L. H. Cohen, W. L. Claiborn, & G. A. Spector (Eds.), *Crisis intervention* (pp. 165–185). New York: Human Sciences Press.

Kilpatrick, D. G., & Veronen, L. J. (1984, February). *Treatment of fear and anxiety in victims of rape.* Final report of NIMH grant no. MH29602.

Kilpatrick, D. G., Veronen, L. J., & Best, C. L. (1985). Factors predicting psychological distress among rape victims. In C. R. Figley (Ed.), *Trauma and its wake* (pp. 113–141). New York: Brunner/Mazel.

Kilpatrick, D. G., Veronen, L. J., & Resick, P. A. (1979). The aftermath of rape: Recent empirical findings. *American Journal of Orthopsychiatry, 49,* 658–669.

Kilpatrick, D. G., Veronen, L. J., & Resick, P. A. (1982). Psychological sequelae to rape: Assessment and treatment strategies. In D. M. Dolays & R. L. Meredith (Eds.), *Behavioral medicine: Assessment and treatment strategies* (pp. 473–497). New York: Plenum Press.

Kilpatrick, D. G., Veronen, L. J., Saunders, B. E., Best, C. L., Amick-McMullen, A., & Paduhovich, J. (1987, March). *The psychological impact of crime: A study of randomly surveyed crime victims.* Final report for the National Institute of Justice grant no. 84-IJ-CX-0039.

Koss, M. P. (1988). Hidden rape: Sexual aggression and victimization in a national sample of students in higher education. In A. W. Burgess (Ed.)., *Rape and sexual assault* (Vol. 2, pp. 3–25). New York: Garland.

Koss, M. P. (1992). The underdetection of rape. *Journal of Social Issues, 48*, 63–75.

Koss, M. P., Dinero, T. E., Seibel, C., & Cox, S. (1988). Stranger and acquaintance rape: Are there differences in the victim's experience? *Psychology of Women Quarterly, 12*, 1–24.

Koss, M. P., & Gidycz, C. A. (1985). Sexual Experiences Survey: Reliability and validity. *Journal of Consulting and Clinical Psychology, 53*, 422–423.

Koss, M. P., Gidycz, C. A., & Wisniewski, N. (1987). The scope of rape: Incidence and prevalence of sexual aggression and victimization in a national sample of higher education students. *Journal of Consulting and Clinical Psychology, 55*, 162–170.

Koss, M. P., & Harvey, M. R. (1987). *The rape victim: Clinical and community approaches to treatment.* Lexington, MA: Stephen Green Press.

Koss, M. P., & Heslet, L. (In press). Somatic consequences of violence against women. *Archives of Family Medicine.*

Koss, M. P., Koss, P. G., & Woodruff, W. J. (1991). Deleterious effects of criminal victimization on women's health and medical utilization. *Archives of Internal Medicine, 151*, 342–357.

Koss, M. P., Woodruff, W. J., & Koss, P. (1991). Criminal victimization among primary care medical patients: Prevalence, incidence, and physician usage. *Behavioral Sciences and the Law, 9*, 85–96.

Lang, P. J. (1977). Imagery in therapy: An information-processing analysis of fear. *Behavior Therapy, 8*, 862–886.

Lang, P. J. (1979). A bio-informational theory of emotional imagery. *Psychophysiology, 16*, 495–512.

Lange, A. J., & Jakubowski, P. (1976). *Responsible assertive behavior.* Champaign, IL: Research Press.

Lazarus, R. S., & Folkman, S. (1984). *Stress, appraisal, and coping.* New York: Springer.

Libow, J. A., & Doty, D. W. (1979). An exploratory approach to self-blame and self-derogation by rape victims. *American Journal of Orthopsychiatry, 49*, 670–679.

Lurigio, A. J., & Resick, P. A. (1990). Healing the psychological wounds of criminal victimization: Predicting postcrime distress and recovery. In A. J. Lurigio, W. G. Skogan, & R. C. Davis (Eds.), *Victims of crime: Problems, policies, and programs* (pp. 51–67). Newbury Park, CA: Sage.

Masters, W. H. (1986). Sexual dysfunction as an aftermath of sexual assault of men by women. *Journal of Sex and Marital Therapy, 12*, 35–45.

McCahill, T. W., Meyer, L. C., & Fishman, A. M. (1979). *The aftermath of rape.* Lexington, MA: Lexington Books.

McCann, I. L., & Pearlman, L. A. (1990). *Psychological trauma and the adult survivor: Theory, therapy, and transformation.* New York: Brunner/Mazel.

McNair, D., Lorr, M., & Droppleman, L. (1971). *Manual Profile of Mood States.* San Diego: Education and Industrial Testing Service.

Meichenbaum, D. (1974). *Cognitive behavior modification.* Morristown, NJ: General Learning Press.

Meyer, C. B., & Taylor, S. E. (1986). Adjustment to rape. *Journal of Personality and Social Psychology, 50*, 1226–1234.

Minisek, N. A. (1984). *Flooding as a supplemental treatment for Vietnam veterans.*

Paper presented at the Third National Conference on Post-Traumatic Stress Disorders, Baltimore, MD.

Moore, K. A., Nord, C. W., & Peterson, J. L. (1989). Nonvoluntary sexual activity among adolescents. *Family Planning Perspectives, 21,* 110–114.

Murphy S. M. (1990). Rape, sexually transmitted diseases and human immunodeficiency virus infection. *International Journal of STD and AIDS, 1,* 79–82.

National Victims Center (NVC). (April 23, 1992). *Rape in America: A report to the nation.* Arlington, VA: Author.

Norris, F. H. (1992). Epidemiology of trauma: Frequency and impact of different potentially traumatic events on different demographic groups. *Journal of Consulting and Clinical Psychology, 60,* 409–418.

Norris, J., & Feldman-Summers, S. (1981). Factors related to the psychological impacts of rape on the victim. *Journal of Abnormal Psychology, 90,* 562–567.

Orlando, J. A., & Koss, M. P. (1983). The effect of sexual victimization on sexual satisfaction: A study of the negative-association hypothesis. *Journal of Abnormal Psychology, 92,* 104–106.

Peal, M., Westin, A. B., & Peterson, L. G. (1985). The female rape survivor: Time-limited group therapy with female-male co-therapists. *Journal of Psychosomatic Obstetrics and Gynecology, 4,* 197–205.

Perloff, L. S. (1983). Perceptions of vulnerability to victimization. *Journal of Social Issues, 39,* 41–61.

Peterson, D. L., Olasov, B., & Foa, E. B. (1987, July). *Response patterns in sexual assault survivors.* Paper presented at the Third World Congress on Victimology, San Francisco.

Rachman, S. (1980). Emotional processing. *Behavior Research and Therapy, 18,* 51–60.

Reiff, R. (1979). *The invisible victim: The criminal justice system's forgotten responsibility.* New York: Basic Books.

Reiker, P. P., & Carmen, E. H. (1986). The victim-to-patient process: The disconfirmation and transformation of abuse. *American Journal of Orthopsychiatry, 56,* 360–370.

Resick, P. A. (1986, May). *Reactions of female and male victims of rape or robbery.* Final report of NIMH grant no. MH37296.

Resick, P. A. (1987). *Reactions of female and male victims of rape or robbery.* Final report NIJ grant no. 85-IJ-CX-0042.

Resick, P. A. (1990). Victims of sexual assault. In A. J. Lurigio, W. G. Skogan, & R. C. Davis (Eds.), *Victims of crime: Problems, policies, and programs* (pp. 69–85). Newbury Park, CA: Sage.

Resick, P. A. (In press). Cognitive treatment of crime-related PTSD. In R. Peters & R. McMahon (Eds.), *Violence and aggression throughout the lifespan.* Newbury Park, CA: Sage.

Resick, P. A., Calhoun, K. S., Atkeson, B. M., & Ellis, E. M. (1981). Social adjustment in victims of sexual assault. *Journal of Consulting and Clinical Psychology, 49,* 705–712.

Resick, P. A., Jordan, C. G., Girelli, S. A., Hutter, C. K., and Marhoefer-Dvorak, S. (1989). A comparative outcome study of behavioral group therapy for sexual assault victims. *Behavior Therapy, 19,* 385–401.

Resick, P. A., & Markaway, B. E. (1991). Clinical treatment of adult female victims of sexual assault. In C. R. Hollin & K. Howells (Eds.), *Clinical approaches to sex offenders and their victims*. New York: Wiley.

Resick, P. A., & Schnicke, M. K. (1991). Treating symptoms in adult victims of sexual assault. *Journal of Interpersonal Violence, 5*, 488–506.

Resick, P. A., & Schnicke, M. K. (1992). Cognitive processing therapy for sexual assault victims. *Journal of Consulting and Clinical Psychology, 60*, 748–756.

Riger, S., & Gordon, M. T. (1988). The impact of crime on urban women. In A. W. Burgess (Ed.), *Rape and sexual assault Vol II* (pp. 139–156). New York: Garland Publishing Co.

Roth, S., & Lebowitz, L. (1988). The experience of sexual trauma. *Journal of Traumatic Stress, 1*, 79–107.

Rothbaum, B. O., Foa, E. B., Riggs, D. S., Murdock, T., & Walsh, W. (1992). A prospective examination of post-traumatic stress disorder in rape victims. *Journal of Traumatic Stress, 5*, 455–475.

Rubin, D. C. (Ed.). (1986). *Autobiographical memory*. Cambridge, England: Cambridge University Press.

Ruch, L. O., & Chandler, S. M. (1980, September). *The impact of sexual assault on three victim groups receiving crisis intervention services at a rape treatment center: Adult rape victims, child rape victims and incest victims*. Paper presented at the American Sociological Meetings, New York.

Ruch, L. O., Chandler, S. M., & Harter, R. A. (1980). Life change and rape impact. *Journal of Health and Social Behavior, 21*, 248–260.

Ruch, L. O., Gartrell, J. W., Amedeo, S., & Coyne, B. J. (1991). The sexual assault symptom scale: Measuring self-reported sexual assault trauma in the emergency room. *Psychological Assessment, 3*, 3–8.

Ruch, L. O., Gartrell, J. W., Ramelli, A., & Coyne, B. J. (1991). The Clinical Trauma Assessment: Evaluating sexual assault victims in the emergency room. *Psychological Assessment, 3*, 405–411.

Ruch, L. O., & Leon, J. J. (1983). Sexual assault trauma and trauma change. *Women and Health, 8*, 5–21.

Russell, D.E.H. (1982). The prevalence and incidence of forcible rape and attempted rape of females. *Victimology: An International Journal, 7*, 81–93.

Russell, D.E.H. (1984). *Sexual exploitation: Rape, child sexual abuse, and workplace harassment*. Beverly Hills, CA: Sage.

Russell, D.E.H. (1990). *Rape in marriage* (rev. ed.). Bloomington: Indiana University Press.

Rychtarik, R. G., Silverman, W. K., Van Landingham, W. P., & Prue, D. M. (1984). Treatment of an incest victim with implosive therapy: A case study. *Behavior Therapy, 15*, 410–420.

Sales, E., Baum, M., & Shore, B. (1984). Victim readjustment following assault. *Journal of Social Issues, 40*, 117–136.

Sanders, W. (1980). *Rape and women's identity*. Beverly Hills, CA: Sage.

Scheppele, K. L., & Bart, P. B. (1983). Through women's eyes: Defining danger in the wake of sexual assault. *Journal of Social Issues, 39*, 63–80.

Shapiro, F. (1991). Eye movement desensitization and reprocessing procedure: From EMD to EMD/R: A new treatment model for anxiety and related trauma. *The Behavior Therapist, 14*, 133–135.

Shore, B. (1980). An examination of critical process and outcome factors in rape. NIMH Grant No. 17114-8194, Final Report.

Siegel, J. M., Sorenson, S. B., Golding, J. M., Burnam, M. A., & Stein, J. A. (1989). Resistance to sexual assault: Who resists and what happens? *American Journal of Public Health, 79*(1), 27–31.

Silver, R. L., Boon, C., & Stones, M. H. (1983). Searching for meaning in misfortune: Making sense of incest. *Journal of Social Issues, 39,* 81–101.

Skogan, W. G. (1981). *Issues in the measurement of victimization.* (NCJ-74682). Washington, DC: U.S. Government Printing Office.

Sorenson, S. B., & Siegel, J. M. (1992). Gender, ethnicity, and sexual assault: Findings from a Los Angeles study. *Journal of Social Issues, 48,* 93–104.

Sorenson, S. B., Stein, J. A., Siegel, J. M. Golding, J. M., & Burnam, M. A. (1987). Prevalence of adult sexual assault: The Los Angeles Epidemiologic Catchment Area Study. *American Journal of Epidemiology, 126,* 1154–1164.

Sparks, R. F. (1982). *Research on victims of crime: Accomplishments, issues, and new directions.* (DHHS Publication No. [ADM] 82-1091). Washington, DC: U.S. Department of Health and Human Services.

Spielberger, C. D., Gorsuch, R. L., & Luchene, R. E. (1970). *The State-Trait Anxiety Inventory.* Palo Alto, CA: Counsulting Psychologists Press.

Stewart, B. D., Hughes, C., Frank, E. Anderson, B., Kendall, K., & West, D. (1987). The aftermath of rape: Profiles of immediate and delayed treatment seekers. *Journal of Nervous and Mental Disease, 175,* 90–94.

Storaska, F. (1975). *How to say no to a rapist and survive.* New York: Random House.

Sudman, S., & Bradburn, N. M. (1974). *Response effects in surveys: A review and synthesis.* Chicago, IL: Aldine.

Summit, R. L. (1983). The child sexual abuse accommodation syndrome. *Child Abuse and Neglect, 7,* 177–193.

Taylor, S. E. (1983). Adjustment to threatening events: A theory of cognitive adaptation. *American Psychologist, 38,* 1161–1173.

Turner, S. M., & Frank, E. (1981). Behavior therapy in the treatment of rape victims. In L. Michelson, M. Hersen, & S. M. Turner (Eds.), *Future perspectives in behavior therapy* (pp. 862–886). New York: Plenum Press.

Veronen, L. J., & Kilpatrick, D. G. (1980). Self-reported fears of rape victims: A preliminary investigation. *Behavior Modification, 4,* 383–396.

Warr, M. (1985). Fear of rape among urban women. *Social Problems, 32,* 239–250.

Williams, J. E., & Holmes, K. A. (1981). *The second assault: Rape and public attitudes.* Westport, CT: Greenwood Press.

Winfield, I., George, L. K., Schwartz, M., & Blazer, D. G. (1990). Sexual assault and psychiatric disorders among a community sample of women. *American Journal of Psychiatry, 147,* 335–341.

Wolpe, J. (1958). *Psychotherapy by reciprocal inhibition.* Stanford: Stanford University Press.

Wyatt, G. E. (1992). The sociocultural context of African American and White American women's rape. *Journal of Social Issues, 48,* 77–92.

14

Research on Battered Women and Their Assailants

Maureen C. McHugh, Irene Hanson Frieze, and Angela Browne

In the past two decades there has been an explosion of information on wife battering and other forms of physical and emotional abuse. Much of this awareness was engendered by the women's movement, which, in the 1960s, began to examine violence against women in the form of rape. Such examinations revealed a prevalence of women experiencing sexual assaults by male partners as well as by strangers and provided a forum for the identification of the physical assault of wives as a problem of previously unrecognized proportions. Starting at the grass-roots level, feminists have named the problem, developed a network of shelters and centers to aid abused women and their children, and demanded research and other resources for assisting women victims. Many of the researchers who have conducted research or developed theories about wife abuse define themselves as feminists and perceive their work as directly or indirectly advocating for women. However, there are important controversies in the field between feminists and nonfeminists and among feminists themselves. A feminist analysis of the research conducted to date—a careful examination of the questions asked, of the methods used, of the samples studied, and of the conclusions reached—highlights serious limitations in the professional literature.

Much of the research on wife abuse or "domestic violence" has been guided by a series of questions raised by researchers. In many ways, these questions mirror the concerns of those in the general public. When raising questions about why wife battering occurs, many people blame the battered woman herself. She may be perceived as provoking her husband in some way that leads to his being violent, or she may be seen as having a personality disorder or liking to be

beaten. Particularly in the early work, some researchers shared these precon-
ceptions (Kleckner, 1978; Shainess, 1977; Snell, Rosenwald & Robey, 1964).
Other attributions for wife battering found in the general public involve men—
often that they could not control themselves because of unusual stress or being
drunk (Frieze, 1979). A more recent viewpoint sees the couple at fault (Margolin,
1979). In the following sections, we review some of the major questions and
how they have shaped our definitions of the issue and the types of information
gained.

IS WIFE ABUSE A COMMON PHENOMENON?

Naming the Violence

Feminists have stressed that names are essential to constructing reality
(Spender, 1980), and that not having names/terms for our experiences has si-
lenced women (Rich, 1979) and has made our experiences invisible (Daly, 1979).
A major contribution of feminist social action around sexual violence has been
to provide words with which to name our experience (Kelly, 1988). *Battered
women*, *sexual harassment*, *marital rape*, and *date rape* are all terms developed
within the past 20 years to enable women to talk about their experiences.

Even if a name exists and is known, the way it is understood can vary greatly.
Researchers recognize that the boundaries of a phenomenon are set by the definitions of terms and that these definitions can influence incidence rates and other
findings. Typically, researchers have disagreed with each other about definitions
of terms on methodological and conceptual grounds (Browne & Dutton, 1990).
Some of the definitional issues with regard to wife abuse are reviewed here.

Much of the research on marital violence focuses on the "battered woman."
However, the term *battering* and the related terms of *abuse* and *violence* are
used in quite varying ways across studies. Sonkin, Martin, and Walker (1985)
outline four types of marital violence: physical, sexual, property, and psychological. For physical violence, it is important to consider the types of violent
actions, the potential for the infliction of injury, and the harm done by these
actions (Frieze & Browne, 1989). Forced sexual acts and marital rape are associated with sexual forms of marital violence. The destruction of property
belonging to the abused is another form of violence. Marital violence also includes psychological abuse such as threats of violence, pathological jealousy,
mental degradation, and controlling the freedom of movement of the spouse so
that she is not free to go or do what she wants.

Regardless of its form, any use of violence in a relationship can alter the
nature of interaction within the couple. Being a victim of violence from a loved
one can destroy a sense of openness and trust, resulting in a permanent sense
of inequality, threat, and loss (Browne, 1987; Dobash & Dobash, 1984; Pagelow,
1984; Straus & Gelles, 1986; Walker, 1979).

Incidence of Domestic Violence

It is now clear from numerous studies that physical assaults between married and/or cohabiting partners are a serious problem that occurs among blacks and whites and all SES (socioeconomic status) groups (Coley & Beckett, 1988; Frieze & Browne, 1989). In a national survey of over 2,000 homes conducted in 1975, Straus, Gelles, and Steinmetz (1980) asked married couples about assaults directed toward one another and found that more than one-quarter (28%) of those interviewed reported at least one instance of physical assault in their relationships; 16% reported violent incidents in the year just prior to the study. Of these incidents, over a third were serious assaults involving such acts as punching, kicking, hitting with an object, beating up, and assaults with a knife or gun. Estimates based on the Straus et al. (1980) study suggest that over 1.5 million women are the victims of such major assaults by a partner each year (Straus & Gelles, 1986).

Early estimates of incidence and prevalence were based on reports from intact couples and applied only to abuse occurring within the current relationship. Urban samples in the United States during the late 1970s yielded higher estimates, at least for woman abuse when respondents were asked if they had ever been assaulted by a male partner. In a random sample of women in San Francisco, 21% of the women who had been or were currently married reported at least one occasion of physical abuse by their mates (Russell, 1982). A telephone survey of Long Island, New York, residents yielded lower figures of 16% of men and 11% of women having "hit" their spouse (Nisonoff & Bitman, 1979). In another study conducted in Pittsburgh, researchers found that 34% of a general comparison group of ever-married women (chosen as battered women's matches) reported being attacked at least once by a male partner (Frieze, Knoble, Washburn & Zomnir, 1980). These data all suggest that domestic violence affects a large proportion of couples. It is not a rare event.

Marital Violence or Wife Abuse

One of the secondary questions within the literature on incidence of domestic violence is whether this phenomenon is better described as "marital violence" or "wife abuse." Many sociologists tend to use gender-neutral terms such as family violence and to view violence as a problem of both sexes (Straus et al., 1980; Straus & Gelles, 1986). This emphasis on abuse as a family issue has affected the methods employed in research, as well as the subsequent findings.

We would argue that such terminology is misleading. When wife abuse is subsumed under the rubric of family violence or "spouse abuse," the dimensions of gender and power that are fundamental to understanding the abuse of women are obscured (Breines & Gorden, 1983; Schecter, 1982). These generic terms ignore the context of the violence, its nature and consequences, the role obligations of each family member, and the sequences that lead to abuse. When gender-neutral terms mask the dimension of gender, they can lead to biases in how the causes and solutions of wife abuse are conceptualized and treated (Bograd, 1988).

Misconceptions about the nature of assaults by men and women partners spring in part from a careless use of the term *violence* (Browne & Dutton, 1990). In reflecting the general meaning, Webster's *New World Dictionary* (Guralnik, 1984) defines "violence" as "physical force used so as to injure, damage, or destroy; *extreme* roughness of action; intense, often devastatingly or explosively powerful force or energy, as of a hurricane or volcano; *great* force or strength" (p. 1581, emphasis added). By this definition—and based on findings on patterns of abuse and outcomes such as injuries—violence between intimates is primarily directed by parents toward children and by men toward women. Definitions of terms and the appropriate use of these terms, once defined, become especially important in an area in which information is so widely disseminated to the general public and the "results" of empirical research are used to guide legal and social policy and interventions (Browne, 1989, 1990).

Too often in reporting on "spouse abuse," the words *assaultive, aggressive,* and *violent* have been used interchangeably. This lack of definitional clarity has led to ambiguity, both in the collection of empirical data and in how results of the research are interpreted. This can lead to erroneous reports that women are as "violent" as men in partner relationships (Brush, 1990).

In their study of American families, Straus et al. (1980) did find that half (49%) of those who reported assaultive behavior said that both partners had used some kind of force; in 27% of the cases, only the husband had been assaultive, and in 24%, only the wife had been assaultive. However, the 1980 Straus et al. survey was not designed to ask about injuries sustained from the violence, nor about what proportion of the acts were in response to violence initiated by the other or in self-defense. Further, questions about violence were set in a context of settling disputes in a conflict situation and therefore may not have elicited information about attacks that seemed to come "out of the blue."

Another factor in assessing the mutuality of violence is whether or not injuries result. Partners may "trade punches," but they rarely "exchange" injuries (Berk, Berk, Loseke & Rauma, 1983). Even when both partners are injured in an altercation, the woman's injuries are usually more serious (Berk & Loseke, 1981; Stark et al., 1981). Straus and his colleagues noted that, because of men's greater average size and physical strength and their tendency toward greater aggressivity, the same acts frequently have quite a different effect when done by a woman and a man in terms of pain, injury, and threat (Straus et al., 1980). For many of the same reasons, men are also more able to avoid physical victimization than are women. As Pagelow (1984) observed: "Men are, on the average, larger and muscularly stronger than women, so if they choose to strike back they can do greater physical harm than is done to them, they can nonviolently protect themselves from physical harm, or they can leave the premises without being forcibly restrained" (p. 274).

In the Straus et al. studies, assaultive actions were divided into categories of relatively "minor" (threw something at the other; pushed, grabbed, or shoved; and slapped) and "severe" violence (kicked, bit, punched, hit with object, beat up, threatened with a knife or gun, and used a knife or gun). Despite the seemingly equal appearance of assaultive behavior by men and women when looked at in isolation, Straus and his colleagues (1980, 1986) found that men had a higher rate of using the most dangerous and injurious forms of violence—such as physically beating up their partner or using a knife or gun. Another analysis of the same data indicated that the average number of severely violent assaults by a husband against a nonviolent wife was three times greater than wives' assaults on nonviolent husbands (Straus, 1980).

Other evidence, too, supports the idea of high levels of aggressive behavior by men toward women. In the Bureau of Justice Statistics report on family violence (Klaus & Rand, 1984), for instance, 91% of all reported violent crimes between spouses were victimizations of women by husbands or ex-husbands, while only 5% were victimizations of husbands by wives or ex-wives. Studies of severely battered women suggest that they are not typically violent toward their spouses or partners. For these women, the physical danger is too great (Browne, 1987). It appears to be the "mildly battered" women who fight back, whereas more severely battered women are less likely to use violence. Interview studies of battered women have found that, for those women who do fight back, the husbands' level of violence is typically higher than that of their wives (Frieze et al., 1980; Saunders, 1986).

The Subjectivity of Incidence Rates

To date, most of the debate over terminology has focused on differences among researchers in how the violence has been conceptualized and measured. Little or no attention has been focused on the way in which the women themselves define, conceptualize, or label their experiences. How a woman labels or defines the situation may determine the extent and direction of her help-seeking behaviors (Kelly, 1988). How acts are defined also influences public attitudes, agency practice, and legal decisions (Borkowski, Murch & Walker, 1983; Radford, 1987). But most importantly, it is a primary value of feminist researchers to elucidate women's experiences from their own perspectives (Bograd, 1988).

Women experiencing similar acts of assault against them by men often defined these experiences in very different ways. Kelly (1988) reports that the terms typically used to label domestic violence caused problems for some of the women in her study. For example, *wife beating* implied that violence happens only to married women, and *battering* tended to be understood in terms of severe, frequent physical violence. "Battering" was not seen as including more minor forms of physical violence or psychological abuse.

Typically, researchers have employed social, legal, conceptual, or method-ological perspectives in deciding what constitutes wife abuse. Women's definitions and conceptualizations of violence have not been investigated. This is one of the ways in which we have not taken seriously the perspectives of respondents. In research on battered women, as in other areas of research, the responses of participants are challenged, discounted, and discredited. The feminist researcher is caught in a dilemma between validating women's experiences and recognizing that distortions in perceptions are likely. Researchers have typically been criticized because information on violent acts is gathered from only one member of a couple, without corroboration from the other partner or other sources (Szinovacz, 1983).

The identity of the person doing the reporting also seems to be important in assessing what weight to give responses. Studies of crime victims show that they have a surprising tendency to forget or not to report even fairly serious attacks (Block & Block, 1984; Schneider, 1980). Experience with women victims of a partner's violence confirms this. Battered women, especially those who have been victimized over a long period of time, tend to underestimate both the frequency and the severity of the violence they experience when their reports are compared with the reports of witnesses or hospital and other records. Denial that anything at all has happened has also been observed. Chandler (1986) argues that such denial may be a factor in why women marry men who have already been violent during courtship.

Kelly (1988), like other researchers, has noted that many women forget experiences of abuse and have vague and sketchy memories of the actual incidents of abuse. She argues that such responses shouldn't be interpreted as evidence of deception, resistance, or manipulation, but as the result of two common adaptive coping strategies to experiences of victimization: forgetting and minimizing. Kelly also noted that women changed their definitions of their experiences over time as the abuse continued. Almost always, this change was in the direction of relabeling an incident as abuse.

There may be a special problem for women with sexual forms of violence. Researchers have noted that women have great difficulty in responding to questions about violent or forced sex in marriage (Frieze, 1983). Even when they ask specific questions, researchers observe that the extreme sense of shame and humiliation that many victims experience makes it difficult for them to disclose the existence of rape by a partner, even when assured anonymity (Finkelhor & Yllo, 1983; Gelles, 1979; Pagelow, 1984; Russell, 1982; Walker, 1984). Based on her random sample study in San Francisco, Russell (1982) concluded that obtaining "honest disclosure of unwanted sexual experiences in marriage was more difficult . . . than disclosure of sexual abuse by all other categories of people, including the victims of incestuous abuse" (p. 39).

Similarly, experts working with abusive men note that they greatly underreport their violent actions, minimizing or denying assaultive behavior against their wives and claiming more involvement by the victim in justification of their violence than witness or police reports would support (Deschner, 1984; Ewing,

Lindsey, & Pomerantz, 1984; Ganley & Harris, 1978; Sonkin & Durphy, 1982, 1985; Szinovacz, 1983). In a study combining estimations of violence by male perpetrators and women victims, one is thus faced with the possibility that the male perpetrators will sound less violent and more victimized, while their victims will appear to have been less assaulted and more likely to victimize their partners than an observer would corroborate.

What Do Answers to This Question Tell Us?

Why is it important to assess or document the prevalence of assault of women by male partners? Why was this one of the first questions addressed, and why do incidence estimates continue to be important today? Incidence rates are important for the individuals who set mental health and family policy and for those who make decisions about the distribution of resources. By providing statistical evidence of the extent of wife abuse, researchers have played a critical role in making this a social issue. How much abuse occurs is important information when determining what levels of societal responses (i.e., legal, police, physician, mental health, and so on) are needed. The incidence and prevalence rates have been used as the basis for obtaining resources to cope with the issue on a societal level. Funding for police training, shelters, and additional research is dependent on our ability to demonstrate the severity of the problem.

Incidence rates also have important etiological implications. The perspective that abuse of women by their partners is the result of individual pathology is less convincing as an explanation for a phenomenon that occurs in a relatively high proportion of relationships. Higher incidence rates are typically interpreted as indicating the existence of structural or societal causes, such as societal tolerance of male aggression. Paradoxically, the same high incidence rates that suggest a structural component have been used to obtain resources to intervene at the individual level.

Thus, the incidence rate research conducted to date can be seen as making important contributions to our understanding of wife abuse. This research helped us name the phenomenon, forced us to see it as both a local and a national problem, served as the basis for obtaining resources, and encouraged us to consider certain etiological perspectives. However, we need to ask if this is the research that a battered woman might find most helpful. Is the information that a large percentage of one's neighbors are also being battered comforting or helpful? The incidence rates may encourage battered women, along with the rest of us, to see wife battering as a societal problem that is culturally produced or at least tolerated. Such a perspective might modify the degree to which she blames herself. But research in other areas suggests that knowing that others also suffer does not reduce the pain or anguish (Fiske & Taylor, 1984) and does not suggest a solution.

WHAT'S WRONG WITH HER?

Masochism and the Acceptance of Violence

One of the common beliefs found in early writings on battered women is that they were masochists (Snell et. al., 1964). Although such research (and treatment) approaches have been repeatedly criticized as being victim blaming and androcentric (e.g., Wardell, Gillespie & Leffler, 1983; Yllo & Bograd, 1988), Rosewater (1988) reports examples of recent studies that used the MMPI to examine masochism in abused wives (Palau, 1981) and to conclude that women in abusive relationships have disordered personalities (Gellman, Hoffman, Jones & Stone, 1984). Critics of the revised manual of the American Psychiatric Association (Rosewater, 1988) argue that the new diagnosis of "self-defeating personality disorder" (originally termed masochistic personality disorder) may perpetuate this view of battered women and cause therapists to confuse the effects of violence in women victims with symptoms of mental illness. The view of abused women as masochistic has been especially evident in clinical studies or discussions. Shainess (1977) has elaborated on the psychoanalytic notion that women are masochistic. She contends that women contribute to their own victimization by acting indecisive and vulnerable.

Until recently, almost all psychological interventions focused on the women. This may be a function of the fact that it is typically the woman who enters psychological treatment (Star, 1983). It may also come from the beliefs that the woman has provoked the violence or should somehow be responsible for stopping it.

Masochistic views take many different forms. One form of treatment has aimed at helping the battered wife understand her masochistic needs for a violent relationship. In this type of treatment, the woman is urged to examine her family of origin, to understand her supposed "need" to be treated badly. She is also led to review the maneuvers she employs that (supposedly) provoke the violence (Rounsaville, 1978). The view that some women are "destined" to be attracted to and/or desperately in love with abusive men has been popularized (Forward & Torres, 1986) as a contemporary version of female masochism. Others, too, have suggested love as the reason for accepting abuse. Interview studies of battered women indicate that there is generally less affectionate behavior (physical affection, giving presents, having a good sexual relationship, and so on) in their marriages than in those of nonviolent comparisons (Frieze et al., 1980). At the same time, clinicians working with battered women have observed that they often appear to love their abusive husbands and very much value signs of love and affection from them (Walker, 1983). Others have described a strong emotional attachment in the form of a "traumatic bond" (Dutton & Painter, 1983).

The fact that many battered women do maintain positive feelings toward their husbands may be a result of feelings generated for them before the relationships became violent (Browne, 1987). In most of the studies of long-term battering relationships, the majority of battered women—73 to 85%—do not experience physical assault until after they have made a major commitment to and/or married their abuser (Bowker, 1983; Dobash & Dobash, 1978; Mason & Blankenship, 1987; Pagelow, 1981; Rosenbaum & O'Leary, 1981). On the basis of clinical observations, Browne (1987) and Walker (1984) note that abused women report that their partners were extremely attentive and affectionate early in the relationship, before the onset of violence. They showed great interest in the woman's whereabouts and activities, a desire to be with them all the time, and intense expressions of affection and wanted an early commitment to a long-term relationship. Such behaviors may be difficult to distinguish from idealized romantic interactions. Over time, though, such behavior is increasingly seen by the woman as intrusive, possessive, and controlling. She begins to feel isolated as she becomes separated from former friends and family networks. At the same time, she does not know how to interpret her growing sense of discomfort. By the onset of the first violence, strong emotional bonds have typically been formed between the partners. The woman's social isolation by this time makes her especially vulnerable and unable to get help (Browne, 1987; Pagelow, 1984; Walker, 1979, 1984).

Over time, behaviors that battered women initially viewed as evidence of affection can become the triggers that lead to their assaults. Abused women report that the men's constant desire to know their whereabouts may escalate into a requirement that they account for every hour of their time. Violent reprisals may occur if their explanations do not satisfy their partners. Further, battered women frequently report extreme and delusional jealousy on the part of their partners, leading to increasing levels of isolation and risk in contacts with others (Frieze et al., 1980; Hotaling & Sugarman, 1986).

Helplessness in Battered Women

Another form of masochism or victim-blame theories is that battered women are helpless. Dobash and Dobash (1988) argue that concentrating on the victim and positing that she learns to be helpless or helps to perpetuate the violence against her are similar in their implications to the older notions of masochism. However, this view of battered women is still widely held. The image of the passive, self-deprecating, helpless, and depressed battered woman is one of the common images in the media today and one that is being labeled as the "stereotypic battered woman profile" by researchers in the field (Walker, 1979, 1984). In fact, there are clearly battered women who do not show evidence of a generalized feeling of helplessness. Shaud's (1983) study of Minneapolis battered women indicated that, when asked to respond to a scale measuring generalized feelings of helplessness, there was very low interitem consistency. Thus, although battered women may have felt helpless to control some aspects of their lives, this was not a pervasive reaction to all aspects of their lives.

However, there is empirical evidence that at least some battered women do display helplessness. Clinical studies have identified such feelings in battered women. With repeated unsuccessful attempts to control the battering, some battered women begin to demonstrate many of the signs of generalized feelings of helplessness and a perception of being unable to control their lives (Walker, 1979, 1984). As this occurs, they become less and less able to change their situations for the better.

Consistent with the idea of helplessness in battered women, Finn (1985) reported that these women are less likely than the general female population to utilize active, problem-solving behaviors. Finn describes these women as ignoring their problems or using other passive coping strategies. However, as discussed in the next section, such reactions are not unique to abused women.

Why Does She Stay?

Given the abusiveness of violent marriages, many ask why battered women remain in such relationships. Remaining in the relationship is often seen as yet another manifestation of helplessness in battered women. If one examines the data, however, it becomes clear that there are many reasons that battered women stay with their abusers or leave (Browne, 1987; Frieze & Browne, 1989; Gelles, 1976).

Leaving behavior in battered women tends to take one of two forms. First, the woman may leave for a brief period of time and then return to her violent mate. Or, she may leave permanently and establish a new life-style. The battered women who feel in immediate danger may be most likely to use temporary leave-taking. This would be especially likely in those women who blame the husband for the violence (rather than themselves) and feel that they have no way of controlling an immediate outburst of violence. The decision about leaving is affected by whether the woman has somewhere to go. Having money, a car, nearby friends or family who could shelter her, or a "safe house" or woman's shelter nearby facilitates the option of leaving. Isolated rural women may have the most difficulty in finding somewhere to go. Leaving on a temporary basis would also be a more likely response if the woman fears that the next violent incident will consist of extreme violence (Frieze, 1979).

A number of factors may prohibit women from leaving permanently. Some women cannot leave because of economic dependence upon their husbands; others have nowhere to go because they lack the resources of their own simply to pack up and drive to a motel, and they have no other source of shelter that would not require money (Frieze et al., 1980; Pagelow, 1981). For economically disadvantaged women, leaving an abusive relationship may mean temporary, if not permanent, homelessness. This situation is further complicated if the woman has children she would want to take with her. Other factors that might make it difficult for her to leave would be loss of her job and her social status and fear of disapproval from family or friends (Pagelow, 1977). By leaving, a woman gives up her identity as a wife, risks social disapproval, loses economic support, and loses any love she feels from her husband (Waites, 1978).

Another factor that keeps women in abusive relationships is fear about retaliation from her violent husband (Ridington, 1978). The battered wife may fear that her husband will retaliate against her, their children, or her other family if she tries to leave. This fear of her abuser finding her or others he has threatened is a reasonable concern. Some women who have left an abusive partner have been followed and harassed for months or even years, and some have been killed (Browne, 1987; Jones, 1980; Pagelow, 1980). Evidence suggests that, in many cases, the man's violence continues to escalate after a separation (Fields, 1978; Fiora-Gormally, 1978; Lewin, 1979; Pagelow, 1980).

In spite of these dangers, one of the best empirical predictors of women leaving is the severity of the violence. The women themselves also cite this as one of the major factors in wanting to leave (Frieze et al., 1980). The severely battered woman may leave her husband because she is in fear of her life or that of her children if she stays (Frieze, 1979; Walker, 1978). Women who are battered and raped by their husbands suffer some of the strongest negative reactions; it is not surprising, therefore, that this group is most likely to leave their abusive mates (Frieze, 1983).

Battered Women: Victims or Survivors?

In assessing helplessness in battered women, one must first consider whether this characteristic is the cause of their being battered or is a consequence of the battering. Masochistic theories assume the former, but empirical research is more supportive of the latter explanation. Studies of victims of crimes, accidents, environmental disasters, and harassment have all found common emotional stress reactions (Bard & Sangrey, 1979; Frieze, Hymer & Greenberg, 1987). Psychiatrists have identified these reactions in the DSM-III as "posttraumatic stress disorder." Common manifestations of this stress include feelings of anger, shock, disbelief, confusion, fear, and anxiety. It is not uncommon for any type of victim to feel helpless and insecure as well (Figley, 1985). Long-term victims may become dependent and suggestible or passive and demonstrate difficulty making decisions or functioning alone. Normal recoveries from a single assault can take months or even years and can be characterized by continued anxiety or confusion and lapses into helplessness and fear (Bard & Sangrey, 1979; Figley, 1985).

As would be expected, women assaulted by a male partner evidence reactions similar to those noted for other types of victims. But a battered woman's emotional reactions to an assault may be greater than those of some other victim of stranger crime or natural disaster. For the battered woman, the victimization is often repeated (Miller & Porter, 1983). Her situation may be more analogous to that of the prisoner of war (Romero, 1985) or torture victim (Chandler, 1986) than to victims of other crimes. Chandler's phenomenological analysis of battered women's experiences suggests that overriding fear and a loss of a sense of self characterize the severely battered woman. Other empirical data show elevated anxiety scores and high levels of depression for these women (Hughes & Barad, 1983).

Furthermore, for battered women, the experience of assault is compounded by the fact that the assailant is an intimate—someone they may love, someone they are supposed to be able to trust, and someone on whom they may depend for many of the necessities of daily life. In such cases, perceptions of vulnerability, loss, and helplessness may be especially severe. For abused women who are married to their assailants, their legal, social, financial, and emotional connection to their victimizer makes alternatives such as escape or help seeking especially complex. Decisions are clouded by family ties, fears of reprisal, and issues relating to children. Abused women's perceptions of alternatives may also be influenced by societal expectations related to gender and role relationships that encourage women to be self-sacrificing and adaptive and and to care for and protect those close to them, regardless of the cost to self (Browne, 1987; Walker & Browne, 1985).

In spite of their repeated victimization, however, many battered women do not demonstrate helplessness. An important feminist concern involves the extent to which research and theory developed over the past decades have focused on women's oppression and victimization while ignoring women's strengths and assets. Although battered women are certainly victims, research may have focused too much on their passivity and helplessness rather than their help seeking, coping mechanisms, survival skills, and other strengths.

Self-Blame

There are a number of coping mechanisms that have been identified as important for battered women (Frieze & Browne, 1989). One form of the search for meaning in the battered woman is for her to see herself as somehow to blame for the violence. It is this tendency in battered women that may have led to some of the early masochism theories. Research dealing with the reactions of all types of victims shows a general tendency for victims to blame themselves. Thus a battered woman may say to herself, "If only I had gotten dinner ready on time."

Battered women have often been cited as blaming themselves for the violence (Frieze, 1979; Miller & Porter, 1983). This is not always maladaptive. Self-blame may give battered women a feeling of control and hopefulness for the future. Rather than asking the "Why me?" question posed by other victims, they may instead ask, "What did I do tonight that set him off?" (Miller & Porter, 1983). Once they answer this question, battered women may go to great ends to change their behaviors so that they will not trigger violence again. Although this may make them feel that they have some control over their mate's aggression, the reality is that they often do not. Thus, behavioral self-blame as a coping response for battered women does not appear to be a successful long-term strategy.

Taking Action

Along with psychological coping, battered women frequently demonstrate active coping responses. This is clearly more consistent with seeing the battered woman as survivor than with seeing her as a victim. Gondolf and Fisher (1988) view battered women as survivors, acting assertively and logically in response to the abuse. They document the extent to which these individuals have contacted a variety of help sources and suggest that battered women increase their help seeking in the face of increased violence, rather than decreasing help seeking, as a theory of learned helplessness would suggest. Walker (1984) also reports data consistent with the perspective that battered women are survivors, noting, "As the violence escalated, so did the probability that the battered would seek help" (p. 27). In Walker's (1984) sample, abused women did not score lower on psychological tests for self-esteem, depression, or external locus of control than did a control group of women.

Far from complete passivity, most battered women do seek help for the violence or for marital problems (Frieze, 1979; Pagelow, 1981). Bowker (1983) found that formerly battered women had persistently sought help from a wide range of sources and that the more intensified and prolonged the abuse, the greater the variety and extent of their help seeking. In Schulman's (1979) Kentucky sample, 57% of the respondents who had been abused had told someone. Forty-three percent of the 146 battered women in a Milwaukee study received help from family members, and 52% received help from friends (Bowker, 1984). Similar findings were reported by Frieze et al. (1980), who found that 55% of the self-identified battered women in their sample had sought help from relatives, 52% from friends, and 39% from ministers or priests. Forty-two percent of the women had sought psychological help.

Although sometimes adding to her frustrations, social support and other types of help can be quite important for the battered woman in trying to cope with her victimization and in avoiding future battering (Mitchell & Hodson, 1982). According to Bowker (1983), material assistance was given to battered women by family members in 50% of the cases in his sample. Friends were also likely to give such concrete forms of help. Both of these groups also allowed the battered woman to talk about her situation and to problem-solve.

Probably one of the most important sources of community help for battered women is shelters. Ten percent of the women in Bowker's sample went to a shelter after the first incidence of abuse; with repeated abuse, 29% took refuge in shelters (Bowker, 1983). Shelters provide physical protection as well as other services. One important service of shelters is self-help groups in which women share common experiences. Others who have dealt with the same problems provide encouragement (Bowker, 1983) and serve as a basis of social comparison (Coates & Winston, 1983). A study of 20 residents of a New Haven, Connecticut, shelter showed clear evidence of less depression and more hopefulness in the women after living two weeks in the shelter (Sedlak, 1983).

Another form of help seeking is to call the police. In Bowker's (1983) sample of women who had "beaten wife beating," 9% had called the police after the first violent incident. This number rose to 38% after the worst violence occurred. But, several studies have found that abused women have not found the police to be as helpful as they might be (Bowker, 1983; Frieze et al., 1980; Pagelow, 1981). Both Bowker and Frieze et al. found that abused wives rated the police as the least helpful of various potential help providers. There are a number of reasons for this. Police officers may not define battered women as the victims of violent crime, and they may refuse to arrest the abusive husband even when the wife requests them to do so (Bowker, 1983). Women reporting assaults or threats by partners are familiar with being referred for personal mental health counseling or being asked why they don't leave their homes, rather than being offered effective alternatives. But such police reactions may be changing. Some social science evidence suggests that arrest can be an effective mechanism for reducing marital violence, at least in some circumstances (Langan & Innes, 1986; Sherman & Berk, 1984).

Besides seeking help, some battered women may physically attack their batterers in an attempt to defend themselves or retaliate (Saunders, 1986). Physical retaliation was used by the women in the Bowker (1983) sample (after 29% of the battering incidents). About one-quarter of the women in the Walker (1984) sample pushed or shoved the batterer, and one-fifth clawed or scratched him during the worst incident. Although battered women may fight back, most do not inflict serious injury on their mates. For example, note the discrepancy in types of actions and potential for injury. The "worst incident" in the Walker study involved kicking, punching, beating up, sexual abuse, choking, and using a knife by the men, whereas the women's responses typically involved very mild aggression.

Some women do eventually kill their abusers in defense of themselves or a child (Browne, 1987; Jones, 1980; Totman, 1978). In analyzing all one-on-one cases of homicide in the United States, Browne and Williams (in press) noted that, although neglected as an area of inquiry until recently, the number of individuals at risk for partner homicide is quite high. From 1976 through 1987, the deaths of approximately 38,648 people over the age of 15 resulted from one partner killing another (including homicide by dating, common-law, married, exmarried). Of these deaths, 61% of the victims were women killed by male partners and 39% were men killed by women partners (Browne & Williams, in press). Women in the United States are more at risk of homicide victimization from a male partner than from all other categories of persons combined: over half (52%) of women murdered during this time period were killed by their male partners. Black women are even more likely than whites to be killed by a spouse (Plass & Straus, 1987).

National homicide figures do not give us information on the histories of individual couples, so it is impossible to determine how many of these partner homicides were the culmination of an ongoing history of abuse and threat.

However, homicide studies beginning with Wolfgang's (1958, 1967) early research on criminal homicide indicate the frequency with which women who kill male partners are responding to the partner's aggression and threat (Chimbos, 1978; Totman, 1978; Wilbanks, 1982, 1983). In analyzing trends in partner homicide from 1976 through 1980, Browne and Williams (1989) found over a 25% decrease in the number of homicides perpetrated by women against their male partners. This decline began in 1979, at about the time that domestic violence legislation and other resources for abused women were coming into place. Browne and Williams further noted that those states having more domestic violence legislation and other resources for abused women, such as shelters, crisis lines, and support groups, had lower rates of female-perpetrated partner homicide in general and that the presence of such resources was associated with the decline in these homicides from 1979 through 1984.

Unfortunately, findings on homicides by men were not as encouraging. On average, across the 50 states, men were killing their female partners more in the first half of the 1980s than in the 1970s. In spite of the fact that domestic violence legislation has been designed to sanction and deter those who assault family members and to offer protection and relief to victims, there was no correlation between the presence of domestic violence statutes in a state and the rates or changes in rates of men killing female partners (Browne & Williams, in press). Again, this is an example of the important differences between men's and women's patterns of violence in couple relationships.

Implications of Victim-Focused Questions

Much of the research on wife abuse has focused on the supposed inadequacies of the battered woman. Original formulations of the battered woman as masochistic have been challenged repeatedly. Yet, as our review suggests, this perspective and other victim-blaming perspectives continue to influence both the research and the treatment of wife abuse. For example, a widely held formulation is that battered women are suffering from helplessness; but the evidence suggests that abused wives actively seek help from family and from social agencies. Some research suggests that it is the responses of others to the battered woman's request for assistance that are inadequate. More systematic study of resources and effective interventions may be more important than adding to our list of the "problems" of battered women.

Why has the research focused so heavily on the inadequacies of the battered woman? Some critics have argued that the focus on the female victim as responsible for the violence directed at her is the legacy of Freud (Caplan, 1984). Alternatively, it has been argued that viewing the batttered woman as inadequate is a result of the fact that victimized women are the ones who have most typically sought professional help. Thus, women's help-seeking behaviors—a positive coping response—might ironically have led to them being labeled as inadequate or pathological. Not only does their entry into shelters and therapy make them more accessible to the researcher, but women's presentation as a client makes them available for intervention strategies by professionals. Since it is the woman's behavior and personality that we can measure and possibly change, it must therefore be her behavior and personality that are viewed as problematic. A feminist analysis suggests that we challenge both the view of women as passive victim and our tendency to focus our research and intervention efforts on them.

WHAT'S WRONG WITH THIS COUPLE?

A Family Systems Approach to Marital Violence

The work of Straus, Gelles, and Steinmetz (Gelles, 1974, 1979; Steinmetz, 1977; Straus et al., 1980) is the most widely published and cited perspective on battering as family violence. Although not strictly a systems approach, Straus and his colleagues are often classified within this framework. Their work tends to emphasize the fact that both men and women are violent toward their spouses. In their work, the family is the central unit of analysis. They believe all family members carry out and are victims of violence (Kurz, 1989) and that violence is an all-pervasive feature of family life. Gelles and Straus (1988) tie spouse abuse to the structure of the family. But they also look outside the family for explanations of marital violence. They see underlying causes as the stress experienced by family members and the emphasis on family privacy in our society. The acceptance and socialization of violence as a means of conflict resolution are also cited.

The emphasis on external stress as a primary causal factor for family violence has been utilized as an explanation for higher rates of violence in black families (Coley & Beckett, 1988; Kurz, 1989; Plass & Straus, 1987). Although there is some disagreement about whether rates are truly higher for blacks (see Coley & Beckett, 1988), there seems to be general agreement that black men in particular live in highly stressful environments and that such stresses may lead to their being violent in the home.

Systems theory has increasingly become an accepted theory both in explaining and in intervening in situations of marital abuse (McIntyre, 1984). This approach does not focus on the individual, but relocates the "blame" onto the interaction within the couple. Thus, the interpersonal relationship becomes the system of concern. This perspective, like the victim-blame theories, is of special interest to counselors, since the larger social system is not open to intervention by marriage counselors (Patterson, 1982).

In the systems approach, the wife is seen as a coparticipant in the violence, even if the violence is unidirectional. For example, a family systems theorist might examine the way that family arguments develop and escalate, assuming that both spouses play a role in this process. The wife might be held accountable for the escalation of the anger and conflict (Neidig & Friedman, 1984). Alternatively, the systems approach tends to view the wife as the overadequate partner and the one able to provide leverage in the system. Family interaction approaches to marital violence emphasize the rules of the system, power imbalances in the system, or resources that underlie the interaction (Giles-Sims, 1983; Neidig & Friedman, 1984). Giles-Sims (1983) suggests that wives inadvertently reinforce violent behavior in their mates by capitulating to them.

Employing the systems perspective, the family therapist is encouraged to reframe the situation for the wife so that getting the husband into treatment is an act of caring. Once in treatment, intervention strategies continue to emphasize the wife as the leverage (Cook & Cook, 1984). Particular types of intervention techniques follow from this systemic analysis of domestic violence. They reflect the assumption that the violence is mutually constructed. The first task of the therapist is to reattribute the violence as a mutual problem, rather than the fault of one partner (Margolin, 1979). Intervention focuses then on changing relationship patterns that maintain violence and preventing conflict from escalating to physical violence. Couples are helped to see how they trigger each other's "anger buttons," how to reframe violence-provoking situations more positively, how to see violence as a form of weakness rather than strength, and how to switch to alternative methods of dealing with aggressive feelings (Margolin, 1979). McIntyre (1984) criticizes these techniques as merely repeating the violence against the woman at an emotional and sociopolitical level.

Power and Decision Making

Although based on different theoretical assumptions, research on the power dynamics of violent couples also asks the question of what's wrong with the couple. On a very basic level, use of violence or the threat of violence is an effective mechanism for controlling other people. It is clear that violence is used in this way among family members (Straus et al., 1980). Straus (1978) argues that having been violent toward his wife only once causes a permanent change in the balance of marital power toward a strongly husband-dominant pattern. Other researchers have also noted the instrumental nature of husband violence. Hilberman and Munson (1978) found in their study of battered women that their husbands were likely to become violent whenever they did not get their way.

One measure of power is the possession of resources such as money, education, social status, and friends. Violent men sometimes appear to lack resources outside the home (Dvoskin, 1981; Finkelhor, 1983; Frieze & McHugh, 1981; Straus et al., 1980). They may use violence against weaker family members as a way of compensating for their own feelings of inadequacy (Finkelhor, 1983). Walker (1983) and Hotaling and Sugarman (1986) also cite differences in resources as a causal factor in violence. Presumably, the husband, with fewer of these status-related resources, feels a need to use violence to assert his power in the family.

In one study of relative resources, Hornung, McCullough, and Sugimoto (1981), in an analysis of a random sample of Kentucky women (Schulman, 1979), found that the risk of physical abuse was 1.3 times greater for women married to men who were underachievers in relation to their education level. Risk rates of 1.5 and 1.2 were associated, respectively, with women whose occupational attainments were low relative to their husbands or whose relative attainments were high. Similar patterns of risk were found for psychological abuse as well.

Another measure of family power is decision making. Frieze and McHugh (1981) found that such decision making was highly related to the level of violence in the husbands. The most violent husbands also tended to make most of the decisions about where the couple went together, whose friends they would see, and what major household purchases they should make. In this study, the most egalitarian marriages were found in the control group, where there was no marital violence. Coleman and Straus (1986) concur. In an analysis of the national household study data, they found that egalitarian and divided-power marriages were the least violent. Such relationships may be similar to the low-violence marriages reported by Frieze et al. (1980) in which there was relatively equal low-level violence between husbands and wives. In these marriages, there appeared to be more equality within the couple than in the severely violent marriages, which were much more husband-dominant.

Another way in which physically abusive men exert power is through controlling the freedom of movement of their wives. Frieze and McHugh (1981) found that battered wives had less freedom to go where they wanted and that they tended to remain at home much more than women married to nonviolent men. The severe batterers also controlled family finances the most closely. Walker (1983) also found that abusing men closely monitor where their wives are. Her explanation for such behavior is that violent men are basically insecure and feel a need for this type of control over their wives. Of course, it is their violence or the threat of such violence that allows them to exert this type of dominance. Other men who felt similarly insecure would not have the same means of enforcing these restrictions on their wives.

As this brief review has indicated, the issues surrounding power and violence are quite complex. It is never clear how much the use of physical force changes the power dynamics of the marriage and the characteristics of the man and woman involved. Do battered women have less influence over marital decision making because they are fearful of repeated violence, or is it the less assertive women who are more likely to be beaten? Such questions cannot truly be answered without longitudinal data.

What Do Answers to This Question Tell Us?

Both of these couple-focused perspectives—family systems and familial power dynamics—suggest that the problem or pathology occurs at the dyadic level. Spouses in violent marriages are seen as having inadequate conflict resolution strategies or as failing to establish an appropriate power equilibrium. Intervention strategies based on these perspectives typically focus on the acquisition of skills by both partners or on altering the perspectives (reframing) of both spouses. Both the research and the interventions avoid blaming the perpetrators for the violence. The family systems approach also fails to examine the dimensions of gender involved (McIntyre, 1984). Although the familial power perspective does explicitly consider gender as an important variable, more could be done to develop the implications of differential power held by men and women.

More consideration should also be given to the fact that the violence may serve instrumental purposes for the perpetrator. Adams (1988) argues that many researchers fail to acknowledge the utility and the purposeful nature of violence. Goode (1971), in his exchange theory analysis of family violence, interprets male violence as directed toward maintaining the husband's power within the family. Similarly, Gelles (1979) contends that family violence occurs because there are few social sanctions against it and numerous rewards or gains.

WHY DOES OUR SOCIETY ALLOW WIFE BATTERING?

Feminist scholars have argued that wife abuse and other forms of violence against women are rooted in patriarchy (Daly, 1979; Dobash & Dobash, 1979; Kaufman, 1987; Koss, 1990; Kurz, 1989; Rhodes & McNeill, 1985; Yllo & Bograd, 1988). Male dominance within the family, social institutions, and society itself is seen as providing the structural and ideological foundation for violence against women. As discussed earlier, this perspective is implicitly supported by the high prevalence rates that have been documented for wife abuse and other forms of male-to-female violence. However, there have been only a few systematic attempts to demonstrate quantitatively a relationship between patriarchy and violence against women. Dobash and Dobash (1979), using responses obtained from interviews with 109 working-class victims in Scottish shelters, relate wife beating to patriarchal attitudes. Yllo (1983, 1984, 1988) has conducted a series of studies examining how women's status affects violence in the family, using quantitative analysis of secondary data on wife abuse. Yllo constructed a Status of Women index and used it to rank 30 American states regarding the economic, political, educational, and legal status of women. This index was then correlated with the state rates of wife beating drawn from a nationally representative survey on family violence. Yllo's research indicates that there is a curvilinear relationship between the status of women and wife abuse. Violence against wives was highest in states where women had low status and was lower as women's status improved. However, rates of abuse increased in those states in which women's status was highest relative to men's.

In a related study, Yllo (1984) examined the association among structural inequality, interpersonal inequality, and wife beating. Interpersonal inequality, in this study, referred to one partner's having the final say in marital decision making. The highest rates of violence were found for husband-dominant couples in high-status-of-women states. Wife-dominant couples in low-status-of-women states also experienced high levels of wife beating.

Other studies have examined the relationship between traditional sex-role attitudes and wife abuse. In a review of these studies, Hotaling and Sugarman (1986) report that only two of eight studies found a statistically significant relationship between traditional sex-role attitudes and wife abuse. They concluded that nonviolent men are as likely as violent men to hold a patriarchal set of beliefs. However, Saunders and his colleagues (Saunders, Lynch, Grayson & Linz, 1987) developed a scale of attitudes specifically about wife beating and, using it, found that male batterers in treatment were more likely than male college students to believe that wife beating is justified under some circumstances.

Societal encouragement of violence against women is also discussed by Bowker (1983, 1984). Bowker (1983) suggests that male members of some subcultures socialize their peers into the ideology of male dominance and support wife beating as a method of maintaining that dominance.

What Do Answers to This Question Tell Us?

Why have we focused our research and intervention efforts on the individual and failed to examine the societal context in which violence occurs? Social psychologists would argue that there is a natural tendency to place an emphasis on individuals as the causes of behavior; they have termed this the "fundamental attribution error" (Fiske & Taylor, 1984). This research suggests that our visual focus influences our attributions. Thus, since we have traditionally interviewed and treated female victims, we have focused on them, rather than on other possible causes of the violence. A second explanation for our failure to examine societal or structural-level explanations is that interventions based on such perspectives are more difficult to conceptualize and to conduct. If patriarchy and patriarchal attitudes are the basis for wife abuse, it will be much more difficult to alleviate the problem.

WHY DO MEN BEAT THEIR WIVES?

Only recently have researchers asked the more obvious question, Why does he beat her? Failure to demonstrate empirically that abused wives were characterologically different from their nonabused counterparts has helped to shift research focus to the characteristics of the abusive husband (Rosenbaum & O'Leary, 1981). The feminist criticism of the victim-blaming focus on the woman contributed to this movement to consider the personality and the motives of the batterer.

Personality of Batterers

In a major review of previous research findings, Hotaling and Sugarman (1986) noted that the characteristics associated with the violent man were much better predictors of his violence than were the characteristics of the woman predictive of her being victimized. Personality profiles of male spouse abusers reported by Hamberger and Hastings (1986) indicated that abusers were asocial/borderline, narcissistic/antisocial, and dependent/compulsive. More recently, Hastings and Hamberger (1988) depict the batterer as a psychologically rigid and unstable individual who is so self-absorbed that empathy and reciprocity are impossible for him. Abusive men have been reported to have low self-esteem and to be vulnerable to criticism (Goldstein & Rosenbaum, 1985; Rouse, 1984) and to be unassertive (Dutton & Strachan, 1987). Waldo (1987) describes the batterers as confused, guilt-ridden, and frightened. On the other hand, batterers have been depicted as domineering (Caesar, 1986) and controlling (Gondolf, 1985). Dutton (1988) concludes that the depictions of wife assaulters in the literature are contradictory. Explanations for such discrepancies are differences in sampling and the fact that batterers are actually quite heterogeneous (Dutton, 1988).

Exposure to Violence

Violence in the batterer's family of origin is frequently cited as a factor in wife beating (Hotaling & Sugarman, 1986). Rosenbaum and O'Leary (1981) reported that abusive husbands were more likely to have witnessed parental spouse abuse in their family or to have been victims of child abuse than their nonabusive counterparts. Roy (1982) reported that 80% of the abusive partners in her study had experienced or witnessed abuse as children. Caesar (1988) also noted that batterers were more likely than comparison subjects to have been abused as children, to have witnessed their father beating their mother, and to have been disciplined with corporal punishment as children. However, within this study, 38% of the batterers denied having witnessed or experienced abuse as a child. Some nonbattering men also reported witnessing (17%) or experiencing (11%) violence as children.

In spite of the many studies showing early family effects, there is still uncertainty about the mechanism by which this translates into adult violence. Kalmuss and Seltzer (1986) conclude that the batterer's repertoire of aggressive behaviors may not be learned in his family of origin, but that batterers have learned that violence is an appropriate and effective way to exert authority. Evidence for this idea is seen in the fact that violence developed in a first marriage was maintained in subsequent relationships.

Recently, the association between exposure to violence as a child and later marital violence has been questioned. Early studies reporting a relationship between exposure to violence as a child and subsequent wife abuse as an adult relied on wives as informants or failed to compare batterers with nonviolent men (Caesar, 1988).

Batterers as Out of Control

Clinical descriptions of batterers often describe them as out of control. Their violence is seen as "uncontrollable rage" or "uncontrollable aggression"

(Deschner, 1984; Walker, 1979). Other researchers hypothesize that the violence is a man's desperate attempt to maintain control when he feels as if he is losing it (Dutton & Strachan, 1987; Gondolf, 1985). The abusive men themselves are seen as having "irrational aggressive impulses" or as having "poor impulse control" (Deschner, 1984; Star, 1983). Ptacek (1988) points out that the language used by clinicians to describe male violence and male batterers is similar to the accounts given by the batterers themselves. In a qualitative analysis of batterers' attributions, Ptacek concludes that their accounts consist of more excuses than explanations; they tended to excuse themselves of full responsibility and at the same time offered justifications for their actions. Common excuses included loss of control and victim blaming; justifications included denial of "real" injury and the wife's failure to fulfill the obligations of a good wife. Ptacek (1988) suggests that such a view is often endorsed by clinicians, who view the male violence as beyond his control and in many cases provoked by his wife.

Many researchers and clinicians working with abusive men strongly disagree with the view that men who assault their wives are acting in a random manner and are simply "out of control." Browne and Dutton (1990) contend that men who assault their wives gain from their use of violence through personal feelings of power and through having gained control of a situation that may have felt unmanageable to them, prior to the violence (see also Novaco, 1976; Sonkin, Martin & Walker, 1985). Dutton and Browning (1988) theorize that abusive men fear intimacy and use physical and verbal assaults—as well as other hurtful behaviors such as emotional withdrawal, verbal criticism, and extramarital affairs—to control the emotional distance between themselves and a significant other. These men are characterized as continually attempting to move closer and farther away. Power issues are typically described by abusive men as a need to control or dominate the woman, feelings of powerlessness vis-à-vis the woman, and descriptions of female independence as a male loss of control (Dutton & Browning, 1988; Hamberger & Hastings, 1986).

Alcohol and Drug Abuse

A common scenario in fiction is a drunken husband coming home and severely beating his wife. Such behavior on the part of the man is at least partially excused because he was drinking. Many feel that his drinking causes his violence. Alcohol consumption on the part of the wife is also seen as important in understanding the dynamics of family violence. A woman who is beaten when she has been drinking is more likely to be blamed for the violence. Her drunken behavior is seen as provoking the violence, whereas a woman who is sober is less likely to be blamed for the violence of her husband (Richardson & Campbell, 1980).

Research does indicate that abusive men with severe alcohol or drug problems are apt to abuse their partners both when drunk and when sober, are violent more frequently, and inflict more serious injuries on their partners than abusive men who do not have a history of alcohol or drug problems. They are also more apt to attack their partners sexually and are more likely to be violent outside the home (Browne, 1987; Frieze & Knoble, 1980; Roy, 1977; Walker, 1984). Seven of nine studies that investigated this question using some sort of a comparison group found that abusive men were more likely to abuse alcohol than nonviolent men (Hotaling & Sugarman, 1986). Coleman and Straus (1983) analyzed the National Survey data to determine the relationship of marital violence and alcohol abuse. A general correlation of "drunkenness" and spousal violence was found. However, those who showed evidence of extreme alcohol abuse were not the most violent. This finding was interpreted as indicating that those who were most often drunk were "anesthetized" to an intolerable world. This finding that the men who most often drank alcohol were not the most violent husbands was also found by Frieze and Knoble (1980). These researchers suggested that alcoholics may show diminished violence because of having less physical control over their bodies.

It is not surprising that alcohol should be linked to marital violence in our culture, since there is a good deal of evidence that alcohol use is related to physically aggressive behavior in men. Alcohol use is reported to be common in cases of assault (Mayfield, 1976; Nicol, Gunn, Gristwood, Foggitt & Watson, 1973) and homicide (Virkkunen, 1974; Wolfgang & Strohm, 1957), as well as in crimes in general (Fitzpatrick, 1974; Sobell & Sobell, 1975).

Although a strong association has consistently been found between substance abuse and the use of violence, some have argued that alcohol should be viewed as a disinhibiting, but not a causal factor (Pagelow, 1981; Sonkin et al., 1985; Walker, 1984). Gelles (1974) has speculated that perpetrators of violence may drink to excuse their own conduct. This may be particularly effective when the excuse of intoxication is also accepted by others. A number of researchers have discussed the tendency of abused women to blame the drinking, rather than their violent assailant, for abusive incidents (Bowker, 1983; Frieze & Knoble, 1980; Pagelow, 1981; Roy, 1977; Russell, 1982). By saying that the violence is caused by alcohol use, family members do not have to admit that they are engaging in socially unacceptable or deviant behavior. Many people believe that people who are intoxicated have a period of "time-out" during which they are not expected to follow normal social rules (Richardson & Campbell, 1980). Along with giving abused wives an explanation for their husband's violence, the alcohol attribution also gives them hope that, if their mates could stop drinking, the violence would also cease (Browne, 1987; Frieze & Knoble, 1980; Walker, 1984).

Sonkin and Durphy (1985), in their work with violent men, also suggest that aggressive men may use substances such as alcohol or recreational drugs in part to dull the guilt and sadness they feel for their abuse of loved ones, but this connection is hard to establish since other evidence of contrition appears to decrease over time (Walker, 1984).

Treatment Programs for Abusive Men

Social learning theory has been the approach used by most treatment groups for assaultive men. In part, these groups operate by challenging the abuser's rationalization system that excuses or denies the violence. While acknowledging the formative role of background and situational events in shaping personal response patterns, it also stresses choice and responsibility for individual action (Browne & Dutton, 1990). This emphasis creates a therapeutic imperative for the counselor to repeatedly challenge statements by the abuser that his violence was caused by an external force (such as his wife), a short-term circumstance, or an uncontrollable predisposition. In addition, most treatment groups attempt to identify and confront more ingrained beliefs such as general attitudes toward women, beliefs about power in intimate relationships, and beliefs about partriarchy (Edelson, Syers & Brygger, 1987).

Psychologically based treatment for men who abuse their intimates has also been more recently undertaken. Although much of the current literature has pointed to the importance of social and cultural factors, the focus of most treatment has been on the personality or skill deficits of the batterer. This focus has come in spite of the lack of clear evidence for a personality profile that can be attributed to all batterers (Pence & Shepard, 1988). Many practitioners have concluded that a supportive environment that allows for the sharing of feelings and for teaching interpersonal skills is an important element of treatment for batterers (Ganley, 1981; Purdy & Nickle, 1981; Star, 1983). Waldo (1987) describes a treatment group for male batterers: the group attempts to overcome resistance to treatment, trains members in basic anger management, covers methods for improving personal adjustment, and focuses on the development of relationship skills.

Of course, participation in a treatment group does not guarantee a successful change in each individual. The hazard of such groups is that, if men remain at risk for violence despite treatment, their partners may be imperiled while falsely believing that the abuser is "cured" (Browne & Dutton, 1990; Sonkin, 1986). It is imperative that the facilitators of treatment programs for male abusers (1) make it clear to both the men and their partners that the risk of assaultive behavior may still exist; (2) provide linkages for the women with resources for safety and support; and (3) remain in contact with the women victims as a means of knowing if the violence has truly ended or if other coercive behaviors have taken its place.

Several recent studies on the effectiveness of treatment programs for abusive men have been completed (Dutton, 1987; Edelson et al., 1987; Saunders & Hanusa, 1984). In general, nonviolence after treatment is reported for from 64% to 85% of the men. However, treatment groups reach only a small proportion of men who abuse female partners. Much more work needs to be done on understanding and intervening with abusers, if we are ever effectively to alleviate intimate violence against women.

What Do Answers to This Question Tell Us?

In a recent special issue of *Violence and Victims* on wife assaulters, the editors (Sonkin & Dutton, 1988) note that research on men who assault their wives is in an infancy stage and suffers from a lack of organization. Compared with the research available on battered women, this is certainly true. Possible explanations for this discrepancy are the relative inaccessibility of the batterer and the feminist researcher's reluctance to interact with batterers in a nonjudgmental manner.

The research that has been done suggests that different questions need to be asked as we continue to explore the motivations of the batterer and the causes of his behavior. First, it is clear that there is more than one type of batterer. Given the prevalence of wife abuse, it would be surprising if all men who assault their partners shared a distinctive personality or came from a single type of family background. Some researchers have attempted to delineate types of batterers on the basis of clinical interviews or statistical analyses (Caesar, 1986; Elbow, 1977). Others have differentiated men who were violent toward their wives from men who were generally violent (Dutton, 1988; Gondolf, 1984; Hanneke, Shields & McCall, 1981).

Three types of assaulters were described by Saunders (1987). The most severely violent abuser was violent inside and outside the home and abused alcohol as well. A second type had high scores on depression, jealousy, and anger, while a third type was characterized by moderate levels of anger and depression and denial of these emotions.

Hastings and Hamberger (1988) suggest that batterers may be differentiated on the basis of alcohol use. In their data, the alcohol-abusive batterers were more moody, sullen, and psychologically isolated than nonalcoholic batterers. Abusers with alcohol problems were also more likely to have witnessed or experienced abuse as a child than were the nonalcoholic batterers.

As with research on battered women, research on the men is based on different underlying questions. Early studies of incarcerated batterers focused on psychopathology. Studies relying on reports of women in shelters focus more on the lack of control and the use of alcohol by the men—variables that are directly observable by the women. Studies of court-mandated treatment groups may overrepresent severely violent men (Dutton, 1988). Future work needs to consider more carefully the effects of the sample and the underlying questions and assumptions being made.

CHALLENGES TO EXISTING QUESTIONS

Should We Be Asking Other Questions?

Although most of this chapter has discussed violence within marriages and battered or abused wives, there are many other situations in which interpersonal violence occurs. These include violence in dating relationships, postmarital violence, and violence within homosexual couples. The recent "discovery" of high levels of violence in nonmarital, intimate relationships suggests that previous perspectives on marital violence have not allowed us to understand this phenomenon fully.

Violence in Nonmarital, Heterosexual Relationships

Many of the studies of battered wives have found that the violence within the couple started before the marriage ceremony took place, during the dating or courtship period (Pagelow, 1984; Walker, 1983). However, such research often relies on retrospective reports of events occurring many years ago.

Other research has focused more specifically on violence occurring in non-marital intimate relationships. In an early, often-cited study, Makepeace (1981) called attention to previously unexamined levels of violence in premarital het-erosexual relationships. An expanding literature on dating violence confirms Makepeace's (1981) contention that dating violence is as extensive as marital violence. In one study in the southern part of the United States, Deal and Wampler (1986) found that 47% of their college sample had some experience with violence in dating relationships. Many of this group had been involved in a series of violent relationships. Drawing upon another southern U.S. sample, Rose and Marshall (1985) and Marshall and Rose (1987) also found that high percentages of college students had been recipients of violence or had been aggressors with dates. In their sample, 52% of the respondents had had some experience with dating violence, and 38% had engaged in violence with their current dating partner. Slightly lower percentages of students from New York reported dating violence (Arias, Samios, & O'Leary, 1987), as have those from other parts of the country (Cate, Henton, Koval, Christopher, & Lloyd, 1982; Makepeace, 1981; Stets & Pirog-Good, 1987). The prevalence rates for experience of inter-personal violence range from 12% among high school students (Henton et al., 1983) to the 57% reported by Rose and Marshall (1985). High levels of inter-personal violence appear to exist among high school and college students.

In addition to estimating the incidence of premarital violence, research has investigated the direction and the type of violence. Carlson (1987) concluded that both males and females are perpetrators and recipients of violent acts. A high percentage of the aggressive acts occurring in a dating couple are recip-rocated (Bernard & Bernard, 1983). Billingham and Sack (1986) argue that the violence should be viewed in terms of abusive relationships rather than abusive individuals and that violence within courtship should be viewed as a breakdown in attempts at conflict resolution, rather than as a phenomenon in and of itself. However, others have concluded, based on empirical data, that violence against women—rather than violence against men—is a serious problem in dating re-lationships (Stets & Pirog-Good, 1987). Makepeace (1983) argues that questions regarding the reciprocity of violence and the prevalence of female-perpetrated violence are not relevant in dating relationships. In his research, males were more likely to have used every specific type of violent tactic than were females. The rate of expressed (as opposed to received) violence was over 2.5 times higher in males than in females.

The "discovery" of premarital violence in couples raises several important issues. Many of our ideas about when and why intimate violence occurs are challenged by these findings. Makepeace (1983) argues that the dating violence literature raises important questions about our previous interpretations of intimate violence and about our existing theories of causation of family violence.

Others have similarly observed that studies of marital abuse may have limited utility for understanding dating violence (Firestein, 1988). For example, Makepeace (1983) discussed the fact that the specific life events that are associated with spouse abuse (i.e., in-law problems, children-related conflict) are relevant not to college dating relations, but to other life events (i.e., academic problems, peer rejection) and may influence levels of expressive violence in males. Makepeace (1983) reported a significant direct relationship between the amount of undesirable life change and courtship violence for males only. Jealousy has been frequently cited by both respondents and theorists as an explanation for dating violence. In another example, research focusing on the psychology of battered wives suggested that they are socially isolated and that they have low levels of self-esteem. Based on her clinical experience, Goodwin (1988) questions whether college women involved with abusive boyfriends have low levels of self-esteem or suffer from social isolation. In an empirical investigation, Firestein (1988) found that women who had experienced violence in their dating relationships did not differ in perceived support from women reporting no relationship violence. Violence was somewhat associated, however, with lower self-esteem and with higher levels of psychological distress.

Not surprisingly, women who experience violence in their dating relationships report less satisfaction with the quality of that relationship and more frequent conflict (Firestein, 1988). These findings suggest the need to reexamine the question, Why does she stay? Many of the reasons theorized or documented for staying in an abusive marriage do not logically extend to staying in an abusive dating relationship. Most specifically, the arguments involving the sanctity of marriage or the stigma of divorce are not applicable. Further, individuals involved in dating relationships are not typically financially dependent on their partners and, in most cases, have another residence and/or someplace to stay. Typically, children and concerns about child custody would not be involved. Thus, reasons for staying, such as love, having a boyfriend, investment in relationship, and difficulties terminating the relationship, need to become the focus of future research.

The existence of high levels of dating and cohabiting violence suggests the need to examine relationship investment as an explanation for relationship continuation. Researchers have found that violence and male sexual aggression were more likely to occur in serious courtship relationships (Cate et al., 1982; Laner & Thompson, 1982; Russell, 1982; Stets & Pirog-Good, 1987) or to occur more frequently in relationships of longer duration (Firestein, 1988; Stets & Pirog-Good, 1987). For example, Cate and her colleagues (1982) found that 47% of their respondents first experienced violence during serious dating, 25% during engagement or cohabitation, and 28% during casual dating. Billingham and Sack (1986) interpreted their results as indicating that a certain degree of intimacy had to be present in a dating relationship before significant increases in verbal aggression occurred. Although most of their respondents were not physically violent, those most likely to resort to violence were those subjects with some emotional involvement and those who had discussed marriage but had no definite plans. Mason and Blankenship (1987) also found abuse to occur most frequently between more committed couples.

Lesbian Battering

Recent research has suggested that we have ignored other victims of relationship violence—battered lesbians. Because research to date has been limited to a few studies (Kelly & Warshafsky, 1987; Renzetti, 1987) and articles in gay and lesbian newsletters, the incidence rates of abuse in lesbian relationships has been difficult to determine. Bologna and his colleagues (1987) have estimated that physical aggression occurs in 40% of lesbian relationships. The recent documentation that lesbian women are often abused by other women (Bologna, Waterman & Dawson, 1987; Lobel, 1986; Renzetti, 1987) raises new questions for researchers and requires us to readdress old questions.

Why has previous research on intimate abuse ignored homosexual populations? Several reasons for the lack of information on lesbian battering have been proposed. Lobel (1986) suggests that battered lesbians, like battered women in general, are reluctant to admit the abuse and may feel ashamed, frightened, and unable to seek help. Abuse may be particularly difficult to admit in a community that views itself as feminist, nonviolent, and/or utopian (Hart, 1989). Lesbians also may be loath to report the problem to a "helping" community that they already perceive as homophobic. Concerns that heterosexuals would associate lesbianism with violence and abuse have also been raised (Kelly & Warshafsky, 1987).

Thus, there are some plausible explanations for why lesbian abuse victims have not sought clinical intervention and research attention. But why did it not occur to clinicians and researchers to explore the incidence of abuse in lesbian relationships or to seek out lesbians as a comparison group for heterosexual relationships? One explanation is the operation of heterosexism in the selection of research questions and populations. Lesbians have remained "invisible" in the psychological literature, even as we have attempted to study women's experiences. The problems experienced by lesbians are not seen as important as those experienced by heterosexual women, and they are not seen as "informing" us about the nature of human relationships. The failure to investigate abuse in lesbian relationships also exposes some assumptions of researchers about the nature of perpetrators and victims and challenges many of our theoretical explanations for sexual violence.

Misconceptions about battered lesbians seem to parallel those of battered wives (Myers, 1989). Lesbian women who belong to minority groups, who are uneducated, and who are unemployed are perceived to be more likely to be involved in abusive relationships. Research to date suggests that this perception is not accurate. Battered lesbians come from all races, educational levels, and employment statuses (Renzetti, 1987). The existence of battered lesbians also challenges our view of the battered woman as one who subscribes to traditional gender and marital roles. It would be interesting to investigate the gender role and relationship role perspectives of battered lesbians relative to other lesbians and to heterosexual women in nonviolent relationships.

Lesbian battering is a hidden phenomenon due, in part, to the stereotypic beliefs we have about batterers. Since the vast majority of batterers among heterosexual couples are men and women are more often overpowered physically by their abusers, one is led to believe that battering among females would be nonexistent. Unlike abuse within the heterosexual community, the lesbian batterer is often of equal size and strength as her victim (Lobel, 1986; Myers, 1989). Further, Bologna et al. (1987) reported that lesbians in their sample were more likely than gay men to be perpetrators of violence.

Many of our theories and popular conceptions about the factors causing or contributing to wife abuse do not hold up as explanations for lesbian battering. For example, explaining wife abuse in terms of the aggressive nature of males or in terms of the institutional or legal aspects of marriage cannot be applied to abuse in lesbian relationships.

Battered Women Research: Asking the Right Questions?

As we have attempted to demonstrate in this chapter, the questions that researchers ask channel the data they look at and the conclusions that they will be able to draw. No one set of questions is right or wrong. In writing this chapter, we found that the three authors disagreed about which of the approaches outlined was the most productive or most correct. Although we cannot make recommendations about the best way to do good research on battered women, we do agree that researchers need to be aware of the implications of the questions being asked and the underlying assumptions being made about the phenomenon being investigated.

The review also suggests that the research process and the questions researchers investigate are strongly influenced by societal assumptions, by the accessibility and accuracy of respondents, by priorities of the funding sources, and by personal biases and perspectives. Only a small portion of the research conducted has investigated questions that battered women themselves might ask. Few studies have investigated battered women's own conceptions of their experience.

Recent research suggests that battered women are not homogeneous, but diverse, not only in age, class, race, and ethnicity, but also in marital status and sexual orientation. More attention needs to be given to these differences. Each of these variables provides an additional context to the violence that must be identified and interpreted as we attempt to better understand the battering experiences of women.

Assumptions about women and gender roles have also kept us from ''seeing'' some women who are battered by their intimates. The "discovery" of dating violence and battered lesbians not only exposes our conceptual blinders, but also reiterates the prevalence of battering in close relationships. Despite overwhelming evidence of the widespread nature of woman battering, many researchers have resisted moving to a structural or cultural perspective. Few studies have investigated woman battering in relation to patriarchal ideology or status inequalities.

Intervention efforts continue to be focused on the individual or dyad. Research has typically not examined the effectiveness of the different intervention strategies. The only outcome of interest to researchers has been the battered women's departure from the domicile or relationship. Recently this focus has been questioned (Bennett, Silver & Ellard, in press). Some research has indicated that the batterer continues his assaults on the same/or another woman even after termination of the relationship, divorce, and physical relocation efforts.

As court-mandated treatment programs have made samples of batterers available for research, more research and intervention effort have become focused on the batterer. Until recently, the design of clinical interventions has been based primarily on theory since little research on the batterer had been conducted. This is changing, but the research needs to become more sophisticated. Like battered women, batterers have been viewed as a homogeneous group. But, unlike the recipients of their assaults, batterers have not been held responsible; researchers have examined a variety of excuses for male violence, including prior victimization and alcohol use. Only a small portion of the existing literature views battering as an intentional behavior designed to achieve the goals of the assailant.

Thus, the research on battered women has not been particularly feminist. Feminist research examines women's experiences from the perspective of women themselves. The questions and the responses of women are central to the research endeavor. The feminist researcher advocates for woman rather than blaming her; feminist research is used to improve the conditions and status of women. McHugh, Koeske, and Frieze (1986) also suggest that nonsexist research should consider multiple and complex models of causation. Research on battered women has typically been conducted within a single explanatory framework (i.e., family systems or individual pathology) and has not examined complex interactive models.

This review of the battered women research demonstrates the extensiveness of the literature and the broad range of questions addressed. Today we know a lot more about battering, but we have not yet been able to effectively address the problem.

Perhaps there are new questions, too, that need to be addressed. Some that we find especially exciting are the relationship of nonphysical violence and abuse to physical aggression. Are these two aspects of the same basic behavior, or is psychological abuse fundamentally different from physical abuse? A related issue is whether sexual violence and physical violence against women are related, and if so, in what ways. Researchers are just beginning to look seriously at both of these types of violence together (Frieze, 1987; Koss, 1990). We also need to know more about how violence begins in an intimate relationship. How do relationships change as violence becomes a part of the interaction style of the couple? Does violence come from certain types of love feelings for the partner? How does the presence of violence early in a relationship affect the feelings of the participants for one another?

REFERENCES

Adams, D. (1988). Treatment models of men who batter: A profeminist analysis. In K. Yllo & M. Bograd (Eds.), *Feminist perspectives on wife abuse* (pp. 176–200). Beverly Hills: Sage.

Arias, I., Samios, M., & O'Leary, D. (1987). Prevalence and correlates of physical aggression during courtship. *Journal of Interpersonal Violence, 2*, 82–90.

Bard, M., & Sangrey, D. (1979). *The crime victim's book.* New York: Basic Books.

Bennett, T. L., Silver, R. C., & Ellard, J. H. (in press). Coping with an abusive relationship: I. How and why do women stay? *Journal of Marriage and the Family.*

Berk, R. A., Berk, S. F., Loseke, D. R., & Rauma, D. (1983). Mutual combat and other family violence myths. In D. Finkelhor, R. J. Gelles, G. T. Hotaling, & M. A. Straus (Eds.), *The dark side of families: Current family violence research* (pp. 197–212). Beverly Hills: Sage.

Berk, S., & Loseke, D. (1981). Handling family violence: Situational determinants of police arrest in domestic disturbances. *Law and Society Review, 15*(2), 317–344.

Bernard, M. L., & Bernard, J. L. (1983). Violent intimacy: The family as a model for love relationships. *Family Relations, 32*, 283–286.

Billingham, R. E., & Sack, A. R. (1986). Courtship violence and the interactive status of the relationship. *Journal of Adolescent Research, 1*, 315–325.

Block, C. R., & Block, R. L. (1984). Crime definition, crime measurement, and victim surveys. *Journal of Social Issues, 40*(1), 137–160.

Bograd, M. (1988). Feminist perspectives on wife abuse: An introduction. In K. Yllo & M. Bograd (Eds.), *Feminist perspectives on wife abuse.* Beverly Hills: Sage.

Bologna, M. J., Waterman, C. K., & Dawson, L. J. (1987, July). *Violence in gay male and lesbian relationships: Implications for practitioners and policy makers.* Paper presented at the Third National Conference for Family Violence Researchers, Durham, NH.

Borkowski, M., Murch, M., & Walker, V. (1983). *Marital violence: The community response.* London: Tavistock.

Bowker, L. H. (1983). *Beating wife-beating.* Lexington, MA: Lexington Books.

Bowker, L. H. (1984). Coping with wife abuse: Personal and social networks. In A. R. Roberts (Ed.) *Battered women and their families* (pp. 168–191). New York: Springer.

Breines, W., & Gorden, L. (1983). The new scholarship on family violence. *Signs: Journal of Women in Culture and Society, 8*(3), 490–531.

Browne, A. (1987). *When battered women kill.* New York: Macmillan.

Browne, A. (1989, November). *Are women as violent as men?* Response to gender differences in violence as a function of context and method by M. A. Straus. Commentary at the meeting of the American Society of Criminology, Reno, NV.

Browne, A., & Dutton, D. G. (1990). Escape from violence: Risks and alternatives for abused women. In R. Roesch, D. G. Dutton, & V. F. Sacco (Eds.), *Family violence: Perspectives in research and practice* (pp. 67–91). Simon Fraser University Press.

Browne, A., & Williams, K. R. (1989). Exploring the effect of resource availability and the likelihood of female-perpetrated homicides. *Law and Society Review, 23*, 75–94.

Browne, A., & Williams, K. R. (in press). Gender, intimacy, and lethal violence: Trends from 1976–1987. *Gender & Society.*

Brush, L. D. (1990). Violent acts and injurious outcomes in married couples: Methodological issues in the National Survey of Families and Households. *Gender & Society, 4*, 56–67.

Caesar, P. L. (1986). Men who batter: A heterogeneous group. In L. K. Hamberger (Chair), *The male batterer: Characteristics of a heterogeneous population.* Symposium conducted at the meeting of the American Psychological Association, Washington, DC.

Caesar, P. L. (1988). Exposure to violence in the families-of-origin among wife abusers and maritally nonviolent men. *Violence and Victims, 3*, 49–64.

Caplan, P. (1984). The myth of women's masochism. *American Psychologist, 39*, 130–139.

Carlson, B. E. (1987). Dating violence: A research review and comparison with spouse abuse. *Social Casework: The Journal of Contemporary Social Work, 68*, 16–23.

Cate, R., Henton, J. M., Koval, J., Christopher, F. S., & Lloyd, S. (1982). Premarital abuse: A social psychological perspective. *Journal of Family Issues, 3*, 74–90.

Chandler, S. (1986). *The psychology of battered women.* Unpublished doctoral dissertation, Department of Education, University of California, Berkeley.

Chimbos, P. D. (1978). *Marital violence: A study of interspousal homicide.* San Francisco: R & E Research Associates.

Coates, D., & Winston, T. (1983). Counteracting the deviance of depression: Peer support groups for victims. *Journal of Social Issues, 39*(2), 169–194.

Coleman, D. H., & Straus, M. A. (1983). Alcohol abuse and family violence. In E. Gottheil, A. Durley, I. E. Skolada, & H. M. Waxman (Eds.), *Alcohol, drug abuse and aggression* (pp. 104–123). Springfield, MA: C. C. Thomas.

Coleman, D. H., & Straus, M. A. (1986). Marital power, conflict, and violence in a nationally representative sample of American couples. *Violence and Victims, 1*, 141–157.

Coley, S. A., & Beckett, J. O. (1988). Black battered women: A review of empirical literature. *Journal of Counseling and Development, 66*, 266–270.

Cook, O. R., & Cook, A. (1984). A systematic treatment approach to wife battering. *Journal of Marriage and Family Therapy, 10*, 83–93.

Daly, M. (1979). *Gyn/Ecology.* London: Women's Press.

Deal, J. E., & Wampler, K. S. (1986). Dating violence: The primacy of previous experience. *Journal of Social and Personal Relationships, 3*, 457–471.

Deschner, J. P. (1984). *The hitting habit.* New York: Free Press.

Dobash, R. E., & Dobash, R. P. (1978). Wives: The "appropriate" victims of marital violence. *Victimology, 2*, 426–442.

Dobash, R. E., & Dobash, R. P. (1979). *Violence against wives.* New York: Free Press.

Dobash, R. E., & Dobash, R. P. (1984). The nature and antecedents of violent events. *British Journal of Criminology, 24*, 269–288.

Dobash, R. E., & Dobash, R. P. (1988). Research as social action: The struggle for battered women. In K. Yllo & M. Bograd (Eds.), *Feminist perspectives on wife abuse* (pp. 51–74). Newbury Park, CA: Sage.

Dutton, D. G. (1987). The criminal justice response to wife assault. *Law and Human Behavior, 2,* 189–206.

Dutton, D. G. (1988). Profiling of wife assaulters: Preliminary evidence for a trimodal analysis. *Violence and Victims, 3,* 5–30.

Dutton, D. G., & Browning, J. J. (1988). Concern for power, fear of intimacy and wife abuse. In G. T. Hotaling, D. Finkelhor, J. T. Kirkpatrick, & M. Straus (Eds.), *New directions in family violence research*. Beverly Hills: Sage.

Dutton, D., & Painter, S. L. (1983). Traumatic bonding: The development of emotional attachments in battered women and other relationships of intermittent abuse. *Victimology, 6,* 139–155.

Dutton, D. G., & Strachan, C. E. (1987). Motivational needs for power and spouse-specific assertiveness in assaultive and nonassaultive men. *Violence and Victims, 2,* 145–156.

Dvoskin, J. A. (1981). *Battered women—An epidemiological study of spousal violence.* Unpublished doctoral dissertation, University of Arizona.

Edelson, J. L., Syers, M., & Brygger, M. P. (1987, July). *Comparative effectiveness of group treatment for men who batter.* Paper presented at the Third National Family Violence Conference, Durham, NH.

Elbow, M. (1977). Theoretical considerations of violent marriages. *Social Casework, 58,* 515–526.

Ewing, W., Lindsey, M., & Pomerantz, J. (1984). *Battering: An AMEND Manual for Helpers.* Denver, CO: Littleton Heights College.

Fields, M. D. (1978). Does this vow include wife-beating? *Human Rights, 7*(20), 40–45.

Figley, C. R. (Ed.). (1985). *Trauma and its wake: The study and treatment of post-traumatic stress disorder.* New York: Brunner/Mazel.

Finkelhor, D. (1983). Common features of family abuse. In D. Finkelhor, R. J. Gelles, G. T. Hotaling, & M. A. Straus (Eds.), *The dark side of families: Current family violence research* (pp. 11–16). Beverly Hills: Sage.

Finkelhor, D., & Yllo, K. (1983). Rape in marriage: A sociological view. In D. Finkelhor, R. J. Gelles, G. T. Hotaling, & M. A. Straus (Eds.), *The dark side of families: Current family violence research* (pp. 119–131). Beverly Hills: Sage.

Finn, J. (1985). The stresses and coping behavior of battered women. *Social Casework: Journal of Contemporary Social Work, 66,* 341–349.

Fiora-Gormally, N. (1978). Battered wives who kill. Double standard out of court, single standard in? *Law and Human Behavior, 2,* 133–165.

Firestein, B. A. (1988). *The relationship of abuse and social support to the psychological health of college women in dating relationships.* Paper presented at the annual meeting of the Association for Women in Psychology, Bethesda, MD.

Fiske, S. T., & Taylor, S. E. (1984). *Social cognition.* Reading, MA: Addison-Wesley.

Fitzpatrick, J. P. (1974). Drugs, alcohol, and violent crime. *Addictive Disorders, 1,* 353–367.

Forward, S., & Torres, J. (1986). *Men who hate women and the women who love them.* New York: Bantam.

Frieze, I. H. (1979). Perceptions of battered wives. In I. H. Frieze, D. Bar-Tal, & J. S.

Carroll (Eds.), *New approaches to social problems: Applications of attribution theory* (pp. 79–108). San Francisco: Jossey-Bass.

Frieze, I. H., (1983). Investigating the causes and consequences of marital rape. *Signs*, *8*, 532–553.

Frieze, I. H. (1987). The female victim: Rape, wife beating, and incest. In Gary R. VandenBos & Brenda K. Bryant (Eds.), *Cataclysms, crises, and catastrophes*: *Psychology in action* (pp. 109–146). Washington, DC: American Psychological Association.

Frieze, I. H., & Browne, A. (1989). Violence in marriage. In L. Ohlin & M. H. Tonrey (Eds.), *Crime and justice—An annual review of research* (pp. 163–218). Chicago: University of Chicago Press.

Frieze, I. H., Hymer, S., & Greenberg, M. S. (1987). Describing the crime victim: Psychological reactions to victimization. *Professional Psychology*, *18*, 299–315.

Frieze, I. H., & Knoble, J. (1980). *The effects of alcohol on marital violence*. Paper presented at the annual meeting of the American Psychological Association, Montreal.

Frieze, I. H., Knoble, J., Washburn, C., & Zomnir, G. (1980). *Types of battered women*. Paper presented at the Annual Research Conference of the Association for Women in Psychology, Santa Monica, CA.

Frieze, I. H., & McHugh, M. C. (1981). *Violence in relation to power in marriage*. Paper presented at the annual meeting of the American Psychological Association, Los Angeles.

Ganley, A. (1981). *Court-mandated counseling for men who batter*. Washington, DC: Center for Women Policy Studies.

Ganley, A. L., & Harris, L. (1978). *Domestic violence: Issues in designing and implementing programs for male batterers*. Paper presented at the annual meeting of the American Psychological Association, Toronto.

Gelles, R. J. (1974). *The violent home: A study of physical aggression between husbands and wives*. Beverly Hills: Sage.

Gelles, R. J. (1976). Abused wives: Why do they stay? *Journal of Marriage and the Family*, *38*(4), 659–668.

Gelles, R. J. (1979). *Family violence*. Beverly Hills: Sage.

Gelles, R. J., & Straus, M. A. (1988). *Intimate violence*. New York: Simon & Schuster.

Gellman, M. T., Hoffman, R. A., Jones, M., & Stone, M. (1984). Abused and nonabused women: MMPI profile differences. *Personnel and Guidance Journal*, *62*, 601–604.

Giles-Sims, J. (1983). *Wife battering: A systems theory approach*. New York: Guilford Press.

Goldstein, D., & Rosenbaum, A. (1985). An evaluation of the self-esteem of maritally violent men. *Family Relations*, *34*, 425–428.

Gondolf, E. (1984). *Men who batter: How to stop abusing their wives*. Paper presented at the Family Violence Researchers Conference, University of New Hampshire, Durham.

Gondolf, E. (1985). *Men who batter: An integrated approach for stopping wife abuse*. Holmes Beach, FL: Learning.

Gondolf, E., & Fisher, E. R. (1988). *Battered women as survivors: An alternative to treating learned helplessness*. Lexington, MA: Lexington Books.

Goode, W. J. (1971). Force and violence in the family. *Journal of Marriage and the Family*, *33*, 624–636.

Goodwin, B. (1988). *Unlearning victimization: Working with victims in a college counseling center.* Paper presented at the meeting of the Association for Women in Psychology, Bethesda, MD.

Guerney, B. (1987). Wife battering: A theoretical construct and case report. *American Journal of Family Therapy*, *15*, 34–43.

Guralnik, D. B. (Ed.). (1984). *Webster's New World Dictionary.* New York: New American Library.

Hamberger, L. K., & Hastings, J. E. (1986, November). *Characteristics of male spouse abusers: Is psychopathology part of the picture?* Paper presented at the meeting of the American Society of Criminology, Atlanta, GA.

Hanneke, C. R., Shields, N. M., & McCall, G. J. (1981). *Patterns of family and non-family violence: An approach to the study of violent husbands.* Paper presented at the First Conference for Family Violence Research, Durham, NH.

Hart, B. (1989). *Assessing lethality.* Paper presented to the Domestic Violence Conference, Pittsburgh.

Hastings, J. E., & Hamberger, L. K. (1988). Personality characteristics of spouse abusers: A controlled comparison. *Violence and Victims*, *3*, 31–48.

Henton, J., Cate, R., Koval, J., Lloyd, S., & Christopher, F. S. (1983). Romance and violence in dating relationships. *Journal of Family Issues*, *4*, 467–482.

Hilberman, E., & Munson, K. (1978). Sixty battered women. *Victimology*, *2*, 460–471.

Hornung, C. A., McCullough, B. C., & Sugimoto, T. (1981). Status relationships in marriage: Risk factors in spouse abuse. *Journal of Marriage and the Family*, *43*, 675–692.

Hotaling, G. T., & Sugarman, D. B. (1986). An analysis of risk markers in husband to wife violence: The current state of knowledge. *Violence and Victims*, *1*, 101–124.

Hughes, H. M., & Barad, S. J. (1983). *Psychological functioning of battered women and their children: A preliminary investigation.* Paper presented at the 91st Annual Meeting of the American Psychological Association, Anaheim, CA.

Jones, A. (1980). *Women who kill.* New York: Fawcett Columbine Books.

Kalmuss, D. S., & Seltzer, J. A. (1986). Continuity of marital behavior in remarriage: The case of spouse abuse. *Journal of Marriage and the Family*, *48*, 113–120.

Kaufman, M. (1987). *Beyond patriarchy: Essays by men on pleasure, power and change.* Toronto: Oxford.

Kelly, L. (1988). How women define their experiences of violence. In K. Yllo & M. Bograd (Eds.), *Feminist perspectives on wife abuse* (pp. 114–132). Newbury Park: Sage.

Kelly, C., & Warshafsky, L. (1987, July). *Partner abuse in gay and lesbian couples.* Paper presented at the Third National Conference for Family Violence Researchers, Durham, NH.

Klaus, P. A., & Rand, M. R. (1984). *Family violence.* Washington, DC: Bureau of Justice Statistics, U.S. Department of Justice.

Kleckner, J. H. (1978). Wife beaters and beaten wives: Co-conspirators in crimes of violence. *Psychology*, *15*(1), 54–56.

Koss, M. P. (1990). The women's mental health research agenda. *American Psychologist*, *45*, 374–380.

Kurz, D. (1989). Social science perspectives on wife abuse: Current debates and future directions. *Gender and Society*, *3*, 489–505.

Laner, M. R., & Thompson, J. (1982). Abuse and aggression in courting couples. *Deviant Behavior: An Interdisciplinary Journal*, *3*, 229–244.

Langan, P. A., & Innes, C. A. (1986). *Preventing domestic violence against women*. Washington, DC: Bureau of Justice Statistics, U.S. Department of Justice.

Lewin, T. (1979). When victims kill. *National Law Journal*, *2*, 2–4, 11.

Lobel, K. (Ed.). (1986). *Naming the violence: Speaking out about lesbian battering*. Seattle, WA: Seal Press.

Lystad, M. (1986). Interdisciplinary perspectives on family violence: An overview. In M. Lystad (Ed.), *Violence in the home: Interdisciplinary perspectives* (pp. xi-xxxv). New York: Brunner/Mazel.

Makepeace, J. M. (1981). Courtship violence among college students. *Family Relations*, *30*, 97–102.

Makepeace, J. M. (1983). Life events stress and courtship violence. *Family Relations*, *32*, 101–109.

Margolin, G. (1979). Conjoint marital therapy to enhance anger management and reduce spouse abuse. *American Journal of Family Therapy*, *7*, 13–23.

Marshall, L. L., & Rose, P. (1987). Gender, stress and violence in the adult relationships of a sample of college students. *Journal of Social and Personal Relationships*, *4*, 299–316.

Mason, A., & Blankenship, V. (1987). Power and affiliation motivation, stress, and abuse in intimate relationships. *Journal of Personality and Social Psychology*, *52*, 203–210.

Mayfield, D. (1976). Alcoholism, alcohol, intoxication, and assaultive behavior. *Diseases of the Nervous System*, *37*, 288–291.

McHugh, M. C., Koeske, R. D., & Frieze, I. H. (1986). Issues to consider in conducting nonsexist psychological research: A guide for researchers. *American Psychologist*, *41*, 879–890.

McIntyre, D. (1984). Domestic violence: A case of the disappearing victim? *Australian Journal of Family Therapy*, *5*(4), 249–258.

Miller, D. T., & Porter, C. A. (1983). Self-blame in victims of violence. *Journal of Social Issues*, *39*(2), 139–152.

Mitchell, R. E., & Hodson, C. A. (1982). *Battered women: The relationship of stress, support, and coping to adjustment*. Paper presented at the meeting of the American Psychological Association, Washington, DC.

Myers, B. A. (1989). *Lesbian battering: An analysis of power inequality and conflict in lesbian relationships*. Unpublished doctoral dissertation, Department of Psychology, Indiana University, Indiana, PA.

Neidig, P. H., & Friedman, D. H. (1984). *Spouse abuse: A treatment program for couples*. Champaign, IL: Research Press.

Nicol, A. R., Gunn, J. C., Gristwood, J., Foggitt, R. H., & Watson, J. P. (1973). The relationship of alcoholism to violent behavior resulting in long-term imprisonment. *British Journal of Psychiatry*, *123*, 47–51.

Nisonoff, L. & Bitman, I. (1979). Spouse abuse: Incidence and relationship to selected demographic variables. *Victimology*, 4, 131–140.

Novaco, R. (1976). The functions and regulation of the arousal of anger. *American Journal of Psychiatry*, *133*(1), 1124–1128.

Pagelow, M. D. (1977). *Secondary battering: Breaking the cycle of domestic violence.* Paper presented at the annual meeting for the Sociologists for Women in Society Section of the American Sociological Association, California.

Pagelow, M. D. (1980). *Double victimization of battered women: Victimized by spouses and the legal system.* Paper presented at the annual meeting of the American Society of Criminology, San Francisco.

Pagelow, M. D. (1981). *Woman-battering: Victims and their experiences.* Beverly Hills: Sage.

Pagelow, M. D. (1984). *Family violence.* New York: Praeger.

Palau, N. (1981). *Battered women: A homogenous group? Theoretical considerations and MMPI data interpretation.* Paper presented at the annual meeting of the American Psychological Association, Los Angeles.

Patterson, G. (1982). *Coercive family processes.* Eugene, OR: Cataglia Press.

Pence, E., & Shepard, M. (1988). Integrating feminist theory and practice: The challenge of the battered women's movement. In K. Yllo & M. Bograd (Eds.), *Feminist perspectives on wife abuse* (pp. 282–298). Beverly Hills: Sage.

Plass, P. S., & Straus, M. A. (1987). *Intra-family homicide in the United States: Incidence, trends, and differences by religion, race, and gender.* Paper presented at the Third National Family Violence Research Conference, University of New Hampshire, Durham.

Porter, C. A. (1983). *Coping and perceived control in battered women.* Unpublished doctoral dissertation, Department of Psychology, University of British Columbia, Vancouver.

Ptacek, J. (1988). Why do men batter their wives? In K. Yllo & M. Bograd (Eds.), *Feminist perspectives on wife abuse* (pp. 133–157). Beverly Hills: Sage.

Purdy, F., & Nickle, N. (1981). Practice principles for working with groups of men who batter. *Social Work with Groups, 4,* 111–112.

Radford, L. (1987). Legalizing woman abuse. In J. Hanmer & M. Maynard (Eds.), *Women, violence and social control.* London: Macmillan.

Renzetti, C. (1987). *Violence in lesbian relationships: A preliminary analysis of causal factors.* Paper presented at the Annual Meeting of the American Society of Criminology, Montreal.

Rhodes, D., & McNeill, S. (1985). *Women against violence against women.* London: Onlywomen Press.

Rich, A. (1979). *On lies, secrets, and silence.* New York: Norton.

Richardson, D. C., & Campbell, J. L. (1980). Alcohol and wife abuse: The effects of alcohol on attributions of blame for wife abuse. *Personality and Social Psychology Bulletin, 6,* 51–56.

Ridington, J. (1978). The transition process: A feminist environment as reconstructive milieu. *Victimology, 3,* 563–575.

Romero, M. (1985). A comparison between strategies used on prisoners of war and battered wives. *Sex Roles, 13,* 537–547.

Rose, P., & Marshall, L. L. (1985). *Gender differences: Effects of stress on expressed and received abuse.* Paper presented at the annual meeting of the American Psychological Association, Los Angeles.

Rosenbaum, A., & O'Leary, K. D. (1981). Marital violence: Characteristics of abusive couples. *Journal of Consulting and Clinical Psychology, 49,* 63-71.

Rosewater, L. B. (1988). Battered or schizophrenic: Psychological tests can't tell. In K. Yllo and M. Bograd (Eds.), *Feminist perspectives on wife abuse* (pp. 200–216). Newbury Park, CA: Sage.

Rounsaville, B. (1978). Theories in marital violence: Evidence from a study of battered women. *Victimology: An International Journal, 3*, 11–31.

Rouse, L. P. (1984). Models of self-esteem, and locus of control as factors contributing to spouse abuse. *Victimology, 9*(1), 130–144.

Roy, M. (1977). Research project probing a cross-section of battered women. In M. Roy (Ed.), *Battered Women: A Psychosociological Study of Domestic Violence*. New York: Van Nostrand Reinhold Co.

Roy, M. (1982). *The abusive partner: An analysis of domestic battering*. New York: Van Nostrand Reinhold Co.

Russell, E. H. (1982). *Rape in Marriage*. New York: MacMillan.

Saunders, D. G. (1986). When battered women use violence: Husband-abuse or self-defense? *Victims and Violence, 1*, 47–60.

Saunders, D. G. (1987). *Are there different types of men who batter? An empirical study with possible implications for treatment*. Paper presented at the Third National Conference for Family Violence Researchers, Durham, NH.

Saunders, D. G., & Hanusa, D. R. (1984). *Cognitive-behavioral treatment for abusive husbands: The short term effects of group therapy*. Paper presented at the Second National Conference on Family Violence Research, Durham, NH.

Saunders, D. G., Lynch, A. B., Grayson, M., & Linz, D. (1987). The inventory of beliefs about wife beating: The construction and initial validation of a measure of beliefs and attitudes. *Violence and Victims, 2*, 39–57.

Schecter, S. (1982). *Women and male violence: The visions and struggles of the battered women's movement*. Boston: South End.

Schneider, A. (1980). Methodological problems in victim surveys and their implications. In J. Dahman & J. Sasty (Eds.), *Victimology Research Agenda Development (Vol. 1)*. McLean, VA: The Mitre Corporation.

Schulman, M (1979). *A survey of spousal violence against women in Kentucky*. (Study #792701 for the Kentucky Commission on Women). Washington. DC: U. S. Department of Justice—LEAA.

Sedlak, A. J. (1983). The use and psychosocial impact of a battered women's shelter. Paper presented at the Annual Meeting of the American Psychological Association, Anaheim, CA.

Shainess, N. (1977). Psychological aspects of wife-battering. In M. Roy (Ed.), *Battered Women* (pp. 111–119). New York: Van Nostrand Reinhold Co.

Shaud, K. A. (1983). *The bind of the battering relationship: A study of learned helplessness and no-win binds in battered women*. Paper presented at the Annual Meeting of the American Society of Criminology, Denver.

Sherman, L. W., & Berk, R. A. (1984). The specific deterrent effects of arrest for domestic assault. *American Sociological Review, 49*, 261–272.

Snell, J., Rosenweld, R., & Robey, A. (1964). The wife beater's wife: A study of family interaction. *Archives of General Psychology, 11*, 107–112.

Sobell, L. C., & Sobell, M. B. (1975). Drunkenness, a special circumstance in crime and violence, sometimes. *International Journal of the Addictions, 10*, 869–882.

Sonkin, D. J. (1986). Clairvoyance vs. common sense: Therapist's duty to warn and protect. *Violence and Victims*, *1*(1), 7–22.

Sonkin, D. J. (1988). The male batterer: Clinical and research issues. *Violence and Victims*, *3*, 65–g79.

Sonkin, D. J., & Dutton, D. G. (Eds.). (1988). Special issue on wife assaulters. *Violence and Victims*, *3*.

Sonkin, D., & Durphy, M. (1982). *Learning to live without violence: A handbook for men*. San Francisco: Volcano Press.

Sonkin, D., & Durphy, M. (1985). *Learning to live without violence: A handbook for men* (Rev. ed.). San Francisco: Volcano Press.

Sonkin, D. J., Martin, D., & Walker, L. E. A. (Eds.). (1985). *The male batterer: A treatment approach*. New York: Springer.

Spender, D. (1980). *Manmade language*. London: Routledge & Kegan Paul.

Star, B. (1983). *Helping the abuser: Intervening effectively in family violence*. New York: Family Service Association.

Stark, E., Flintcraft, A., Zuckerman, D., Grey, A., Robinson, J., & Frazier, W. (1981). *Wife abuse in the medical setting: An introduction in health personnel*. (National Clearinghouse on Domestic Violence Monograph Series No. 7). Washington, DC: National Clearinghouse on Domestic Violence.

Steinmetz, S. (1977). *The cycle of violence: Assertive, aggressive and abusive family interaction*. New York: Praeger.

Stets, J. E., & Pirog-Good, M. A. (1987). Violence in dating relationships. *Social Psychology Quarterly*, *50*, 237–246.

Straus, M. A. (1978). Wife beating: How common and why? *Victimology*, *2*, 443–458.

Straus, M. A. (1979). Measuring intrafamily conflict and violence: The Conflict Tactics (CT) scales. *Journal of Marriage and the Family*, *41*, 75–88.

Straus, M. A. (1980). Victims and aggressors in marital violence. *American Behavioral Scientist*, *23*, 681–704.

Straus, M. A., & Gelles, R. J. (1986). Societal change and change in family violence from 1975 to 1985. *Journal of Marriage and the Family*, *48*, 465–479.

Straus, M. A., Gelles, R. J., & Steinmetz, S. K. (1980). *Behind closed doors: Violence in the American family*. Garden City, NY: Doubleday.

Szinovacz, M. E. (1983). Using couple data as a methodological tool: The case of marital violence. *Journal of Marriage and the Family*, *45*, 633–644.

Totman, J. (1978). *The murderess: A psychosocial study of criminal homicide*. San Francisco: R & E Research Associates.

Virkkunen, M. (1974). Alcohol as a factor precipitating aggression and conflict behavior leading to homicide. *British Journal of Addictions*, *69*, 149–154.

Waites, R. E. (1978). Female masochism and the enforced *restriction* of choice. *Victimology*, *3*, 535–544.

Waldo, M. (1987). Also victims: Understanding and treating men arrested for spouse abuse. *Journal of Counseling and Development*, *65*, 385–388.

Walker, L. E. (1978). Battered women and learned helplessness. *Victimology*, *3*, 525–534.

Walker, L. E. (1979). *The battered woman*. New York: Harper & Row.

Walker, L. E. (1983). The battered woman syndrome study. In D. Finkelhor, R. J. Gelles, G. T. Hotaling, & M. A. Straus (Eds.), *The dark side of families: Current family violence research* (pp. 31–48). Beverly Hills: Sage.

Walker, L. E. (1984). *The battered woman syndrome*. New York: Springer.

Walker, L. E., & Browne, A. (1985). Gender and victimization by intimates. *Journal of Personality, 53*(2), 179–195.

Wardell, L., Gillespie, D., & Leffler, A. (1983). Science and violence against women. In D. Finkelhor, R. J. Gelles, G. T. Hotaling, & M. A. Straus (Eds.), *The dark side of families: Current family violence research* (pp. 69–84). Beverly Hills: Sage.

Wilbanks, W. (1982). Murdered women and women who murder. In N. H. Rafter & E. A. Stanko (Eds.), *Judge, lawyer, victim, thief: Women, gender roles and criminal justice*. Boston: Northeastern University Press.

Wilbanks, W. (1983). The female homicide offender in Dade County, Florida. *Criminal Justice Review, 8*(2), 9–14.

Wolfgang, M. E. (1958). *Patterns in criminal homicide*. New York: John Wiley and Sons.

Wolfgang, M. E. (1967). A sociological analysis of criminal homicide. In M. E. Wolfgang (Ed.), *Studies in homicide*. New York: Harper & Row.

Wolfgang, M. E., & Strohm, R. B. (1957). The relationship between alcohol and criminal homicide. *Quarterly Journal of Studies on Alcohol, 17*, 411–425.

Yllo, K. (1983). Sexual equality and violence against wives in American states. *Journal of Comparative Family Studies, 14*, 67–86.

Yllo, K. (1984). The status of women, marital equality, and violence against wives. *Journal of Family Issues, 5*, 307–320.

Yllo, K. (1988). Political and methodological debates in wife abuse research. In K. Yllo & M. Bograd (Eds.), *Feminist perspectives on wife abuse* (pp. 28–50). Newbury Park, CA: Sage.

Yllo, K., & Bograd, M. (Eds.). (1988). *Feminist perspectives on wife abuse*. Newbury Park, CA: Sage.

15

Breaking Silence: The Sexual Harassment of Women in Academia and the Workplace

Louise F. Fitzgerald and Alayne J. Ormerod

> The sound of silence breaking makes us understand what we could not hear before. But the fact that we could not hear does not prove that no pain existed.
>
> —Sheila Rowbotham,
> "Women's Consciousness, Man's World"

In a society where the sexual victimization of women is so widespread as to have been effectively invisible, sexual harassment is the last great open secret. Although all women know of it and most will experience it, until recently it had no name, a situation that contributed to its continuation, for it is not possible to complain of that for which there are no words. In its broadest terms, sexual harassment refers to the "imposition of sexual requirements in the context of a relationship of unequal power" (MacKinnon, 1979, p. 1). Originally thought to be limited to those relatively rare situations where women are threatened with their jobs to extort sexual cooperation, it is now understood more broadly as the inappropriate sexualization of an otherwise nonsexual relationship, an assertion by men of the primacy of a woman's sexuality over her role as worker or student.

In these pages, we review what is known about this particularly pernicious form of sexual exploitation, noting throughout our discussion the many similarities between sexual harassment and other forms of sexual victimization, not only in the secrecy that surrounds them but in the mythology that supports them. As with acquaintance rape, the phenomenon to which it bears perhaps the closest resemblance, we shall see that sexual harassment has been mystified as natural sexual or romantic attraction, society has blamed women for its occurrence, and, most insidiously, women have blamed themselves.

We begin our discussion by reviewing the extensive debate on definitional issues and the consequences of this debate for measurement and the development of sound epidemiological studies. We consider the various theories advanced to explain sexual harassment, as well as victim characteristics, that is, the factors that place women at highest risk for this form of victimization, and the contexts in which harassment is most likely to occur. Finally, we examine the ways in which women have responded to harassment and review the research on the outcomes or consequences of this process for the women who experience it. We conclude our discussion with a consideration of methodological issues and suggestions for future research, attempting to balance the tension between traditional social science research and the feminist understanding that seeks to transform it while producing an analysis that is true to both.

THE EXPERIENCE OF SEXUAL HARASSMENT

Definitions

Definitional issues have plagued the study of sexual harassment since its inception. The sources of this ambiguity are many and varied, but share at their core a deeply rooted societal reluctance to acknowledge the pervasive victimization of women or to accept women's accounts and descriptions of these experiences. Women who claim to have been harassed are discounted in many ways, often on the basis that they are overly sensitive; for example, the man involved didn't mean to offend them, they can't take a joke, or they didn't suffer any negative consequences. Such issues of severity, intentionality, and outcomes are raised, not just in casual or informal discussions, but in scholarly ones as well. Thus, one of the original tasks in this area was to create a shared definition that could then be used as the basis for theory building and research. Although progress has been made, such a shared definition is still not completely within our grasp. Since definitions are the source of operationalizations, each new study has tended to develop its own methodology, yielding a literature that is littered with conflicting estimates of incidence rates, behaviors, and other forms of noncomparable data. Among the problems that this has created has been the diminished credibility of these studies within the legal system and a lessening of the impact of this research as a vehicle for social change.

Definitions developed to date have been of two varieties, those that are stated a priori (theoretical definitions) and those that are constructed from investigation of individuals' judgments or perceptions of sexual harassment, that is, empirical definitions (Fitzgerald, 1990). A priori definitions are not data-based, but rather are derived from theoretical propositions about harassment. Such efforts generally consist of descriptive statements concerning the nature of harassment and the status relationships of the persons involved or consist of a list of specific actions thought to constitute the behavioral domain. This type of definition is most often offered by legal and regulatory bodies or by women's political or professional organizations. Examples include the extremely influential guidelines published by the United States Equal Employment Opportunity Commission (U.S. Equal Opportunity Commission [EEOC], 1980), which have guided much subsequent sexual harassment litigation, as well as statements from various influential professional organizations. Harassment on the basis of sex is a violation of Sec. 703 of Title VII of the United States Civil Rights Act. According to the EEOC guidelines, unwelcome sexual advances, requests for sexual favors, and other verbal or physical conduct of a sexual nature constitute sexual harassment when

1. submission to such conduct is made either explicitly or implicitly a term or condition of an individual's employment,

2. submission to or rejection of such conduct by an individual is used as the basis for employment decisions affecting such individual, or

3. such conduct has the purpose or effect of unreasonably interfering with an individual's work performance or creating an intimidating, hostile or offensive working environment. (EEOC, 1980)

Empirical definitions, on the other hand, are, as the name implies, data-based and most generally developed and used by researchers. They are derived from women's descriptions of their experiences of harassment, which are then categorized, and the categories are used as the elements of the definition. An alternate empirical approach utilizes data from consensus ratings concerning whether a given behavior constitutes sexual harassment. This latter method can be generally thought of as a policy-capturing approach, the most elaborate of which has recently been offered by York (1989).

The most complete and influential definition of the empirical sort was developed by Till (1980), who classified the responses to an open-ended sexual harassment survey of college women and derived five categories of generally increasing severity:

1. *Gender Harassment*: generalized sexist remarks and behavior

2. *Seductive Behavior*: inappropriate and inoffensive, but essentially sanction-free behavior; that is, there is no penalty attached to noncompliance

3. *Sexual Bribery*: solicitation of sexual activity or other sex-linked behavior by promise of rewards

4. *Sexual Coercion*: coercion of sexual activity by threat of punishment

5. *Sexual Imposition or Assault*: gross sexual imposition (e.g., touching, fondling, grabbing) or assault

As can be determined from the above discussion, neither of these types of definitions is entirely satisfactory. The theoretical, or a priori, definitions usually identify the conditions under which a behavior may constitute harassment, but generally do not give "pointatable" examples. Empirical definitions, on the other hand, rely on the responses of individuals asked for either their experiences or their perceptions of various events. Such definitions are limited to the data provided by a particular sample and thus often lack important principles or elements, such as the issues of consent, status differential, and sexuality that are necessary for identification and classification. Further, given the pervasive denial of the reality of sexual harassment, social consensus or policy-capturing approaches are often quite limited. At best, such definitions are overly influenced by various demographic and attitudinal characteristics, the best example being the large and reliable gender differences in social perceptions of harassment.

In an attempt to address some of these issues, Fitzgerald (1990) has offered a rational-empirical definition drawn both from theory and from Till's data-based classification system. This definition states:

Sexual harassment consists of the sexualization of an instrumental relationship through the introduction or imposition of sexist or sexual remarks, requests or requirements, in the context of a formal power differential. Harassment can also occur where no such formal differential exists, if the behavior is unwanted by or offensive to the woman. Instances of harassment can be classified into the following general categories: gender harassment, seductive behavior, solicitation of sexual activity by promise of reward or threat of punishment, and sexual imposition or assault. (Fitzgerald & Ormerod, 1991)

This definition includes both a rational, theoretical description of the nature and elements of harassment and an enumeration of types of harassment based on an empirically derived classification scheme. It addresses contextual issues by assuming that all sexist or sexual behaviors constitute harassment when they occur within the framework of a formal power differential, since the woman is not considered able either to consent or to resist freely. When the participants are of equal formal power, it is the recipient's reactions that constitute the defining factor.

Measurement

Given that measurement devices are inherently a form of definition, it is not surprising that attempts to actually collect data on sexual harassment have been burdened with many of the difficulties experienced by the definitional efforts described above. In addition, the seriousness of sexual harassment as a social problem created a critical need for data that could serve as the basis for policy decisions by government, university, and other decision makers. Thus, early studies were concerned with developing estimates of the extent and severity of the problem and afforded little attention to traditional measurement issues that would be necessary for more controlled and fine-grained analysis. More recently, these issues have been receiving increased attention in the literature (Fitzgerald, 1990) and have resulted in at least one inventory that attempts to meet standard psychometric criteria of reliability and validity (Fitzgerald & Shullman, 1985; Fitzgerald et al., 1988). Known as the Sexual Experiences Questionnaire (SEQ), this inventory provides data on each of Till's (1980) categories of sexual harassment based solely on the individual's endorsement of behaviorally based items without reference to the words *sexual harassment*. Three forms of the SEQ are currently available (one version for use with students, and the other two for use with employed women); a complete description of the development of the SEQ is available in Fitzgerald et al. (1988).

Dimensions

In addition to developing definitions of harassment, researchers have attempted to examine its structure and to identify the various dimensions that are encompassed by the construct. It has been widely accepted, although only rarely tested, that sexually harassing behaviors exist on a continuum of severity beginning with sexist or sexual comments and extending through actual sexual assault. Till's data reported above appear to conform to this model, although no formal test was performed. An alternative structure was suggested some years ago by MacKinnon (1979), who made the distinction between quid pro quo behaviors— those that are based on the notion of required sexual exchange—and those that constitute conditions of work—unwanted and offensive sexual behavior that is present in the workplace but that is not attached to punishment or reward.

Early attempts to confirm Till's (1980) five-level severity model were not successful (Fitzgerald et al., 1988), as factor analyses of SEQ data—which are explicitly derived from the Till model—yielded not five factors, but three: gender harassment, sexual harassment (seductive behavior and sexual imposition), and sexual coercion (bribery and threat). More recently, we were able to confirm the five-factor model in a large sample of faculty and graduate students, using data based on ratings of behavior rather than incidence reports (Fitzgerald & Ormerod, 1991).

Padgitt and Padgitt (1986) explicitly tested the continuum hypothesis and reported that their data (ratings of eight sexually harassing behaviors) did not conform to such a structure until three items were removed, thus implicitly disconfirming the continuum model. Recently, Fitzgerald and Hesson-McInnis (1989) criticized this model as too simplistic and explicitly tested the hypothesis that sexual harassment is a multidimensional construct. Using pair-comparison data of 20 situations drawn from the SEQ, this multidimensional scaling analysis yielded a two-dimensional solution: severity of harassment and type of harassment, where type conformed to MacKinnon's distinction between quid pro quo and conditions of work. In addition, gender harassment emerged as a clearly distinct construct, which was related to, but separate from, other forms of harassment.

Incidence Rates

By far the great majority of research on sexual harassment has investigated the issue of prevalence, addressing such questions as how widespread the phenomenon is, what types of harassment are experienced most frequently, and so forth. Although our previous discussions imply that harassment is a relatively common experience for women, it has been difficult to ascertain exactly how widespread it is. In this respect, it is similar to other forms of victimization such as rape and childhood sexual abuse, in which various factors combine to produce underreporting and underestimates. In addition, the lack of a clear definition and sexual harassment's multidimensional nature have added further complexity to this issue.

Despite such difficulties in converging on a reliable estimate, several major studies and numerous smaller ones suggest that the parameters of such an estimate are not entirely unknown. The present discussion will focus on three major investigations, each of which samples a different population of interest.

In what is clearly the largest and probably the best-known study conducted so far, the United States Merit Systems Protection Board (U.S. Merit Systems Protection Board [Merit Systems], 1981) investigated harassment in the federal workplace and indicated that 42% of all female employees reported being sexually harassed. Merit Systems noted that many incidents occurred repeatedly, were of long duration, and had a sizable practical impact, costing the government an estimated minimum of $189 million over the two-year period covered by the study. When explicit behaviors were examined, 33% of the women reported receiving unwanted sexual remarks, 28% reported suggestive looks, and 26% reported being deliberately touched. These behaviors were classified as less severe forms of harassment. When more severe incidents were examined, 15% of the women reported experiencing pressure for dates, 9% reported being directly pressured for sexual favors, and 9% had received unwanted letters and telephone calls. One percent of the sample had experienced actual or attempted rape or assault. Merit Systems repeated their study in 1987 and reported essentially identical results.

The most extensive study of the civilian workplace was conducted by Gutek (1985). Based on telephone interviews generated through random digit-dialing procedures, Gutek reported that 53% of her women subjects had experienced at least one incident that they considered harassing during their working lives, including insulting comments (19.8%); insulting looks and gestures (15.4%); sexual touching (24.2%); socializing expected as part of the job (10.9%); and expected sexual activity (7.6%). The actual incidence rates for these behaviors were considerably higher; our discussion utilizes figures only for those behaviors that the women considered to be harassing. Although the differences between the Gutek and Merit Systems methodology make comparisons difficult, their overall estimates are fairly comparable, that is, (very) approximately half the female work force has been harassed during their working lives.

With respect to the harassment of university women, an extensive study of academia was recently completed by our research group (Fitzgerald et al., 1988), in which we studied nearly 2,000 women at two major state universities. Once again, nearly half of the women reported experiencing some form of sexually harassing behavior. With respect to particular types of experiences, approximately 35% of these students had experienced some form of gender harassment by their professors or instructors; 15% reported being the targets of seductive behavior; approximately 5% had been either bribed or threatened to induce sexual cooperation; and 9% reported some form of sexual imposition, from unwanted touching and fondling to outright sexual assault. As with the two studies reported previously, methodological differences render any but the most general of comparisons untenable.

In summary, although generalizations are extremely difficult given the nature of the available data, it seems reasonable (if not conservative) to estimate that one out of every two women will be harassed at some point during her academic or working life, thus indicating that sexual harassment is the most widespread of all forms of sexual victimization studied to date.

Perceptions

There is a relatively well-developed literature concerning what might best be thought of as the appraisal process (Lazarus & Folkman, 1984); that is, by whom and when will a particular incident be perceived and labeled as sexual harassment? In our first study, we found that although approximately 50% of women endorsed items indicative of harassment, less than 10% of the subjects reported that they had been sexually harassed. Similar, if less extreme, results were reported by Gutek (1985).

Perceptions of this phenomenon have been found to be influenced by the gender of the perceiver; the severity and explicitness of the behavior; the status of the initiator; the degree of prior relationship between the individuals involved; the behavior of the victim; and various attitudes of the perceiver, most notably his or her attitudes about feminism. Of these variables, gender has clearly proven to be the most robust (Collins & Blodgett, 1981; Fitzgerald & Ormerod, 1991; Padgitt & Padgitt, 1986; Powell, 1986), with women universally more likely to label a given situation as harassing than men. Lee and Heppner's (1991) study found no gender differences in perceptions of sexual harassment, but the authors do note that this finding could be attributed to the fact that women comprised less than 20% of their sample.

Gender is not always the main determinant, however; the severity of the behavior has been shown to influence individual reactions regardless of gender. Not surprisingly, the more extreme and explicit the situation, the more likely it is to be viewed as harassment. Those behaviors previously labeled as quid pro quo, involving threats of retaliation for noncompliance, as well as sexual imposition or assault, are clearly viewed as harassment by both women and men

(Fitzgerald & Ormerod, 1991; Reilly, Carpenter, Dull, & Bartlett, 1982). In one study, we surveyed a large sample of faculty and graduate students and found that the mean ratings of situations depicting quid pro quo behaviors averaged 6.56 on a 7-point scale (where 7 indicated "definitely is sexual harassment"), with no rating falling below 6.00. Similarly, Konrad and Gutek (1986) reported that 94% of the men and 98% of the women in their sample agreed that "being asked to have sexual relations with the understanding that it would hurt your job situation if you refused or help if you accepted" was harassment.

When the situation is less explicit, however, or when the behaviors are portrayed as more "romantic" or seductive, both men and women become much less certain in their reactions. The same is true for situations of gender harassment. It is here that contextual variables such as the status of the initiator, the degree of prior relationships, and any so-called suggestive behavior on the part of the woman come into play, influencing the interpretation of these more ambiguous conditions of work. In our perceptions study, we found that the mean ratings of gender harassment items fell into the "uncertain" range of the scale.

Although most individuals are uncertain about these behaviors, gender differences remain remarked, with women consistently more likely to view them as harassing (Koenig & Ryan, 1986; Fitzgerald & Ormerod, 1991), offensive (Padgitt & Padgitt, 1986), or both. We noted that women appear to be more sensitive to issues of sexism in the classroom, offensive and suggestive jokes, and other incidents of gender harassment; they are also more likely to consider romantic or sexual attention directed at a student to be harassment even when there is no suggestion that refusing such overtures would lead to negative consequences.

Merit Systems (1981) analyzed their data on this topic by gender and other status characteristics and found that men and supervisors react similarly to each other, but differently than women and victims about expressions of sexual interest and the responsibility of victims for their own harassment. Men and supervisors showed more of a tendency to blame the victim and to believe that people shouldn't take offense so quickly about sexual attention at work. This is not surprising, given that most supervisors are men and most victims are women; it is, however, somewhat discouraging when one considers the fact that it is supervisors who are often responsible for responding to the woman's complaint or for sanctioning the harasser.

Federal workers in the Merit Systems studies (1981, 1987) also believed that supervisory status should influence sexually oriented behavior at work. Both men and women were more likely to consider a behavior harassment if it was initiated by a supervisor and felt that supervisors should be held to a higher standard of conduct than other workers. The influence of this variable has also been demonstrated by other investigators; Gutek, Morasch, and Cohen (1983), for example, found that behavior that might be tolerated from a coworker was considered harassing when initiated by a supervisor. These findings are apparently related to the widespread agreement concerning incidents of quid pro quo harassment, since supervisors presumably have the power to impose sanctions for noncooperation.

An additional, consistently powerful influence on individual perceptions of possibly harassing situations is the behavior of the woman involved. For example, Reilly et al. (1982) showed that any "suggestive" behavior on the part of a woman student consistently lowered harassment ratings of interactions that were otherwise identical; a similar effect was found when the parties were described as having been involved in a prior relationship. Thus, behavior that is otherwise inappropriate is seen as more acceptable if the woman has previously consented to intimacy or has in some way "asked for it" by her dress or behavior. The parallels with attitudes toward rape are quite striking here.

Brooks and Perot (1991) demonstrated that the frequency of low-level harassing behaviors, as well as the raters' degree of feminist ideology, predicted the likelihood of perceiving those behaviors as offensive. The finding that profeminist attitudes increase the likelihood that a given behavior will be perceived as harassing has also been demonstrated by other researchers (Pryor & Day, 1988; Schneider, 1982).

Finally, Lee and Heppner (1991) found that a sample of mostly male city supervisors and managers were more likely to rate sexual rather than nonsexual behaviors as harassing, and these ratings may be strongest for the most severe sexually harassing behaviors. Although Lee and Heppner developed their inventory to measure perceptions of whether behaviors meet the legal definition (e.g., EEOC criteria) of sexual harassment.

Theoretical Formulations

Although it is obvious that recent years have seen an explosion of interest in the topic of sexual harassment, most of this work has been strictly empirical in nature, and little in the way of formal theory has emerged. However, a few studies have attempted to test theoretical frameworks, and some progress has been made. This section of the chapter begins the examination of this theoretical work.

Tangri, Burt, and Johnson (1982) identified three broad models of sexual harassment from their review of the literature and attempted a partial test based on the initial Merit Systems (1981) data set. The natural/biological model suggests that sexual behavior in the workplace is simply a natural extension of human sexuality. Its assumptions include a natural, mutual attraction between men and women, a stronger male sex drive, and men in the role of sexual initiators. According to this position, harassing behavior is not meant to be offensive or discriminatory, but is merely the result of biological urges. Tangri et al. (1982) suggest that if this model is correct, women victims should be similar to their harassers in age, race, and other socially relevant characteristics; both parties should be unmarried or eligible as partners; the behaviors exhibited should closely resemble typical "courtship" behaviors; and, of course, the harasser should desist if the woman shows disinterest. Thus, this model implies that the concept of sexual harassment is a mistaken one; the relevant interactions are most appropriately viewed as courtship behavior.

The organizational model posits that sexual harassment is a "result of aspects of the workplace infrastructure that provide opportunities for sexual aggression" (Tangri et al., 1982, p. 38). From this perspective, harassment is a power issue, with power defined as formal and organizational in nature. Opportunities for harassment arise from the hierarchical manner in which organizations are structured and are unrelated to gender. According to this theory, powerful women may harass subordinate men, and such occurrences are rare only because women are generally employed in subordinate positions. If this theory is accurate, it is individuals in positions of little power, either men or women, who are most likely to be targets of harassing behavior (e.g., trainees, temporary or part-time workers, those on probation, low-income individuals, and so on).

Finally, the sociocultural model conceptualizes sexual harassment as the male domination of women in the workplace, a domination that reflects the more general patriarchal system in which men are the preeminent political and economic group. According to this model, victims of sexual harassment will, overwhelmingly, be female workers, particularly those in traditionally male-dominated occupations. From this perspective, harassment is conceptualized as the assertion of personal power, with power explicitly deriving from gender rather than from organizational status.

Tangri and her colleagues tested various predictions from these three models and reported that their analyses provided some support for both the organizational and sociocultural models. Given the usual confounding of gender and organizational status, it is probably not possible to obtain a completely clear-cut test of these competing explanations; in addition, as the authors point out, it is likely that sexual harassment is multidetermined. Further, as they discuss, the base rates for harassment are so high that it may not be possible to develop reliable predictors. However, as these authors' analyses make clear, the central issue is one of power rather than biology.

Another major theoretical effort has been that of Gutek (Gutek, 1985; Gutek & Morasch, 1982; Konrad & Gutek, 1986), whose sex-role spillover model suggests that when occupations are dominated by one sex or the other, the sex role of the dominant gender influences (i.e., "spills over") the work role expectations for that job. Gutek proposes that sexual harassment is more likely to occur in such occupations than in those that are more gender-balanced, but that the form of the harassment and the women's reactions to it differ depending upon which sex is numerically dominant.

For example, she suggests that when women predominate in an occupation, the sexual aspects of the female role may spill over into the work role; obvious examples would be in the occupation of flight attendant or cocktail waitress. According to this model, both men and the women themselves expect men to treat traditionally employed women primarily as women, not as workers. Thus, the theory predicts that sexual harassment, particularly of the seductive variety, will be high, but that the women will not label it as such nor consider it a problem because of the confounding of their sex role with their work role. In other words, sexuality is just a part of the job.

For the nontraditionally employed woman, on the other hand, sex role and work role conflict. When men respond to her sexually, she is likely to consider such treatment to be problematic. Sexuality is definitely not perceived as part of her job, and the woman is able to recognize that she is being treated differently than her (male) colleagues. Although Gutek draws on Kanter's (1977) seminal work concerning the behavior and treatment of tokens in developing her model, Baker (1989) has noted that one can actually derive different predictions concerning harassment from these two formulations. For example, Kanter's work leads to predictions that women in nontraditional blue-collar occupations will experience more sexually harassing behaviors than women in traditional jobs, whereas Gutek's model suggests that the frequency of the behaviors will either be the same for all gender-skewed groups or actually greater for traditionally employed women. In addition, Kanter's model implies that the woman's recognition of harassment should be directly related to the amount of sexually harassing behaviors experienced, whereas Gutek's theory predicts that the sex ratio of the job should be the determining factor in predicting recognition and labeling. Baker tested these competing predictions and reported that Kanter's formulations were more successful in accounting for the data among a sample of industrially employed women (Baker, 1989); this study is discussed in more detail below.

In her discussion, Baker (1989) points out:

Increasingly, researchers and theorists in the area are recognizing that no one factor or variable can account for or explain all of the aspects of how, why and when sexual harassment occurs. Simple assertions that harassment is an expression of male power which serves to keep women in subordinate positions are being replaced with efforts to determine the relative impact of various factors and types of factors (i.e., situational, societal or individual) on the occurrence and effects of sexual harassment. (p. 38)

Reviewing theoretical frameworks that attempt meta-explanations of sexual harassment has brought home the wisdom of this statement to us rather clearly.

THE VICTIMS OF SEXUAL HARASSMENT

Gender

A large proportion of the early sexual harassment research was directed at identifying factors that placed individuals at risk for sexual harassment. Although much of this work is confusing and contradictory, it had the effect of clearly establishing that sexual harassment is overwhelmingly a woman's problem. The original Merit Systems (1981) report found that of the 462,000 individuals in their sample of the federal work force who had experienced sexual harassment, over two-thirds were women; other studies make clear that this is a serious underestimate. For example, we (Fitzgerald et al., 1988) demonstrated that, with the exception of gender harassment (e.g., sexist comments, jokes, and so on), virtually all the harassment reported by our sample of over 3,000 college students was reported by women. Given the way the items were phrased, it is not clear whether the gender harassment that was reported by the male subjects was directed at them personally or was actually directed at women and observed by the men.

This is not to deny that occasional instances of reverse harassment do occur and are very distressing to the individual men involved. Still, it is clear that this is a highly unusual event (not surprising in a culture where women are directly socialized not to be sexually assertive and deviations from this norm are subject to considerable levity and even ridicule). It is, in fact, exactly the extreme counter-normativeness of such behavior that makes it the focus of such extensive attention. Far more common than these occurrences, however, are studies showing that men interpret women's behaviors as sexual when, in fact, they are not. For example, Saal, Johnson, and Weber (1989) recently replicated and extended Abbey's (1982) research demonstrating that male observers see more "sexiness" in women's behavior than do female observers; women observers were more likely to interpret a particular behavior as "friendly," an interpretation similar to that given by the women "targets" themselves when they were asked to describe the characteristics they were attempting to project. These authors suggest that this difference in social perceptions may account for some incidents of sexual harassment, in that men may misinterpret a woman's behavior as being a sexual invitation. It seems to us equally reasonable to suggest that this tendency to sexualize women's behavior may also account for many instances where men report being sexually harassed by women, a suggestion similar to that made by Gutek (1985).

Age

In the workplace, it appears that younger women are more often the target of harassment (Gutek, 1985; Merit Systems, 1981, 1987), and the younger the worker, the more likely she is to be harassed. Gutek (1985) reported that the women targets she studied were often younger than the average worker; of the women in her sample who had experienced sexual harassment, over half were less than 35 years old. Similar findings are reported in both Merit Systems (1981, 1987) studies, with workers less than 34 years of age most often the targets of harassment. Other studies report similar results (Baker, 1989; LaFontaine & Tredeau, 1986).

Despite the relative consistency of the data indicating that younger women are at greater risk for harassment, we believe that this may represent somewhat of an oversimplification. Despite the apparent importance of age as a risk factor, it is clear that the experience of sexual harassment is not limited to younger women. Not only do all age groups report experiencing harassment, but the practice of utilizing the median to divide the sample into younger and older workers renders the data sample-specific and thus somewhat arbitrary. More informative practice would be simply to sort subjects into a priori categories (e.g., less than 25, 26–30, 31–35, 36–40, and so on), the procedure followed by the Merit System researchers. Probably more importantly, studies rarely examine what sorts of harassment are experienced by which groups of women. For example, gender harassment would reasonably be expected to demonstrate a weaker relationship to age. Finally, most investigations confound the experience of sexual harassment with the recognition or labeling of harassment, variables that likely bear differential relationships to age. Thus, although younger women do appear to be at greater risk for sexual harassment, to conclude that the problem is limited to this group is erroneous.

Marital Status

Marital status also appears to be related to the experience of sexual harassment, with unmarried (divorced, separated, never-married, and cohabiting) women more often experiencing harassment than other (married, widowed) women. As with the variable of age, it is easy to overinterpret such data. Marital status is most likely a "dummy variable," representing one or more factors that are influential, for example, perceived "availability"; lack of the protected status of wife, particularly if the husband or partner is a powerful male; or, most likely, age itself.

Race

Few attempts have been made to examine whether and to what degree race and ethnic status influence a woman's risk of being sexually harassed. DeFour (1990) has speculated that various myths concerning the sexuality of ethnic women (for example, that Hispanic women are "fiery" or passionate, or that black women are sexually promiscuous) may place them at greater risk than other women by providing the harasser with a rationale for his approach. Similarly, she argues that the economic vulnerability of many ethnic women makes it more difficult for them to resist unwelcome advances. Despite the intuitive appeal of these arguments, at this point they remain largely unexamined, most likely because most samples have not contained enough women of ethnic minority status to allow them to be tested.

Gutek's (1985) report of harassment in a large, scientifically selected sample of the Los Angeles County work force provides the best data so far available on this question, as approximately one-third of her 824 women respondents were non-Caucasians. Gutek reported that, in this group, the minority women were no more vulnerable to harassment than other women and, in fact, were actually less likely to report quitting a job because of it. However, as she points out, "A variety of factors may contribute to these findings; minority women may report fewer of their experiences and Caucasian women may represent the cultural standard of attractiveness" (p. 56). Clearly, this is still a largely unexplored area.

Sexual Orientation

If studies of the sexual harassment of minority women are rare, those examining harassment of lesbian women are practically nonexistent. In this respect, the sexual harassment literature parallels other areas of psychology, including all too often the psychology of women. This is an unfortunate state of affairs, as even informal observation suggests that lesbian women (to the degree they are known) are quite likely at high risk for harassment. For example, D'Augelli (1988) notes the extremely high levels of harassment and sexual and other assault of homosexual individuals simply on the grounds that they are homosexual. Among the incidents he reports is that of a woman who was sexually assaulted by assailants attempting to "rescue" her from her life-style (see also the report of the National Gay and Lesbian Task Force, 1986). Thus, it is reasonable to suggest that lesbian women are also at greater risk of other forms of victimization, such as sexual harassment. In the one study that addresses this issue directly, Schneider (1982) reported that the lesbian women in her sample indeed reported higher levels of all types of sexual approaches at work than did the heterosexual women. However, she cautions that in this case, age and sexual orientation were seriously confounded, with age also being a strong risk factor; thus, the causative factors are unclear. As with the issue of race, this is a critical area for further research.

Attitudes

Although most attitudinal studies in this area have examined individual beliefs about harassment and its nature and causes, a few efforts have been made to examine the attitudes and behaviors of the victim herself. The most extensive effort of this sort was that of Gutek (1985).

Gutek found that both men and women believe that women who are the target of sexual behavior in the workplace find such experiences flattering and complimentary. She also reported that the majority of individuals in her survey believed that these women encouraged advances by seductive dress or behavior and that they could prevent advances if they wanted to. However, women who had actually had such experiences reported that they found them insulting. In particular, women who had experienced various negative consequences of harassment, such as quitting or losing their job, had different attitudes about women's responsibility for sexual advances. They were less likely to believe that women caused overtures or to think that women dress or act seductively; rather, they were more likely to believe that sex-role expectations cause men to seek sex at work. (This parallels the finding of Brooks & Perot (1991), who reported that women who had experienced sexually harassing behavior more frequently were more likely to label such experiences as harassment.) Both targets and nontargets, however, did tend to hold women (other than themselves) responsible for propositions received at work.

Highly educated women (those with a college degree or higher) also tended to hold more liberal attitudes about social and sexual behavior at work. These women were more likely to report being insulted by propositions at work and to indicate that both men and women contributed equally to sexual overtures. It also appeared that divorced, separated, and cohabiting women were likely to view sex at work more traditionally, that is, as somewhat complimentary.

Finally, as might be expected, attitudes toward feminism and attitudes toward sexual harassment (i.e., personal definitions of harassment) also influence the ways in which women structure their experiences. Women with profeminist attitudes seem more likely to label behaviors that they have experienced as sexual harassment or as personally offensive (Brooks & Perot, 1991; Pryor & Day, 1988) especially when these behaviors occur within the framework of seduction or gender harassment (Schneider, 1982).

Summary

It appears that although certain characteristics appear to be stronger predictors of harassment than others, women of all ages, races, marital statuses, and so forth are harassed. Gender is by far the most powerful predictor of victimization; other characteristics pale by comparison and may or may not be present in any given case. As previously discussed, sexual harassment is an extensive phenomenon in both the workplace and academic environment; as with any extremely high-frequency behavior, the best prediction is simply that it will occur. Tangri, et al. (1982) have noted, "[Sexual harassment] may approximate a random event in women's working lives—something which is highly likely to happen at some time, with just when, where and how being so multi-determined that prediction is difficult" (p. 52).

This being so, we are disturbed by what appears to us to be a tendency in the literature to inappropriately conceptualize victim characteristics as explanations for sexual harassment, rather than as risk factors. Research that asks, "Was she young?" or "Was she attractive?" runs the risk of misportraying harassment as legitimate sexual or romantic interest, although it is by now clear that the great majority of harassment is not of this type. Most harassment is not designed to elicit sexual cooperation, but rather to insult, exploit, and degrade; approaches that are indeed sexual in nature are experienced as offensive, humiliating, and frightening by the women who receive them. Similarly, studies that focus on what the recipient was wearing or how she responded (e.g., "Did she appear to be flattered?'') not only perpetuate sexual mythology but in addition place responsibility for the behavior on the victim. We are not suggesting that research on victim characteristics and reactions is not important; it should be very clear from this review that we believe that it is critical. However, we are concerned that such variables not be erroneously conceptualized as explanations for harassment. From a feminist perspective, it seems very important that these variables be conceptualized, labeled, and discussed very carefully as the risk factors that they are.

THE ORGANIZATIONAL/INSTITUTIONAL CONTEXT OF SEXUAL HARASSMENT

Even before the data on incidence rates were well understood, the research on sexual harassment generally subscribed to the view that the phenomenon is a social issue of serious, if as yet unclear, proportions. Thus, most writers on this topic have demonstrated, at least implicitly, a concern with understanding causal influences so that they can be altered or eradicated. As we noted previously, early studies focused on defining the phenomenon and demonstrating its existence and extent; other investigations examined possible causes that had been proposed, such as human nature (what Tangri et al., 1982, called ''the natural/ biological model''), biology (i.e., men's supposedly ''naturally'' greater sexual interest or assertiveness), or socialization. However, as Baker (1989) pointed out, theories subscribing to the causative influence of such macrovariables as biology or socialization of necessity imply that the phenomenon is not easily amenable to intervention. Thus, some researchers turned their attention to situational or environmental factors that may serve to sustain harassing behaviors. ''This . . . asserts that it is necessary neither to change human nature, nor to raise a whole new generation of women and men. Instead, such explanations suggest that we can reduce or eliminate the target behavior [by] changing organizational rules or laws, altering sex ratios in various settings, altering the distribution of power, and so forth'' (Baker, 1989). Consistent with this concern with women's practical and political reality, this section of the chapter examines what is presently known about various contextual or structural factors and the effect they have on women's experiences.

Occupational Group Differences

Some studies have attempted to examine group differences in the experience of harassment; however, until recently, the results of these efforts have been difficult to interpret. In one study (Fitzgerald et al., 1988), we reported that women who were employed in a university setting (faculty, staff, and administrative women) were more likely to experience harassment than were women students in the same institution. In addition, we pointed out that these incidence rates were considerably lower than those generally found in the nonacademic workplace, although reasons for the differential incidence rates were not intuitively evident. Gold (1987), using similar SEQ methodology, reported that her sample of blue-collar tradeswomen experienced significantly and substantially higher levels of all types of harassment than did either white-collar professional women or pink-collar clerical women. LaFontaine and Tredeau (1986), using a different questionnaire, reported similar results for a sample of 160 women, all college graduates employed in what the authors described as traditionally male-dominated occupations (mostly engineering and management).

The majority of this research appears to have been guided by the assumption discussed above, that women in nontraditional occupations will experience greater harassment than other women. Unfortunately, much of this work has not operationalized the variable of nontraditionality in a systematic or careful way. For example, LaFontaine and Tredeau (1986) examined mainly managers and engineers, whereas Gold (1987) compared tradeswomen with secretaries and (mostly) lawyers and accountants. Although there is nothing problematic in such designs in and of themselves, it is difficult to compare them and impossible to identify the structural or environmental variables that are implicated without a clear specification of the rationale for the grouping (occupational) variable.

One study that has directly addressed these issues is that of Baker (1989), who studied a sample of 100 women employed in either traditional or nontraditional occupations, where traditionality was defined by the gender distribution in the work group. The traditional group was further divided into pink- and blue-collar workers, the pink-collar group consisting of secretaries and similar clerical workers, whereas the blue-collar group was composed of industrial workers. Thus, the final sample included nontraditional blue-collar workers (machinists), traditional blue-collar workers (production workers), and pink-collar workers (clerical). This design effectively separates the influence of gender representation (i.e., the relative number of women in the work group) from that of type of work (blue-collar or pink-collar) and is unique in its recognition that not all blue-collar occupations are nontraditional for women. The results clearly demonstrated that high levels of sexual harassment are associated with having low numbers of women in the work group. The machinists reported extremely high frequencies of all types of harassment, whereas the traditional blue-collar workers reported very low levels. The clerical women reported experiences that, while more extensive, were more similar to those of the traditional blue-collar workers than the nontraditional blue-collar workers. Interestingly, high levels of sexual harassment were not related to the number of men encountered in the workplace, but only to being part of a male-dominated work group, thus lending support to Kanter's (1977) theories concerning the treatment of tokens in the workplace. The women in the pink-collar and traditional blue-collar groups encountered just as many men as the machinists during the workday, but were treated differently. Baker's research suggests that as women approach numerical parity in various segments of the work force, harassment may decline, a prediction also made by sex-role spillover theory (Gutek, 1985).

Environmental Context and Organizational Norms

Although it is intuitively reasonable to suppose that institutional or organizational norms exert an important effect on individuals' behavior within that organization, this assumption is almost completely unexamined in the present case. To our knowledge, no published research has examined the effect of institutional policy on incidence or reporting rates, and little is actually known concerning the influence of what is generally referred to as organizational climate. One study that begins to examine these variables is that of Bond (1988), who studied the graduate school experiences of 229 female community psychologists. In addition to collecting frequency data on the occurrence of 15 sexually harassing events, Bond attempted to "better understand what qualities of the educational environment contribute to or inhibit sexual harassment" (p. 8). She collected data on six potentially important environmental variables: departmental norms concerning sexual relationships between faculty and students; formal acknowledgment of sexual harassment as an ethical issue, through such media as course coverage; the availability of formal complaint mechanisms; the percentage of women faculty; the percentage of women students; and the general supportiveness of the program to women's professional development. Using these variables as predictors, multiple regression procedures were used to predict the occurrence of both subtle and overt forms of harassment. Although other factors were marginally influential (e.g., percentage of women students, supportive professional environment), the most important predictor of both types of sexual harassment was departmental norms concerning sexual contact between faculty and students. Thus, organizational norms that communicate disapproval of such relationships may also serve to inhibit harassment of women students. Although accounting for only a small amount of the variance, these data do provide beginning evidence of the importance of ecological factors in supporting or inhibiting harassment, thus providing possible avenues for intervention.

Summary

Research on the role of environmental factors in maintaining the harassment of women is in its infancy, and most investigators still employ an individual level of analysis. The characteristics of individuals, both victim and harasser, have received much more attention than ecological or structural variables. Yet, as Fuehrer and Maitland-Schilling (1988) have pointed out, such analyses belie the prevalence data indicating the enormous number of women who experience this behavior. These writers propose that sociocultural explanations may be more powerful, suggesting as they do that harassment functions as a means of social control to keep women in a subordinate position (cf. Russell, 1984). They note:

This limiting of women's status in the workplace is seen as a natural response on the part of men to women's attempts to gain more power by leaving their appropriate places in the home, in order to achieve equality in the workplace. *By sexualizing interactions with women in the workplace, men call attention to women's sexuality, thereby detracting from women's work.* Ultimately, women's ambitions are curtailed. . . . Sexual harassment is viewed as an appropriate behavior for men within the context of typical patterns of relationships between powerful men and powerless women. And organizations, by advocating most strongly for the rights of their most powerful individual members, condone such actions. (p. 12, emphasis added)

The data that have been reviewed here concerning the high levels of harassment of women in occupations traditionally reserved to men, as well as the inhibiting effect of normative disapproval of the sexualization of the faculty-student relationship, are consistent with such an explanation. More critically, they suggest specific avenues for intervention, thus implying the practical importance of such research for improving women's educational and occupational lives.

RESPONSES TO SEXUAL HARASSMENT

Given the extent of sexual harassment, in both academia and the workplace, surprisingly little formal attention has been paid to the ways in which women respond to, and cope with, various forms of abuse, although it seems reasonable to suppose that such responses may mediate outcomes for the victim, possibly influencing both her immediate and her long-term well-being. Merit Systems (1987) reported that the majority of victims in their most recent study of the federal workplace either ignored the behavior or did nothing (53%), a strategy that was generally viewed as ineffective, whereas 61% of the women who asked or told the harasser to stop reported that this response "made things better." Fifteen percent of the victims reported the harasser to their supervisor, but less than half felt that this was an effective strategy. In Reilly, Lott, and Gallogly's (1986) study of college students, 61% of women victims ignored the behavior or did nothing, and 16% asked or told the person to stop, whereas only a tiny proportion sought any formal relief. Jennings and Metha (1981) report that their interviews of harassment victims indicated that those who reacted to the incident with anger were more likely to take external action; those whose primary emotional response was fear were more likely to ignore the behavior, blame themselves, and so on.

Even this brief review reveals that the research in this area remains in a rudimentary stage. With the exception of Jennings and Metha's study, what little data there are consist of responses to checklists of "commonsense" actions that might logically be considered reasonable responses to harassment, lists that have no particular rationale and that furthermore vary from study to study. Although many papers speculate on the role of self-blame, fear of retaliation, and so forth in influencing women's coping behaviors, only Jennings and Metha (1987) show any link between emotional and instrumental responses, and no study has yet examined the relationship between particular types or levels of harassment and victim response. This is a particularly important omission as the link between type of harassment and labeling or recognition of harassment is well established, whereas the stress and coping literature has equally firmly linked the appraisal of a stressor with subsequent coping responses.

Attempting to develop a more systematic approach, Ormerod and Gold (1988) constructed an empirically based system for classifying responses to sexually harassing events. Based on the experiences of a large sample of both working and university women, they noted that responses can be broadly classified as internal or external in nature. External strategies focus on the harassing situation itself (e.g., "I told him to leave me alone," "I reported it to my supervisor") whereas internal strategies represent attempts to manage the cognitions and emotions associated with the event ("I told myself that it wasn't important and that he didn't mean to upset me"). Their classification system, as revised by Fitzgerald, Gold, and Brock (1990), is as follows.

Internally Focused Strategies

Detachment

The individual utilizes a distancing strategy, which includes such things as minimizing the situation, treating it like a joke, telling herself it's not really important, and so on.

Denial

The individual denies that the harassment is occurring; she pretends that nothing is happening or that she doesn't notice; she assumes that it won't continue; she tries to forget about it.

Relabeling

The individual reappraises the situation as less threatening; she offers excuses for the harasser (e.g., "He didn't mean to upset me") or interprets the behavior as flattering.

Illusory Control

The individual attempts to gain a sense of control by taking responsibility for the incident, through attributing the harassment to her behavior or attire.

Endurance

The individual essentially does nothing; she "puts up with" the behavior; either through fear (of retaliation, of hurting the harasser, of not being believed, of being blamed, or of embarrassment) or because she believes that there are no resources available for help.

Externally Focused Strategies

Avoidance

The individual attempts to avoid the situation by staying away from the harasser (e.g., dropping the class, changing advisors, quitting a job, etc.).

Assertion/Confrontation

The individual refuses sexual or social offers; verbally confronts the harasser; or otherwise makes clear that the behavior is unwelcome.

Seeking Institutional/Organizational Relief

The individual reports the incident, consults with an appropriate administrator, files a grievance, etc.

Social Support

The individual seeks the support of significant others; seeks validation of her perceptions, or acknowledgement of the reality of the occurrence.

Appeasement

The individual attempts to evade the harassment, but without confrontation or assertion. She offers an excuse, or otherwise attempts to placate the harasser.

Readers will notice the similarity to the two general strategies identified by Lazarus and Folkman (1984), that is, emotion-focused versus problem-focused coping; a conceptually similar system was reported earlier by Schaffer and Shoben (1956). Ormerod and Gold noted that although internal strategies represented by far the most common response overall, the employed women were more likely to adopt external strategies than were women students. Fitzgerald, Gold, and Brock (1990) have recently reported a validation study of this classification system, as well as the development of a paper-and-pencil inventory based on its categories.

As with research on acquaintance rape, there has been considerable interest shown in women's reluctance to confront or report their harassers. Gold (1989) reported that women students in her analogue study were significantly more likely to recommend more assertive strategies to others than they would employ themselves. Ormerod (1989) applied a self-efficacy framework to understanding women's external coping responses and demonstrated that such responding was inhibited by high levels of negative outcome expectations; that is, the women believed that they would suffer negative consequences if they responded assertively or reported the harasser to some appropriate authority. Malovich and Stake (1990) found that women students who were high in performance self-esteem and who held nontraditional sex-role attitudes were more likely to report incidents of sexual harassment than women who were high in self-esteem and who held traditional sex-role attitudes, or women who were low in self-esteem. Finally, Brooks and Perot (1991) showed that reporting behavior was predicted both by the severity of the offense and by feminist attitudes on the part of the subject. Although the underreporting of sexual harassment continues to be a serious problem, most such incidents will likely continue to be handled informally; thus, research on other forms of coping are an important area of future study.

THE CONSEQUENCES OF SEXUAL HARASSMENT

Several studies have attempted to document the impact of harassment on women's lives and well-being. Such impact, which we have labeled the outcomes of the sexual harassment/victimization process, can be examined from three main perspectives: educational/work-related, psychological, or physical/health-related. In the original Merit Systems study (1981), nearly 1 in 10 women who were harassed reported changing jobs as a result; more recently, Merit Systems (1987) noted that over 36,000 federal employees left their jobs due to harassment in the two-year period covered by the study, including victims who quit, were fired from their jobs, or were transferred or reassigned because of unwanted sexual attention. Incredibly, one California study (Coles, 1986), noted that half of those who filed a formal sexual harassment complaint were fired; an additional 25% resigned due to psychological pressures associated with either the harassment or the complaint. Crull (1982) reports a similar level of job loss among a sample of self-identified victims of harassment who sought assistance from the Working Women's Institute. In addition to outright job loss, many women report other negative work-related outcomes, including decreased morale and absenteeism (Merit Systems, 1981), changes in work quantity and quality, and deleterious effects on interpersonal relationships at work (Bandy, 1989). Nor are such effects limited to working women; university students report dropping courses and changing majors, academic departments, and programs (Fitzgerald et al., 1988).

It is difficult to overestimate the toll that harassment takes on women's lives. In addition to the obvious damage done to careers, jobs, educational plans, and so forth, the psychological costs are enormous, and many women suffer serious physiological or health-related reactions as well. In her review of the literature, Koss (1990) notes that victims describe fear, anger, anxiety, and depression; self-questioning and self-blame are common in clinical or self-selected samples (the only ones so far available). In an early study (Silverman, 1976–1977), victims reported feelings of anger, upset, fear, helplessness, guilt, and alienation. More recent research (Crull, 1982; Gutek, 1985) describes similar outcomes, as well as (sometimes severe) physical symptoms (e.g., anxiety attacks, headaches, sleep disturbance, disordered eating, gastrointestinal disorders, nausea, weight loss or gain, and crying spells).

Noting that research on impact and outcome is still in a descriptive mode and depends heavily on samples of self-identified victims, Koss (1990) reviews related areas of sexual victimization, arguing that the similarities among all forms of victimization point to the likelihood of similar outcomes. She concludes, "To the extent that sexual harassment resembles the trauma of rape or incest, these studies suggest that it could be a stressor which poses significant obstacles to women's achievement of mental health," and she calls for a state-of-the-art prospective study of the impact of harassment on women's well-being. We now turn to this suggestion.

FUTURE RESEARCH

The preceding sections of this chapter have reviewed various issues in, and factors influencing, the sexual harassment of women, as well as women's responses to such harassment and the various psychological and work- and health-related consequences of sexual harassment victimization. The following summary examines those factors that have been the focus of previous study and suggests several observations.

Characteristics of the Event or Process of Sexual Harassment
- Definitions of sexual harassment
- Incidence rates (i.e., frequency and type of incident)
- Context of incident (e.g., supervisory relationship)
- Perceptions of sexual harassment
- Theories concerning the nature or causes of sexual harassment

Characteristics of the Victim
- Demographic (e.g., age, marital status, attractiveness)
- Behavioral (e.g., dress, behavior)
- Attitudinal (e.g., toward feminism, harassment, and so on)

Characteristics of the Organization/Work Environment
- Nature of work (e.g., traditional/nontraditional)
- Gender distribution in the work group
- Organizational/institutional norms
- Presence/absence of sexual harassment policies and procedures

Characteristics of Response Strategies
- Internal
- External

Characteristics of Outcomes (i.e., Impact and Consequences)
- Educational/work-related
- Psychological
- Physiological or health-related

Even a cursory review reveals that some of these variables have been much more thoroughly studied than others. The great majority of the research conducted so far has focused on definitions, perceptions, and incidence rates, with much less attention paid to other factors. In particular, although clinical samples suggest that sexual harassment victimization poses a severe threat to women's psychological well-being, as well as to their educational and career development, most studies have seriously neglected these factors, and no formal prospective studies exist.

In addition, the manner in which these numerous variables interact and the relative importance of their effects are not well understood and require much additional study. Typically, each factor is studied in isolation (e.g., perceptions, attitudes, organizational context), although in reality they occur simultaneously and in interaction with one another. A clear understanding of sexual harassment victimization, its predictors, correlates, and consequences will not be possible until researchers begin to utilize more comprehensive research designs and more sophisticated statistical analysis capable of contemplating multiple variables simultaneously. As has been pointed out by others, the complexity of women's lives and the processes that affect them require correspondingly complex research design and analysis (see Betz & Fitzgerald, 1987, Chapter 9; Fassinger, 1985; for a similar discussion concerning research on women's career development).

The present discussion suggests, then, that the study of sexual harassment would benefit from the introduction of more integrative, explanatory investigations, as well as those that take a prospective approach to examining important outcome variables. One possible approach to such research appears in Figure 1. Figure 1 presents a heuristic model, encompassing the various factors displayed in the previous list and designed specifically to predict the outcomes of the sexual harassment victimization process. The model is capable of empirical examination through covariance structure modeling (Bentler, 1980; Fassinger, 1987; Long, 1983), a technique capable of simultaneous examination of multiple (potentially) causal variables. The circles represent hypothetical constructs (known in this context as latent variables) that are inferred from various indicators, or operational definitions; the arrows represent the type and direction of hypothesized causal relationships among the latent variables.

The model in Figure 1 is designed to predict the outcomes or consequences of the sexual harassment process for the women who experience it. Thus, sexual harassment, victim characteristics, and organizational/institutional context are hypothesized to affect victim response mode (coping strategy), which in turn predicts outcome. In addition, sexual harassment and organizational/institutional context are hypothesized to directly affect outcome as well as response mode, both directly and indirectly through their effect on the victim. The causal ordering of the model is designed to reflect the assumption that the outcomes of sexual harassment are influenced by all of the variables previously depicted. Figure 1 thus contains three exogenous (independent) and two endogenous (dependent) variables, which appear to be critical to the study of sexual harassment based on the research conducted to date.

Constructions such as those depicted in Figure 1 are known as theoretical models; actually to test such a model, it would be necessary to identify one or more indicators (operational definitions) for each of the latent variables, such indicators constituting the corresponding measurement model. Possible indicators for the latent variables in Figure 1 might include the SEQ (Fitzgerald et al., 1988), as well as a composite indicator of harasser characteristics (supervisory status, degree of authority, and so on). Victim characteristics could be assessed both by demographic markers indicative of her relative power, for example, age and occupational level, and by attitudinal ones (personal definition of sexual harassment [Perceptions of Sexual Harassment Questionnaire (PSHQ); Fitzgerald & Ormerod, 1991]; attitudes about sexual harassment [Tolerance for Sexual Harassment Inventory (TSHI); Reilly, Lott, & Gallogly, 1986]; and some mea-

Figure 1
Theoretical Model of the Outcomes of Sexual Harassment for College and Working Women

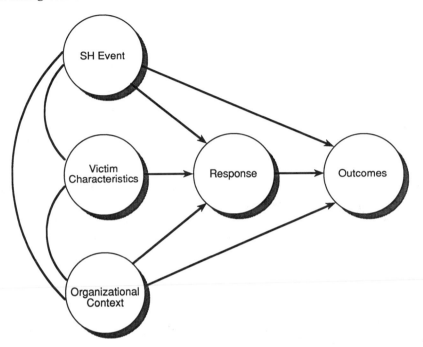

sure of attitudes toward feminism). Context could be assessed by such variables as the traditionality of the occupation, the gender distribution in the proximate workplace, and presence and rated effectiveness of sexual harassment policies. Response mode might be assessed by scores for internal and external strategies on the Coping with Harassment Questionnaire (CHQ) (Fitzgerald, Gold & Brock, 1990). Finally, multiple indicators for outcome should include variables such as occupational stress (Personal Strain Questionnaire, Osipow & Spokane, 1983), psychological well-being (SCL-90; Derogatis, 1983), physical health status (e.g., the Cornell Medical Index), and some measure of withdrawal behavior (quitting, changing major or program, being fired, absenteeism, and so on). The promise of such multivariate studies has recently been demonstrated in the investigation by Brooks and Perot (1991) described above that successfully utilized a path model to predict reporting behavior (what the present authors have labeled seeking institutional/organizational relief).

The design described above is, of course, essentially cross-sectional in nature; an alternative approach would be to select a representative sample of university or working women and follow them for some period of time, possibly with interview data being collected on a subsample. Such an approach would be particularly suited to the university environment, where widely differing departmental contexts and the time-limited nature of a complete cohort cycle offer ideal conditions for a longitudinal effort.

CONCLUSION

The study of sexual harassment is currently moving from a disconnected series of exploratory studies toward a unified body of knowledge, bringing with it a cohesive understanding of an often subtle, always pernicious form of sexual victimization that has plagued the lives of women in both academia and the workplace. This pervasive, yet often trivialized, behavior is best conceptualized in terms of feminist theory and best studied through the methods of traditional social science, as transformed by such theory. This chapter has attempted to form a working understanding of sexual harassment, to critique the literature that has accumulated thus far, and to suggest future directions for its study. It is our hope that this literature will continue to grow and that the examination and knowledge of sexual harassment will contribute to the changes needed for women to receive truly equitable treatment in both the workplace and academic environments.

NOTE

This chapter was completed before the Anita Hill/Clarence Thomas controversy precipitated a veritable explosion of research in the area of sexual harassment. For comprehensive updates, see L. F. Fitzgerald (in press), ''No Safe Haven: Violence Against Women in the Workplace.'' In APA Taskforce on Male Violence Against Women (Eds.), *No Safe Haven: Violence Against Women at Home, at Work, and in the Community* (Washington, DC: American Psychological Association).

REFERENCES

Abbey, A. (1982). Sex differences in attributions for friendly behavior: Do males misperceive females' friendliness? *Journal of Personality and Social Psychology, 47,* 830–838.

Baker, N. L. (1989). *Sexual harassment and job satisfaction in traditional and nontraditional industrial occupations.* Unpublished doctoral dissertation, California School of Professional Psychology, Los Angeles.

Bandy, N. (1989). *Relationships between male and female employees at Southern Illinois University.* Unpublished doctoral dissertation, College of Education, Southern Illinois University, Carbondale.

Bentler, P. M. (1980). Multivariate analysis with latent variables: Causal modeling. *Annual Review of Psychology, 31,* 419–456.

Betz, N. E., & Fitzgerald, L. F. (1987). *The career psychology of women.* New York: Academic Press.

Bond, M. E. (1988). Division 27 sexual harassment survey: Definition, impact and environmental context. *Community Psychologist, 21*, 7–10.

Brooks, L., & Perot, A. (1991). Reporting sexual harassment: Exploring a predictive model. *Psychology of Women Quarterly, 15*, 31–47.

Coles, F. S. (1986). Forced to quit: Sexual harassment complaints and agency response. *Sex Roles, 14*, 81–95.

Collins, E. G., & Blodgett, T. B. (1981). Sexual harassment: Some see it . . . some won't. *Harvard Business Review, 59*, 76–95.

Crull, P. (1982). Stress effects of sexual harassment on the job: Implications for counseling. *American Journal of Orthopsychiatry, 52*, 539–544.

D'Augelli, A. R. (1988). Sexual harassment and affectional status: The hidden discrimination. *Community Psychologist, 21*, 11–12.

DeFour, D. C. (1990). The interface of racism and sexism on college campuses. In M. Paludi (Ed.), *Ivory Power: Sexual harassment on campus* (pp. 45–52). Albany, NY: SUNY Press.

Derogatis, L. R. (1983). *SCL-90-R: Administration, scoring, and procedures manual-II*. Towson, MD: Clinical Psychometric Research.

Fassinger, R. E. (1985). A causal model of career choice in college women. *Journal of Vocational Behavior, 27*, 123–153.

Fassinger, R. E. (1987). Use of structural equation modeling in counseling psychology research. *Journal of Counseling Psychology, 34*, 425–436.

Fitzgerald, L. F. (1990). Sexual harassment: The definition and measurement of a construct. In M. Paludi (Ed.), *Ivory power: Sexual harassment on campus* (pp. 21–44). New York: SUNY Press.

Fitzgerald, L. F., Gold, Y., & Brock, K. F. (1990). Responses to victimization: Validation of an objective policy. *Journal of College Student Personnel, 27*, 34–39.

Fitzgerald, L. F., & Hesson-McInnis, M. (1989). The dimensions of sexual harassment: A structural analysis. *Journal of Vocational Behavior, 35*, 309–326.

Fitzgerald, L. F., & Ormerod, A. J. (1991). Perceptions of sexual harassment: The influence of gender and context. *Psychology of Women Quarterly, 15*, 281–294.

Fitzgerald, L. F., & Shullman, S. L. (1985). *The development and validation of an objectively scored measure of sexual harassment*. Paper presented at the annual conference of the American Psychological Association, Los Angeles.

Fitzgerald, L. F., Shullman, S. L., Bailey, N., Richards, M., Swecker, J., Gold, A., Ormerod, A. J., & Weitzman, L. (1988). The incidence and dimensions of sexual harassment in academia and the workplace. *Journal of Vocational Behavior, 32*, 152–175.

Fuehrer, A., & Maitland-Schilling, K. (1988). Sexual harassment of women graduate students: The impact of institutional factors. *Community Psychologist, 21*, 12–13.

Gold, Y. (1987, August). *The sexualization of the workplace: Sexual harassment of pink-, white- and blue-collar workers*. Paper presented to the annual conference of the American Psychological Association, New York.

Gold, Y. (1989, August). *Women's ways of coping: Strategies for dealing with sexual harassment*. Paper presented to the annual conference of the American Psychological Association, New Orleans.

Gutek, B. (1985). *Sex and the workplace*. San Francisco: Jossey-Bass.

Gutek, B., & Morasch, B. (1982). Sex ratios, sex role spillover, and sexual harassment of women at work. *Journal of Social Issues, 38*, 55–74.

Gutek, B., Morasch, B., & Cohen, A. G. (1983). Interpreting social-sexual behavior in a work setting. *Journal of Vocational Behavior, 22*, 30–48.

Jennings, A. C., & Metha, A. (1981). *Sexual harassment: An in-depth approach*. Unpublished manuscript, Arizona State University College of Education, Tempe.

Kanter, R. M. (1977). *Men and women of the organization*. New York: Basic Books.

Koenig, S., & Ryan, J. (1986). Sex differences in levels of tolerance and attribution of blame for sexual harassment on a university campus. *Sex Roles, 15*, 535–549.

Konrad, A. M., & Gutek, B. (1986). Impact of work experiences on attitudes toward sexual harassment. *Administrative Science Quarterly, 31*, 422–438.

Koss, M. P. (1990). Changed lives: The psychological impact of sexual harassment. In M. Paludi (Ed.), *Ivory power: Sexual harassment on campus* (pp. 73–92). New York: SUNY Press.

LaFontaine, E., & Tredeau, L. (1986). The frequency, sources and correlates of sexual harassment among women in traditional male occupations. *Sex Roles, 15*, 423–432.

Lazarus, R. S., & Folkman, S. (1984). *Stress, appraisal and coping*. New York: Springer.

Lee, L. A., & Heppner, P. (1991). The development and evaluation of a sexual harassment inventory. *Journal of Counseling & Development, 69*, 512–517.

Long, J. S. (1983). *Covariance structure models: An introduction to LISREL*. Beverly Hills: Sage.

MacKinnon, C. A. (1979). *Sexual harassment of working women*. New Haven, CT: Yale University Press.

Malovich, N. J., & Stake, J. E. (1990). Sexual harassment on campus: Individual differences in attitude and beliefs. *Psychology of Women Quarterly, 14*, 63–81.

National Gay and Lesbian Task Force. (1986). *Anti-gay violence: Causes, consequences, responses*. Washington, DC: Author.

Ormerod, A. J. (1989, August). *Women students' self-efficacy expectations about coping with sexual harassment*. Paper presented to the annual conference of the American Psychological Association, New Orleans.

Ormerod, A. J., & Gold, Y. (1988, March). *Coping with sexual harassment: Internal and external strategies for coping with stress*. Paper presented to the annual conference of the Association for Women in Psychology, Bethesda, MD.

Osipow, S. H., & Spokane, A. R. (1983). *A manual for measures of occupational stress, strain and coping*. Columbus, OH: Marathon Consulting & Press.

Padgitt, S. C., & Padgitt, J. S. (1986). Cognitive structure of sexual harassment: Implications for university policy. *Journal of College Student Personnel, 27*, 34–39.

Powell, G. N. (1986). Effects of sex-role identity and sex on definitions of sexual harassment. *Sex Roles, 14*, 9–19.

Pryor, J. B., & Day, J. D. (1988). Interpretations of sexual harassment: An attributional analysis. *Sex Roles, 18*, 405–417.

Reilly, M. E., Lott, B., & Gallogly, S. M. (1986). Sexual harassment of university students. *Sex Roles, 15*, 333–358.

Reilly, T., Carpenter, S., Dull, V., & Bartlett, K. (1982). The factorial survey technique: An approach to defining sexual harassment on campus. *Journal of Social Issues, 38*, 99–110.

Russell, D. (1984). *Sexual exploitation: Rape, child sexual abuse and workplace harassment*. Beverly Hills: Sage.

Saal, F. E., Johnson, C. B., & Weber, N. (1989). Friendly or sexy? It may depend on whom you ask. *Psychology of Women Quarterly, 13*, 263–276.

Schaffer, L. F., & Shoben, E. J., Jr. (1956). *The psychology of adjustment*. Boston: Houghton-Mifflin.

Schneider, B. E. (1982). Consciousness about sexual harassment among heterosexual and lesbian women workers. *Journal of Social Issues, 38*, 75–98.

Silverman, D. (1976–1977). Sexual harassment: Working women's dilemma. *Quest: A Feminist Quarterly, 3*, 15–24.

Tangri, S. S., Burt, M. R., & Johnson, L. B. (1982). Sexual harassment at work: Three explanatory models. *Journal of Social Issues, 38*, 33–54.

Till, F. J. (1980). *Sexual harassment: A report on the sexual harassment of students*. Washington, DC: National Advisory Council on Women's Educational Programs.

U. S. Equal Employment Opportunity Commission. (1980). Discrimination because of sex under Title VII of the 1964 Civil Rights Act as amended: Adoption of interim guidelines—Sexual harassment. *Federal Register, 45*, 25024–25025.

U.S. Merit Systems Protection Board. (1981). *Sexual harassment of federal workers: Is it a problem?* Washington, DC: U.S. Government Printing Office.

U.S. Merit Systems Protection Board. (1987). *Sexual harassment of federal workers: An update*. Washington, DC: U.S. Government Printing Office.

York, K. M. (1989). Defining sexual harassment in workplaces: A policy-capturing approach. *Academy of Management Journal, 32*, 830–850.

Part VI

Achievement Motivation, Career Development, and Work

16

Women and the Psychology of Achievement: A View from the Eighties

Martha T. Mednick and Veronica G. Thomas

INTRODUCTION

There is a long history of concern about women and the why (usually the why not) of their achievement, and we do not here undertake to review an entire century or more of writing on this topic. Yet, in order to provide a proper context for talking about and thinking about psychology's study of achievement, we took a brief look at the reviews, analyses, and critiques that began to appear as a feminist psychology of women developed. Social change and a social movement spurred psychologists to take "a new look" (Mednick & Tangri, 1972; Mednick & Weissman, 1975) at the psychological study of women, offering new theories, methods, and techniques, and innovative perspectives on women's experiences, circumstances, and development.

As this handbook attests, an enormous amount of research and discussion on a broad range of psychological topics was thus catalyzed. It is important to remember the larger context of this surge of work; the feminist movement spurred intellectual ferment and reevaluation in most disciplines, and psychology was no exception. Thus the research evolved within the framework of efforts to create a feminist psychology, suggesting that one consequence of the work was to have been social change. During the sixties, psychologists had become increasingly aware that accumulated knowledge and the knowledge being generated were not value-free. Feminist psychology added a further level of analysis, specific to gender in the context of the social system that was its creator (Mednick, 1978; Sherman & Beck, 1977).

The study of women's achievement in the new vein received—aside from the fact that the world was clamoring for it—a boost with Horner's (1972) now very familiar work on the motive to avoid success, popularly referred to as fear of success (FOS). Horner's work was presented within the dominant model of social motivation, as articulated by McClelland (1961) and Atkinson (1958). It was a model that had stimulated an immense body of research on achievement motivation since World War II, and Horner's work drew attention to the inadequacy of that body of work with respect to understanding sex differences in achievement motivation. Her catalytic idea forced motivation researchers at least to consider the external validity of their measures. While the value of the FOS work is still being debated, and a revisionist review by Stewart and Chester (1982) forces some reevaluation of where things stood in the first place, surely it marked an important turning point.

Reviews documenting the surge of interest in women and achievement appeared throughout the seventies and into the very early eighties (Mednick & Weissman, 1975; Mednick, 1978; Mednick, Tangri & Hoffman, 1975; Mednick, 1982; Nieva & Gutek, 1981), and it is not our intent to re-review. We focus on the decade of the eighties, assess the content of current research, the extent of continuing interest, the kinds of questions being asked, and attempt to make projections for the nineties.

Mednick and Tangri (1972) considered the area of achievement to be one of several that were to be reevaluated in discussing new approaches. They raised concerns about the kinds of questions that were being asked and those that were not being asked regarding women and careers and women and work: ''[We are not saying] that more women should work—virtually *all* adult women [except heiresses] work at least one job [housekeeper], most combine this within a second job [childcare], and a growing proportion of these, plus all other women, hold still a third job [employment outside the home]'' (1972, pp. 11–12). Mednick and Tangri framed their discussion in sex equity terms, noting that ''fair employment for equal pay is the greatest equalizer of the sexes. There is a change in climate about sex roles and stereotypes, sex difference research, and sexism'' (1972, pp. 11–12).

By 1975, Mednick and Weissman found that achievement had become a preeminent concern of researchers on the psychology of women. The major concepts dealt with in their review were achievement motivation and fear of success, expectancies, and causal attribution. In addition, there was considerable focus on the question of the intersection of sex-role and sex identity issues (variously defined) with the psychological factors in women's achievement.

By the early eighties, as women, married and single, with children, without children, and beyond children, flooded into the workplace, it was realized that a new question had to be considered. Earlier concern with the determinants of career aspirations and commitment (Tangri, 1972; Mednick et al., 1975) was broadened to the question of why, in spite of years of rhetoric, legislation, and EEO suits, women's economic level and status in the workplace continued to lag. While sociologists of occupations focused on macro variables such as the sex-segregated marketplace, psychologists began to relate their findings about psychological factors to these larger social questions. Thus a symposium on women and work (Bernardin, 1982) included research on the psychology of achievement (Mednick, 1982; O'Leary & Hansen, 1982), and in an important book published in that era, *Women and Work: A Psychological Perspective*, Nieva and Gutek (1981) similarly extended their discussion to such larger questions.

The questions that we raise now address the research concerns of the eighties with respect to the achievement domain. What are we trying to explain, and what kinds of concepts are being examined? In what ways has a feminist perspective affected the questions being asked?

CURRENT RESEARCH ON THE PSYCHOLOGY OF ACHIEVEMENT

Looking at the issue of women's accomplishments from a purely psychological perspective has always been difficult. It is frustrating to speak of these as though outcomes depend only on the personal factors that psychologists tend to study, while ignoring social structure and social forces. It is glib to speak of the interaction of such factors in the absence of meaningful study of the interaction. Yet, it is very difficult to study such interaction, and most of the work reviewed continues to exist in a social context vacuum (see exceptions: Helson, Mitchell & Moane, 1986; Tangri & Jenkins, 1986; Jenkins, 1987; Helson, 1987). The view of Nieva and Gutek (1981) is pertinent:

Our analytic emphasis will be the individual woman, and the environment will be considered to the extent that it influences her options and decisions, . . . After all it is her actions that form the basis of the larger macrolevel processes. Nevertheless, we cannot ignore the larger context in which her actions are based. . . . [We] will try therefore to bridge part of the gap between the macrolevel processes that concern economists, sociologists, and legislators, and the psychological processes within individual women. (p. vii)

Such concerns have been frequently reiterated (see, e.g., Mednick, 1982; Sherif, 1977). But, as we have examined the major portion of the research of the eighties, such a concern with broader contextual variables does not appear to be the way most psychologists think about, and carry out, research.

Constraints on Review

The major topics of our review are confined to what we have found by searching through the late eighties. We depended to a large extent on computer searching, but also wrote to active researchers in the area asking for reports of their recent work and placed an announcement in the newsletter of the Division of the Psychology of Women of the American Psychological Association. We have included all relevant materials obtained in these ways. Though most of the references are to published studies, preprints are also included, though generally only if in press. Other constraints include a focus mainly on adult research, with a few exceptions for particularly relevant research on adolescents. We eliminated cross-cultural research, though such efforts are in fact very important; a full treatment was simply not feasible. However, we consider cultural diversity very important and have attended to race, ethnicity, and class, insofar as the research makes that possible. Our review focuses only on empirical and theoretical articles; clinical literature is not included.

Overview

What is our overall impression? There is continued study of what has been studied before, both in terms of explanatory concepts and what is being explained. Setting aside for the moment the question of whether there has been a meaningful advance since the feminist-inspired shift of the late sixties and the early seventies, we turn to look at the psychological constructs that have been offered as explanation for either sex differences in achievement behavior or for variations among women. The major constructs have been around for a while, though some have ascended in their popularity with researchers, while others have declined.

Achievement motivation as formulated by McClelland (1961) and Atkinson (1958) and developed further by Feather (1981), Heckhausen, Schmalt, and Schneider (1985), and others is still a theory around which there is much discourse. Even though the major discoursers seem to have little to say about gender as a fundamental question (e.g., see Heckhausen et al., 1985), concern about gender and achievement motivation continues to be much studied in other contexts. We will therefore turn first to a review of current studies of achievement motives/motivation and to an examination of success avoidance as a motive.

In keeping with social and personality psychology's concern with cognitive variables, expectancy for success and failure—that is, self-confidence about achievement—has been much examined, as well as the related issues of causal attributions about success and failure and the behavioral consequences of these cognitions. A review of these concepts will be followed by a look at self-efficacy and self-esteem. Another major explanatory construct is sex or gender roles and gender identity. This is a concept that has eluded all efforts by psychologists to unmuddy the definitional waters. However, it is part of this literature, so we will try to make sense of how it is implicated in achievement behavior.

We turn next to the question of what is being predicted. In most earlier work, achievement had been viewed as a variable on a continuum from performance on achievement tasks, to risk taking in experimental situations, to school-related achievement, to aspirations to work and careers (including the level of aspiration concept), to career development. We still view the domain as a continuum, but since (due, of course, to the expansion of the field) this handbook contains chapters on work, on career development, and on women in management and leadership roles, much will be elsewhere reviewed. Nevertheless, theory and research in this area are directed at prediction of the very same areas of behavior as they always have been, so some overlap is unavoidable.

Next we will consider methodology; we have gone through a period of serious feminist critique of methods used to "study women" and need therefore to ask what new approaches have emerged. Finally, we will assess and make recommendations for future concerns of a viable feminist scholarship in this area.

Achievement Motivation

It was sobering and stimulating to read Stewart and Chester's (1982) revisionist analysis of the sex difference studies conducted by achievement motivation researchers working within the McClelland-Atkinson expectancy value theory. They reviewed every study of sex differences in achievement motivation and concluded that no systematic or programmatic study of sex differences had ever been undertaken in the study of motives. By the time the issue of gender was seriously raised, the basic measurement work had already been done, and the later work, which did consider gender, was more like a graft than a basic reanalysis. So, as Stewart and Chester (1982) point out, "Questions about sex differences have been generated ad hoc" (p. 174). Their review is worth detailed attention here because the issues they raised had not been raised before and have not yet had an impact on researchers in the field.

They report that the studies that had looked at gender effects on imagery had not found differences, nor did those that looked at whether different stimuli (i.e., male versus female) or those that are gender-role–related elicit different responses from men and women. The question of arousal is one that has been even more central in the achievement motivation literature. The received wisdom has been that the kind of arousal manipulation used in traditional research was inappropriate for women, hence the great difficulties in arousing the motive. According to Stewart and Chester, the answer to the question of whether there are sex differences in arousal of achievement motivation has never been adequately tested. They point to methodological problems that led to conclusions of no difference or of differences due to sex, when results were actually due to design factors. One example is the operational definition of a "relaxed" condition in achievement studies conducted in a college setting. Generally, two groups, one in a neutral condition and one in an arousal condition, are compared. However, they note, "the context of university research, especially with college students, includes so many achievement cues that it may be quite difficult to control them" (p. 180). Further, they suggest that the validity of the "arousal" conditions is open to question for both men and women. Finally (this is probably where stereotypes about gender had more subtle impact that we had previously supposed):

Failures to arouse the motive have been readily and consistently interpreted as reflecting a real phenomenon in women, rather than as reflecting aspects of the research design or procedure. It is hard to resist the interpretation that researchers were eager to see the arousal of the achievement motive in women as especially problematic . . . . Thus it was generally assumed that "achievement," even broadly defined as "a concern for excellence," was consonant only with the male sex role. (p. 181)

This line of thinking was pursued, beginning as early as 1951 (Field, cited by Stewart & Chester, 1982), by researchers looking for conditions under which women would become aroused; it is interesting that similar searches were not undertaken for men. Most studies included only women, since they proceeded on the assumption that women's roles, but not men's, had a constraining effect on arousal, and thus focused on an examination of the interaction of arousal conditions with gender role related values. Gralewski and Rodgon (1980) found that traditionally role-oriented women displayed greater achievement motivation on a projective measure under affiliative conditions, while nontraditional women showed more arousal under achievement arousal conditions. Stewart and Chester (1982) argue that research such as this, which assumes that only the female role constrains achievement, has led investigators to ignore data showing that women are aroused by traditional achievement manipulations, as well as to avoid hypotheses about male constraints. For example, there is some evidence that women strive for excellence in a wide range of domains, while men seem incapable of similar breadth; this is a rarely studied hypothesis. Such issues raise the question of whether the research on psychology of women has perhaps occassionally erred when it has focused only on women.

The question of behavioral correlates of need for achievement (Nach) was also tackled by Stewart and Chester (1982). They concluded that there is evidence that for women, just as for men, Nach predicts laboratory performance and career aspirations. Still, results are contradictory, and they argue that some of the contradictions may be due to inadequate attention to the value of achievement to the individual. Stewart and Chester conclude again that the designs used have precluded answering such questions and are saying that assumed sex differences are perhaps not there or may be different from what was expected. In this connection the point made by Deaux and Kite (1987) that beliefs about sex differences are in general far greater than actual differences is affirmed.

The Stewart and Chester review was of the classic Nach motive model. However, our search has revealed very little research on women that adhered to this framework; it seems that there has been a shift of methods and definitions.

Redefining Achievement Motivation

Spence and Helmreich (1983) criticized the conceptualization and measurement of motivation in the Nach tradition. Arguing against a unidimensional view as well as against projective measurement, they developed a self-report, multidimensional measure, the work and family orientation questionnaire (WOFO)

(Spence & Helmreich, 1983; Adams, Priest & Prince, 1985). Indeed, the projective/imagery measure has been criticized as unreliable (but see Fleming, 1982 for a response) and unstable. Objective measures of Nach within the expectancy value framework have been developed (e.g., Mehrabian, cited by Spence & Helmreich, 1983), but the WOFO is unique. According to Spence and Helmreich (1983), the WOFO measures several dispositions to strive for excellence, dispositions that remain latent until engaged (aroused) by a particular event.

With respect to sex differences, Spence, Helmreich, and their coworkers (Spence & Helmreich 1983) have found that in general men score higher than women on the competitiveness and mastery subscales of the WOFO, but that women score higher on work. These investigators have consistently found that the personality traits of instrumentality and expressivity, which have been traditionally tied to gender identity, are mediators of the sex differences. Instrumentality and expressiveness accounted for the sex differences in work and mastery scores, though not in competitiveness, with men scoring higher on competitiveness independent of their trait levels. Summarizing a variety of studies, Spence and Helmreich (1983) concluded, ''In general, males have an edge in mastery and competitiveness motives and in related instrumental personality characteristics'' (p. 47). Spence and Helmreich stress the great overlap of male and female characteristics in this area and are skeptical about attributing women's lesser vocational achievement to basic differences in personality and related characteristics. Further, they argue that there is little evidence that affiliative motivation can be invoked, since it has been found that expressiveness is not apparently incompatible with achievement. Spence, Helmreich, and their colleagues have confirmed this general point of view in studies of businesspeople, academic psychologists, and varsity athletes. In a recent study they even addressed themselves to the issue of health and achievement striving and found that the consequences of achievement striving are similar for men and women (Spence, Helmreich, & Pred, 1987).

Related to the multidimensional nature of achievement motivation is the issue of the implications of such motivations for activities not directly associated with school and vocational accomplishment and success. Several studies reported by Spence and Helmreich (1983) appear to indicate that striving for excellence is related to other areas of life as well and that this is true for both men and women. Gaeddert's (1987) research also suggests that when individuals are asked for subjective definitions of areas of achievement, gender differences disappear. Travis, McKenzie, Wiley, and Kahn (1988) also found that the achievement domain was a better predictor of achievement-related cognitive variables than sex. They, like others, call for a ''broader'' definition of achievement.

Other theorists and investigators have addressed the issue of different achievement styles; Lipman-Blumen, Handley-Isaksen, and Leavitt (1983) present some confirmatory data for a model of achieving styles that combines the notion of personality traits with a role theory analysis. Of interest here is that while homemakers and other women appear to differ in instrumental and relational achieving styles, when occupational groups were studied (e.g., managers), no consistent gender differences in styles were found. Stewart (1980) also addressed the question of women's varying stylistically in her study of self and socially defined women.

The concern with motive interaction led Horner (1972) to do her classic study examining sex differences in achievement motivation and its effects. The differential effects of achievement and affiliation motive arousal continue to be a subject of research and discussion. A theoretical discussion by Griffin-Pierson (1986) brings the issue back, though in different terms. Like Gilligan (1982), she argues that women are, in contrast to men, more relational and also, curiously enough, cites the Spence and Helmreich work described above to support her claim that women and men are affiliatively "different." Several studies have appeared that have argued back and forth about the kind of imagery—imagery per se is the dependent variable—men and women express when they are confronted with achievement cues or intimacy (affiliative) cues. Pollak and Gilligan (1982) found that male imagery to intimacy cues was more hostile than female imagery; the converse of that is that women have trouble with achievement imagery, and men don't. The study failed to replicate (Benton et al., 1983), but Helgeson and Sharpsteen (1987) did find marginally significant differences in men's and women's perception of danger in achievement and affiliation conditions. These studies reflect the preoccupation with supposed conflicts between these two domains. Paludi and Fankell-Hauser's (1986) study of women's achievement striving also addressed similar issues. These studies seem to circle back to the issues discussed by Stewart and Chester—is it deja vu all over again?

Achievement motivation and gender have also been examined in relation to the issues of intrinsic versus extrinsic motivation (see Spence & Helmreich, 1983, for review). There is no evidence that women are more extrinsically motivated than men; it depends on the circumstances and the individual. Koestner, Zuckerman, and Koestner (1987) found that women showed more intrinsic motivation when they were praised than when they were not praised, while men showed the reverse pattern. The authors note that praise must have different meaning for different people, an idea that is hardly surprising, but worth pursuing.

Heaven (1987) found some interesting sex differences in his look at the extent to which authoritarians are achievement-motivated. The prediction was upheld only for men, and he incidentally found that high achievement women had high self-esteem.

Fear of Success

It is perhaps more a measure of the tenacity of metaphor than of conceptual value that fear of success studies continued to appear throughout the eighties. While hundreds of studies discredited the notion that such an avoidance motive can explain sex differences in achievement, the idea seems to live on (Mednick, 1989a). A significant number of dissertations continued to appear throughout the decade. The concept has been measured in a variety of ways, with mixed outcomes. The questions being asked are about measurement, about sex differences, about background and other correlates, and about whether FOS is indeed a motivational construct that predicts achievement behavior.

As far as measurement is concerned, very few of the studies conducted in the period under review have used the traditional imagery approach. The original FOS cues about medical school have been rendered useless in the face of social change, but adherents of the use of imagery (generally expectancy value theorists) continue to maintain that the original approach, if not the original cue, is best. They are willing to live with low reliability, taking comfort from their construct's construct validity. Fleming (1982) has addressed the issue of projective versus objective measurement in greatest depth. She reports on Horner's ''new'' projective measure developed in an arousal experiment and concludes that the measure is useful. Fleming's (1982) review is a good source of references to this particular method. Paludi (1984) presented a review of the available objective measures; she concluded that none had demonstrably better psychometric properties than the projective measure. Paludi and Fankell-Hauser (1986) used a biographical interview procedure and coded responses to an open-ended interview for various positive and negative aspects of achievement striving. Although the authors concluded that fear of success was measured via this method, they do not present clear-cut psychometric support for this assertion (see also Gravenkemper & Paludi, 1983).

MacDonald and Hyde (1980) conducted a factor analytic study of several measures of FOS, fear of failure (FOF), and Nach, in an effort to clarify some of the measurement issues. They included both objective and projective measures of each concept. Horner's original FOS cues and later cues and methods were included, including a measure developed by Cohen (1974, cited by MacDonald & Hyde, 1980) and the Zuckerman and Allison Fear of Success Scale (FOSS; 1976, cited by MacDonald & Hyde, 1980). Reliabilities ranged from .22 to .83; as might be expected, the projective measures were the least reliable. The Cohen scale loaded on an anxiety factor, and not on other FOS measures, which, as the authors note, is to be expected from the Freudian-based origin of the scale. The two projective measures of FOS did not load on the same factor. With regard to the other FOS measures, each of these seems to be measuring different constructs. Mulig, Haggerty, Carbollosa, Cinnick, and Madden (1985) found that FOS and FOF were significantly related, for both men and women. Orlofsky (1981) compared objective and projective measures of FOS and found low- or zero-order correlations; moreover, he reported that the different measures were related to different outcome variables. It makes sense to keep such findings in mind as we review the studies using various measures.

One of the ostensibly most damaging criticisms of FOS raised in the earlier reviews was that sex differences were not found. The meaning of that finding was hotly debated (Hoffman, 1975). The current search did not turn up very much testing of that question; the study of the construct in the eighties appears to have been largely confined to women. MacDonald and Hyde (1980) found that men and women produced similar factor structures; however, there were consistent differences for all FOS measures, with women showing consistently more negative attitudes about success than men. However, at the same time, none of the FOS scores predicted to GPA or ACT scores for either men or women. It is worth noting parenthetically that generalized anxiety did predict to these achievement measures for both men and women. Incidental to a study of how relationships affect outcomes of fear of success, Kronberger (1983) reported finding no sex differences in either an objective measure or with Horner's revised projective measure. Janman (1984) found that men and women were very similar in their responses to projective cues, as did Bremer and Wittig (1980) in an earlier study.

With respect to studies exploring the meaning of the construct, investigators in the eighties continued to raise the question of whether FOS is a motive or whether it is a response to perceptions of deviance and violations of gender-role stereotypes. Bremer and Wittig (1980) found that both men and women wrote stories with negative themes in response to cues that manipulated the two situational factors of role overload and role deviance. Since they used only female cues, it was not possible to test the question of whether similar responses would be obtained when male cues are used. Janman (1984) found that the effect of role overload and occupational deviance was very much dependent on the sex of the cue character. Kirshbaum (1984) found that FOS, measured objectively, correlated with traditional gender-role attitudes, providing indirect support for a situational, rather than a motive, interpretation. On the other hand, Lentz (1982) manipulated the gender and role of an anticipated evaluator and found no difference in projectively measured fear of success. With a similar manipulation, however, Wernikoff (1980) did show an effect of role.

A pivotal question in this area, and probably one that has not been sufficiently studied, is how FOS affects the kinds of performance variables generally studied by motivation researchers. Horner (see Fleming, 1982) consistently argued that in order for the construct to be acceptable as a motivational one, a performance decline had to be shown to be a function of level of FOS, particularly in the face of competition with a male competitor. Horner presented such data with her 1973 scoring system (Fleming, 1982). These results were confirmed by Karabenick (cited by Heckhausen, Schmalt & Schneider, 1985), but not by Cook and Chandler (1984). The latter study of adolescents found boys more affected by competition with a girl than with a boy. Further studies have not been forthcoming. Lentz (1982) found that performance level on an anagram task was not related to projectively measured FOS. Situational manipulations of sex and role of anticipated evaluator in an evaluation situation did affect performance in a manner that ran counter to the author's predictions. Although Lentz argued for a situational explanation of the performance decrement found, the study did not control for other personality variables that may have served as mediators, so the conclusion is premature. It must also be noted that Lentz did not manipulate competition.

Wernikoff (1980), using the FOSS, in a design that might in a way be regarded as the opposite of a competition manipulation, found that high FOS women were less confident about their performance when they were expecting to receive male evaluation than when such evaluation was not expected. In general, high FOS women were less confident about their performance than low FOS women were, regardless of other factors.

Other reported correlates of FOS include learned helplessness (Ris & Woods, 1983), career salience and role traditionality (Illfelder, 1980), race (Fleming, 1983), mother's attitudes and birth order (Kripke, 1980), Type A traits (Loewenstine & Paludi, 1982), and age and Eriksonian identity status (Freilino & Hummel, 1985).

It is difficult to sum up. Clearly, the amount of research conducted on FOS per se has declined; its heyday is past. Yet there is a sense that some regard the story as incomplete, with various issues unresolved. Heckhausen et al. (1985) argue that it is a complex motive that cannot be studied independently of its relation to affiliation motivation, a hypothesis that has not been addressed in the time period reviewed. A recent effort by Piedmont (1988) also refocuses the argument in theory development. In this study there was some support for a motive interaction explanation, in this case of Nach and FOS for women, but not for men. Piedmont used self-report measures and does not help sort out the measurement problems, which as Heckhausen et al. (1985) point out, continue to plague the area, a fact that our review has clearly confirmed.

Cognitive Variables Affecting Gender and Achievement

In this section we review studies of self-confidence, that is, expectancies for achievement, self-efficacy, and causal attributions. These cognitive variables have been front and center in the achievement area for many years and have been prominently utilized in explanatory efforts (e.g., see later discussion of Eccles's work). It is important to note that major theories of achievement and social learning theories have long utilized expectancy variables.

Achievement Expectancies

Earlier reviews consistently concluded that women had lower self-confidence about ability than men. They had been found to expect to do less well than their male counterparts and to underestimate their ability. These findings were repeated in many studies, in a wide variety of situations (see Nieva & Gutek, 1981; Mednick, 1982, for reviews of earlier work) and developmentally (Gold, Brush & Sprotzer, 1980). Although sex differences were not found in all situations, standard achievement settings elicited lower self-confidence on the part of women. In some instances men overestimate their ability, while women are realistic, or modest. In any event while it is true that under some circumstances women may raise their expectations, they rarely surpass men. Lenney's (1977) important work in this area showed that differences disappear when women and men are asked to rate themselves on interpersonal and social skills. She also found that women's expectancies are raised in a noncompetitive and nonevaluative atmosphere and when immediate and clear-cut feedback is given. Thus there are situational effects. But if we focus on the problem of achievement in school and work arenas, it is important to note that, much as one would wish to create nonevaluative and noncompetitive atmospheres and immediate feedback, this does not reflect the worlds of education and work as they are now structured.

Macro issues aside, and though Frieze, Whitley, Hanusa, and McHugh (1982) have concluded from a meta-analysis that overall expectancy differences are insignificant, studies continued to focus on the question of the conditions under which sex differences are obtained. Stake (1983) confirmed Lenney's (1977) finding that clear, unambiguous feedback obviates sex differences; however, this was so only when the feedback was bogus. Under the condition of accurate feedback based on their own performance, she found that male college students overestimated their performance even more than they had in their initial expectancy statements, while women continued to make lower expectancy statements. It is also of interest that male inaccuracy in goal setting was related to overestimation, while women were more likely to fall short of their actual performance. Vollmer (1986) found that expectancy differences were accounted for by controlling perceived ability; the trait of instrumentality was implicated as a mediator in this study. Vollmer's findings were based on a real examination situation, while the Lenney (1977) and Stake (1983) studies used experimental manipulations. It should be noted that Vollmer measured perceived ability with a seven-item scale, with items such as, "If I have worked hard in preparation, I am usually optimistic and expect to do well." The psychometric data are not readily available, but such items appear very much like expectancy or academic self-confidence statements, so it is not clear that the study explained anything. In any event, men were higher than women in both perceived ability and their expectations for course grades. Erkut (1983) also found college men to have higher expectancies in future course grades than women, though no actual performance (grades in school) differences.

McMahan (1982) found that women stated lower expectancies than men in a role-play situation, in which sex linkage of a group of cognitive tasks was manipulated. The effect of sex linkage was significant, with men having highest expectations for male-linked tasks. With ability level controlled, men overestimated and women underestimated their future successes. While Gitelson, Peterson, and Tobin-Richards (1982) also found sex differences in expectancies, their results were similar for both spatial and verbal tasks. Their adolescent subjects appeared to have a generalized set of expectations about achievement. Similar findings in a nonachievement setting were reported by Carr, Thomas, and Mednick (1985). Men in two field studies were more self-confident than women about driving or fixing a car and about shopping. This difference was maintained even when past experience with these tasks was controlled.

Other situational variables have been examined. Lenney and Gold (1982), following upon Lenney (1981), used a social comparison variable and found that women were more affected by being compared with competent others than men were (see also LaNoue & Curtis, 1985). Completion of the task also made a difference, but only when some information (feedback) was available. Task completion without feedback was evidently not enough. Alagna (1982) also found that women responded more to social approval than to disapproval, while for men it made no difference. Monahan (1983) used high school students and reported also that success feedback affected female, but not male, expectancies. Her findings held for both average and superior students. McMahan's (1982) study also speaks to the feedback factor; his findings suggest that in the absence of feedback, people may assume that their expectancies are confirmed, thus bolstering Lenney's argument for specific, immediate feedback. Bridges (1988) manipulated public versus private disclosure, sex linkage of occupations, and sex of social comparison person. Her findings did not confirm earlier findings and predictions: situational factors had no clear-cut effects. Her study, it must be noted, was indirect, in that subjects were asked to state expectations about hypothetical occupations, not the ones they actually aspired to.

Karabenick, Sweeney, and Penrose (1983) showed that women preferred skill rather than chance on tasks that were feminine more than for masculine sex-typed tasks. However, these skill-chance preferences were a function of expectancies for success on the skill task and not of sex typing or gender. Tangentially related here is Hackett and Campbell's (1987) finding that performance on a gender-neutral task was not different for men and women. Finally, Travis et al. (1988) have found that achievement domain overrides sex differences in initial expectancies.

Personality variables have also been implicated. Stake (1983) found that performance self-esteem had no effect on expectancies. The trait of instrumentality influenced expectancies in the aforementioned study by Vollmer (1986), albeit indirectly. Alagna (1982) also reported that masculinity and androgyny, as measured by the PAQ (Personal Attributes Questionnaire) (Spence & Helmreich, 1978), resulted in higher performance expectancies. The actual performance as well as perceived success of masculine individuals, was also higher than for feminine individuals. Kranser (1987) found that high school girls with a masculine self-schema had higher expectations for success, which also predicted their mathematics achievement. The latter finding fits with the work of Eccles and her colleagues in the area of mathematics achievement. Eccles (1983) also found that sex differences in confidence in one's mathematics abilities consistently emerged past age 12, along with a decline, for girls, in valuing of mathematics. Yount's (1986) theory of work-emergent traits would argue that gender-related traits are created by the sexual division of labor and serve the social function of maintaining such division.

In sum, sex differences are obtained in expectations for success at traditional achievement tasks, but under certain conditions these differences disappear. Further, there is some evidence (Kranser, 1987) that all women are not the same in this regard and that personality characteristics such as instrumentality (defined as masculinity on most gender identity measures) may be implicated. It has also been shown that others' expectations follow suit and in fact may reflect more consistently held and stronger stereotypes than actual behavior. This literature has been well reviewed (O'Leary & Hansen, 1982; Deaux & Kite, 1987).

Causal Attributions for Success and Failure

Even though it is clear that expectations influence goal setting and aspirations and even performance (Nieva & Gutek, 1981; Mednick, 1982), it is less clear how expectancy change takes place and how it operates to affect performance.

Self-attributions for the causes of success and failure have been found to be an important factor in this process. The question of whether there are gender differences in causal attributions remains an open question, apparently one of those "now you see it, now you don't" phenomena. In all probability, inconsistent findings are due to the same kind of factors that impede replication in general, but in this area in particular, they are probably, to a great extent, the result of looking at men and women as homogenous groups. As already indicated, it is becoming clear that there are different types of people within each gender; the research that takes this into account is beginning to move us to a more sophisticated stage of the development of the field.

A brief summary of causal attribution theory will be presented, but the reader is cautioned to read theoretical work by Weiner (1972; see also Heckhausen et al., 1985) and early reviews of the area (Frieze, 1975) for background. Most of the study of causal attribution in the achievement area has focused on four major factors: ability, effort, luck, and task difficulty. These vary along two dimensions: the cause may be classified as internal or external or as stable or unstable in origin. Thus a cause such as ability is internal and stable, while effort is internal, but unstable. The nature of the attributions made for success and failure affects achievement behavior in specific ways. For example, it has been shown that attributing failure to (poor) ability is associated with low expectations and with low persistence (Dweck, Goetz & Strauss, 1980). Failure attributed to lack of effort, on the other hand, while internal, is also unstable, and thus its effects are not as debilitating.

Since Frieze (1975; see also Frieze, Whitley, Hanusa & McHugh, 1982) did her pioneering work on gender differences in this area, a great deal of interest has been maintained (Mednick, 1982; Nieva & Gutek, 1981). Two reviews of the early eighties (Frieze et al., 1982; Sohn, 1982) concluded that sex differences are not consistently found and, when they are found, explain very little of the variance. Frieze, Francis, and Hanusa (1983) have suggested that gender differences in defining success may be related to gender stereotypes and that the subjective definition of success may vary. This point, which has not been taken into account in most of the research on sex differences in causal attribution, may explain some of the inconsistencies. Past experience with the task, a factor no doubt frequently confounded with sex typing of the task (see Carr et al., 1985), is another variable that McHugh, Frieze, and Hanusa (1983) suggest be controlled for better understanding of the inconsistencies that have been found. It has rarely been controlled.

Such concerns did not deter researchers of the eighties. A number of the expectancy studies previously cited also included causal attribution measures. McMahan (1982) found that men made more ability attributions than women and tended to be less internal for failure; these findings, as he noted, are weak and in any event were obtained only on the neutral and male-linked tasks in his study. The pattern for women was greater externality for success and greater internality for failure. Past experience with the tasks was not controlled. Gitelson et al. (1982) also found sex differences in attributions, with girls attributing to themselves less ability than boys, though only on the male-linked (i.e., spatial relations) tasks. Hackett and Betz (1981), using a gender-neutral task, found that women were more likely to attribute their successes to luck and their failures to low ability. In their study, task neutrality may have inadvertently served as a control for past experience.

McMahan (1982), in line with our previous comments, suggested that individual difference factors should be considered. A popular personality variable has been instrumentality, the personality trait most associated with masculinity as assessed by gender identity measures such as the Bem Sex Role Inventory (BSRI) (Bem, 1974) or the Personal Attribute Questionnaire (PAQ) (Spence & Helmreich, 1978). Levine, Gillman, and Reiss (1982) found that gender differences in attributions—such that men were more likely to attribute outcomes to ability, while women used effort and luck—were explained by differences in a measure of masculinity. Welch, Gerrard, and Huston (1986), comparing high and low instrumental women, as measured by the PAQ, found that high instrumental women attributed their successes to internal factors and their failures to external factors, that is, an ''egotistical'' attributional profile. On the other hand, low instrumental women revealed the opposite profile. These findings, confirming Welch and Huston (1982), were independent of gender appropriateness of the task (see also Erkut, 1983).

LaNoue and Curtis (1985) examined the issue, also raised by McHugh, Frieze, and Hanusa (1982), of the importance of social context of the task. They manipulated sex composition of the setting in which their subjects worked. They found that an experimentally induced effort attribution resulted in raised expectancies, performance, and self-reward only in a mixed-sex condition for women. Women in a like-sexed condition were not affected, nor did men show any change with condition. Finally, very little support for attributional differences was found by Eccles, Adler, and Meece (1984) in their study of high schoolers' attitudes toward, and performance on, mathematics and English. Their study did highlight the importance of another factor, perceived task value.

In sum, though the inconsistencies are duly noted by recent reviewers, there remains a conviction that the value of these concepts is not yet fully understood. Future research must explore personal factors such as instrumentality, situational factors such as task familiarity, and contextual variables such as mixed versus like-sexed conditions.

Self-Concept, Self-Esteem, Self-Efficacy

These concepts are grouped in one section since they are conceptually similar and there were so few studies of each one.

As we noted in the review of expectancy research, girls and women are fairly consistently found to have lower estimates of their ability. This is less consistent in the self-concept/self-esteem literature. One of the more useful and interesting contributions has been that of Stake (1979, 1983), who has defined self-esteem in terms of two factors, social self-esteem and performance self-esteem. Bailey and Mednick (1988) showed that the two scales differentially predicted level of career aspiration for black women.

Heilman and Kram (1983) asked working men and women about their colleagues' views of them. Women anticipated more negative reactions from both male and female coworkers than men did. Other studies of gender and self-esteem have shown that the association is moderated by relationships (Holthe, 1986), traditionality and group counseling (Grottkau, 1986), social roles (Donnelly, 1986), and achievement motivation (Heaven, 1987).

Bandura's concept of self-efficacy (Bandura, 1977, 1982, 1986) has been applied to the study of sex differences in aspiration and achievement by Hackett and her colleagues (Hackett & Campbell, 1987; Betz & Hackett, 1981, 1987; Campbell & Hackett, 1986; Hackett & Betz, 1981). Hackett and Campbell (1987) found that both men and women were similarly affected in their ratings of self-efficacy following success and failure experiences on a gender-neutral task. Campbell and Hackett (1986) found strong gender differences in self-efficacy effects on a mathematics task. They concluded from these and other studies (see Hackett & Campbell, 1987) that gender-role considerations are important modifiers of the predictive success of self-efficacy. An examination of the measures of self-efficacy does raise the question of how different the concept is from expectancies or ability self-confidence. Some comparisons of the concepts' differential predictive power are in order. Keeping this in mind, it comes as no surprise that gender differences, depending, of course, on conditions, are found. However, a pattern has emerged, in this and previously discussed areas, that sex per se is a weak predictor. Gender role and gender identity are among the person variables that need to be, and are being, considered.

Lent, Brown, and Larkin (1986) found that self-efficacy was a strong predictor of grades and perceived career options. However, they did not find a sex difference in level of self-efficacy for their sample of men and women enrolled in a career planning course for students wishing to consider science careers. This sample may be regarded as a self-selected group with "masculine" interests; thus, the lack of a sex difference makes sense in the light of findings regarding instrumentality. It is also of interest that they found that self-efficacy was not related to a measure of general self-esteem. Nevill and Schlecker (1988) found efficacy to be related to willingness to engage in harder career choices. Self-concept of masculinity and femininity, as defined by the PAQ, had no effect on anagram performance, nor did competition with a male or female competitor (Couts, 1987).

An interesting finding that brings up the question of emotionality and how it might interact with self-perceptions of efficacy was reported by Kavanaugh (1987), who looked at mood. He found that "happy" women showed greater persistence and worked more efficiently at an anagrams task than "sad" women, regardless of efficacy level. The issue of affect has been infrequently raised by investigators during the cognitive eighties and is worth pursuing.

A concept related to self-esteem and anxiety (Topping & Kimmel, 1985) is the "impostor phenomenon" (IP). It is defined as a feeling of intellectual phoniness. Like fear of success, it is alleged to be observed in very high-achieving women (Clance & Imes, 1978; Imes, 1980). As Topping and Kimmel (1985) noted, the construct is one of those attractive ones that have great face validity, but little serious research support. Topping and Kimmel (1985) in their analytic study of the construct validity of IP, found it to be higher in men than in women and moderately correlated with self-esteem and anxiety. Its usefulness as a concept applied to the general population and as one useful for the understanding of women's achievement behavior has yet to be established.

Occupational Aspirations and Career Development

This section will examine women's occupational aspirations and career development. We begin with an overview of the work on women's occupational aspirations, followed by an examination of recent theories of women's career development. Since there has been increased attention regarding women's participation, or lack of participation, in math and science-related fields, this area is given special consideration. We then address some methodological issues in the study of women's occupational aspirations; last, to the extent that empirical data are available, a review of the achievement strivings of minority women is included.

Overview

While the research on basic concepts is proceeding, some investigators have attempted to apply theories generated in the laboratory to the study of real life behavior. Performance on an anagram task or sex-stereotyped tasks of various sorts, for example, is of importance only insofar as it can be eventually generalized to the real world. A prime real world concern has been occupational aspirations and career development of women. The concepts of achievement motivation, fear of success, self-esteem, and causal attribution have been applied to the study of occupational aspirations of girls and young women. In this section, we review research on occupation aspirations and career development of women within the context of the achievement motivation literature. While the studies cited in this section are primarily limited to the 1980s, because of the limited availability of published data on achievement of minority women, discussion relies also upon many earlier publications.

During the past 20 years, there has been a substantial increase in the amount of research focusing on achievement-related strivings and concerns of women (Baruch, 1967; Tangri, 1972; Harmon, 1971; Farmer, 1976, 1985; Tangri & Jenkins, 1986; Eccles, 1987; Osipow, 1987). Psychological research on women and work has primarily been cross-sectional, sampling mostly white, middle-class young women, with less focus on the occupational aspirations of lower-class, minority, or older women. In addition, much of the psychological research over the last two decades on women and work dealt with the increasing influx of women into nontraditional, white-collar professions such as law, medicine, and business. Much less work focused on the participation of women in traditionally male-dominated blue-collar jobs. Notable exceptions include the work of Deaux and Ullman (1982), Palmer and Lee (1988), and Douglass (1981) on problems women experience while employed in traditionally blue-collar jobs.

In general, the research utilizes many different, yet oftentimes overlapping, concepts. All of the psychological variables reviewed above (e.g., self-esteem, fear of success, expectancies), as well as external or institutional barriers (e.g., access discrimination, treatment discrimination, tokenism), are often included as predictors. Since many women develop and pursue their aspirations within the context of marital, homemaking, and childrearing responsibilities, much of the research on women and achievement has also examined various situational factors such as the influence of family background (e.g., marital status, length of marriage, number and age of children), husband's supportiveness, and work-family conflict on women's employment aspirations. Jenkins (1987) noted that there has been more research emphasis on these and other situational facilitators (e.g., mentoring, mother's role modeling, father's support) in studies of women than in similar studies of men. The latter more often focus on predictors that emphasize characteristics such as individuality and agentic capacities, as well as work-related values and attitudes, achievement and power motivation, career plans, and pursuit of opportunities. Such variables are often omitted from studies of women.

Despite the extent of women's occupational involvement, it has been generally accepted that men's goals and aspirations exceed those of women. Fitzgerald and Crites (1980) noted that, even considering men and women of comparable ability levels, the career aspirations of women are often noticeably lower than are the aspirations of men. While women are increasingly entering traditionally "male-dominated" fields, they are still considerably underrepresented in such fields. Furthermore, recent surveys of the career aspirations of children and adolescents suggest that sex-segregation will continue to characterize the work environment into the future despite women's growing interest in traditionally male-dominated occupations and professions.

The "homogenization of women," a term coined by Bem and Bem (1976), suggests a pattern of socialization of girls and young women that is detrimental to the establishment of equal opportunity in the job market. These socialization experiences impinge upon the processes that shape girls' perceptions of the viable options for occupations. Thus, certain career options are not considered because they do not fit well into the female gender-role schema (Eccles, 1987). As a result, many women, despite their abilities and talents, do not consider the full range of objectively available options in making their career decisions (Eccles, 1987; Harmon, 1981; Nieva & Gutek, 1981). The large gaps in wages and earning potential between male and female workers are thus, in large degree, a direct reflection of their differential choices of occupational roles determined by gender-role perceptions.

During the decade under review, new and exciting approaches to career development and occupational choice have been presented to explain women's occupation and career decisions (Astin, 1984; Eccles, 1987; Betz & Fitzgerald, 1987; Betz & Hackett, 1981; Farmer, 1985). These innovative approaches do not simply attempt to focus on the applicability of existing theoretical perspectives of career development, but instead suggest a meaningful approach to understanding women's career choices in the achievement arena.

Theories of Career Development and Career Choice

In an extensive review of the literature from 1960 to 1985, Betz and Fitzgerald (1987) concluded that there was no adequate theory of the career development of women, although they pointed to several promising beginnings. As evident from the following discussion, the new approaches to career development and preference among women rely upon many of the concepts we have previously discussed (e.g., expectancy, self-efficacy, attributions, values). The primary distinguishing feature among these approaches is which concept is given the central role as predictor of vocational preference.

Hackett and Betz (1981) applied self-efficacy theory (Bandura, 1977) to career behavior. In particular, they proposed that self-efficacy, or individuals' beliefs concerning their ability to successfully perform a given task or behavior, has particular relevance for the understanding of women's career development because their gender-role socialization is less likely than that of men to facilitate the development of strong career-related self-efficacy expectations. Hackett and Betz argue that women's failure to fully utilize their capabilities and talents in certain male-dominated professions, such as engineering, medicine, and various skilled trades, is due, in large part, to their low or weak self-efficacy expectations, with regard to behaviors required for successful pursuit and performance in those occupations. In a test of their theory, Hackett and Betz (1981) found that women reported higher levels of self-efficacy with regard to traditional female occupations and lower self-efficacy in relation to nontraditional occupations. Numerous studies (Ayres, 1980; Betz & Hackett, 1983; Layton, 1984; Lent et al., 1986; Nevill & Schlecker, 1988; Post-Kammer & Smith 1985; Taylor & Betz, 1983; Wheeler, 1983) have demonstrated that self-efficacy beliefs predict a wide range of career choice behavior.

Astin (1984) formulated a sociopsychological model of women's career choice and work behavior. Drawing upon empirical evidence and past theoretical formulations (Roe, 1956; Bandura, 1977; Hackett & Betz, 1981), Astin's model incorporates psychological variables, as well as contextual-sociological variables, or social forces and the interaction of the two, as shapers of career aspirations. Astin proposed that basic work motivation is the same for men and women but they make different choices because their early socialization experiences, as well as structural opportunities, are different. This sociopsychological model is primarily intended to deal with two important issues: (1) gender differences in career choice and (2) recent changes in women's career aspirations and occupational behavior.

While Astin supports Hackett and Betz's focus on self-efficacy as an important intrapsychic variable in explaining the career development of women, she also pointed to the limited capacity of such a model in increasing our understanding of how changes in social-structural factors are also involved in such behavior. Astin's model is a need-based sociological model that incorporates the concepts of motivation, expectations, gender-role socialization, and the structure of opportunity. It is also a developmental model intended to explain changes in career choice and work behavior, changes observed not only in the lives of individuals but also in groups (e.g., women) over time. In a critique of Astin's model, Fitzgerald and Betz (1984) pointed out that it was inadequate on scientific grounds. However, Astin's approach is one of the few psychological models that at least recognize the significance of social context.

Farmer (1985) developed a multidimensional model of career development and achievement motivation for women. This model, like that of Betz and Hackett (1981), was also heavily influenced by Bandura's (1977) social learning theory. Farmer incorporated Bandura's principles that learning and related behavior result from three sets of interacting influences, namely, (1) background factors (e.g., gender, ethnicity, ability), (2) psychological or personal self-concept factors (e.g., attitudes, beliefs, previous experiences), and (3) environmental or social factors that affect the individual. She argues that this wide range of influences affects three motivational dimensions: (1) aspirations, (2) mastery, and (3) career commitment. In this multidimensional model, Farmer noted that the combined influences of the several factors are expected to account for substantial variance in achievement-related outcomes. Farmer stressed that the multidimensional nature of her model was especially applicable when studying women and persons of different social status or ethnic background because of the wide array of personal and cultural influences studied.

Farmer tested her theory and found that all three sets of influences were significantly related to each of the three motivation dimensions. In particular, career motivation was influenced approximately three times as much by personal factors (e.g., expressiveness and independence, homemaking commitment, personal unconcern) as by background and environment factors. With respect to gender differences, she found that homemaking commitment was negatively and significantly related to long-range career motivation for young women but not for young men. Androgynous self-concept also more often related to long-range career motivation for women than for men. Farmer believes that her model, unlike the dominant career motivation models of Holland (1985) and Super and colleagues (Super, 1957; Super, Stareshevskey, Matlin & Jordan, 1963), is more comprehensive since it takes into account the powerful influence of the changing environment on career and achievement motivation for women.

Eccles (1987) postulated that occupational choices are influenced most directly by the value individuals place on each of an array of choices perceived as appropriate and by their subjective estimate of the probability of success at these various options. In her theory, Eccles does not focus on why women do not achieve like men, a deficiency model, but instead postulates positive factors that motivate women to make certain achievement-related choices, a subjective choice model. This approach views occupational choice as heavily influenced by socialization pressure, gender-role beliefs, and cultural norms. Also, expectation for occupational success is viewed as being influenced by confidence in one's abilities, as well as by the dynamics of various institutional constraints such as discrimination and tokenism.

Eccles proposed that occupational choices are determined by four major factors: (1) an individual's expectations for success on various options perceived as being appropriate, (2) an individual's values or the relation of these options to the individual's short- and long-range goals and to his or her core self-identity and basic psychological needs, (3) the individual's gender role and more general self-schema, and (4) the potential cost of investing time in one activity rather than another. Integrating the notion of subjective task value, Eccles suggests that differences in male and female career choices result from the fact that, oftentimes, men and women have different, but equally important, goals for their lives and that these goals influence occupational aspirations. She did note, however, that men's and women's goals may change over their lifetime as their roles and obligations change.

In summary, recent theories of career development make concerted efforts to integrate the occupational aspirations and development of women within a theoretical framework. In their book, *The Career Psychology of Women,* Betz and Fitzgerald (1987) pointed out that further advances in our knowledge of women's career development will require both theoretical innovation and synthesis. For the most part, however, newer theories of career development and occupational aspirations recognize the importance of personality factors, individual interests, values, the availability of desired rewards, perceived capabilities or self-efficacy, as well as a variety of external factors such as sexism and tokenism within the workplace. The role of a changing society is also given some attention in newer theories. The increased use of a multidimensional approach (Farmer, 1985; Tinsley & Faunce, 1980) is thus apparent, as well as a concern regarding the formulation of testable models of women's career development and the use of a multivariate methodology such as structural equation modeling (e.g., Fassinger, 1985). While better theories of women's career development are emerging, there is still a need for the development and elaboration of theories with a view toward integrating existing knowledge, generating testable hypotheses, and guiding vocational counseling approaches to ensure that girls and young women are encouraged to consider a broad range of occupational options based not on their sex, but instead, upon their values, talents, and abilities.

Women's Achievement in Math and Science-Related Fields

There are numerous occupational areas that have a relatively small proportion of women. Among professional fields, however, the limited participation of women in mathematics and scientifically related jobs is quite evident. Over the past 20 years, there has been considerable empirical interest in women's capability and education in mathematics and their subsequent participation in math-related careers (Benbow & Stanley, 1980; Chipman, Brush, & Wilson, 1985; Chipman & Thomas, 1987; Eccles & Jacobs, 1986; Hyde et al., 1989; Jagacinski, 1987; Lips & Temple, 1988; Singer & Stake, 1986). While most research generated by social scientists and educators is seldom considered newsworthy by the popular media, the issue of gender differences in mathematical ability was extensively covered by the media in the late 1970s and early 1980s (Jacobs & Eccles, 1985).

Chipman and Thomas (1987) noted that since scientific and technical experts play a critical role in shaping the future of our society, it is important that the gender and racial composition of our scientific and technical work force be broadly representative. In the 1970s, the issue of women and mathematics was examined by both the popular and scholarly press. During this time, math anxiety and math avoidance were considered women's issues. Programs, clinics, and workshops for overcoming math anxiety were designed with young women as the target audience.

Newspaper and magazine accounts of the eighties were somewhat misleading. While these sources suggested that the major reason women were poorly represented in many highly paid professional occupations was that they lacked the prerequisite mathematical knowledge, it came as quite a surprise to many to know that throughout the period of 1950 to 1976, women averaged 30% of all bachelor's degrees in mathematics; they received 38 to 42% of all bachelor's degrees in mathematics between 1971 and 1976; and, in 1987, women received

46% of bachelor's degrees in mathematics. In terms of the high school years, the College Entrance Examination Board (1985) reported that as of 1985, 45% of students reporting four or more years of high school mathematics courses and who were taking the Scholastic Entrance Examination (SAT) were women. Thus, mathematics as a "critical filter" or the problem of females' participation in high school mathematics courses and as an undergraduate mathematics major is not as severe as many had assumed.

Based upon a review of empirical studies, Chipman and Thomas (1985) concluded that sex differences in mathematics course enrollment are largely confined to the very advanced courses (e.g., calculus, trigonometry). However, gender differences do exist in aspirations to a life career in which mathematics is essential. An array of biological, attitudinal, and affective variables has been studied to explain these differences.

From a biological perspective, Benbow and Stanley (1980) argued that genetically based superior male mathematical ability is the best explanation for sex differences in mathematics aptitude and attitudes toward mathematics. These conclusions, however, have been strongly challenged by other investigators (Eccles & Jacobs, 1986; Schafer, 1981; Slack & Porter, 1980; Jackson, 1980), who posited experiential factors of various sorts.

Social influences that have been demonstrated to have an effect on girls' and women's pursuit of and persistence in mathematics-related endeavors include parental and teacher encouragement, peer influence, role models, and family background (e.g., socioeconomic status, parents' occupational status, and parents' sex-stereotyped beliefs; see, e.g., Armstrong, 1985; Eccles & Jacobs, 1986). In an overview of the empirical literature, Chipman and Thomas (1987) concluded that a weak positive relation exists between parental encouragement and continued enrollment in mathematics; a somewhat stronger relationship, especially for older students, exists between teacher encouragement and continued enrollment in mathematics.

A number of attitudinal factors have been found to be related to women's persistence in mathematics. For example, Eccles, Adler, and Meece (1984) concluded that sex differences in math participation are mediated by individuals' attitudes regarding the value of mathematics for their future lives. Boswell (1985) pointed out that stereotypes associated with mathematics are learned by children at a very young age and that knowledge of such stereotypes affects their participation and performance in mathematics. These findings are not always consistent. For example, Singer and Stake (1986), in a study of male and female college students, did not find that women, compared with men, had greater math anxiety, lower self-assessments of math ability, or lower endorsement of mathematics as useful. While these investigators noted that women may now be more positive in their math attitudes than may have been the case in the past, Singer and Stake did acknowledge that the bulk of the research findings indicates that women's math attitudes are still somewhat less positive than those of males.

Jacobs and Eccles (1985) found that exposure to media reports affects parents' attitudes toward their children's math abilities. For example, these investigators found that mothers who were exposed to the media reports of Benbow and Stanley's (1980) research that indicated a major sex difference in mathematical reasoning ability thought that their daughters had less math ability, were less likely to succeed in math in the future, and had to work harder to succeed in math than those mothers who were not exposed to the Benbow and Stanley report; exposure to media reports also increased the gender-role stereotyping of fathers of daughters, but to a lesser extent than it did for fathers of sons. Thus, the influence of the media on math attitudes is evident. It is also noteworthy that the print media continue to find even the most trivial research reporting sex differences in mathematics newsworthy, even though results of meta-analyses of gender differences and mathematics performance and attitudes are at most small to moderate (Hyde et al., 1990).

Methodological Issues

A number of methodological concerns need to be raised in relation to the study of women's career and occupational aspirations. Three issues discussed in this section are (1) defining career aspirations, (2) research design, and (3) generalizability.

Defining Career Aspirations

Career aspirations and career choice are the most widely examined dependent variables studied in field research of women's achievement strivings and behavior. The bulk of this research has examined how motivational, cognitive, and situational factors relate to women's achievement striving in the workplace. In general, the study of career aspirations and choice of women has focused on their desire to pursue traditional or nontraditional occupations. Most of the research has utilized a statistical definition in operationalizing a career as "traditional" or "nontraditional." That is, nontraditional careers are those employing less than 30% of women according to either U.S. census data or statistics reported by the U.S. Department of Labor; traditional fields are defined as those employing more than 50% women. Tangri (1972) referred to nontraditional women as role innovators. In addition to the role innovators and the traditionals, Tangri included another category in her earlier and follow-up (Tangri & Jenkins, 1986) research. These women, referred to as moderates, were employed in fields consisting of a 30 to 50% concentration of women.

While the statistical definition of career traditionality and nontraditionality is consistently used in current research, there are some inadequacies in relying solely upon such an approach. Bailey and Mednick (1988) noted that occupations usually statistically defined as nontraditional may have subspecialties or other characteristics that may conform to the demands and characteristics of women's traditional role and thus may be viewed in traditional terms by the aspirant. Thus, the perception or image of the occupation held by the individual is a critical element. This is especially the case for minority women since there are still career options that may be statistically defined as traditional for women in general, but are viewed as nontraditional by black or other ethnic minority women (e.g., ballet dancer, flight attendant). Some investigators focusing on minority women have measured perceived traditionality of career choices (Bailey, 1982; Bailey & Mednick, 1988; Thomas, 1983).

Another aspect of job traditionality that is not often examined in studies of minority women is the traditionality of a job for the gender and racial group simultaneously. In her 1982 study, Malveaux (cited in Malveaux & Wallace, 1987) explored the dual division of occupational segregation for black women and developed the concept, "black women's crowding" to measure the extent to which black women work in occupations that are "crowded" by black women. Within Malveaux's framework, "typically black female jobs" are those in which black women are four or more times their labor proportion in that particular occupation. We argue that studies of traditionality of work aspirations, when studying minority populations, should examine the interaction between occupations that are traditional for women and those that are traditional for specific ethnic groups. No psychological studies were found that examined this interaction.

Some investigators (e.g., Bailey, 1982; Bailey & Mednick, 1988) suggest that the utilization of a combination of the statistical and subjective methods of defining occupations provides a more useful approach than either method in isolation. Career aspirations are complex; thus, women aspiring to nontraditional occupations may be traditional in other respects and vice versa. For example, Mednick (1982) reported that many women who aspired to a nontraditional field, such as pharmacy, gave traditional reasons for wanting to enter this field. These reasons centered around the pharmacy's occupational structure, such as the availability of part-time employment and the availability of employment close to one's home; such characteristics permit the coordination of family and work life. Thus, the classification of women as "nontraditional" or "traditional" based solely on the percent of women in a given field may be misleading and lead to inappropriate and incorrect conclusions regarding such women's achievement and affiliative values. This may also explain some of the inconsistencies and contradictions of prediction in this area.

The work of Helson and her colleagues (Helson, 1987; Helson, Elliot & Leigh, 1990; Helson, Mitchell & Moane, 1984) presents an innovative approach to defining women's career aspirations. In contrast to traditional measures that simply classify occupations as female (traditional)- or male (nontraditional)-dominated, these investigators ranked occupations in terms of within-field characteristics such as opportunity for advancement, need for advanced degree, level of sustained success, level of responsibility, leadership, and specialization. For example, the ranking of a nurse or social worker would be higher if the individual had advanced training or had managerial functions in this position. Helson, Mitchell, and Moane (1984) also introduced the concepts of masculine occupational clock (MOC) and feminine social clock (FSC). These investigators view MOC and FSC as social clock patterns that deal with the life schedules of particular individuals in particular societies and cohorts. Social clock patterns organize the study of lives in terms of patterned movement along, or away from, adherence to active social norms. The FSC pattern was used to describe women who got married and started a family in their early or middle twenties. On the other hand, women were classified as having started on the MOC if by age 28, they had chosen a field of work with status potential and had shown evidence of persistence and advancement in their field. This approach has the potential to channel the research in this area to a useful and fruitful integration of social context into the equation.

Research Design

As stated earlier, most of the psychological studies conducted on women's career aspirations and career development have been cross-sectional, as is the case for most research in our field. Only three longitudinal studies are available at this time. Clearly, our understanding of women's career and work aspirations and how these change during women's lives cannot be fully understood only through cross-sectional research (Stewart, Lykes & LaFrance, 1982). Tangri and Jenkins (1986), in a longitudinal study, examined the career and life development of women (Tangri, 1972) who had finished college. These women were studied first in 1967, again in 1970, and most recently in 1981. Tangri and Jenkins (1986) compared the plans these women had made about careers and family with the directions they actually took and were thus able to detect general trends in the occupational attainment, marriage, and childbearing patterns over time, conflict experienced over combining these roles, and the relationship of these patterns with the larger social changes of which this cohort was a part. Harmon's (1981) work included a follow-up study of the life and career paths of 391 women six years after they had entered college. Helson, et al. (1984) conducted a longitudinal study of 132 women who had graduated from college in 1958 and 1960. These women were contacted again in 1981 to ascertain the timing of life events and their fit with societal norms. While the results of these studies are enlightening, much more longitudinal research is needed to further increase our understanding of changes and development in women's aspirations over time. The focus of most cross-sectional research is also on college students, and it is clear from the adult development literature (Troll, 1982) that adulthood is best understood via longitudinal research. Thus, our knowledge of influencers of women's choices is incomplete. Further studies will be invaluable in demonstrating how environmental, sociocultural, and personality developmental factors influence women's achievement strivings and behavior.

Generalizability

Most of the psychological research on women, achievement, and career aspirations has utilized white, middle-class college students. This raises questions regarding the generalizability of these findings to other socioeconomic groups. Nieva and Gutek (1981) noted that there are talented women of lower-class socioeconomic status who do not attend college and are certainly worth studying. Also, psychological research has almost exclusively omitted empirical investigation of nonprofessional women. Given that the majority of women in the labor force are in nonprofessional white-collar, clerical, and sales jobs, there is obviously a large segment of the female population being ignored in studies of achievement strivings within the work environment.

Generalizability of current research to women of ethnic or minority background is also problematic since few studies focus on minority women. As a result of cultural differences in the socialization patterns, as well as the additional institutional barriers experienced by minority women, there is no real justification for the expectation that the findings of research based on white women are generalizable to women of color. Similarly, most of the research has focused on women residing in an urban environment, with little research geared toward southern and/or rural women. Turner (1983) noted the paucity of research on southern women, particularly southern black women. Her investigation was one of the few studies that examined achievement among young, southern black women. A concerted effort should be made to ensure that future research includes women from different ethnic, racial, and socioeconomic statuses.

Minority Women

Though the psychological literature on minority women and achievement is quite sparse, it is well worth reviewing. However, the present overview of the literature relies heavily upon research conducted prior to the 1980s and a synthesis and review of the few recent studies. It must also be noted that the bulk of the psychological research available on minority women has focused on black women.

Murray and Mednick (1977) reviewed the literature on motivational and cognitive factors related to achievement orientation of black women. These investigators concluded that no specific patterns emerge regarding determinants of achievement orientation in black women. Murray and Mednick did note that data revealed that black women do not consistently hold expectancies and make causal attributions in a manner that is predictable from traditional role considerations; in fact, their behavior in these areas oftentimes resembles that of achievement-oriented men. Similarly, Weiner and Kukla (1970) suggested that black women with high achievement motivation employ both ability and effort attributions. Murray and Mednick's (1977) review of fear of success (FOS) studies (Bright, 1970; Mednick & Puryear, 1975; Weston & Mednick, 1970) indicated that black women consistently exhibited lower levels of FOS imagery than their white counterparts. Research focusing on black women reported by Fleming (1977) indicated that the behavior of middle-class women supported the notion that black women, in comparison with white women, are more achievement-oriented and that FOS does not inhibit their performance on competitive tasks. For working-class black women, however, Fleming found that FOS exerted a strong influence on behavior and inhibited performance. Fleming also found that FOS among black, middle-class women was associated with a father who encouraged behavior consonant with achievement while no such relationship was observed among their working-class counterparts. Thus, it becomes apparent that under certain conditions the achievement behavior of black women parallels that of their white counterparts, whereas in other conditions different patterns of behavior emerge.

Career Aspirations of Minority Women

Historically, minority women have been more likely to be in the labor force than white women. From 1978 to the present, however, the rate of labor force participation of white women grew much more rapidly than for minority women. In most recent years, there was little difference between white women's overall employment rate (57.2%) and that of black women (58.7%) and Hispanic women (53.5%) (U.S. Department of Labor, 1990). The fact that minority women historically participated in the labor force as a result of financial necessity rather than for self-development probably has some psychological implications for how minority women view work. That is, minority women's career aspirations may be influenced, in large part, by a sense of responsibility rather than simply by their need to achieve.

Black Women

Fleming (1983) notes that there are two conflicting images of black women in the social science literature. These images affect black women's, as well as society's, perception of appropriate occupational aspirations for them. One image portrays black women as strong, competent, self-reliant, and dominant. The opposing view depicts them as victims who suffer the double jeopardy of being female and black in a sexist and racist society. In reality, these views may not represent opposing dimensions, since black women, as victims of double discrimination, may develop qualities such as strength, competence, self-reliance, and dominance in order to survive in a society that is both racist and sexist.

While there is a perception that black women have an advantage over black men in the work world (Puryear, 1980; Thomas, 1990), statistics indicate that black women are more likely than black men or white women to be in low-paying jobs, to be single head of households, and to account for a larger proportion of those living in poverty (U.S. Department of Commerce, 1990). Despite the multiple negatives, there is a small, but growing, segment of black women pursuing professional careers. Black women's educational achievements and actual wage earnings are closer to those of black men than are those of white women to white men. In fact, in 1989, the median income of full-time black women workers was $17,908, which represented 86% of black men's total earnings. Comparatively, white women's median income of $19,873 was 67%, of white men's earnings. Of course, it is important to note that none of these groups has caught up to the top earner—white men. In terms of higher educational achievement, black women received 60% of all bachelor's degrees awarded to blacks (cited in Horton & Smith, 1990). This advantage for black women does drop considerably at the doctoral and first professional degree level (Chipman & Thomas, 1987).

Studies suggest that the psychological barriers that may impede white women from pursuing certain career options may be less of an inhibiting factor for black women. For example, earlier work on fear of success suggested that some black women have low levels of fear of success imagery relative to that generally found in white women (Bright, 1970; Mednick & Puryear, 1975; Mednick & Weissman, 1975; Weston & Mednick, 1970). It has been argued that sex-role stereotyping and fear of rejection by men may not be as salient a factor in the lives of black women when considering a career, because black men are generally more supportive of working wives (Axelson, 1970), have less stereotypic views of the female role (Crovitz & Steinmann, 1980), and tend to make accommodations to the special needs of working wives (Scanozi, 1975).

It should also be noted, however, that motivational and personality factors have similarly differentiated black women aspiring to traditional and nontraditional careers. For example, Thomas (1983) found that black women who were high in risk taking, high in preference for delayed gratification, and low in fear of success perceived their careers to be more nontraditional than black women who were low in risk taking, low in preference for delayed gratification, and high in fear of success. Mednick (1981) found that perceived causal attributions distinguished two groups of black women such that traditionals were more likely than nontraditionals to be external and to make unstable attributions for success and more internal attributions for failure. Research (e.g., Thomas, 1986) also has shown that most young, black, female adolescents still aspire to traditionally female-dominated occupations. While the psychological research on black women is growing, considerably more research is clearly needed before broad generalizations can be made. We are also totally unaware of how the interaction of age, social change, and family life choices has affected black women since there has not been one longitudinal study conducted with black women as the target group.

Other Ethnic Women

Data reported by the U.S. Census (1990) indicate that approximately 13% of Hispanic women are employed in managerial professional occupations. Amaro, Russo, and Johnson (1987) noted that with relatively few exceptions (e.g., Ash, 1972; Cooney, 1975), studies examining the occupational pursuits of Hispanic women have relied upon a gender model, or one that uses personal characteristics and family situations as predictor variables. While Hispanic women grow up with rigid, traditional gender-role norms and expectations (Canino, 1982) that influence achievement strivings, there is not much empirical research to evaluate how this translates into achievement behavior.

Similar to some of the assumptions regarding Hispanic culture, researchers (e.g., Chow, 1987) suggest that Asian American women have been generally confined to traditional sex roles and are perceived as subservient to men. Chow further notes that Asian culture tends to reinforce affiliation, altruism, adaptiveness, and timidity for both sexes, while especially discouraging women from acquiring masculine traits such as activism, independence, and competitiveness. Studies relating how these values influence achievement behavior among Asian women are also needed.

No empirical studies were found in the psychological literature on achievement behavior among American Indian women. It is noteworthy to mention, however, that in the late seventies, the Women's Research Program at the National Institute of Education developed a program initiative to address the occupational and educational needs of American Indian women, as well as black, Hispanic, Asian-Pacific Island, and white ethnic women.

Summary

A review of the literature certainly points to the need for empirical studies of achievement and minority women. While numerous influences and hypotheses can be made based on cultural patterns, more laboratory and field studies are necessary to confirm such speculations. As research in this field is expanded to include minority women, the nature of achievement among women and the conditions under which there are some systematic variations in achievement strivings can be more readily discerned.

CONCLUSIONS

When we started this review, we posed a set of "big questions." Has the research on women and achievement fulfilled expectations, particularly those based on a feminist view of research? Have the phenomena being studied changed? What is the nature of the change? Have important, useful theories been developed? How have we dealt with the problems of integrating race, class, and ethnicity into this work? Indeed, has the goal of understanding all kinds of women been achieved, or even approached?

Of course, these are the kinds of questions that are very difficult to answer with a review of the research that appears in journals, books, and papers published by psychologists. There are a number of reasons for this; one is that we are method-bound, so a huge amount of research is done simply because an easily administered instrument is available. Another is that psychology responds to fashion in ideas, and ideas become fashionable for a variety of reasons (Mednick, 1989a), in addition to the legitimate questions in an area. Also, there are perceived social need and the politics of funding. Psychologists, like most scientists, are not generally in positions where they can do unfunded research. This may be more true of psychologists who are feminist researchers than of others. There is also little evidence that the research gatekeepers have welcomed feminist, or any kind of innovative, research.

If one were to search for a word to characterize the research we have reviewed, *mainstream* would serve quite well for the bulk of it. However, since the social context of the study of women and achievement has undergone great change, the meaning of the research takes on a different hue. In the eighties, there was less questioning about whether women ought to achieve or can achieve, but instead there was a realization that women are in the workplace because they need to be and, moreover, because they are needed. In view of these facts, the questions we ask, even in laboratory studies of such concepts as motivation or expectancies, have entirely different implications for life in the real world. This is most strongly reflected in interpretations of findings, particularly in a continued questioning of stereotypic assumptions about gender identity and roles.

Certain old issues are absent, at least from the literature we surveyed, for example, the complete absence of questions about career commitment, an often-asked question in earlier days. It does not seem to be an interesting concern anymore; at least one reason is that asking the question earlier was due to the assumption that women did not have commitment to careers. We, of course, are also no longer assuming that women are not motivated to achieve; the review demonstrates very clearly that they are. The only argument appears to be around the questions of whether there are different arenas of achievement (Travis et al., 1988) or different types or styles of achievement motivation (Spence & Helm-reich, 1983; Lipman-Blumen et al., 1983) and whether women behave differently from men in this regard.

Certainly it is also no longer assumed that women who pursue careers are neurotic, an often-expressed view in prefeminist days. However, the move away from such a view began in the early seventies, and the question we have tried to answer is what has changed during the past decade. We are very much inclined to say, not enough. The vast amount of literature reviewed has continued on the same track. This is evident in the variables studied, the methods used, and the questions asked by researchers. Also, for the most part, current trends in research in psychology are reflected in the study of women and achievement. There are a few exceptions to this assessment, for example, the longitudinal studies we reviewed, particularly those that used conceptions that integrated social context and person variables. Longitudinal research in general seems to be moving us to a type of analysis and theory that should be fruitful to guide future work. The goal of looking at women's lives developmentally and in social context holds the greatest promise for a feminist approach to achievement.

A number of investigators have recognized and addressed the complexity issue as well. In particular, these are in the domains of occupational aspiration and math achievement, work that indicates that a complete understanding of women's achievement behavior awaits further efforts at multivariate analysis. It is to be hoped that feminist psychologists working on these questions will also deal with contextual issues such as power and status differentials between the genders.

It is probably more controversial to assert that sex differences are few, that is, sex is a very weak predictor. The studies we reviewed demonstrated again and again that other characteristics, though they may be gender-related, explain apparent differences. This was true in the achievement motivation research, the expectancy research, the causal attribution research, and even in a variable created for women, fear of success. Future researchers, particularly those who wish to address the question of apparent differences, must be very careful to rule out alternative explanations. We would argue very strongly for the latter point and urge that journals do not accept a mere sex difference finding, no matter how robust it appears to be. The "women are different" hypothesis has not been demonstrated in the achievement arena.

On the other hand, it is also clear that what might be dubbed "the heterogeneity factor" continues to be ignored. There has been much rhetoric since the late sixties about the need to study all types of women. Most notable, as we have seen in this review, is the issue of race and ethnic variation. We still have to write about the *absence* of research on these women. Although there is more awareness of the need, there has not been a commensurate increase in published research or in dissertation research. We also have not done much with socio-economic class; as we noted, studies of working-class women are notable by their absence. And, of course, little has been done to address the interaction of race, class, and gender. Another term in such an interaction is age; only a few longitudinal studies have addressed what happens to women as they grow older and pass through various social times (Troll, 1982). Most research conventionally continues to use college-aged samples, and that is intrinsically limiting, not only to generalizability, but to the framing of the questions we need to address.

Finally, it is no longer true that the topic of women and achievement are an unstudied topic. There is a continuing, lively interest in the area, and it is to be hoped that creative feminist researchers will bring new theory and new approaches to the field. As we move through the nineties, the key words need to be theory, social context, and heterogeneity.

REFERENCES

Adams, J., Priest, R. F., & Prince, H. T., II. (1985). Achievement motive: Analyzing the validity of the WOFO. *Psychology of Women Quarterly, 9*, 357–370.
Alagna, S. W. (1982). Sex role identity, peer evaluation of competition, and the responses of women and men in a competitive situation. *Journal of Personality and Social Psychology 43*, 546–554.
Amaro, H., Russo, N. F., & Johnson, J. (1987). Family and work predictors of psy-

chological well-being among Hispanic women professionals. *Psychology of Women Quarterly, 11*, 505–532.

Armstrong, J. M. (1985). A national assessment of participation and achievement of women in mathematics. In S. F. Chipman, L. R. Brush, & D. M. Wilson (Eds.), *Women and mathematics: Balancing the equation* (pp. 59–94). Hillsdale, NJ: Lawrence Erlbaum Associates.

Ash, P. (1972). Job satisfaction differences among women of different ethnic groups. *Journal of Vocational Behavior, 2*, 495–587.

Astin, H. S. (1984). The meaning of women's lives: A sociopsychological model of career choice and work behavior. *Counseling Psychologist, 12*, 117–126.

Atkinson, J. W. (1958). *Motives in fantasy, action and society*. Princeton, NJ: Van Nostrand.

Atkinson, J. W., & Feather, N. T. (1966). *A theory of achievement motivation*. New York: Wiley.

Axelson, L. J. (1970). The working wife: Differences in perception among Negro and white males. *Journal of Marriage and the Family, 32*, 457–467.

Ayres, A. L. (1980). *Self-efficacy theory: Implications for the career development of women*. Unpublished doctoral dissertation, Ohio State University, Columbus.

Bailey, C. (1982). *Career aspirations and commitment in black college women: An examination of background, attitudinal and cognitive factors*. Unpublished doctoral dissertation, Howard University, Washington, DC.

Bailey, C., & Mednick, M. (1988). Career aspiration in black college women: An examination of performance and social esteem. *Women in Therapy, 6*, 65–75.

Bandura, A. (1977). Self-efficacy: Toward a unifying theory of behavior change. *Psychological Review, 84*, 191–215.

Bandura, A. (1982). Self-efficacy mechanism in human agency. *American Psychologist, 37*, 122–147.

Bandura, A. (1986). *Social foundations of thought and action: A social theory*. Englewood Cliffs, NJ: Prentice-Hall.

Baruch, R. (1967). The achievement motive in women: Implications for career development. *Journal of Personality and Social Psychology, 5*, 260–267.

Baruch, G., Barnett, R., & Rivers, C. (1983). *Lifeprints: New patterns of love and work for today's women*. New York: McGraw-Hill.

Bem, S. L. (1974). The measurement of psychological androgyny. *Journal of Consulting and Clinical Psychology, 42*, 155–162.

Bem, S. L., & Bem, D. J. (1976). Training the woman to know her place: The power of a nonconscious ideology. In S. Cox (Ed.), *Female psychology: The emerging self* (180–191). Chicago: Science Research Associates.

Benbow, C. P., & Stanley, J. C. (1980). Sex differences in mathematics: Fact or artifact? *Science, 210*, 1262–1264.

Benton, C., Hernanadez, A., Schmidt, A., Schmidt, M., Stone, A., & Weiner, B. (1983). Is hostility linked with affiliation among males and with achievement among females? A critique of Pollack & Gilligan. *Journal of Personality and Social Psychology, 45*, 1167–1171.

Bernardin, J. J. (1982). *Women in the workforce*. New York: Praeger.

Betz, N. E., & Fitzgerald, L. F. (1987). *The career psychology of women*. Orlando, FL: Academic Press.

Betz, N. E., & Hackett, G. (1981). The relationship of career-related self-efficacy expectations to perceived career options in college women and men. *Journal of Counseling Psychology, 28*, 399–410.

Betz, N. E., & Hackett, G. (1983). The relationship of mathematics self-efficacy expectations to the selection of science-based college majors. *Journal of Vocational Behavior, 23*, 329–345.

Betz, N. E., & Hackett, G. (1987). Concepts of agency in educational and career development. *Journal of Counseling Psychology, 34*, 299–308.

Boswell, S. L. (1985). The influence of sex-role stereotyping on women's attitudes and achievements in mathematics. In S. F. Chipman, L. R. Brush, & D. M. Wilson (Eds.), *Women and mathematics: Balancing the equation* (pp. 175–198). Hillsdale, NJ: Lawrence Erlbaum Associates.

Bremer, T. H., & Wittig, M. A. (1980). Fear of success: A personality trait or a response to occupational deviance and role overload? *Sex Roles, 6*, 27–46.

Bridges, J. S. (1988). Sex differences in occupational performance expectations. *Psychology of Women Quarterly, 12*, 75–90.

Bright, M. F. (1970). *Fear of success and traditionality of occupational choice.* Unpublished master's thesis, Howard University, Washington, DC.

Campbell, N. K., & Hackett, G. (1986). The effects of mathematics task performance on math self-efficacy and task interest. *Journal of Vocational Behavior, 28*, 149–162.

Canino, G. (1982). The Hispanic woman: Sociocultural influences on diagnoses and treatment. In R. Bercerra, M. Karno, & J. Escobar (Eds.), *The Hispanic: Mental health issues and strategies* (pp. 117–138). New York: Grune & Stratton.

Carr, P. G., Thomas, V. G., & Mednick, M. T. (1985). Evaluations of sex-typed tasks by black men and women. *Sex Roles, 13*, 311–316.

Chipman, S. F., Brush, L. R., & Wilson, D. M. (Eds.). (1985). *Women and mathematics: Balancing the equation.* Hillsdale, NJ: Erlbaum.

Chipman, S. F., & Thomas, V. G. (1985). Women's participation in mathematics: Outlining the problem. In S. F. Chipman, L. R. Brush, & D. M. Wilson (Eds.), *Women and mathematics: Balancing the equation* (pp. 1–24). Hillsdale, NJ: Lawrence Erlbaum Associates.

Chipman, S. F., & Thomas, V. G. (1987). The participation of women and minorities in mathematical, scientific, and technical fields. In E. Z. Rothkoph (Ed.), *Review of research in education* (pp. 387–430). Washington, DC: American Educational Research Association.

Chow, E. N. (1987). The influence of role identity and occupational attainment on the psychological well-being of Asian-American women. *Psychology of Women Quarterly, 11*, 69–81.

Clance, P. R., & Imes, S. A. (1978). The imposter phenomenon in high achieving women: Dynamics and therapeutic intervention. *Psychotherapy: Therapy, Research and Practice, 15*, 241–247.

College Entrance Examination Board. (1985). *National college bound seniors.* Princeton, NJ: Admissions Testing Program of the College Board.

Cook, E. A., & Chandler, T. A. (1984). Is fear of success a motive? An attempt to answer criticisms. *Adolescence, 19*, 667–674.

Cooney, R. S. (1975). Changing labor force participation of Mexican-American wives: A comparison with Anglos and blacks. *Social Science Quarterly, 56*, 252–261.

Coutts, J. S. (1987). Masculinity of self-concept: Its effect on the achievement behavior of women. *Sex Roles, 16*, 9–17.

Crovitz, E., & Steinmann, A. (1980). A decade later: Black-white attitudes toward women's familial role. *Psychology of Women Quarterly, 5*, 170–176.

Daubman, K. A., Heatherington, L., & Ahn, A. (1982). Gender and the self presentation of academic achievement. *Sex Roles, 27*, 187–204.

Deaux, K. (1984). Individual differences to social categories: Analysis of a decade's research on gender. *American Psychologist, 39*, 105–116.

Deaux, K., & Kite, M. E. (1987). Thinking about gender. In B. B. Hess & M. M. Ferree (Eds.), *Analyzing gender: A handbook of social science research* (pp. 92–117). Beverly Hills: Sage Press.

Deaux, K., & Ullman, J. (1982). Hard-hatted women. Reflections of blue-collar employment. In H. Bernardin (Ed.), *Women in the Workforce* (pp. 29–47). New York: Praeger.

Donnelly, S. C. (1986). An analysis of themes related to gender identity, social role, and achievement for women writing doctoral dissertations. *Dissertation Abstracts International, 46* (12-A. Pt 1).

Douglass, P. H. (1981). *Black working women.* Cambridge, MA: Harvard University Press.

Dweck, C. S., Goetz, T. E., & Strauss, N. C. (1980). Sex differences in learned helplessness: IV. An experimental and naturalistic study of failure generalization and its mediators. *Journal of Personality and Social Psychology, 38*, 441–452.

Eccles, J. S. (1983). Expectancies, values and academic behaviors. In J. T. Spence (Ed.), *Achievement and achievement motives: Psychological and sociological approaches* (pp. 75–146). San Francisco: Freeman.

Eccles, J. S. (1987). Gender roles and achievement-related decisions. *Psychology of Women Quarterly, 11*, 135–171.

Eccles, J. S., Adler, T. F., & Meece, J. L. (1984). Sex differences in achievement: A test of alternative theories. *Journal of Personality and Social Psychology, 46*, 26–43.

Eccles, J. S., & Jacobs, J. (1986). Social forces shape math participation. *Signs, 11*, 367–380.

Erkut, S. (1983). Exploring sex differences in expectancy, attributions, and academic performance. *Sex Roles, 9*, 217–231.

Farmer, H. (1976). What inhibits career and achievement motivation in women? *Counseling Psychologist, 6*, 12–14.

Farmer, H. S. (1980). Environmental, background and psychological variables related to optimizing achievement and career motivation of high school girls. *Journal of Vocational Behavior, 17*, 58–70.

Farmer, H. S. (1985). Model of career and achievement motivation for women and men. *Journal of Counseling Psychology, 32*, 363–390.

Farmer, H. S. (1987). Female motivation and achievement: Implications for intervention. In M. L. Maehr & D. A. Klecher (Eds.), *Advances in motivation and achievement Vol. 5: Enhancing motivation.* Greenwich, CT: JAI Press.

Fassinger, R. E. (1985). A causal model of college women's career choice. *Journal of Vocational Behavior, 27*, 123–153.

Feather, N. T. (1981). *Expectations and actions: Expectancy-value models in psychology.* Hillsdale, NJ: Erlbaum.

Fitzgerald, L. F., & Betz, N. E. (1984). Astin's model in theory and practice: A technical and philosophical critique. *Counseling Psychologist, 12*, 135–138.

Fitzgerald, L. F., & Crites, J. O. (1980). Toward a career psychology of women: What do we know? What do we need to know? *Journal of Counseling Psychology, 27*, 44–62.

Fleming, J. (1977). Predictive validity and the motive to avoid success in black women. *Humanities, 12*, 225–244.

Fleming, J. (1982). Projective and psychometric approaches to measurement: The case of fear of success. In A. J. Stewart (Ed.), *Motivation and society* (pp. 63–96). San Francisco: Jossey-Bass.

Fleming, J. (1983). Black women in black and white college environments: The making of a matriarch. *Journal of Social Issues, 39*, 41–54.

Freilino, M. K., & Hummel, R. (1985). Achievement and identity in college-age vs. adult women students. *Journal of Youth & Adolescence, 14*, 1–10.

Frieze, I. H. (1975). Women's expectations for, and causal attributions of, success and failure. In M.T.S. Mednick, S. S. Tangri, & L. W. Hoffman (Eds.), *Women and achievement: Social and motivational analyses* (pp. 158–171). Washington, DC: Hemisphere.

Frieze, I. H., Francis, W. D., & Hanusa, B. H. (1983). Defining success in the classroom. In J. M. Levine & M. C. Wang (Eds.), *Teacher and student perceptions: Implications for learning*. Hillsdale, NJ: Erlbaum.

Frieze, I. H., Whitley, B. E., Hanusa, B. H., & McHugh, M. C. (1982). Assessing the theoretical models for sex differences in causal attributions for success and failure. *Sex Roles, 8*, 333–343.

Gaeddert, W. P. (1987). The relationship of gender, gender-related traits, and achievement orientation to achievement attributions: A study of subject-selected accomplishments. *Journal of Personality, 55*, 687–710.

Gilligan, C. (1982). *In a different voice: Psychological theory and women's development*. Cambridge, MA: Harvard University Press.

Gitelson, I. B., Peterson, A. C., & Tobin-Richards, M. H. (1982). Adolescents' expectancies of success, self-evaluation, and attribution about performance on spatial and verbal tasks. *Sex Roles, 8*, 411–419.

Gold, A. K., Brush, C. K., & Sprotzer, E. R. (1980). Developmental changes in self-perceptions of intelligence and self-confidence. *Psychology of Women Quarterly, 5*, 670–678.

Gralewski, C., & Rodgon, M. M. (1980). Effects of social and intellectual instruction on achievement motivation as a function of role orientation. *Sex Roles, 6*, 301–309.

Gravenkemper, A. S., & Paludi, M. A. (1983). Fear of success revisited: Introducing an ambiguous cue. *Sex Roles, 9*, 897–900.

Griffin-Pierson, S. (1986, July). A new look at achievement motivation in women. *Journal of College Student Personnel*, 313–317.

Grottkau, B. J. (1986). The effects of a group counseling intervention on self-concept, self-esteem, anxiety and grade point average of female, nontraditional students. *Dissertation Abstracts International, 47* (2-A).

Hackett, G., & Betz, N. E. (1981). A self-efficacy approach to the career development of women. *Journal of Vocational Behavior, 18*, 326–339.

Hackett, G., & Campbell, N. T. (1987). Task self-efficacy and task interest as a function of performance on a gender-neutral task. *Journal of Vocational Behavior, 30*, 203–211.

Harmon, L. W. (1971). The childhood and adolescent plans of college women. *Journal of Vocational Behavior, 1*, 45–56.

Harmon, L. W. (1981). The life career plans of young adult college women: A follow-up study. *Journal of Counseling Psychology, 28*, 416–427.

Heaven, P.C.L. (1987). Authoritarianism, dominance, and need for achievement. *Australian Journal of Psychology, 39*, 331–357.

Heckhausen, H., Schmalt, H. I., & Schneider, K. (1985). *Achievement motivation in perspective.* New York: Academic Press.

Heilman, M. E., & Kram, K. C. (1983). Male and female assumptions about colleagues' views of their competence. *Psychology of Women Quarterly, 7*, 329–337.

Helgeson, V. S., & Sharpsteen, D. J. (1987). Perceptions of danger in achievement and affiliation situations: An extension of the Pollak vs. Benton et al. debate. *Journal of Personality and Social Psychology, 53*, 727–733.

Helson, R. (1987). Which of those young women with creative potential became productive: From college to midlife. In R. Hogan & W. H. Jones (Eds.), *Perspectives in personality*, Vol. 2 (pp. 51–92). Greenwich, CT: JAI Press.

Helson, R., Elliott, T., & Leigh, J. (1990). Number and quality of roles: A longitudinal personality view. *Psychology of Women Quarterly, 14*, 83–101.

Helson, R., Mitchell, V., & Moane, G. (1984). Personality and patterns of adherence and nonadherence to the social clock. *Journal of Personality and Social Psychology 46*, 1079–1096.

Hoffman, L. W. (1975). Fear of success in males and females: 1965 and 1971. In M.T.S. Mednick, S. S. Tangri, & L. W. Hoffman (Eds.), *Women and achievement: Social and motivational analyses.* Washington, DC: Hemisphere.

Holland, J. (1985). Making vocational choices: *A theory of vocational personalities and work environments.* New York: Prentice-Hall.

Holthe, I. (1986). The relationship between self-concept, significant partner support, and academic achievement of adult female students. *Dissertation Abstracts International, 47* (2-A).

Horner, M. S. (1972). Toward an understanding of achievement-related conflicts in women. *Journal of Social Issues, 28*(2), 157–176.

Horton, C. P., & Smith, J. C. (Eds.). (1990). *Statistical record of Black Americans.* Detroit, MI: Gale Research.

Hyde, J. S., Fennema, E., Ryan, M., Frost, L. A., & Hopp, C. (1990). Gender comparison of mathematics attitudes and affect: A meta-analysis. *Psychology of Women Quarterly, 14*, 295–324.

Illfelder, J. K. (1980). Fear of success, sex-role attitudes, career salience and anxiety levels of college women. *Journal of Vocational Behavior, 16*, 17.

Imes, S. (1980). The imposter phenomenon as a function of attribution patterns and internalized femininity/masculinity in high achieving women and men. *Dissertation Abstracts International, 40* (12-B).

Jackson, R. (1980). The Scholastic Aptitude Test: A response to Slack and Porter's critical appraisal. *Harvard Educational Review, 50*, 382–391.

Jacobs, J., & Eccles, J. S. (1985). Science and the media: Benbow and Stanley revisited. *Educational Researcher, 14*, 20–25.

Jagacinski, C. (1987). Engineering careers: Women in a male-dominated field. *Psychology of Women Quarterly, 11*, 97–110.

Janman, K. (1984). Gender dependency of occupational deviance and role overload as determinants of fear of success imagery. *European Journal of Social Psychology, 14*, 421–429.

Jenkins, S. R. (1987). Need for achievement and women's careers over 14 years: Evidence of occupational structure effects. *Journal of Personality and Social Psychology, 53*, 922–932.

Karabenick, S. A., Sweeney, C., & Penrose, G. (1983). Preference for skill versus chance-determined activities: The influence of gender and task sex-typing. *Journal of Research in Personality, 17*, 125–142.

Kavanaugh, D. J. (1987). Mood, persistence and success. *Australian Journal of Psychology, 39*, 309–318.

Kirshbaum, K. R. (1984). Differentiation of fear of success of gender-role inappropriate behavior in females. *Dissertation Abstracts International, 46*, 305.

Koestner, R., Zuckerman, M., & Koestner, J. (1987). Praise, involvement, and intrinsic motivation. *Journal of Personality and Social Psychology, 53*, 383–390.

Kranser, V. Z. (1987). Adolescent females' self-schemas for gender, expectancy of success, achievement level, and achievement attribution in a masculine domain. *Dissertation Abstracts International, 47*, 3162.

Kripke, C. K. (1980). The motive to avoid success and its impact on vocational choice of senior college women. *Dissertation Abstracts International, 41*, 2016–2017.

Kronberger, C. V. (1983). Fear of success, a relationship between competition, and achievement performance of women. *Dissertation Abstracts International, 43*, 3775.

LaNoue, J. B., & Curtis, R. C. (1985). Improving women's performance in mixed-sex situations by effort attributions. *Psychology of Women Quarterly, 9*, 337–356.

Layton, P. L. (1984). *Self-efficacy, locus of control, career salience, and women's career choice*. Unpublished doctoral dissertation, University of Minnesota.

Leder, G. C. (1990). Gender differences in mathematics: An overview. In E. Fennema & G. C. Leder (Eds.), *Mathematics and gender*. New York: Teachers College, Columbia University.

Lenney, E. (1977). Women's self-confidence in achievement settings. *Psychological Bulletin, 84*, 1–13.

Lenney, E. (1981). What's fine for the gander isn't always good for the goose: Sex differences in self-confidence as a function of ability area and comparison with others. *Sex Roles, 7*, 905–924.

Lenney, E., & Gold, J. (1982). Sex difference in self-confidence: The effects of task completion and comparison to competent other. *Personality and Social Psychology Bulletin, 8*, 74–80.

Lenney, E., Mitchell, L., & Browning, C. (1983). The effect of clear evaluation criteria on sex bias in judgments of performance. *Psychology of Women Quarterly, 7*, 313–328.

Lent, R. W., Brown, S. D., & Larkin, K. C. (1986). Self-efficacy in the prediction of academic performance and perceived career options. *Journal of Counseling Psychology, 33*, 265–269.

Lentz, M. E. (1982). Fear of success as a situational phenomenon. *Sex Roles, 8*, 987–997.

Levine, K., Gillman, M., & Reiss, H. (1982). Individual differences or sex differences in achievement attributions. *Sex Roles, 4,* 455–466.

Lipman-Blumen, J., Handley-Isaksen, A., & Leavitt, H. J. (1983). Achieving styles in men and women: A model, an instrument, and some findings. In J. T. Spence (Ed.), *Achievement and achievement-related motives: Psychological and sociological approaches* (pp. 147–204). San Francisco: Freeman.

Lips, H. M., & Temple, L. (1988). *Majoring in computer science: Causal models for women and men.* Paper presented at the 96th Annual Meeting of the American Psychological Association, Atlanta, GA.

Loewenstine, H. V., & Paludi, M. A. (1982). Women's Type A/B behavior patterns and fear of success. *Perceptual and Motor Skills, 54,* 891–894.

MacDonald, N. E., & Hyde, J. S. (1980). Fear of success, need achievement, and fear of failure: A factor analytic study. *Sex Roles, 6,* 695–711.

Malveaux, J., & Wallace, P. (1987). Minority women in the workforce. In K. S. Koziara, M. H. Moskow, & L. D. Tanner (Eds.), *Working women: Past, present and future* (pp. 265–298). Washington, DC: Bureau of National Affairs.

McClelland, D. (1961). *The achieving society.* Princeton, NJ: Van Nostrand.

McHugh, M., Frieze, I. H., & Hanusa, B. (1983). Attributions and sex differences in achievement: Problems and new perspectives. *Sex Roles, 8,* 467–479.

McMahan, I. D. (1982). Expectancy of success on sex-linked tasks. *Sex Roles, 8,* 949–958.

Mednick, M. T. (1978). Psychology of women: Research issues and trends. *New York Academy of Science Small Annals, 309,* 77–92.

Mednick, M. T. (1982). Women and the psychology of achievement: Implications for personal and social change. In H. J. Bernardin (Ed.), *Women in the workforce* (pp. 48–65). New York: Praeger.

Mednick, M. T. (1989a). Fear of success. In H. Tierney (Ed.), *Women's studies encyclopedia.* Westport, CT: Greenwood.

Mednick, M. T. (1989b). On the politics of psychological constructs: Stop the bandwagon, I want to get off. *American Psychologist, 44,* 1118–1123.

Mednick, M. T., & Puryear, G. R. (1975). Motivational and personality factors related to career goals of black college women. *Journal of Social and Behavioral Sciences, 21,* 1–30.

Mednick, M. T. & Tangri, S. S. (Eds.). (1972). New perspectives on women. *Journal of Social Issues, 29.*

Mednick, M. T., Tangri, S. S., & Hoffman, L. W. (Eds.). (1975). *Women and achievement: Social and motivational analyses.* Washington, DC: Hemisphere.

Mednick, M. T., & Weissman, H. J. (1975). The psychology of women: Selected topics. *Annual Review of Psychology, 26,* 1–18.

Monahan, L. (1983). The effects of sex differences and evaluation on task performance and aspiration. *Sex Roles, 9,* 205–215.

Mulig, J. C., Haggerty, M. E., Carbollosa, A. B., Cinnick, W. J., & Madden, J. M. (1985). Relationships among fear of success, fear of failure, and androgyny. *Psychology of Women Quarterly, 9,* 284–287.

Murray, S. R., & Mednick, M. T. (1977). Black women's achievement orientation: Motivational and cognitive factors. *Psychology of Women Quarterly, 1,* 247–259.

Nevill, D. D., & Schlecker, D. I. (1988). The relation of self-efficacy and assertiveness to willingness to engage in traditional/nontraditional career activities. *Psychology of Women Quarterly, 12,* 91–98.

Nieva, V. R., & Gutek, B. A. (1981). *Women and work: A psychological perspective.* New York: Praeger.

O'Farrell, B. (1982). Women and nontraditional blue collar jobs in the 1980's: An overview. In P. Wallace (Ed.), *Women in the workplace* (pp. 135–165). Boston: Auburn House.

O'Leary, V. E., & Hansen, R. D. (1982). Trying hurts women, helps men: The meaning of effort. In J. H. Bernardin (Ed.), *Women in the workforce* (pp. 100–123). New York: Praeger.

Orlofsky, J. L. (1981). A comparison of projective & objective measures as predictors of women's performance on masculine & feminine tasks. *Sex Roles, 7,* 999–1018.

Osipow, S. H. (1987). Career counseling. *Annual Review of Psychology, 38,* 257–278.

Palmer, H. T., & Lee, J. A. (1988). *Female workers and acceptance in traditionally male-dominated blue collar jobs.* Paper presented at the 96th Annual Convention of the American Psychological Association, Atlanta, GA.

Paludi, M. A., (1984). Psychometric properties and underlying assumptions of four objective measures of fear of success. *Sex Roles, 10,* 765–781.

Paludi, M. A., & Fankell-Hauser, J. (1986). An idiographic approach to the study of women's achievement striving. *Psychology of Women Quarterly, 10,* 89–100.

Piedmont, R. L. (1988). An interactional model of achievement motivation and fear of success. *Sex Roles, 19,* 467–490.

Pollak, S., & Gilligan, C. (1982). Images of violence in Thematic Apperception Test stories. *Journal of Personality and Social Psychology, 42,* 159–167.

Pollak, S., & Gilligan, C. (1983). Differing about difference: The incidence and interpretation of violent fantasies in women and men. *Journal of Personality and Social Psychology, 45,* 1172–1175.

Post-Kammer, P., & Smith, P. L. (1985). Sex differences in career self-efficacy consideration, and interests of eighth and ninth graders. *Journal of Counseling Psychology, 32,* 551–559.

Puryear, G. R. (1980). The black woman: Liberated or oppressed? In B. Lindsay (Ed.), *Comparative perspectives of third world women: The impact of race, sex, and class* (pp. 251–275). New York: Praeger.

Ris, M. D., & Woods, D. J. (1983). Learned helplessness and fear of success in college women. *Sex Roles, 9,* 1067–1072.

Roe, A. (1956). *The psychology of occupations.* New York: Wiley Press.

Scanzoni, J. (1975). Sex roles, economic factors, and marital solidarity in Black and White marriage. *Journal of Marriage and the Family, 37,* 130–144.

Schafer, A. (1981). Sex and mathematics. *Science, 211,* 392.

Scott, J. W. (1988). Deconstructing equality versus difference: On the uses of post-structuralist theory. *Feminist Studies, 14*(1), 33–50.

Sherif, C. W. (1977). Bias in psychology. In J. A. Sherman & E. T. Beck (Eds.), *The prism of sex: Essays on the sociology of knowledge* (pp. 93–133). Madison: University of Wisconsin Press.

Sherman, J. A., & Beck, E. T. (Eds.). (1977). *The prism of sex: Essays in the sociology of knowledge.* Madison: University of Wisconsin Press.

Singer, J. M., & Stake, J. E. (1986). Mathematics and self-esteem: Implications for women's career choice. *Psychology of Women Quarterly, 10,* 339–352.

Slack, W., & Porter, D. (1980). Training, validity, and the issue of aptitude: A reply to Jackson. *Harvard Educational Review, 50*, 392–401.

Sohn, D. (1982). Sex differences in achievement self attributions: An effect-size analysis. *Sex Roles, 8*, 345–357.

Spence, J. T., & Helmreich, R. L. (1978). *Masculinity and femininity: Their psychological dimensions, correlates, and antecedents.* Austin, TX: University of Texas Press.

Spence, J. T., & Helmreich, R. L. (1983). Achievement-related motives and behaviors. In J. T. Spence (Ed.), *Achievement and achievement motives: Psychological & sociological approaches* (pp. 7–74). San Francisco: Freeman.

Spence, J. T., Helmreich, R. L., & Pred, R. S. (1987). Impatience versus achievement strivings in the Type A pattern: Differential effects on students' health and academic achievement. *Journal of Applied Psychology, 72*, 522–528.

Stake, J. E. (1979). The ability/performance dimension of self-esteem: Implications for women's achievement behavior. *Psychology of Women Quarterly, 3*, 365–377.

Stake, J. E. (1983). Ability level, evaluative feedback, and sex differences in performance expectancy. *Psychology of Women Quarterly, 8*, 48–58.

Stewart, A. J. (1980). Personality and situation in the prediction of women's life patterns. *Psychology of Women Quarterly, 5*, 195–206.

Stewart, A. J., & Chester, N. L. (1982). The exploration of sex differences in human social motives: Achievement, affiliation & power. In A. J. Stewart (Ed.), *Motivation and society* (pp. 172–218). San Francisco: Jossey-Bass.

Stewart, A. J., & Healy, J. M., Jr. (1989). Linking individual development and social change. *American Psychologist, 44*, 30–42.

Stewart, A. J., Lykes, M. B., & LaFrance, M. (1982). Educated women's career patterns: Separating social and developmental changes. *Journal of Social Issues, 38*(1), 97–118.

Super, D. (1957). *The psychology of careers.* New York: Harper & Row.

Super, D., Stareshevskey, R., Matlin, N., & Jordan, J. (1963). *Career development: Self-concept theory.* New York: College Entrance Examination Board.

Tangri, S. S. (1972). Determinants of occupational role innovation among college women. *Journal of Social Issues, 29*(2), 177–200.

Tangri, S. S., & Jenkins, S. R. (1986). Stability and change in role innovation and life plans. *Sex Roles, 14*, 647–662.

Taylor, K. M., & Betz, N. E. (1983). Applications of self-efficacy theory to the understanding and treatment of career indecision. *Journal of Vocational Behavior, 22*, 63–81.

Thomas, V. G. (1983). Perceived traditionality and nontraditionality of career aspirations of black college women. *Perceptual and Motor Skills, 57*, 979–982.

Thomas, V. G. (1986). Career aspirations, parental support and work values among black female adolescents. *Journal of Multicultural Counseling and Development, 14*, 117–185.

Thomas, V. G. (1990). Problems of dual-career Black couples: Identification and implications for family interventions. *Journal of Multicultural Counseling and Development, 18*, 58–67.

Tinsley, D., & Faunce, P. (1980). Enabling, facilitating, and precipitating factors associated with women's career orientation. *Journal of Vocational Behavior, 17*, 183–194.

Topping, M.E.H., & Kimmel, E. B. (1985). The imposter phenomenon: Feeling phony. *Academic Psychology Bulletin, 1*, 213–226.

Travis, C. B., McKenzie, B. J., Wiley, D. C., & Kahn, A. S. (1988). Sex and achievement domain: Cognitive patterns of success and failure. *Sex Roles, 19*, 509–525.

Troll, L. (1982). *Continuations: Adult development and aging.* Monterey, CA: Brooks-Cole.

Turner, H. (1983). *Factors influencing persistence/achievement in the sciences and health professions by black high school and college women.* Final report submitted to the National Institute of Education, Washington, DC.

U. S. Department of Commerce, Bureau of the Census. (1990). *Money, income and poverty status in the United States.* Data from the March 1990 Current Population Survey.

U. S. Department of Labor. (1990, September). *20 facts on working women.* Washington, DC: Women's Bureau.

Vollmer, F. (1986). Why do men have higher expectancy than women? *Sex Roles, 14*, 351–362.

Weiner, B. (1972). *Theories of motivation: From mechanism to cognition.* Chicago: Markham.

Weiner, B., & Kukla, A. (1970). An attributional analysis of achievement motivation. *Journal of Personality and Social Psychology, 15*, 1–20.

Welch, R., Gerrard, M., & Huston, A. (1986). Gender-related personality attribute and reactions to success-failure: An examination of mediating variables. *Psychology of Women Quarterly, 10*, 221–233.

Welch, R. L., & Huston, A. C. (1982). Effects of induced success/failure and attributions on the problem-solving behavior of psychologically high instrumental and low instrumental women. *Journal of Personality, 50*, 81–97.

Wernikoff, I. N. (1980). The effect of fear of success & male attitude towards competency in a mixed decision making situation. *Dissertation Abstracts International, 40*, 4990.

Weston, P., & Mednick, M. T. (1970). Race, social class, and the motive to avoid success in women. *Journal of Cross-Cultural Psychology, 1*, 284–291.

Wheeler, K. G. (1983). Comparisons of self-efficacy and expectancy models of occupational preference for college males and females. *Journal of Occupational Psychology, 56*, 73–78.

White, M. C., de Sanctis, G., & Crino, M. D. (1981). Achievement, self-confidence, personality trait, and leadership ability: A review of literature on sex differences. *Psychological Reports, 48*, 547–569.

Yount, K. R. (1986). A theory of productive activity: The relationships among self-concept, gender, sex role stereotypes, and work-emergent traits. *Psychology of Women Quarterly, 10*, 63–88.

17

Women's Career Development

Nancy Betz

INTRODUCTION

Like many areas of psychology, attention to women in the field of career psychology is a relatively recent phenomenon. Women were essentially ignored for the first 50 or 60 years of the history of vocational or career psychology, because women were not viewed as pursuing careers. Everyone knew that while some women might "hold down jobs" as a temporary expedient until marriage, or permanently for those unlucky few who couldn't snare a man, the idea that women might want to choose and pursue careers was not considered seriously until relatively recently.

In the early 1960s, however, interest in women's career development began to grow, and the field has burgeoned in the last 20 to 25 years. The study of career development (men's as well as women's) can generally be divided into two major topical areas, corresponding to the two major phases of career behavior: career choice and career adjustment. Career choice theory and research attempt to describe the nature and influences of the career choices people make. The most common choice points studied are the educational and career choices made by adolescents and young adults. Although some people do make initial career choices at later ages (e.g., reentry women) and others change their career direction once or more during their adult lives, the focus of theory and research has been on the initial choices made by young adults.

Career adjustment, on the other hand, is the term describing what happens to the individual after career entry. Two major dependent variables, success and satisfaction, have been used in the study of career adjustment (Crites, 1969;

Dawis & Lofquist, 1984). Research and theory on career adjustment are generally also covered under the rubric "women and work," encompassing such traditional topics as gender differences in job performance or success, satisfaction, and motivation, as well as such topics as discrimination, sexual harassment, dual career issues, and the work-family interface.

The present chapter focuses on the nature of, and processes influencing, women's initial career choices, while the topic of career adjustment is covered in chapters 15 and 18. These topics are also covered in more detail by Betz and Fitzgerald (1987), Fitzgerald, Weitzman, Gold, and Ormerod (1988), Gutek and Larwood (1987), Nieva and Gutek (1981), and Larwood, Stromberg, and Gutek's annual reviews of women and work (1985; Gutek, Stromberg, & Larwood, 1988; Stromberg, Larwood, & Gutek, 1987).

This chapter is organized into six sections: (1) basic assumptions, (2) describing women's career participation, (3) barriers to women's career choices, (4) facilitators of women's career development, (5) women of color, and (6) summary and recommendations for research.

BASIC ASSUMPTIONS

Any discussion of a concept as basic as career development to the lives of women requires one to make certain assumptions. For the present chapter, several major assumptions, largely based on research findings, were made.

The first assumption is that women, like men, need a variety of major sources of satisfaction in their lives—as stated by Freud (according to Erikson, 1950), the psychologically well-adjusted human being is able "to love and to work" effectively. Both women and men need the satisfactions of interpersonal relationships, with family and/or friends, but also the satisfaction of achievement in the outside world. Osipow (1983), in his major treatise on theories of career development, states, "It is clear that working holds an important place both in society and in the lives of individuals" (p. vii). As stated by Baruch and Barnett (1980):

It is almost a cliche now for people who work long hours at demanding jobs, aware of what they are missing in terms of time with family, long talks with friends, concerts, and all kinds of opportunities for leisure, to express the sentiment that there is more to life than work. The problem is that life *without* productive work is terrible. We assume this for men in thinking about their unemployment and retirement, but we do not think about the situation of women in this way. (p. 244)

A second major assumption is that the fulfillment of individual potential for achievement is vitally important. Although the roles of homemaker and mother are important and often very satisfying, they do not allow most women to fulfill their unique abilities and talents. These, rather, must be fulfilled through career pursuits or volunteer and avocational activities, just as they are in men. This is not to discount the importance of childrearing, but only its insufficiency as a lifelong answer to the issue of self-realization. Even if a woman spends a number of years creatively rearing children, these children inevitably grow up and begin their own lives, which must of necessity be increasingly independent from the parental home.

The evidence is very strong that homemakers who do not have other outlets for achievement and productivity are highly susceptible to psychological distress, particularly as children grow and leave home. For example, when the women in the Terman gifted sample were followed up in their sixties (Sears & Barbie, 1977), those who reported the highest levels of life satisfaction were employed. Least satisfied with their lives were those who'd been housewives all of their adult lives. The most psychologically disturbed women were those with exceptionally high IQs (above 170) who had not worked outside the home. It seems fairly clear that women with genius-level IQs who did not pursue meaningful careers outside the home suffered psychological consequences for that failure.

More generally, there is strong evidence for the salutary effects of working outside the home on women's psychological adjustment, regardless of marital status. Bernard (1971), in an analysis of the relationship between marital status and psychological health, concluded that the healthiest individuals were the married men and the single women, while married women were at particularly high risk for psychological distress. Further analyses of the relationships of marital status to mental health by Gove and Tudor (1973) and Radloff (1975), among others, led to similar conclusions.

However, it does not seem to be marriage per se that is detrimental to women's psychological adjustment, but rather the lack of meaningful paid employment. In the studies mentioned, the women who were not employed accounted for the surplus of psychological distress among the married women. Ilfeld (1977), in a large-scale study of households in the Chicago area, found that the women who were as psychologically healthy and free from symptoms of distress as the average man were those employed in high-prestige occupations. But both Ilfeld and Ferree (1976) found that even working-class employed women were happier and had higher self-esteem than their nonworking counterparts. Bart (1971), in a study of middle-aged women, found that employed women were much less susceptible to depression in middle age than were women who had concentrated all their attention on the home—women who were overidentified and overinvolved with children who had recently left home (leaving the "empty nest") were the most vulnerable to depression in middle age.

In an important review article, Repetti, Matthews, and Waldron (1989) summarize evidence suggesting that the causal mechanism may go the other way as well; that is, healthier married women are more likely to seek paid employment in the first place than are those with psychological or physical problems. The authors go on, however, to conclude that employment improves the health of unmarried women and of married women who have positive attitudes toward employment.

Given these assumptions, it will not be surprising that I resist suggestions in the literature that marriage and childrearing, because they involve work at home, can by themselves constitute a legitimate "career" option. Although I accept the legitimacy of this as a life-style choice, it has been our premise (Betz & Fitzgerald, 1987) that such work does not constitute a legitimate "career" in the sense used by psychologists because (1) this work is unpaid and is also usually unaccompanied by such benefits as accumulation of retirement income, (2) it has no opportunities for advancement, (3) it has no training requirements or job security, and (4) it would not be considered a legitimate career for a male (males who stay home are generally referred to as "unemployed").

Thus, this chapter is based on the assumption that women should pursue meaningful careers that allow them to utilize their individual abilities and talents fully. They, like men, should be able to "have it all." Accordingly, the focus of this chapter is on factors that prevent women from pursuing such careers and on ways of facilitating that pursuit.

DESCRIBING WOMEN'S CAREER PARTICIPATION

Trends in the Extent of Women's Labor Force Participation: 1900–1990

At the turn of the century, paid employment for women was the exception rather than the rule, and those women who did work outside the home did so only preliminary to marriage and the bearing of children. The chief occupations held by women were domestic service, factory work, and teaching. By and large, the only women working throughout adulthood were those "unfortunate" enough to be without a husband—the unlucky spinsters and the widowed. Thus, when the family life cycle began, the work cycle ended (Perun & Del Vento Bielby, 1981).

Although this pattern remained stable until about 1940, the World War II years were characterized by a dramatic influx of women into the labor force to fill jobs vacated by servicemen. Views of women as the delicate sex were temporarily suspended when women were needed in such dangerous or physically demanding jobs as explosives manufacturing and construction. In the postwar years, the percentages of women working both before and during marriage accelerated markedly. Overall, the percentage of women working has increased threefold since 1940, but, even more dramatically, the percentage of working mothers has increased 10-fold since 1940! In the 1950s, one-third of women were in the labor force (Russo & Denmark, 1984), while in the 1990 census, almost 80% of women reported working outside the home, including 75% of those with children aged 6 to 17 and 62% of those with children under 6.

Thus, a trend that began to accelerate after World War II has now firmly established women's "place" in the labor force and has led to the near-inevitability of work outside the home for American women. The odds that any given woman would work outside the home at some time in her life were about 95 out of 100, and the average woman could expect to spend about 30 years in the labor force, compared with 39 years for the average man. While about one-third of working women are married and have husbands making adequate incomes, the other two-thirds are women who are single, widowed, divorced, or separated or have husbands whose incomes were at or below poverty level.

In summary, women whose adult lives will not include work outside the home are increasingly becoming the exception rather than the rule. As so well summarized by Hyde (1985), the fact that the majority of American women hold jobs outside the home is one of our country's best kept secrets: "The working woman, then, is not a variation from the norm, she *is* the norm" (p. 169).

Paralleling the greatly increased labor force participation of women is dramatic change in the aspirations of young women, with most young women now expressing a preference to combine career and family roles in their adult lives. Since 1964, when Matthews and Tiedeman reported that 60–75% of girls and women aged 11 to 26 planned to be married and not working 10 years from the time of the study, research has shown a consistent decrease in the number of women preferring marriage-only life-styles. Rand and Miller (1972) described what they termed a new cultural imperative, "marriage and a career," in their finding that 95% of their sample of women of junior high through college age expected to both marry and work. Recent data support the trend described by Rand and Miller. Zuckerman (1980), in a study of women in the "seven sisters" colleges, found that 92% were planning to complete education beyond the B.A. degree. Harmon (1980), in a follow-up of women six years after college entry, found that 46% wanted to work most of their lives (versus 27% in 1968) and that only 2% wanted minimal employment (versus 16% in 1968). Indeed, evidence suggests that college women want to "have it all"—career, marriage, and children—even though most are unprepared for the realities of combining career and family (Catalyst, 1987).

Thus, trends over the past 25 years and recent data strongly suggest the importance of occupational pursuits in the plans and lives of women. It is clear that most women will work outside the home and that this work will play an increasingly important role in their lives. However, while the extent of women's labor force participation is approaching that of men, the nature of that participation continues to differ greatly from that of men, keeping working women economically disadvantaged, lower in status, and burdened with multiple role demands. The career and life "choices" that young women make continue to tend toward stereotypically female occupational fields and to represent lower levels of both educational and career achievement compared with equally able males.

Problem: Continued Occupational Sex Segregation

Although some occupational barriers have fallen, the U.S. work force is still sex-segregated—most occupations continue to be dominated by one sex or the other (Ferraro, 1984). The problem of women's low earning power is due to both sex-based wage discrimination and occupational sex segregation (Ferraro, 1984), among other factors. Simply put, women get paid less than men for doing the same job, and the jobs that women tend to be concentrated in are by and large low status and low paying, with few or no opportunities for advancement. More specifically, even though women constitute 44% of the labor force, they continue to be concentrated in a small number of traditionally female jobs and professions. A majority of women workers are in pink-collar jobs (Howe, 1977), for example, clerical work, retail sales, waitress, beautician, and housekeeping services (U.S. Department of Labor, 1984).

Women professionals are concentrated in professions of lower pay and status than the male-dominated professions; and women continue to be seriously underrepresented in many career fields, particularly mathematics, the sciences, and engineering, as well as the skilled trades (Dix, 1987; National Science Foundation, 1990). For example, the proportion of women entering schools of engineering increased from 5% in 1973 to 17% in 1983 but then began to go back down, to 15% in 1986 (Vetter, 1988). In 1985 women accounted for 87% of librarians and 95% of nurses but only 18% of lawyers and judges, 17% of doctors, 11% of architects, and 7% of engineers (U.S. Bureau of Labor Statistics, 1985). Ehrhart and Sandler (1987) and Vetter and Babco (1986) document the way in which the underrepresentation of women in traditionally male careers is mirrored in and, worse, perpetuated by their continued low college and graduate school enrollments in those fields. For example, even though women constituted 39%, 41%, 44%, and 27% of the 1983 bachelor's degrees in agriculture, business, mathematics, and physical sciences, respectively, their share of doctorates in those fields in 1983 was, respectively, 14%, 17%, 16%, and 14% (cf. Ehrhart & Sandler, 1987). On the other hand, women earned 95% of the B.A.'s and 68% of the doctorates in home economics, 76% of the bachelor's degrees in education, and 83% of bachelor's degrees in the allied medical fields of medical technology, physical and occupational therapy, and dental hygiene. Even though more women are now pursuing careers in some previously male-dominated fields such as business and law, their levels of pay and rates of advancement continue to lag behind those of comparably educated and experienced men (Dix, 1987; Moore, 1986; U.S. Department of Labor, 1984).

Further, the career aspirations of young women and girls continue to focus on stereotypically female occupations. Recent evidence suggests that, in comparison with men, women continue to select occupations from a more restricted range of options (Hesse-Biber, 1985), see fewer occupations as suitable (Poole & Clooney, 1985), and choose occupations less consistent with their vocational interests (Knapp, Knapp & Knapp-Lee, 1985; Swaney & Prediger, 1985). While there does seem to be a small proportionate increase in the number of women pursuing nontraditional careers, the predominant pattern among women continues to suggest a limited and sex-stereotypic range of female occupational pursuits.

Problem: Underutilization of Abilities

Related to women's concentration in traditionally female and frequently low-level occupations is the finding that, in contrast to men in general, women's intellectual capacities and talents are not reflected in their educational and occupational achievements; women's career aspirations and choices are frequently far lower in level than are the aspirations of males with comparable levels of ability (Fitzgerald & Crites, 1980).

The oldest and most pervasive model of career choice, the "matching" or trait-factor model, posits that people will be most successful and satisfied in careers that utilize and draw upon their individual abilities, talents, and interests. This is, in essence, a model fostering the nurturance of individual differences in those characteristics relevant to educational and work pursuits, especially abilities and talents. (See Betz, Fitzgerald & Hill, 1989, for an overview of trait-factor theory.) It is a model valuing self-fulfillment and actualization. Within a model of this sort, a relationship between ability level and attained educational and occupational levels is not only expected but desirable for subsequent individual satisfaction and fulfillment.

Among men, the relationship of intellect to obtained educational and occupational level holds reasonably well (Tyler, 1978). Among women, however, the relationship begins to break down in adolescence and by college age and beyond has broken down almost completely for the majority of women. Women fail to use their talents and abilities in educational and career pursuits, resulting in losses both to themselves and to a society that needs their talents.

Ironically, females start out as the higher achievers in comparison with males and as the children more likely to utilize their abilities in educational pursuits. Girls perform better academically than boys at all educational levels. Studies going back as far as 1929 have shown that girls obtain higher school grades than do boys beginning in elementary school and continuing through college (Carnegie Commission on Higher Education, 1973; Hyde, 1985). One study was Project Talent. Project Talent, conducted by researchers at the University of Pittsburgh (Flanagan, 1971), was a large-scale longitudinal study of 440,000 9th through 12th graders carefully sampled from 1,353 secondary schools across the country. Students were originally administered a battery of tests in 1960. Follow-up surveys measuring subjects' educational and occupational attainment 1, 5, and 11 years after subjects' expected high school graduation were also conducted. Among 1,960 Project Talent seniors, 51% of the girls in comparison with 39%

of the boys reported high school averages of mostly A's and B's (Carnegie Commission on Higher Education, 1973).

The school progress of girls is also superior to that of boys. Girls less frequently need to repeat a grade, and girls are more likely than boys to be accelerated and promoted (cf. Hyde, 1985). In college, women consistently receive higher grades than do men in major fields ranging from the humanities and social sciences to the sciences, engineering, and even mathematics. Women's grade point advantage ranges from one-half to one full grade point, depending on the major field.

In addition to obtaining higher school and college grades, women receive higher grades in relationship to their scholastic aptitude test scores and their high school grade point averages (GPAs) than do men. Thus, the predicted college GPA would be higher for a given female than for a male with an equivalent record of test scores and high school grades (Carnegie Commission on Higher Education, 1973).

Women's underutilization of their abilities is even more apparent in the occupational realm. Assuming few or no major gender differences in vocationally relevant abilities, we would assume an approximately equal tendency of women as of men to achieve high occupational levels and to achieve eminence. Unfortunately, this has not been the case, with only negligible representation of women among the eminent throughout history. For example, fewer than 10% of the people who could be characterized as eminent based on having entries in standard biographical dictionaries have been women, and more than half of those women listed were so because they were sovereigns and were thus eminent by birth or were the wives or mistresses of famous men (Anastasi, 1958). (It should also be noted that throughout much of recorded history a women could not get her work recognized unless she adopted a male pseudonym, e.g., George Sand, or used only initials, A. B. Smith, as a hypothetical example. Thus, tallying the number of eminent women by counting female names in biographical dictionaries surely underestimates the contributions of eminent women who could not identify their sex and still get their work recognized.)

An early attempt to study eminence in women (Castle, 1913) found only 868 eminent women across 42 nations and extending from the seventh century B.C. The largest number of these had achieved eminence in literature, but the highest level of eminence (as indicated by the number of lines allocated in the biographical dictionary) was achieved by sovereigns, political leaders, and mothers or mistresses of eminent men. Other nonintellectual ways in which women achieved eminence (or at least the fame necessary to end up in a biographical dictionary) were through great beauty, a tragic fate, or being immortalized in literature (Castle, 1913).

Among the women who would have been likely to achieve eminence had they been born male are the gifted girls-grown-up in the longitudinal studies of gifted children of Terman, Merrill, and Oden. The sample, originally obtained in 1921–1922, consisted of 1,528 children having measured IQs equal to or greater than 135. Of the sample, 671 were girls, and 847 were boys.

The follow-up study of the gifted group at midlife (Terman & Oden, 1959) indicated that, as expected, the great majority of men had achieved prominence in professional and managerial occupations. They had, by their midforties, been exceptionally productive scientists, made literary and artistic contributions, and become prominent lawyers, physicians, psychologists, and college professors. In contrast to the men, the women were primarily housewives or were employed in traditionally female occupations. About 50% of the women had been and continued to be full-time housewives. Of those who were working full-time, 21% were teachers in elementary or secondary schools, 8% were social workers, 20% were secretaries, and 8% were either librarians or nurses. Only 7% of those working were academicians, 5% were physicians, lawyers, or psychologists, 8% were executives, and 9% were writers, artists, or musicians. Two-thirds of the women with IQs equal to or greater than 170 (clearly genius level) were either housewives or office workers. Further, although the girls were judged the most artistically gifted as children, and the seven most talented writers were girls, few of these girls grew up to use their talents professionally (Terman & Oden, 1959).

Thus, ability and talent in gifted girls had almost no relationship to their achievements as women. At least seven talented writers, as well as unknown numbers of artists, musicians, psychologists, biologists, geneticists, and astronomers, were lost to the world. As stated in the report of the Carnegie Commission on Higher Education (1973), "The supply of human intelligence is limited, and the demand for it in society is even greater. The largest unused supply is found among women" (p. 27).

Although the Terman studies are a dramatic illustration of the failure of an individual differences model of career choice within the female half of the population, studies reported in the 1980s continue to show the serious underutilization of female abilities. Card, Steel, and Abeles (1980) reported the results of a long-term follow-up of the ninth grade cohort of the original Project Talent study. They reported that while the female students had higher high school grades and scored higher on a composite of academic ability tests, by 11 years after high school men had obtained significantly more education and were earning significantly more money. Sex differences in realization of potential were found across all SES (socioeconomic status) levels, and differences widened from the 5-year to the 11-year follow-up. The widening of the achievement gap was most apparent for the most talented female students, those in the top quartile as ninth graders. In other words, by age 29 the brightest men are beginning to manifest their intellectual potential while the bright women fall further and further short of their potential for educational and occupational achievement.

Arnold (1987, 1989) reported the results of the Illinois Valedictorian project, a longitudinal study of the lives of 80 students, 46 women and 34 men, who graduated in 1981 as valedictorian or salutatorian of their Illinois high school classes. The students participated in four to five semistructured interviews and responded to questionnaires in the years 1981, 1984, 1985, and 1988. Results indicated that all but four (two male and two female) students finished college and, on the average, performed exceedingly well (mean GPAs of 3.6 and 3.5 for the women and the men, respectively).

Other than the nonsignificant difference in collegiate scholastic performance, gender differences began to emerge immediately after high school. Significant differences that emerged were a decline in the intellectual self-confidence of the women, a persistent concern among the women about combining career and family (with a consequent abandonment of medical school aspirations among six women), and striking gender differences in both the extent and the level of planned labor force participation (Arnold & Denny, 1984, 1985). Two-thirds of the women valedictorians, but none of the men, planned to reduce or interrupt their labor force participation to accommodate child raising. In the most recent follow-up (Arnold, 1989), both male and female valedictorians were pursuing careers in the traditionally male areas of science, business, and the professions (law, medicine, academia), but a substantial proportion of women (but no men) were pursuing traditionally female "helping" professions and, in a few cases, nonprofessional or homeworker roles. Interestingly, differences in educational and career achievements among the men can be predicted by individual differences in ability, motivation, job experience, and college prestige, while the only useful predictor among the women is career versus family priorities (Arnold, 1989).

Thus, the serious problem of underutilization of female abilities in career pursuits has not really diminished, even in the "enlightened eighties." Research and intervention must focus on how to return to women the full range of career options, beyond the gender-stereotypic, to include the extent and variety of options that will make women's choices free in reality as well as in name.

BARRIERS TO WOMEN'S CAREER CHOICES

The major barriers to, and the major facilitators of, women's career choices will be reviewed. Both barriers and facilitators are defined in terms of their effects on women's self-actualization in their career choices. Within this framework, barriers are variables/forces leading or related to the tendency to make gender-stereotypic, traditionally female choices. Facilitators are factors related to broadened career options and higher educational and career achievements. Table 1 shows a summary of some of the major barriers and facilitators to women's career development.

Several points concerning the barrier-facilitator distinction should be made. First, both barriers and facilitators can be environmental or individually based (e.g., socialized barriers such as "math anxiety"). Second, a given factor can be both a barrier and a facilitator, depending on whether it is present or absent. For example, lack of female role models is a significant barrier to women's view of career options, and the presence of role models can be an important facilitator of career development. If we are considering methods of environmental enrich-

Table 1
Summary of Major Barriers to, and Facilitators of, Women's Career Development

BARRIERS	FACILITATORS
Environmental	
Gender role stereotypes	Working Mother
Occupational Stereotypes	Supportive Father
Gender Bias in Education	Highly educated Parents
Barriers in Higher Education	Girls Schools/Women's Colleges
Lack of Role Models	Female Models
The Null Environment	Proactive Encouragement
Gender-Biased Career Counseling	Androgynous Upbringing
	Work Experience
Individual (Socialized)	
Family-Career Conflict	Late Marriage or Single
Math Avoidance	No or Few Children
Self-esteem	High Self-Esteem
Self-Efficacy	Strong Academic Self-Concept
Causal Attributions	Instrumentality
Expectancies for Success	Androgyny

ment/positive intervention, providing role models would be one important source of such enrichment. Third, the nature and effects of barrier and facilitator factors are dynamic rather than static. As O'Connell (1988) states, some factors influencing women's career development are "transhistorical" (p. 362), while others change with historical and social changes. For example, having had a working mother has been consistently shown in research to have a salutary effect on young women's career aspirations and achievements. Yet as more and more children grow up with working mothers (currently about 60% of mothers of children under 18 work outside the home), the differential effects of having a working mother may diminish. Finally, the focus on barriers and facilitators, environmental and individual or socialized, is useful not only for understanding the still-restricted nature of women's career choices but for designing appropriate interventions to broaden those choices.

Environmental Barriers

Gender-Role and Occupational Stereotyping

Certainly the first and most basic barrier to women's career development is societal stereotypes about both life roles and occupational roles. Early childhood socialization, reinforced by parents, teachers, religion, the media, and so on, teaches girls to emphasize home and family pursuits, to expect to assume primary responsibility for childrearing, and to defer her career pursuits to the career priorities of her husband. In terms of personality characteristics, men are expected to develop those associated with competency, instrumentality, and achievement, while women are to develop those comprising a "warmth-expressiveness" cluster, including nurturance, sensitivity, warmth, and emotional expressiveness.

The psychological mechanisms by which children learn gender-role stereotypes, normative expectations for the sexes, and develop gender-typed characteristics include reinforcement and punishment, modeling, and the adoption of rules, schemas, or generalizations based on observation of others or as they are taught by others (Hyde, 1985; Williams, 1977). These mechanisms operate through the influence of parents, teachers, and the media, including literature and television (see Maccoby & Jacklin, 1974; Williams, 1983, for more detailed reviews).

Related to sex-role stereotypes are occupational stereotypes, or normative views of the appropriateness of various occupations for males and females. Although a number of studies have shown that occupational stereotypes are consistent and durable in adult populations (Panek, Rush & Greenwalt, 1977), the study of Shinar (1975) was classic in this area. Shinar asked college students to rate 129 occupations as masculine, feminine, or neutral, using a 7-point rating scale where "masculine" was at the "1" point and "feminine" was at the "7" point. The results indicated that both male and female students consistently stereotyped occupations as masculine or feminine. Mean ratings of masculinity/ femininity ranged from the most masculine-stereotypic job of miner, which received a mean rating of 1.0 with no variability, to the occupations of receptionist (6.3), nurse (6.6), and manicurist (6.7). Other highly masculine stereotypic occupations were highway maintenance worker (1.2), heavy equipment operator (1.2), and U.S. Supreme Court justice (1.3). Among the professions, district attorney (1.6), engineer (1.9), federal judge (1.9), dentist (2.1), surgeon (2.2), physicist (2.3), veterinarian (2.7), and physician (2.7) were clearly masculine-stereotypic, while nurse (6.6), head librarian (5.6), elementary school teacher (5.6), and dietician (5.3) were feminine-typed. A recent study by White and colleagues (1989) replicated the Shinar study.

Not only do adults stereotype occupations as appropriate for males or females, but children appear to learn these stereotypes very early. For example, Gettys and Cann (1981) found that children as young as 2 1/2 were able to distinguish masculine and feminine occupations, while Tremaine and Schau (1979) found that preschoolers identified and agreed with adult job stereotypes. Occupational stereotypes are consistently found in elementary school children (Gettys & Cann, 1981; Rosenthal & Chapman, 1982; Tremaine & Schau, 1979).

One study illustrating the power of occupational stereotypes was that of Drabman et al. (1981). The study utilized a videotaped portrayal of a 7-year-old boy going to visit his doctor. The doctor was a woman (named "Mary Nancy" to double the sex-salience of the name), and she was assisted by a male nurse named "David Gregory." Immediately after viewing the tape, children were given a multiple-choice quiz on which they were asked to recognize the names of the doctor and the nurse. In addition to the correct name, the distractors included a wrong same-sex name, the name of the opposite-sex character in the videotape, and a "wrong" opposite-sex name. In naming the doctor and the nurse, almost all first and fourth grade children assigned a gender-typed name, even if it was a name that hadn't appeared in the videotape at all. Only 4% of the fourth graders chose a male name for the nurse. For the doctor, only 4% of both first and fourth graders chose a female name—41% of first graders chose the wrong male name rather than the correct female name. The authors conclude, distressingly, that children alter their perception or memory of a counterstereotyped videotaped presentation to fit previously learned occupational sex stereotypes and that stereotypic cognitive structures are capable of modifying long-term memory as well.

More optimistically, Alpert and Breen (1989), in their study of occupational stereotyping in children in grades 1 through 12, concluded that children's gender-role attitudes have become more liberal since the 1970s. As in other research on children's occupational stereotyping, girls were more liberal than boys, and older children were more liberal than younger. In the same vein, White, Kruczek, Brown, and White (1989) replicated the Shinar (1975) study and found that although stereotyping was still present, it had moderated somewhat from the earlier study.

Further, children's occupational preferences tend to be consistent with the occupational stereotypes they hold. Both boys and girls tend to choose sex-typed occupations (MacKay & Miller, 1982; Tremaine & Schau, 1979). For example, Kriedberg, Butcher, and White (1978) found that while some second grade girls expressed interest in male-dominated occupations, almost all sixth grade girls were choosing traditionally female occupations. It is unfortunate indeed that occupational stereotypes have limited girls' perceived career options before they finish elementary school. In MacKay and Miller's (1982) study, third and fifth grade boys most frequently chose the occupations of policeman, truck driver, pilot, and architect, while girls chose nurse, teacher, and stewardess. Umstot (1980) found that highly male-stereotyped activities among third through seventh graders included being a soldier, TV service person, and plumber, while highly female-stereotyped activities included knitting, sewing, selling perfume, and being a secretary.

Findings of limited occupational preferences among children as young as first and second grades are consistent with Gottfredson's (1981) theory of circumscription and compromise in career choice. Gottfredson proposes that an individual's occupational aspirations become circumscribed within a range of acceptable sex-typed alternatives and that this acceptable range is normally set by ages 6 to 8. Further, Gottfredson suggests that once set, the range of acceptable alternatives is extremely difficult to modify. While the suggestion of such early constriction in choices is very difficult to accept, it does not seem to be inconsistent with available research data.

Not only do children of all ages hold occupational stereotypes, but these stereotypes are highly resistant to change. For example, in the study of Knell and Winer (1979), preschool-age children were read 12 stories portraying people in each of 12 different occupations. Six male and six female characters were used, and the design varied the extent to which occupations were portrayed with gender-appropriate versus gender-inappropriate characters. Occupational stereotypes were assessed before and after treatment. Although it was hypothesized that nontraditional portrayals in videotapes would reduce stereotyping, no effects for the nontraditional treatments (either half or all 12 of the stories showing a sex-incongruent member of the occupation) were found. The only treatment effect was an increase in stereotyping among girls who had viewed the "traditional" tape (all 12 occupations portrayed by the "appropriate gender"). Boys' responses were highly stereotypic regardless of treatment. Yanico (1978), in a study varying the amount of gender bias in occupational information, also concluded that occupational stereotypes are amazingly resistant to change through treatment. Zuckerman and Sayre (1982), in a sample of middle-class children between ages 4 and 8, found that the children demonstrated less occupational stereotyping than expected but persisted in gender-stereotypic personal choices. Among the girls, 52% chose nurse, 16% chose teacher, 8% chose dancer, and 8% chose veterinarian. Among the boys greater variability in choices was demonstrated, although 83% were gender-stereotypic.

Although attempts have been made to justify the existence of occupational stereotypes on the grounds that certain kinds of job content are more congruent with the skills of males, while others are more congruent with female abilities, there is strong and consistent evidence that the proportion of men and women in the occupation is the best predictor of its job sex-type (Krefting & Berger, 1979; Krefting, Berger & Wallace, 1978). In two studies reported by Krefting et al. (1978) the actual percentage of men versus women in the job explained 48% and 70% of the variance in job sex-types. As stated by Krefting et al., the sex of the job holder is the basis of occupational stereotypes. A disturbing study (Heilman, 1979) reported that high school girls expressed more interest in male-dominated occupations when led to believe that the sex ratios would in the future be more balanced, but high school boys expressed less interest in those occupations when confronted with the prospect of sex balance. Thus, the lack of other women in an occupation serves to deter young women from selecting that occupation, and some males may prefer that the sex ratio in preferred occupations remains unbalanced toward male dominance.

Gender Bias in Education

The early schooling children receive is, of course, critical in terms of transmitting basic cognitive and social skills, but it is also a major source of sex-role socialization, a source of messages concerning appropriate behaviors and roles for girls versus boys and women versus men. Unfortunately, schools have long been communicating to children the same gender biases that characterize society as a whole; see, for example, Ehrhart and Sandler (1987), Klein and Simonson (1984), National Project on Women in Education (1978), among others, for more detailed discussions of the literature on sex discrimination in education.

Wirtenberg and Nakamura (1976) contend, for example, that education plays a dominant role in the ultimate sexual stratification of the labor force through its effects on females' aspirations, expectations, preparation, and occupational attitudes. They discuss several educational practices contributing to the limitation of females' career options. These practices include gender-role stereotyping in textbooks and instructional materials, curricula for males and females, and vocational/career counseling and testing.

Pervasive gender-role stereotyping in school readers and textbooks has been widely documented. For example, several major studies (Howe, 1979; Key, 1975; Scott, 1981) have examined the portrayals of boys and girls and men and women in school readers and textbooks. The portrayals have consistently been stereotypic and, for those interested in equity for women, dismaying. At a very basic level, boys and men appear as story characters far more often than do girls and women, thus implying something about the relative importance and interest of the two sexes. Women portrayed in the readers have almost always been limited to the role of mother, and when they do work (generally as nurses, teachers, or secretaries), it is out of financial necessity rather than through inherent interest or desire to use their talents and abilities. The predominant portrayal of women/females as mommies is well captured by Nilsen's (1971) term "cult of the apron," coined after she noticed that of 58 children's books on display at a book fair, 21 had pictures of women wearing aprons. Even the female animals wore aprons! Men were portrayed as workers and fathers. The message conveyed has been that men work and have families, but women do one or the other.

As dismaying as the differential role portrayals of adults are the portrayals of differential capabilities and personalities of boys and girls. One major difference may be summarized as "Boys do, and girls watch." Boys are portrayed as active, resourceful, brave, creative, and problem solving, while girls are portrayed as passive, helpless, and dull (Scott, 1981). Girls, through stupidity, get into rough spots from which boys rescue them. One children's book entitled *I'm Glad I'm a Boy! I'm Glad I'm a Girl!* taught such differences as "Boys invent things'' and "Girls use what boys invent" (cf. Key, 1975, p. 56). Margaret Mead's quote, "Man is unsexed by failure, woman by success" (cf. Key, 1975), is being taught to children from the first school readers they use.

In addition to elementary school texts and readers, gender-biased content has been demonstrated to characterize texts in all substantive areas and from secondary school to higher education (Key, 1975; Martin, 1982). Women continue to be portrayed primarily in domestic situations. They were absent from history, philosophy, art, and music and were treated in biased and stereotyped ways (when not ignored completely) in psychology, medicine, anthropology, and education (Howe, 1979).

As reviewed by many researchers (Weitzman, 1979; Maccoby & Jacklin, 1974; Sadker & Sadker, 1985) there is also evidence that teachers themselves respond differently to boys and girls. Although much more research is needed to understand teachers' reactions under different conditions, some preliminary generalizations are that boys receive more attention, both positive and negative, from teachers; while they may receive more disapproval, they also receive more positive attention, encouragement, and approval. Second, while there may not be differential encouragement of gender-role appropriate behaviors, gender-role reversals are often punished, particularly if they occur in boys, and are almost never reinforced. What these findings suggest is that a boy, but not a girl, who behaves in stereotypically feminine ways will likely be punished. Given that stereotypic femininity is viewed as less socially desirable and "adultlike" than stereotypic masculinity, teachers are clearly treating the sexes inequitably. In contrast, a girl may be punished or, at a minimum, ignored and so not reinforced for the masculine-stereotypic behaviors traditionally considered socially desirable, adultlike, and mentally healthy, for example, an active and instrumental approach to her world and a mastery-and-achievement-oriented spirit.

Barriers to Women in Higher Education

The enrollment and progress of women in higher education has long been impeded by sex discrimination. It is necessary, of course, to distinguish overt or blatant discriminatory practices from those that are more subtle and, therefore, more pernicious and difficult to address.

Examples of overt discriminatory admissions practices have included higher admissions requirements for female than male applicants, sex quotas for admission, discrimination in the award of financial aid, and age restrictions on enrollment that constitute inadvertent discrimination against women. In terms of financial aid practices, men have traditionally received the bulk of financial aids and awards; obvious examples include athletic scholarships, the GI Bill, ROTC, and many prestigious fellowships reserved for male applicants (e.g., until recently the Rhodes Scholarship program), but the pattern has fitted more general types of loans, fellowships, and graduate assistantships as well. Recent controversy over the differential award of the New York State Regent Scholarships to boys, based on somewhat higher combined SATs, was shown to involve discrimination against women because women's GPAs in high school were higher and because women did better in college (in GPA) than did men with comparable SATs. Thus, if the criterion performance is truly the basis for scholarship awards, predominant use of SAT data is inappropriate and, of course, discriminatory.

In a related vein, the recent proposed policy decision of the trustees of the University of North Carolina (UNC) to shift its admissions emphasis from high school grades (where girls are superior) to SATs (where boys are ahead), so that more men than women would be admitted ("Chapel Hill's Coeds," 1987), is equally discriminatory. Apparently there was concern on the part of the UNC trustees that rich alumni (presumably mostly male) would give more money if they thought they were giving it to young men rather than to young women.

Finally, overtly (as opposed to subtly) discriminatory faculty attitudes and practices include the sexual harassment of women students. The significance and severity of the effects of sexual harassment on women students cannot be overestimated and are the topic of Chapter 15.

As serious and possibly even more pernicious because we can't address them through legislation are the effects on women of subtle forms of discrimination in higher education. Legislation attempts to address discriminatory treatment, but it does not address the prejudices underlying the treatment, in our case, strong and ingrained prejudices against women students. The prejudices remain and, inevitably, exert themselves in ways outside the bounds of legislation. In other words, it is possible to legislate behavior change but far more difficult to bring about attitudinal change (Bernard, 1976). Bernard has long been writing about the nature and deleterious consequences of subtle forms of discrimination against women in higher education. Her descriptions of the "stag effect" and the "putdown" (Bernard, 1976) provided graphic and still useful characterizations of what really happens to women. Her characterization of the effects of such continuing discrimination on women as the "inferiority curriculum" (Bernard, 1988), causing even the most capable women depression, frustration, and damaged self-esteem, provides an apt and poignant portrayal.

The "stag effect" as defined by Bernard, is a "complex of exclusionary customs, practices, attitudes, conventions, and other social forms which protect the male turf from the intrusion of women" (Bernard, 1976, p. 23). At its most blatant, the stag effect took the form of male-only clubs and professional societies and activities, for example, male-only business and faculty clubs and the traditional golf game where major decisions are reached. As related to students, the stag effect is usually reflected in various means of avoiding and failing to encourage and support women students. In three important reports prepared under the auspices of the Project on the Status and Education of Women (Hall & Sandler, 1982, 1984; Ehrhart & Sandler, 1987), the nature and impact of differential treatment of women in the college classroom and the wider campus setting are discussed. Such negative treatments of women as discouraging classroom participation and the informal contact with faculty that is so essential to future professional development and undermining self-confidence are particularly characteristic of male-dominated fields (Ehrhart & Sandler, 1987).

Other problems face "token" women in male-dominated fields. For example, the greater visibility and, hence, scrutiny of tokens can lead to tremendous anxiety and (justifiable) feelings of vulnerability that can impede behavior and undermine self-confidence (Ehrhart & Sandler, 1987; Ware, Streckler & Leserman, 1984). Tokens may also feel (often justifiably) that their performance will reflect well or badly on their entire sex and, in the case of minority women, their entire race as well. Again, the resulting anxiety and perfectionism can be debilitating to performance.

Finally, the stag effect manifests itself in the "old boy network," leaving women as lonely outsiders in their chosen fields. For women in male-dominated fields, the most important ingredient becomes the presence of other women—both students and faculty. What Ehrhart and Sandler (1987) have termed the "comfort factor," the presence of other women, may not only be vital to the retention of women in male-dominated fields but may explain the salutary effect of women's colleges on career development (Tidball, 1980, 1985, 1986).

The "putdown," of course, refers to behaviors that actively disparage, demean, insult, and unfairly criticize women (Bernard, 1976, 1988). Such behaviors include (1) disparaging women's intellectual capabilities or professional potential; (2) using sexist humor; (3) advising women to lower their academic and career goals; (4) responding with surprise when women express demanding career goals; (5) not actively encouraging women to apply for fellowships, grants, and awards; and (6) focusing on marital and parental status as a potential barrier to the career development of women but as an advantage for men (a sign that he's stable, mature, and heterosexual) (Ehrhart & Sandler, 1987). Numerous examples of such treatment are available in the literature. Examples in a medical school setting (see Walsh, 1979) are the use of textbooks such as Williams and Wilkens's *The Anatomical Basis of Medical Practice* (by now forced to withdraw from the market), which contained such insults as pictures of nude females in seductive poses with such captions as "We are sorry that we cannot make available the addresses of the young ladies who grace our pages. Our wives burned our little address books at our last barbecue get-together." And, "If you think that once you have seen the backside of one female, you have seen them all, then you haven't sat in a sidewalk cafe in Italy where girl watching is a cultivated art. Your authors, whose zeal in this regard never flags, refer you to Figures 11–50 and 53 as proof that female backs can keep an interest in anatomy alive." Another medical text available, entitled *Anesthesia for the Uninterested* and in its third printing, used photographs of women in bikinis to demonstrate the use of operating room equipment and, on the cover, showed a male medical student groping a female colleague who is wearing a miniskirt (Walsh, 1979). It would be hard for female medical students to avoid some feeling of devaluation and sexual objectification when confronted by such texts.

Minnich (1988) gives several examples of "modern-day putdowns," including curriculum committees that challenge proposals for women's studies courses, implying that they are "faddish" and/or represent a lowering of academic standards and a "watering down" of the university curriculum.

The especially important point is made (AWIS, 1984) that although individual events of this type may appear trivial when viewed in isolation, their effect is cumulative and more than the sum of the individual incidents. As well stated by Pearson, Shavlik, and Touchton (1988): "The present record of higher education, in spite of some significant efforts, is not particularly good. Female students, on the whole, still experience a loss of personal and career confidence over the period they spend in higher education, even when they make very high grades. For men, the reverse is true."

An additional barrier to women in education has been the lack of female role models throughout the educational system. Beginning with elementary and secondary school, elementary teachers are primarily female, but the principals and administrators are primarily male (currently 81%). High school teachers, while balanced by sex, teach in stereotypic subject matter areas—females predominate in the teaching of literature and the arts, and males predominate in the teaching of math and science (and, of course, the possible existence of a male high school home economics teacher or a female electronics teacher is difficult to imagine). Males also predominate in secondary school administration. Eccles (1987), in her model of the relationship of gender roles to achievement-related behaviors, suggests that the lack of role models for young women may have its most serious effect in reducing their "perceived field of options" (pp. 141–142). As pointed out by Eccles, a reduced field of options will most certainly affect the subsequent career choice.

The situation is even worse in higher education, where there are even fewer female faculty members, so women students must rely on men, as well as the few women, to get the mentoring they need (Paludi & Fankell-Hauser, 1986; Weishaar, Green & Craighead, 1981). In an application of interview methods to the study of women's achievement motives, Paludi and Fankell-Hauser (1986) reported that women predominantly chose cross-sex role models (e.g., relatives, instructors, and professionals), that more male models were named by older rather than younger women, and, most interestingly, that "masculine" personality traits (e.g., competence, intelligence, and ambition) were used to describe the models. O'Connell and Russo (1983, 1988) found that eminent women in psychology reported more male than female mentors, although the proportion of female mentors has increased recently, as more women have been successful in the field.

Even though male professors can serve essential role modeling and mentoring functions for their female students, there is evidence that the relative lack of female faculty is a deterrent to women's educational and career pursuits, particularly in science (McLure & Piel, 1978) and other pioneer fields (O'Donnell & Anderson, 1978). The facilitative effects of same-sex models and mentors were suggested by Goldstein's (1979) report that about 80% of the articles published by recent doctoral degree recipients were by individuals whose faculty advisers were the same sex. Tidball (1980) reported that as the proportion of women faculty relative to the number of women students increases, so does the proportion of women high achievers in professional life.

One of the most basic and most important concepts summarizing the difficulties faced by women in higher education is Freeman's concept of the "null educational environment." A null environment, as defined by Freeman (1989), is an environment that neither encourages nor discourages individuals—it simply ignores them. Its effect is to leave the individual at the mercy of whatever environmental or personal resources to which she or he has access. The effects of null environments on women were first postulated by Freeman following her study of students at the University of Chicago. In this study, students were asked to describe the sources and extent of environmental support they received for their educational and career goals. Although both male and female students reported being ignored by faculty, thus experiencing what Freeman called a null educational environment, male students reported more encouragement and support from others in their environments, for example, parents, friends, relatives, and significant others.

When added to the greater occurrence of negative messages regarding women's roles and, in particular, women's pursuit of careers in fields traditionally dominated by men, the overall effect of the faculty's simply ignoring women students was a form of passive discrimination, through failure to act. As stated by Freeman (1989), "An academic situation that neither encourages nor discourages students of either sex is inherently discriminatory against women because it fails to take into account the differentiating external environments from which women and men students come," where external environments refer to differences in familial, peer, and societal support for career pursuits (p. 221).

In other words, professors don't have to discourage or discriminate overtly against female students. Society has already placed countless negative marks on the female student's "ballot," so a passive approach, a laissez-faire attitude, will probably ensure her failure. Career-oriented female students, to survive, must do so without much support from their environments. (See also N. E. Betz, 1989, for an expanded discussion of the effects of null environments on women.)

Thus, discrimination can result from errors of omission as well as of commission, and both have negative effects on females' progress and success in higher education. The critical aspect of this concept for educators, counselors, parents, and so on, is that if we are not actively supporting and encouraging women, we are, in effect, leaving them at the mercy of gender-role and occupational stereotypes. Eccles (1987) also states it well when she says: "Given the omnipresence of gender-role prescriptions regarding appropriate female life choices, there is little basis for females to develop non-traditional goals if their parents, peers, teachers, and counselors do not encourage them to consider these options" (p. 164). Failure to support women may not be an error of commission, like overt discrimination or sexual harassment, but it is an error of omission because its ultimate effects are the same, that is, limitations in their ability to fully develop and utilize their abilities and talents in educational and career pursuits.

Bias in Career Counseling and Testing

Although a complete review is beyond the scope of this chapter, it is important to note that career counseling and testing have sometimes served to continue the gender-role and occupational stereotyping characteristic of the larger society. For example, research reviewed by Betz and Fitzgerald (1987) has shown that the advice to clients and/or the judgment of career counselors often tended to encourage young women to stay in traditional roles (i.e., those of wife and mother) or to pursue traditionally female-dominated careers, rather than a broader range of career options. Instances of counselor discouragement of career innovation among women were common.

In addition, vocational interest inventories and ability tests have also been biased toward traditional career directions for both sexes (Betz & Fitzgerald, 1987), thus perpetuating societal stereotyping. As a particularly blatant example, which is now of primarily historical interest, the original version of the Strong Vocational Interest Blank (now the Strong Interest Inventory) came in pink and blue forms, the former for women (of course) and the latter for men. The color difference was accompanied, unfortunately, by dramatic differences in the occupational suggestions given to the two sexes. Among the many differences was the suggestion to women (but not to men) of many low-level, pink-collar jobs, in lieu of the largely professional, heavily scientific, and business-oriented occupations suggested to men. In the area of basic activity interests, "numbers" was suggested to women, while "mathematics" was suggested to men.

Thanks to criticism from concerned professional groups (most notably the Association for Measurement and Evaluation in Guidance and the American Psychological Association) and to comprehensive responses from many (although not all) test publishers, some of the biases in both counseling and interest testing have been addressed and corrected. However, continued research and constant awareness of the potential for such bias are very important if some of the interventions designed to help women in their career development are not to be used to perpetuate bias and limitations in perceived range of career options.

Socialized Barriers

Career-Family Conflict

Even though the majority of women now wish to pursue a career, the continued belief that they will need to be the primary homemaker and childraiser causes many young women to downscale their aspirations and accept lower levels of achievement.

In earlier times, it was often assumed that women would choose between career and family, and the prioritization of family roles led to both delay and confusion of young women's career plans. For example, as discussed by Kriger (1972), women's career decisions have been delayed relative to those of men because the former involve two major decisions instead of one. That is, before women decide what occupation or career to pursue, they must decide whether or not and to what degree they wish to make outside employment a focus of their lives. Men, in contrast, are rarely allowed to consider the "whether" and begin instead with the "what," thus getting an earlier start in the process. Angrist (1974; Angrist & Almquist, 1975) suggested that career planning was built into women's socialization as contingency training, which involved strategies to delay career decisions until the other, "more important" decisions of marriage and parenthood have been made or until it becomes apparent that they may not occur. Because of the delay of career decisions, establishment of a vocational role may be delayed until the late thirties and forties for women, versus the expected ages of 20 to 35.

Once a woman has made career decisions, however, the assumption that she is still primarily responsible for maintenance of a home and family, as well as career, creates obstacles in the form of role overload and role conflict. In other words, at the same time as women pursue careers, 90% still expect to have two or more children (Russo & Denmark, 1984). While traditionally the family cycle, when it occurred, was to supersede the work cycle in women's lives, it now most usually occurs concurrently. For women, the major practical implication of these changes is that they are now expected to successfully handle two full-time jobs, that is, one outside the home and the other that of homemaker and mother, the former paid and the latter unpaid.

Recent research indicates that young women, even though more career-oriented than women in years past, do not plan to reduce their assumption of responsibilities at home. Following an analysis of young women's marriage role expectations in 1961, 1972, 1978, and 1984, Weeks and Botkin (1987) concluded that although a trend toward egalitarianism in marital roles was apparent from the 1960s to the 1970s, the late 1970s and 1980s showed the emergence of a new traditionalism and conservatism, with any observable change being backward rather than forward. O'Connell, Betz, and Kurth (1989) reported no differences between women pursuing traditionally female (nursing) versus male-dominated occupations (engineering and veterinary medicine) in their plans for a family life—only about one-fourth of each group indicated a desire to work full-time with preschool children.

One unfortunate implication of the perceived conflict—or, at least, overload—caused by career and family priorities is that women for whom husband and children are a high priority tend to "downscale" their career aspirations, relative to other women and to men (men, of course, have not had to downscale their career aspirations in order to have a family). The research of Arnold (1989) and Arnold and Denny (1984, 1985), following the lives of Illinois valedictorians, provides a particularly vivid illustration of such downscaling in a group of intellectually superior female high school students. As concluded by Gerson (1985) and discussed further by Eccles (1987), women's choices about work continue to be inextricably linked with their decisions about family, and thus family role considerations limit women's investment in the occupational world. Ironically, family involvement has probably served to increase and facilitate men's career involvements because it gives them a strong rationale for achievement-related behavior.

It is important to note that the relationship of marital/familial status to women's career development has been weakening as we have witnessed tremendous increases in work force participation among women in all marital and parental categories. For example, O'Connell (1988), in her analysis of several generations of eminent women in psychology, notes that younger women (those studied in volume 2 of *Models of Achievement*) are much more likely to be married and to have children than were earlier groups of eminent women.

Even so, however, the relationship of marital/parental status to career attainment, commitment, and innovation is still very strong. Theoretically, this relationship has been called the role-conflict approach (O'Connell et al., 1989) to explain gender differences in work-related behavior. This approach assumes that women's work-related behavior is shaped more by family obligations than by the potential rewards associated with occupational activity. Consistent with this approach is a vast array of data showing strong inverse relationships between being married and number of children and every measurable criterion of career involvement and achievement (see Betz & Fitzgerald, 1987, for a comprehensive review.) It is essential to note that this inverse relationship is not true among men—highly achieving men are at least as likely (if not more so) as their less highly achieving male counterparts to be married and to have one or more children. In other words, men do not have to choose, they do not have to downscale, and they can "have it all" (see Gilbert, 1988, for an excellent discussion of this issue). It is, incidentally, with respect to this latter point that I disagree with authors who suggest that lack of career achievement is "OK" for women because they have different "core" values than do men (i.e., interest in people versus interest in achievement)—this stance seems to give too much control to "values," which are the products of gender-role socialization. Women, like men, deserve to have, or at least try for, "it all." My suggestion is that as more men are socialized to have core values including caring for others, men and women can share both the achievement and the nurturance.

Most important may be strategies for dealing with career-family conflict. Much has been written about this, so I will not review it here, but Baber and Monaghan (1988) discuss voluntary childlessness, delayed childbearing, and egalitarian marriages. The extensive works of Gilbert and Sekaran, among others, on coping strategies of dual-career couples are especially important (Gilbert, 1985, 1988; Gilbert & Rachlin, 1987; Sekaran, 1986).

Mathematics: The Critical Filter for Women

The critical importance of mathematics background for entrance to many of the best career opportunities in our society—for example, engineering, scientific and medical careers, computer science, business, and the skilled trades—is now generally agreed upon (Armstrong, 1985; Chipman & Wilson, 1985; Sells, 1982; Sherman, 1982), and lack of math background constitutes one of the major barriers to women's career development.

The classic study of the importance of math to career options was that of Sells (1973). In a study of freshmen at the University of California at Berkeley, Sells found that only 8% of the women, versus 57% of the men, had taken four years of high school math. Four years of high school math were prerequisite to entering the calculus or intermediate statistics courses required in three-fourths of the possible major field areas, and the university did not provide remedial courses to allow a student to complete the prerequisites. Thus, 92% of the freshmen women at Berkeley were prevented by lack of math background from even considering 15 of the 20 major fields at Berkeley! The five remaining "options" were predictable—such traditionally female major areas as education, the humanities, the social sciences, librarianship, and social welfare. Thus, decisions to "choose" these majors may have in many cases been by default, through failure to qualify for any major requiring math background.

Sells (1982) further elaborated the vital importance of math preparation for both career options and future earnings. Four full years of high school math are vital to surviving the standard freshman calculus course, now required for most undergraduate majors in business administration, economics, agriculture, engineering, forestry, resource management and conservation, health sciences, nutrition, food and consumer sciences, and natural, behavioral, physical, and computer sciences. Only the arts, humanities, physical education, and some of the social sciences do not require math background. Further, Sells (1982) shows a strong and direct relationship between college calculus background and both starting salaries and employers' willingness to interview a student for a given job. Mathematics is important even for non-college-degree technical occupations; the U.S. Department of Labor's *Occupational Outlook Handbook* shows that high school math and science are "strongly recommended" for technical and trades occupations. As so well stated by Sells (1982), "Mastery of mathematics and science has become essential for full participation in the world of employment in an increasingly technological society" (p. 7).

Given the importance of math background to career options, rather than to "choices" by default, females' tendency to avoid math course work becomes one of the most serious barriers to their career development. Further, it is fairly clear now that lack of math background, rather than lack of innate ability, is to blame for females' poorer performance on quantitative aptitude and mathematics achievement tests (Chipman & Thomas, 1985; Chipman & Wilson, 1985; Eccles & Jacobs, 1986; Pedro, Wolleat, Fennema & Becker, 1981; Sherman, 1982; Wise, 1985). Thus, the critical issue is females' avoidance of math. The reasons for such avoidance and, by implication, interventions capable of helping young women to be full participants in an increasingly technological society may be one of the most crucial issues in the study of women's career choices (Betz, 1991).

Regarding the first point, females' avoidance of math has been long documented (Eccles, 1983, 1984; Chipman & Thomas, 1985). Girls take fewer math courses than do boys beginning in high school and continuing through college, and even boys who fall into the lower half of the achievement distribution are more likely than their female counterparts to continue the study of math (Sherman & Fennema, 1978).

The breakdown of females' full participation in math begins in adolescence, in about the 9th or 10th grades. Prior to this point, sex differences in math achievement and participation are not generally found. Beginning during the secondary school years, however, girls stop taking math, and, not surprisingly, their math achievement test scores begin to fall below those of boys. Evidence that math course work is vital to math achievement comes from the findings that sex differences do not occur until females stop taking math and that girls who continue the study of math achieve math grades as good as those of the boys (Chipman & Wilson, 1985).

Unfortunately, the performance decrements that follow cessation of math course work create a vicious cycle, since math achievement then becomes an excellent predictor of plans to take additional math (Boswell, 1985; Brush, 1985; Chipman & Wilson, 1985; Wise, 1985). For example, the correlation between 9th grade achievement test scores and later high school math participation in the Project Talent 9th graders was lower in girls than boys, such that there were *no* ·*sex differences* in math achievement test scores; yet by 12th grade there were significant sex differences in math participation. Thus, a girl with a given level of math ability was less likely than a boy of equivalent capability to continue in math. The key question is, Why do girls stop taking math?

The major explanations for females' avoidance of math beginning in adolescence derive from differences in the way female socialization, versus male socialization, influences attitudes toward, and self-confidence with respect to, math learning and performance (Eccles & Jacobs, 1986). Such beliefs as "Math is a male domain," "Girls don't need to study math," and "Females are incompetent in math" have long been part of stereotypic belief systems.

Considerable research has explored the degree to which girls have internalized such societally conveyed beliefs, and there is considerable consistency in research findings. Females have been found to have less confidence in their math ability in comparison with males even when their objectively measured abilities are equal (Chipman & Wilson, 1985). Armstrong (1985) and Chipman and Wilson (1985) concluded that math confidence is a better predictor of further math participation than is actual math achievement, thus implicating girls' lack of confidence as a factor contributing to math avoidance.

Related to the issue of self-confidence is the widespread belief that boys do better than girls in math. Ernest (1976) reported belief of male superiority not only among high school boys and girls but in both male and female teachers. Thus, a self-fulfilling prophecy of male success and female failure in math may be unconsciously set up by teachers.

Just as girls have less confidence in their math abilities, they are also found to be more math-anxious in many (although not all) studies. Boswell (1985) reported greater math anxiety among girls in all school grades, while findings of greater math anxiety in female versus male college students were reported by N. E. Betz (1978), Dew, Galassi, and Galassi (1983), and Llabre and Suarez (1985). In the latter study, women were more math-anxious, even though there were no sex differences in SAT-M scores. On the other hand, Resnick, Viehe, and Segal (1982) did not find sex differences in math anxiety.

Math anxiety, like math achievement, is closely related to amount of math background (N. E. Betz, 1978; Hackett, 1985; Hendel, 1980; Richardson & Woolfolk, 1980). Thus, the vicious cycle is further complicated, with various forces leading to the development of anxiety and the avoidance of math course work sometime in adolescence, both of which hinder subsequent math achievement, thus exacerbating anxiety and solidifying patterns of math avoidance.

Finally, an idea that takes into account both confidence and anxiety is "mathematics self-efficacy expectations," that is, an individual's belief in her capability to successfully engage in various math-related tasks. Basing their research on Bandura's (1977) theory of self-efficacy expectations as a major mediator of behavior and behavior change, Betz and Hackett (1983) developed a three-part measure of mathematics self-efficacy. Using this measure, Betz and Hackett (1983) studied the mathematics self-efficacy expectations of college males and females. As predicted, the math-related self-efficacy expectations of college males were significantly stronger than those of college females on all subscales, and students' math-related self-efficacy expectations contributed significantly to the degree to which students selected science-based college majors. Interestingly, the only items toward which females felt just as efficacious as males were those involving "female" domains such as cooking, grocery shopping, and sewing. (This finding is also supportive of research findings suggesting that the male-oriented content of math tests favors male versus female test performance and that changing test content to include an equal balance of female-oriented, along with male-oriented, domains would be fairer to female test takers than current practices, e.g., Frieze, Parsons, Johnsons, Ruble & Zellman, 1978.)

Another important factor explaining females' avoidance of mathematics may be the lesser perceived utility of math to female versus male students (Chipman & Wilson, 1985). There is considerable evidence both for a relationship of perceived usefulness of math to participation in math (Armstrong, 1985; Lantz, 1985; Pedro et al., 1981; Sherman, 1982; Sherman & Fennema, 1977) and for girls' tendency to perceive math as less useful to them (Sherman & Fennema, 1977; Hilton & Berglund, 1974). Boswell (1985) reported that both males and females perceived math as more useful for men than for women. Eccles, Adler, and Meece (1984) compared several different theoretical explanations for sex differences in math achievement—self-concept theories, attribution theory, learned helplessness versus mastery orientation, and expectancy theory. Eccles et al. (1983) found that the strongest mediator of both academic achievement and math participation was subjective task value, that is, perceptions of the utility and importance of math, interest in math, and perceived worth of effort needed to do well in math. In contrast, there was some evidence for sex differences in ability attributions consistent with the expectancy/self-concept perspective, and there was little support for learned helplessness models.

The influence of traditional life role expectations for females probably also reduces females' likelihood of continuing in math. Evidence of "sex-role strain" in relationship to math was reported by Sherman (1983), who further reported that 29% of girls said they would "play dumb," downplaying their abilities, while 76% perceived other girls as playing dumb. Similarly, Benbow and Stanley (1980) suggest that girls avoid math because they fear social disapproval. Sherman (1983) concludes:

After several years of research, it is my opinion that it is neither anxiety nor lack of ability that keeps women from mathematics. It is a network of sex-role influences which makes mathematics and the careers mathematics are needed in appear incongruent with the female role, especially with motherhood. When girls see that motherhood and demanding careers can be combined, a major source of resistance to mathematics will disappear. Research and action to reduce the perceived and real conflict between demanding careers and motherhood is of crucial importance. (p. 342)

In summary, young women who have continued course work in mathematics and science have a far broader range of career options than do the majority of young women who have avoided such work. An emphasis on changing societal expectations and the expectations of girls and women with regard to the appropriateness and necessity of mathematics for women is essential to the facilitation of women's career development.

Other Socialized Barriers

Chapter 16 covers the important concepts of self-esteem, achievement motivation, fear of success, causal attributions, expectancies for success, and self-efficacy expectations to women's achievements, so these concepts will not be covered here, even though they are important to women's career development. Suffice it to say that issues related to self-esteem, self-perceptions of competence, and attitudes toward, and attributions concerning, success and failure have served as powerful barriers to women's perceived range of career options and their persistence in pursuing desired alternatives. Besides chapter 16, other important reviews of these areas include Sutherland and Veroff (1985).

FACILITATORS OF CAREER DEVELOPMENT

Given all the environmental and socialized barriers to women's career development, what influences allow women to surmount those barriers, to achieve to their fullest educational and occupational potentials, to have important, fulfilling careers just as men have always been able to do? These influences can be discussed under the general rubric of "facilitators" of women's career development. In the discussion to follow, two kinds of facilitators, environmental and individual, will be examined. Some of these facilitators are simply the inverse of the barriers discussed previously. For example, if math avoidance is a barrier, math participation is a facilitator. Similarly, prioritization of family can lead to a downscaling of career aspirations, while remaining single and childless continues to facilitate women's career development. For such facilitators representing the flip side of barriers already reviewed, further review will be unnecessary. Other, new facilitators, however, will receive more attention in the subsequent pages. (Table 1 summarizes the facilitators of women's career development.)

Environmental Facilitators

Family Background

The concept of socioeconomic status (SES) has been variously defined and measured; indices of SES have included the occupational or educational level of the primary breadwinner (usually the father) and family income. While occupational level is the most commonly used index, studies vary in the indices used and, unfortunately, often fail to specify how the index of SES was obtained. In addition, the effects of intelligence on occupational attainments may be difficult to disentangle from the effects of other variables covarying with SES, for example, race and intelligence.

In spite of definitional variation, socioeconomic status is one of the most consistent predictors of the occupational level achieved by males; higher family SES is related to higher achieved occupational levels in sons, while sons of lower-class backgrounds achieve lower occupational levels (Brown, 1970; Hollingshead, 1949; Sewell, Haller & Strauss, 1957). As pointed out by Goodale and Hall (1976), sons are likely to "inherit" their fathers' occupational levels. Sociologists (Stevens, 1986) have consistently reported the tendency for sons to follow in their fathers' occupational footsteps.

In contrast, data regarding the influence of parental SES on women's career development yield an inconsistent pattern of results. In some studies, higher SES was related to stronger career orientation and/or innovation in women. Several studies have found that women pursuing male-dominated professions (e.g., physicians, academics) are significantly more likely than women in general to have fathers who are professionals (Lemkau, 1979; O'Connell, 1988; Russo & O'Connell, 1980; Wertheim, Widom & Wortzel, 1978). O'Connell et al. (1989) conclude that higher SES leads to more egalitarian gender-role beliefs and greater career commitment.

Other studies, however, have reported negative relationships between career orientation and SES (Del Vento Bielby, 1978), and still others have found no relationships between the two variables (Card et al., 1980). Marini (1978) and Stevens (1986) have concluded that while family SES is associated with higher educational aspirations in daughters, the relationship of family SES to girls' occupational aspirations is much weaker (if it exists at all) than the relationship of SES to boys' aspirations.

While studies based on father's occupational level provide a somewhat inconsistent pattern of findings, data regarding father's educational level provide a more consistent pattern of findings and suggest that more highly educated fathers tend to have more career-oriented and innovative daughters. Higher parental education for women compared with men in the same occupations was noted by Lemkau (1979) in a study of Ph.D.'s. Women in pioneer career fields had more highly educated fathers than did women in traditional fields of study (Burlin, 1976; Greenfield, Greiner & Wood, 1980; Russo & O'Connell, 1980).

Even more powerful a predictor of women's career development than father's educational level is maternal employment. Numerous studies have found that daughters of working mothers are more career-oriented (versus home-oriented) than are the daughters of homemakers (Altman & Grossman, 1977; Huth, 1978). Other studies have suggested that daughters of working mothers are more likely to pursue nontraditional occupations in comparison with daughters of homemakers (Crawford, 1978; Haber, 1980). Stephan and Corder (1985) found that girls reared in two-career families were more likely to plan to combine family and work roles than those reared in a traditional family.

While maternal employment may influence women's career development through its provision of a model of female employment and role integration, maternal employment is also related to other variables facilitative of women's career development. Studies have suggested that the daughters of working mothers develop generally more liberal sex-role ideologies (Hoffman, 1984; Hoffman & Nye, 1974), are less stereotypically feminine themselves (Altman & Grossman, 1977; Hansson, Chernovetz & Jones, 1977), and show greater self-esteem and more positive evaluations of female competence (Hoffman, 1984) in comparison with the daughters of homemakers. All of these variables have been shown in other research to be positively related to women's career development.

In addition to maternal employment, maternal level of education, like paternal level of education, appears to be positively related to women's career orientation and choice of nontraditional careers. Harmon (1978) reported that women receiving Ph.D.'s have more highly educated parents than do men receiving Ph.D.'s across academic fields, and Freun, Rothman, and Steiner (1974) reported that female medical school applicants have more highly educated parents than do male applicants. Mother's level of education was found to be related to greater career orientation in daughters in several studies (e.g., Del Vento Bielby, 1978).

Highly educated mothers have been consistently overrepresented in samples of women preferring and pursuing nontraditional professions (Haber, 1980; Harmon, 1978; O'Donnell & Anderson, 1978; Russo & O'Connell, 1980).

Family encouragement was reported as a major facilitator by high school girls planning careers in science (McLure & Piel, 1978) and by samples of women pursuing male-dominated occupations (Haber, 1980; Hackett, Esposito & O'Halloran, 1989; Houser & Garvey, 1985). For example, 72% of Standley and Soule's (1974) architects, lawyers, physicians, and psychologists reported being their father's favorite child. Farmer (1985) found that parent support was one of the strongest predictors of young women's career aspirations and motivation. O'Connell and Russo (1988) found that parental encouragement for achievement and higher education was characteristic of most of the eminent women psychologists studied. Fitzpatrick and Silverman (1989) found that the support of parents and teachers was an important factor in high-ability women's pursuit of engineering careers.

Possibly as important as parental encouragement of daughters' achievements is a concomitant lack of pressure toward the traditional female role. Parents who exert less pressure on their daughters to date, marry, and have children have been found to have more career-oriented daughters (Haber, 1980), as do parents who place less emphasis on the development of stereotypically feminine qualities (Turner & McCaffrey, 1974).

While parental variables, then, appear to be importantly related to women's career development, a major limitation of this research is the assumption that both parents are present while the girl is growing up. Research on father-absent children has focused primarily on boys (e.g., see Bannon & Southern, 1980), and little is known about women raised in single-parent or adoptive homes or with relatives or nonfamily members. Dramatic increases in the number of single-parent families across all racial and ethnic groups (Hoffman, 1977) suggest that research based on nuclear family assumptions will be increasingly irrelevant to an understanding of the career development of many women and men.

Education as Facilitator

It is probably difficult to overestimate the importance of education to career development and achievement. At a very basic level, early schooling serves as a major source of learning and socialization and conveys values regarding work and career that are influential throughout one's life. More specifically, the nature and level of obtained education are importantly related to subsequent career achievements and to adult socioeconomic status and life-style. For example, an undergraduate degree is now a necessary minimum requirement for the pursuit of many occupations, and graduate or professional education is the only route to careers in academe and most other professions. In general, appropriate educational preparation is a major "gate" for occupational entrance. Education creates options, while lack of education closes them; without options, the concept of "choice" itself has no real meaning. Thus, the decisions the individual makes concerning higher education, both the level and major areas of study, will be among the most important career decisions he or she ever makes. Further, success and survival in the educational programs chosen will be critical to the successful implementation of these career decisions.

While education received is an important variable in the study of men's career development, the nature and level of obtained education are strongly related to almost every major dependent variable used in the description of women's career development. Along with marital status and family-related priorities (see Eccles, 1987), education can be considered the most important variable in women's career development (Watley & Kaplan, 1971; Wolfson, 1976). One of the most striking and consistent relationships is that the more education a woman receives, the more likely she is to be working outside the home as an adult, regardless of her marital or parental status (Houseknecht & Spanier, 1980; Vetter, 1980). For example, in 1977 62% of women with bachelor's degrees and 85% of those with master's degrees were in the labor force (Vetter, 1980). The effect of higher education was particularly striking for women with degrees in science and engineering—from 63 to 84% of science B.A.'s, from 78 to 88% of science M.A.'s, and from 90 to 96% of science Ph.D.'s or women with professional degrees were employed. Close to half of B.A.'s and M.A.'s not in the labor force were so because they were working on advanced degrees!

In addition to its relationship to career orientation and achievements, higher education in women is also related to a greater tendency to remain single, to higher rates of marital disruption (e.g., divorce), and to lower fertility rates (Houseknecht & Spanier, 1980). Higher education in women is related to more liberal attitudes toward women's roles and to such characteristics as autonomy and the desire for direct, versus vicarious, achievement (cf. Betz & Fitzgerald, 1987). Thus, educational level is related to a number of other major variables positively related to women's career development. Since few studies have controlled some of these variables while varying others, it is difficult to make conclusions regarding the degree of directness and the relative strength of these variables in influencing women's career orientation and innovation. Further research from which directional inferences can be made is needed in order to clarify the effects of educational level and other related variables on women's career development.

The influence of educational level on career achievements and the pursuit of nontraditional occupations has been even stronger for graduates of women's colleges (Astin, 1977). Graduates of women's colleges are twice as likely to attend medical school as are women graduates of coeducational colleges (Tidball, 1985) and are also twice as likely to have earned research doctorates (Tidball, 1986). Women's colleges have the advantage, first, of providing women with greater opportunities for academic and campus leadership than do coeducational colleges (Astin, 1977). In part, this is because in the absence of the men to whom they have traditionally deferred, women must take leadership roles. But, in addition, many women are more willing to assume leadership and to behave in dominant, assertive ways when they aren't worried about offending men or reducing their femininity in men's view (Tidball, 1986). A second advantage of women's colleges is that they tend to encourage women to pursue nontraditional areas of study and therefore encourage women's pursuits of traditionally male career fields (Tidball, 1980). Even though women's colleges, like coeducational colleges, have been dominated by male faculty, there are at least a few more females in faculty and administrative positions to provide models for female students. It is unfortunate, in my opinion, that a number of well-known women's colleges have "gone coeducational" in the last decade. It remains to be seen whether the move to coeducational education in the Ivy League will compensate for the loss of some of the seven sisters schools as all-women institutions.

Given the importance of education, in conjunction with continuing gender bias and gender-role stereotyping, as well as more subtle barriers such as are summarized by the concept of the null environment, issues of educational fairness and equality and educational enrichment for women are probably among the most crucial we face. Randour, Strasburg, and Lipman-Blumen (1982) suggest that given women's continued lack of equality in higher education, continued monitoring of the level and nature of women's involvement is essential. Further, they suggest the importance of research on the relationship of institutional factors (e.g., degree level, public versus private institutions, full versus part-time study) to subsequent educational and occupational outcomes.

Continued attention to educational equity for women is particularly important given that the 1980s began with a national administration hostile to affirmative action programs and resistant to the enforcement of antidiscrimination legislation. Psychologists, educators, and others committed to facilitating women's career development must ensure that research and positive change within the educational system continue to receive effort and attention and that the 1990s provide a more supportive environment than did the 1980s.

Individual Facilitators

Of the following "individual" facilitators, most, if not all, can be viewed as socialized, just as the internal (as opposed to environmental) barriers were. However, in the case of these facilitators, most go counter to prevailing stereotypes and to prevailing female socialization practices, and thus they might be better termed "unsocialized" or nontraditionally reinforced. In fact, the advantages of nontraditional and androgynous rearing and of a childhood allowing exploration of both traditionally male and traditionally female domains and activities appear to be far-ranging (Lemkau, 1979). Broader views of the meaning of being female in this society are strongly related to higher achievement and stronger career orientation, possibly through their influence on the development of several significant individual facilitators of career development, as discussed below.

Many individual facilitators merely represent the inverse of the barriers discussed in the previous section, and, accordingly, further citations will be avoided. Just as marriage and children often have a "downscaling" effect, later marriage and/or single status and few or no children are strongly associated with career achievement. Just as math avoidance is an impediment to career options, math participation serves to preserve or create options. Just as socialized belief systems such as low self-esteem, low career self-efficacy, or external attributions for success can serve as internal barriers, more adaptive belief systems and characteristics reflective of a transcendence of the traditional female role are important facilitators of women's career development.

An entire chapter could easily be devoted to the concepts of gender-role–related personality characteristics, so the following can be only a brief summary. The study of gender-role–related personality characteristics began, of course, with research on the correlates of "masculinity" and "femininity." Although the terms *masculinity* and *femininity* are no longer used as much, having been replaced in the literature by the terms *instrumentality* and *expressiveness* (Gilbert, 1985; Spence & Helmreich, 1980, 1981), much research exists that used them. The terms *masculinity* and *femininity* have been criticized because they perpetuate stereotypes and assumptions that behavior is gender-based (Lott, 1985), because they imply false dichotomies that overemphasize between-gender and underemphasize within-gender differences (Lott, 1985; Wallston, 1981), and because they aren't descriptive of behavior. Rather, the term *instrumentality*, referring to the capabilities of self-assertion and competence, has been suggested by Spence and Helmreich to descriptively summarize the key aspects of traditional stereotypes of masculinity. The term *expressiveness* best summarizes the central aspects of traditional femininity, that is, nurturance, interpersonal concern, and emotional expressiveness and sensitivity.

Regardless of the labels used to report the results of research in this area, this research has consistently and convincingly shown the importance of these constellations of characteristics, particularly instrumentality or masculinity, to women's career development. More specifically, instrumentality appears to be strongly related to both the extent and nature of women's career pursuits. Higher levels of instrumentality are related to stronger career orientation (Greenglass & Devins, 1982; Marshall & Wijting, 1980), to a greater extent of labor force participation following the birth of the first child (Gaddy, Glass, & Arnkoff, 1983), and to greater career achievement among working women (Wong, Kettlewell & Sproule, 1985). Orlofsky and Stake (1981) reported that masculinity was related to stronger achievement motivation and to greater performance self-esteem and self-perceived capabilities among college women. Metzler-Brennan, Lewis, and Gerrard (1985) found that both masculinity in personality and in childhood activities distinguished career-oriented from home-oriented women.

Most strongly related to instrumentality, however, is pursuit of careers in nontraditional fields for women. Among younger women, masculinity is related to stronger interests in, and greater pursuit of, math and science, more confidence in one's math abilities, and a greater likelihood of selecting a math-related college major (Hackett, 1985). Fassinger (1990) found that instrumentality was related to women's preferences for careers that are science-related, high in prestige, and nontraditional for women. The greater willingness to consider nontraditional college majors, or, alternatively stated, less susceptibility to the limiting influences of traditional female socialization, was the major explanation of Wolfe and Betz's (1981) finding that masculine-typed women were more likely than feminine-typed women to prefer careers congruent with their measured vocational interests. Thus, the trait factor or "matching model" as a basis for career decision making may be more likely to be used among women who have at least in some ways surmounted gender stereotyping.

Several other studies have shown that instrumentality and related characteristics are prevalent among women in male-dominated occupational fields (Bachtold, 1976). Williams and McCullers (1983) reported that women in nontraditional fields scored higher on the Bem Sex Role Inventory (BSRI) masculinity scale than did women in traditional fields; the former group also reported more masculine play patterns and less coercion to fit the feminine stereotype. Helmreich, Spence, Bean, Lucker, and Matthews (1980), in a study of male and female academic psychologists, found no sex differences on instrumentality characteristics that, in the general population, would be found more frequently among males.

Thus, the instrumentality associated with traditional masculinity appears to be importantly and positively related to career innovation and achievement in women. The extent to which the possession of traditionally feminine characteristics is related to career involvement is less clear. While some studies have suggested a relationship between expressiveness (or femininity) and home orientation (Marshall & Wijting, 1980), other studies have suggested that career-oriented women score no differently on measures of femininity than do home-oriented women (Metzler-Brennan et al., 1985). Farmer (1985) reported that highly career-motivated young women tended to be androgynous, possessing relatively high levels of both instrumentality and expressiveness.

The absence of a strong or consistent relationship between femininity and home orientation, coupled with the strong relationship of instrumentality to career orientation, led Spence and Helmreich (1980) to suggest that it may not only be the presence of instrumentality that leads some women to seek career achievements, but the absence of instrumentality that leads home-oriented women to avoid such pursuits. In other words, home-oriented women may be motivated not so much by the desire to nurture but by doubts concerning their capabilities to cope and compete in the larger world. Thus, a "deficit model" of choice of homemaking as the central life pursuit would be suggested.

In addition to an apparent transcendence of gender-stereotypic personality characteristics is transcendence of traditional attitudes toward women's roles as an important predictor of women's career development. One of the most consistent (and, it should be noted, inherently logical) findings in the research literature concerns the greater tendency of career-oriented women to express liberal or feminist attitudes toward women's roles. More liberal gender-role attitudes have been found to characterize career versus home-oriented women (Smith, 1981; Stafford, 1984; Tinsley & Faunce, 1980) and pioneers versus traditionals (Gackenbach, 1978; Orcutt & Walsh, 1979). Stringer and Duncan (1985) found nontraditional gender-role attitudes among women in the skilled crafts, labor, and technical fields. Fassinger (1985) found that responses to the questions "I would label myself a 'feminist' in my beliefs and values" and "I prefer to use the title 'Ms.' when referring to myself" were among the strongest predictors of career orientation and the prestige and nontraditionality of career choices among college women.

Generally, more liberal gender-role attitudes are related to greater labor force participation (Atkinson & Huston, 1984; Dreyer et al., 1981; Stafford, 1984), to higher levels of educational aspiration and attainment (Dreyer, Woods & James, 1981; Lyson & Brown, 1982; Zuckerman, 1981), and to stronger career motivation and higher career aspirations (Komarovsky, 1982; Lyson & Brown, 1982). Fassinger (1985, 1990) found that more liberal gender-role attitudes were the most consistent predictors of high and nontraditional career aspirations among college women.

In considering the strong relationships of liberal or feminist attitudes toward women's career development, it should be noted that feminist orientation and more liberal role attitudes are also strongly related to the tendency to be single or to be childless if married (Dreyer et al., 1981) which, in turn, are also strongly related to career development. Further, more liberal gender-role attitudes are related to perceived self-competence (Stake, 1979) and to higher self-reported and objectively measured intelligence (cf. Williams, 1983). Thus, gender-role attitudes are part of a facilitative constellation of characteristics which Lemkau (1979) postulates are due to an enriched background allowing a girl to grow up with a broadened view of the female role and of her own capabilities and options.

Finally, other personality and attitudinal facilitators of women's career development, as reviewed in chapter 16 of this volume, include high self-esteem, strong expectancies for academic success, adaptive versus maladaptive attributions for success and failure, and high expectations of self-efficacy. Overall, women's career development is facilitated by a constellation of personality and attitudinal characteristics emphasizing positive self-concepts, instrumentality and competence, androgyny, and liberated attitudes toward women's roles. The data clearly fit Almquist and Angrist's (1970) "enrichment" hypothesis, which may be summarized as explaining high achievement and role innovation in women as the result of an enriched background, above-average intellectual and personal assets, and an expanded view of what is possible for women.

In considering these conclusions, a final point should be made: the factors influencing women's career development will almost surely change as societal attitudes and norms change and as increasing numbers of women enter the work force. If girls and women, like boys and men, begin to assume that career pursuits will be an integral part of their lives, we may see changes in the nature of, and influences on, women's career choices. O'Connell (1988) notes changes consistent with historical and social forces in studying the family background, demographic, and life-style patterns characterizing several generations of eminent women psychologists. As so well stated by Osipow (1983), "So much social change is occurring in the area of sex and vocation that any theoretical proposal made now is likely to be premature, as would be any generalization about women's career development" (p. 271). Thus, the study of both barriers to, and facilitators of, these choices will be a continuing and challenging endeavor.

WOMEN OF COLOR

Most studies of the effects of ethnicity on American women's career choices have examined black versus white women; research on Hispanics, Native Americans, and Asian Americans is just beginning (Smith, 1983). Thus, the discussion begins with studies comparing black and white women and ends with work on other groups.

Over the years, one of the most consistent findings regarding black women has been that, in comparison with their white counterparts, the majority of them have expected to work part or all of their adult lives (Smith, 1982). Although the actual labor force participation rate among white women is now catching up to that among black women (Almquist, 1989), the labor force participation rate among black women has traditionally been greater than that among white women (Gump & Rivers, 1975; Almquist, 1989).

The reasons for black women's greater labor force participation stem at least in part from the historical roles played by black women, who have been more likely than white women to be sole support of themselves and/or their families. Black women are far more likely than white women to be heads of households (U.S. Department of Labor, 1984). The incidence of divorce is higher for blacks than whites at every level of education, occupation, and income, and the ratio of males to females is more disproportionate among blacks than whites. While the gender ratio among white adults is about 98 men to 100 women, the gender ratio among blacks has been dropping steadily since 1940 and was less than 75 to 100 in the 1980s. For highly educated black women the disparity of equally well-educated black men is even more serious. Along with the inherent shortage of men, high rates of marital disruption (Houseknecht & Spanier, 1980) help explain why only 38% of black women 14 and over (versus 61% of white women) are married and living with their husbands. Black women learn that they cannot rely on marriage to produce a secure life and, rather, learn the necessity of self-support.

But while black women's expected and actual labor force participation has exceeded that of white women, black women are even more disadvantaged than are white women in the nature of that participation. Black women in particular and ethnic/minority women in general are in a state of what has been referred to as "double jeopardy" (Beale, 1970) because they are both female and minority in a society that has traditionally valued neither group (Almquist, 1989). Thus, on many dimensions they are doubly disadvantaged. Black women are affected not only by sex discrimination but by race discrimination. As so well stated by Almquist (1989), "In their push for freedom, dignity, and equality, black women confront the same barriers that white women do, plus the extra hardships imposed on them by racism" (p. 432). In terms of employment, the barriers of sexism are even more important than the barriers of racism.

Black women, first of all, earn less money than women or men of any ethnic group and earn substantially less than do black men (Smith, 1983; U.S. Department of Labor, 1988). Although black men are clearly disadvantaged relative to white men, males, regardless of race, are better off in terms of earning power than are females. In terms of the nature of labor force participation, proportionately more black women than black men are in professional occupations but proportionately fewer black women are professionally employed (U.S. Department of Labor, 1984). Like white women, black women are concentrated in low-paying professions. In comparison with white women, black women are even more greatly concentrated in traditionally female occupations (Smith, 1982), particularly in domestic and service jobs (U.S. Department of Labor, 1984).

Almquist (1989), on the other hand, points out that the nature, as well as the extent, of black women's labor force participation is becoming increasingly similar to that of white women. More black women are now in white-collar jobs versus service jobs such as private household workers. More black women are now secretaries or clerks. Note that while the nature of black women's labor force participation is increasingly similar to that of white women, both groups of women have remained concentrated in low-level, low-paying, traditionally female occupations (Smith, 1982).

The fact that black women continue to be slightly more highly educated than black men, yet continue to earn far less, is, according to Almquist (1989), a result of sex segregation—that is, the concentration of women into a small number of low-paying professions and occupations—and sex discrimination in pay. Yet Smith (1983) also points out that both blacks and women suffer from the phenomenon of "learning without earning" (Newman et al., 1978), that is, the failure of educational attainments to translate into the higher occupational status and pay that are true of the educational attainments of white males.

In addition to the failure of education to translate into occupational and financial security, higher education remains an especially nonsupportive environment for ethnic/minority women. The problems of being a double token (Zappert & Stansbury, 1984; Loo & Rolison, 1986), the extreme isolation and sense of alienation (Henry, 1985; Loo & Rolison, 1986), and the near-total lack of black female professorial role models (Loo & Rolison, 1986) can make academic survival, not to mention achievement, very difficult. The concept and implications of the null academic environment are doubly applicable to minority women.

Fleming (1986) documents the difficulties of black women in predominantly white universities—their experiences parallel those of women in general in male-dominated universities but, again, they are experiencing a double dose of isolation, lack of role modeling, and lack of social support. Fleming notes that many gifted black women are returning to historically black colleges and universities as a "safe haven"—again such concepts as the null educational environment and the "comfort factor" are doubly important to the understanding of the dilemma of black (and other ethnic minority) women.

Research on Hispanic and Native American women has begun to burgeon in the last few years. In a recent special issue of the *Psychology of Women Quarterly* on Hispanic women and mental health (Amaro & Russo, 1987), an important study of the role that work and family play in the psychological well-being of Hispanic women (Amaro, Russo, & Johnson, 1987) indicated that income and Hispanic group were consistently related to mental health measures, as were discrimination, peer support, and job stress. Hispanic women, like black women, suffer the disadvantages of being both women and a minority, and yet there are some vitally important differences in that Hispanic women are possibly even more subject to rigid and traditional sex-role norms and expectations than are either Anglo or black women (Canino, 1982; Gonzales, 1988). Thus, the Hispanic woman may experience pay discrimination at work and subtle censure at home for work behavior that violates the traditional norms. In addition, perceptions among young Chicanas that Hispanic males will be threatened by their educational accomplishments and that college attainment will cause them to be seen as elitist by the larger Chicano community (Gonzales, 1988) further complicate the picture.

In terms of higher education, Hispanic and Native American women again face the barriers associated with double tokenism—isolation, lack of role models, a feeling that they carry the fate of their race on their shoulders, and outright overt and subtle discrimination (Espin, 1980; Vasquez, 1982; Zeff, 1982). LaFromboise (1986; LaFromboise & Plake, 1983) has written extensively on the educational and counseling needs of American Indian women, pointing out that this group has the lowest level of college attendance and graduation of any group of American ethnic minority women.

Thus, ethnic minority women in this country are very much in need of educational, economic, and counseling assistance because they are at an even greater disadvantage occupationally than is the already disadvantaged Anglo American woman. They deserve much more attention than they have received in the past.

SUMMARY AND RECOMMENDATIONS

This chapter reviewed issues in, and factors influencing, the career choices of women. Problematic aspects of the choices of women included their underutilization of their abilities, their overconcentration in a small number of traditionally female-dominated (and also generally low-paying) occupations and resulting underrepresentation in an extensive variety of traditionally male-dominated (and generally higher-paying) fields, and their avoidance of course work in mathematics, resulting in externally forced limitations in their career options.

As stated in the introduction, there seems ample reason to contend that most women, like most men, should be encouraged to pursue rewarding careers. Men have never had to "choose between home and family," and the possibility of combining important life roles is just as vital to women as it is to men. In their pursuit of careers, women's choices should represent better matching of their individual characteristics to the level and nature of the chosen field. The waste of female talent and ability when women seriously underutilize their abilities in career choices is a significant personal and societal problem and needs to be counteracted. Women's career choices should be made in the context of a broad range of perceived and real options, rather than by default; thus, options should more often include careers in traditionally male-dominated fields, particularly those in mathematical, scientific, and technical areas. Women's career choices, then, should utilize, rather than waste, women's abilities and talents and should represent the full range of occupational possibilities, rather than the restricted range of female-dominated professions and pink-collar jobs. Given these general goals, the final two sections address implications for research and for interventions.

Needs for Further Research

This review has focused primarily on research done since about 1975 and primarily since 1980, and it has been selective. Given this, the sheer volume of research on women's career choices is impressive—even larger than the considerable number of studies reviewed here. We know quite a bit now about the factors, both environmental/institutional and individual or socialized, that affect the career choices of women.

As much as we do know, there is still much to be learned. Probably most important is the issue of contextual validity (see Fine, 1985), a crucial aim of feminist psychology but one that is too easy to violate. Fine (1985) makes a number of suggestions relevant to research in the psychology of women in general and, in my opinion, very important for research on women's career development.

First, the applicability of research findings across groups of women is in serious doubt. As I say to my students in the Psychology of Women course, most of what we know has come from research on white, middle-class, heterosexual women, and we should make no assumptions about other groups of women until we have (as we should) actually studied them. Much needs to be studied about the career development of women of color, of lesbians and bisexual women, of reentry women, and of disabled women. Although the section here on women of color shows some activity in this area, even this has only scratched the surface.

Second, Fine (1985) also urges us to study not only women but those in their interpersonal contexts without whom the women themselves cannot be understood. Probably the best example of this is in the study of women in dual-career couples (particularly those with children), where it is close to impossible to understand the work-related behavior of one without understanding that of the other.

Third, Fine (1985) also urges us to avoid reliance on the traditional "general laws" approach to psychology and, in our case, the psychology of women. It is at least as useful to study why people's behavior is inconsistent with a "general laws" prediction as it is to know the general law. For example, I know a successful female university professor who was the fifth of 10 children raised by a Catholic, nonemployed mother in a blue-collar community. By all rights, she shouldn't have achieved so highly—the "why" of her case is not only fascinating, but vitally important to our understanding. Thus, we should study the predictive "misses," the "long shots" (which may include many readers).

Another promising avenue of research consistent with Fine's recommendation is the idiographic, interview-based approaches of Betz, Hackett, and Doty (1985) and Paludi and Fankell-Hauser (1986). Because they allowed women to define their own meanings of success, the meaningfulness of the reported achievement-related behaviors could have potentially greater validity. More generally, awareness of our own "nonconscious ideologies" (Bem & Bem, 1976) as researchers and of the unchecked assumptions about both the definitions and meanings to our women participants of a given role or behavior is vital to research relevant to the needs of its intended recipients.

Also needed are more investigations simultaneously examining multiple dependent and independent variables. The multivariate causal modeling of variables related to women's career development by Fassinger (1985, 1990) and the models of Eccles (1987), Farmer (1985), and Fitzgerald, Fassinger, and Betz (1989) provide good beginnings.

In addition, the effects of social change and the relationship between personal change and social change are vitally important in the study of career development, as well as other areas of the psychology of women (Harmon, 1989). Most important here are longitudinal studies allowing analysis of both developmental and historical changes in women's career involvements. The studies of Harmon (1981, 1989) and Jenkins (1989; Tangri & Jenkins, 1986) are examples of the kind of research designs needed.

Social change is a vitally important focus of study, especially since the last 20 to 25 years have involved such dramatic changes in norms regarding women, work, and families. As has been mentioned, most research on family background correlates of women's career development assumed two-parent (heterosexual) homes. Today, an increasing number of homes consist of a single parent or, increasingly, two gay or lesbian parents, thus leading to questionable utility of research based on traditional family assumptions. In the past, having an employed mother was something of a novelty (though a fortunate novelty for the development of daughters), but that is now the situation for the majority, rather than the minority, of children in society. There does seem to be a new cultural imperative for women, that of attempting to have a career (or at least a job) as well as a family. It is tempting to postulate that women will increasingly make choices congruent with their abilities, interests, and values, but only time and continuing research will indicate the effects of such changes.

Finally, the mental health implications of societal beliefs about women and work need continued study. For example, the mental health implications of holding two full-time jobs (one's own and that of primary homemaker and child caretaker), when at least the latter one should be shared, are serious and troubling. Also needing study are the problems of conflicts in a society that continues to teach young women that their worth is contingent on the value of a man; this and other detrimental aspects of the female role cannot be assumed to have lessened in impact just because a new role has been introduced. Clearly, further research concerned with factors influencing the development of strong, non-contingent self-concepts is needed. The belief of the present author is that truly free, truly "fitting" career choices are possible only in the context of self-knowledge and positive, noncontingent self-regard.

Recommendations for Interventions

I recommend that interventions into women's career development require attack on both individual and societal levels. At the individual level, this must involve (1) restoring women's options to them, and (2) convincing them that they, like men, not only can, but deserve, to "have it all." At the societal level, this should entail working toward continued change in societal institutions so that women have a better shot at both educational and occupational opportunities and equity.

Beginning with social change, I believe strongly that such change should receive the major portion of our money, time, and effort, and that of all responsible citizens. Fine (1985) appropriately criticizes research that relies on internal explanations for social conditions, not only because this serves to "blame the victim" but because there is then the excuse to focus change efforts on individuals, rather than on social conditions. But it is also essential to help individuals to recover from, and surmount, damage already done, and, further, I contend that a two-pronged attack, one to change society and the other to help individual women, will be more comprehensive and more helpful.

It seems most helpful to view individual women from the framework of the null environment, as discussed previously. We as psychologists are in the best position to both be aware of the differentiating external environments from which women clients and students come and to counteract the limiting effects of these on the development and actualization of individual potential. In career counseling, a counselor should be aware that the choices of women clients may already be seriously constrained by gender-role stereotypes and other barriers to women's career development, for example, home-career conflict and math anxiety. Counselors can accept these limitations as inevitable, as givens, or they can do their best to enrich a woman's environment, to restore some of the options that societal pressures have taken away from her.

Restoring options in career counseling might involve (1) asking a woman client how her beliefs about the abilities and roles of women have influenced her choices and then counteracting restrictive beliefs; (2) encouraging her to make decisions, like continuing in math, which leave her options open until she is ready to reject them for good reasons; (3) using same-sex norms or sex-balanced vocational interest inventories in order to highlight directions in which her interests have developed in spite of sex-role socialization; and (4) suggesting broadening experiences to help her explore previously unexplored areas.

For purposes of increasing interests and competencies in non-traditional areas, Hackett and Betz's (1981) application of Bandura's (1977) theory of self-efficacy expectations to women's career development implies four sources of information useful in increasing women's career-related self-efficacy expectations. Self-efficacy expectations can be strengthened by facilitating performance accomplishments; providing exposure to female role models; assisting girls and women to manage, if not conquer, anxiety with respect to nontraditional domains; and providing active support and encouragement of girls' and women's efforts to develop skills and competencies.

Counselors and educators can also give a woman support and encouragement when she confronts barriers to her goals—we may be the only cheerleader she has, but our support may be enough to enable her to continue the pursuit. Freeman (1989) notes that many women have surmounted the barriers to their career development and a null educational environment by stronger commitment to, and persistence in, their educational and career goals, in comparison with equally able men. O'Connell and Russo (1988) found that determination and perseverance were vitally important to eminent women psychologists in surmounting the numerous barriers they faced. Although this may be a past and current reality, it doesn't seem fair to women—each woman deserves the encouragement, support, and broadening ideas that will enable her to achieve her goals without carrying the entire burden herself.

In addition, a young woman needs help combating stereotypic belief systems that serve to restrict the range of options, for example, "I can't do both," "I can't do math," and "Highly achieving women lose their femininity" and belief systems that perpetuate the likelihood that she will feel completely responsible for home and family work even if she also pursues a career. Only as her self-esteem and the capability of independence and instrumentality in the management of her own life increase will she be able to demand equality and shared responsibility (executive as well as "labor") in her relationships. Only then will she be able to "have it all" without sinking under the weight of fatigue, overwork, and guilt.

Finally, counseling interventions should focus on helping women in these ways: (1) to plan ahead to deal with potentially difficult situations, for example, "But I'll be the only woman in that profession—how will I survive?" and "But I know it's very difficult for women to obtain apprenticeships in that field"; (2) to obtain quality education and/or training and to gain needed skills in job hunting, résumé writing, interviewing, assertion, and information seeking; (3) to locate support systems, role models, and mentors; and (4) to deal with discrimination, sexual harassment, and so on when necessary.

Doubly strong support for women of color is needed because they face the dual barriers of gender and ethnic/minority status.

In addition to these recommendations, there is ample research evidence now to support the contention that education and training are the keys to improving women's place in the labor force. Thus, attention to increasing sex equity in education (see Klein & Simonson, 1984, for a number of suggestions for doing this) is particularly crucial. Finally, further discussion of ways in which counselors and educators can facilitate the career development of women can be found in Betz (1989), Bingham (1992), Brooks (1992), Brooks and Haring-Hidore (1988), Fitzgerald (1986), Hackett (1992), and especially Walsh and Osipow (1993).

REFERENCES

Adams, J. (1984). Women at West Point: A three-year perspective. *Sex Roles, 11,* 525–542.

Almquist, E. M. (1974). Sex stereotypes in occupational choice: The case for college women. *Journal of Vocational Behavior, 5,* 13–21.

Almquist, E. M. (1989). The experiences of minority women in the United States. In J. Freeman (Ed.), *Women: A feminist perspective* (4th ed.) (pp. 414–445). Palo Alto, CA: Mayfield.

Almquist, E. M., & Angrist, S. S. (1970). Career salience and atypicality of occupational choice among college women. *Journal of Marriage and Family, 32,* 242–249.

Alpert, D., & Breen, D. T. (1989). "Liberty" in children and adolescents. *Journal of Vocational Behavior, 34,* 154–160.

Altman, S. L., & Grossman, F. K. (1977). Women's career plans and maternal employment. *Psychology of Women Quarterly, 1,* 365–376.

Amaro, H., & Russo, N. F. (Eds.). (1987). Hispanic women and mental health: Contemporary issues in research and practice [Special issue]. *Psychology of Women Quarterly, 11*(4).

Amaro, H., Russo, N. F., & Johnson, J. (1987). Family and work predictors of psychological well-being among Hispanic women professionals. *Psychology of Women Quarterly, 11,* 505–522.

Amaro, H., Russo, N. F., & Pares-Auila, J. A. (1987). Contemporary research on Hispanic women: A selected bibliography of the social science literature. *Psychology of Women Quarterly, 11,* 523–532.

Anastasi, A. (1958). *Differential psychology* (3rd ed.). New York: Macmillan.

Angrist, S. S. (1974). The study of sex roles. In C. Perucci & D. Targ (Eds.), *Marriage and the family: A critical analysis and proposal for change* (pp. 182–188). New York: McKay.

Angrist, S. S., & Almquist, E. M. (1975). *Careers and contingencies.* New York: Dunellen.

Arkin, R. M., & Johnson, K. S. (1980). Effects of increased occupational participation by women on androgynous and non-androgynous individuals' ratings of occupational attractiveness. *Sex Roles, 6*, 593–606.

Armstrong, J. M. (1985). A national assessment of participation and achievement of courses in mathematics. In S. F. Chipman, L. R. Brush, & D. M. Wilson (Eds.), *Women and mathematics* (pp. 59–94). Hillsdale, NJ: Erlbaum.

Arnold, K. D. (1987). *Values and vocations: The career aspirations of academically gifted females in the first five years after high school.* Paper presented at the annual meeting of the American Educational Research Association, Washington, DC.

Arnold, K. D. (1989). *The Illinois valedictorian project: The careers of academically talented men.* Paper presented at the annual meeting of the American Educational Research Association, San Francisco.

Arnold, K. D., & Denny, T. (1984). *Academic achievement—A view from the top: The lives of high school valedictorians and salutatorians.* Paper presented at the annual meeting of the American Educational Research Association, New Orleans.

Arnold, K. D., & Denny, T. (1985). The lives of academic achievers: The career aspirations of male and female high school valedictorians and salutatorians. (Report No. CE 041 582). *Resources in Education.* (Eric Document Reproduction Service No. Ed 257 951).

Association for Women in Science. (AWIS). (1984, December-January). *Editorial*, p. 2.

Astin, A. W. (1977). *Four critical years*. San Francisco: Jossey-Bass.

Astin, H. S., & Myint, T. (1971). Career development of young women during the post high school years. *Journal of Counseling Psychology Monograph, 18*, 369–393.

Atkinson, J., & Huston, T. L. (1984). Sex role orientation and division of labor early in marriage. *Journal of Personality and Social Psychology, 46*, 330–345.

Baber, K. M., & Monaghan, D. (1988). College women's career and motherhood expectations: New options and dilemmas. *Sex Roles, 19*, 189–204.

Bachtold, L. M. (1976). Personality characteristics of women of distinction. *Psychology of Women Quarterly, 1*, 70–78.

Bandura, A. (1977). Self-efficacy: Toward a unifying theory of behavioral change. *Psychological Review, 84*, 191–215.

Bannon, J. A., & Southern, M. L. (1980). Father-absent women: Self-concept and modes of relating to men. *Sex Roles, 6*, 75–84.

Bart, P. (1971). Depression in middle-aged women. In V. Gornick & B. K. Moran (Eds.), *Women in sexist society* (pp. 163–186). New York: Mentor.

Baruch, G. K., & Barnett, R. C. (1980). On the well-being of adult women. In L. A. Bond & J. C. Rosen (Eds.), *Competence and coping during adulthood* (pp. 240–257). Hanover, NH: University Press of New England.

Basow, S. A., & Howe, K. G. (1978). Model influences in career choices of college students. *Vocational Guidance Quarterly, 27*, 239–243.

Basow, S. A., & Howe, K. G. (1980). Role model influence: Effects of sex and sex-role attitude in college students. *Psychology of Women Quarterly, 4*, 558–572.

Beale, F. (1970). Double jeopardy: To be black and female. In T. Cade (Ed.), *The black woman: An anthology* (pp. 90–100). New York: New American Library.

Bem, S. L. (1981). Gender schema theory: A cognitive account of sex typing. *Psychological Review, 88*, 354–364.

Bem, S. L., & Bem, D. J. (1976). Case study of a nonconscious ideology: Training the woman to know her place. In S. Cox (Ed.), *Female psychology* (pp. 180–191). Chicago: Science Research Associates.

Benbow, C. P., & Stanley, J. C. (1980). Sex differences in mathematical ability: Fact or artifact? *Science, 210,* 1262–1264.

Bernard, J. (1971). The paradox of the happy marriage. In V. Gornick & B. K. Moran (Eds.), *Women in sexist society.* New York: Mentor.

Bernard, J. (1976). Where are we now? Some thoughts on the current scene. *Psychology of Women Quarterly, 1,* 21–37.

Bernard, J. (1988). The inferiority curriculum. *Psychology of Women Quarterly, 12,* 261–268.

Betz, E. L. (1984a). A study of career patterns of college graduates. *Journal of Vocational Behavior, 24,* 249–264.

Betz, E. L. (1984b). Two tests of Maslow's theory of need fulfillment. *Journal of Vocational Behavior, 24,* 204–220.

Betz, N. E. (1978). Prevalence, distribution, and correlates of math anxiety in college students. *Journal of Counseling Psychology, 25,* 441–448.

Betz, N. E. (1989). The null environment and women's career development. *Counseling Psychologist, 17,* 136–144.

Betz, N. E. (1991). *What stops women and minorities from choosing and completing majors in science and engineering.* Washington, DC: Federation of Behavioral, Psychological, and Cognitive Sciences.

Betz, N. E., & Fitzgerald, L. F. (1987). *The career psychology of women.* New York: Academic Press.

Betz, N. E., Fitzgerald, L. F., & Hill, R. E. (1989). Trait factor theories and measures: Foundations of career theory. In M. B. Arthur, D. T. Hall, & B. S. Lawrence (Eds.), *Handbook of career theory* (pp. 26–40). Cambridge, England: Cambridge University Press.

Betz, N. E., & Hackett, G. (1981). The relationship of career-related self-efficacy expectations to perceived career options in college women and men. *Journal of Counseling Psychology, 28,* 399–410.

Betz, N. E., & Hackett, G. (1983). The relationship of mathematics self-efficacy expectations to the selection of science-based college majors. *Journal of Vocational Behavior, 23,* 328–345.

Betz, N. E., Hackett, G., & Doty, M. (1985). The development of a taxonomy of career competencies for professional women. *Sex Roles, 12,* 393–409.

Beutell, N. J., & Brenner, O. C. (1986). Sex differences in work values. *Journal of Vocational Behavior, 28,* 29–41.

Bingham, R. P. (1992). *Career counseling with ethnic minority women.* Paper presented at the Annual Convention of the American Psychological Association, Washington, DC.

Blum, C., & Givant, S. (1982). Increasing the participation of college women in mathematics-related fields. In S. M. Humphreys (Ed.), *Women and minorities in science* (pp. 119–138). Boulder, Co: Westview Press.

Boswell, S. L. (1985). The influence of sex-role stereotyping on women's attitudes and achievement in mathematics. In S. F. Chipman, L. R. Brush, & D. M. Wilson (Eds.), *Women and mathematics* (pp. 175–198). Hillsdale, NJ: Erlbaum.

Brooks, L. (1992, August). *Feminism and career counseling.* Paper presented at the Annual Convention of the American Psychological Association, Washington, DC.

Brooks, L., & Haring-Hidore, M. (Eds.). (1988). Career interventions with women [Special issue]. *Career Development Quarterly, 14*(4).

Brown, D. (1970). *Students' vocational choices: A review and critique*. Boston: Houghton Mifflin.

Brush, L. R. (1985). Cognitive and affective determinants of course preferences in plans. In S. F. Chipman, L. R. Brush, & D. M. Wilson (Eds.), *Women and mathematics: Balancing the equation* (pp. 123–150). Hillsdale, NJ: Erlbaum.

Burlin, F. (1976). The relationship of parental education and maternal work and occupational status to occupational aspiration in adolescent females. *Journal of Vocational Behavior, 9*, 99–106.

Canino, G. (1982). Transactional family patterns: Explanation of Puerto Rican female adolescents. In R. E. Zambrana (Ed.), *Work, family, and health: Latin women in transition* (pp. 27–36). New York: Hispanic Research Center.

Card, J. J., Steel, L., & Abeles, R. P. (1980). Sex differences in realization of individual potential for achievement. *Journal of Vocational Behavior, 17*, 1–21.

Carnegie Commission on Higher Education. (1973). *Opportunities for women in higher education*. New York: McGraw-Hill.

Castle, C. S. (1913). A statistical study of eminent women. *Archives of Psychology, 27*, 20–34.

Catalyst. (1987). *New roles for men and women: A report on an educational intervention with college students*. New York: Author.

Chapel Hill's coeds. (1987, January). Editorial, *Washington Post*.

Chipman, S. F., Brush, L. R., & Wilson, D. M. (1985). *Women and mathematics: Balancing the equation*. Hillsdale, NJ: Erlbaum.

Chipman, S. F., & Thomas, V. G. (1985). Women's participation in mathematics: Outlining the problem. In S. F. Chipman, L. R. Brush, & D. M. Wilson (Eds.), *Women and mathematics* (pp. 1–24). Hillsdale, NJ: Erlbaum.

Chipman, S. F., & Wilson, D. M. (1985). Understanding mathematics course enrollment and mathematics achievement: A synthesis of the research. In S. F. Chipman, L. R. Brush, & D. M. Wilson (Eds.), *Women and mathematics* (pp. 275–328). Hillsdale, NJ: Erlbaum.

Crawford, J. D. (1978). Career development and career choice in pioneer and traditional women. *Journal of Vocational Behavior, 12*, 139–149.

Crites, J. O. (1969). *Vocational psychology*. New York: McGraw-Hill.

Dawis, R. V., & Lofquist, L. H. (1984). *A psychological theory of work adjustment*. Minneapolis: University of Minnesota Press.

Deaux, K. (1984). From individual differences to social categories. Analysis of a decade's research on gender. *American Psychologist, 39*, 105–116.

Del Vento Bielby, D. (1978). Maternal employment and socioeconomic status as factor in daughters' career salience: Some substantive refinements. *Sex Roles, 4*, 249–266.

Dew, K. M. H., Galassi, J. P., & Galassi, M. D. (1983). Math anxiety: Some basic issues. *Journal of Counseling Psychology, 30*, 443–446.

Dix, L. S. (1987). *Women: Their underrepresentation and career differentials in science and engineering*. Washington, DC: National Academy Press.

Douvan, E. (1976). The role of models in women's professional development. *Psychology of Women Quarterly, 1*, 5–20.

Drabman, R. S., Robertson, S. J., Patterson, J. N., Jarvei, G. J., Hammer, D., & Cordua, G. (1981). Children's perceptions of media-portrayed sex roles. *Sex Roles, 7*, 379–390.

Dreyer, N. A., Woods, N. F., & James, S. A. (1981). ISRO: A scale to measure sex-role orientation. *Sex Roles, 7*, 173–182.

Dweck, C., Davidson, W., Nelson, S., & Enna, B. I. (1978). Sex differences in learned helplessness: II. The contingencies of evaluative feedback in the classroom, and III. An experimental analysis. *Developmental Psychology, 14*, 268–276.

Eccles, J. (1983). Sex differences in mathematics participation. In M. Steinkamp & M. Maehr (Eds.), *Women in science* (pp. 80–110). Greenwich, CT: JAI Press.

Eccles, J. (1984). Sex differences in math participation. In M. L. Maehr & W. Steinkamp (Eds.), *Women in science* (pp. 93–138). Greenwich, CT: JAI Press.

Eccles, J. (1987). Gender roles and women's achievement-related decisions. *Psychology of Women Quarterly, 11*, 135–172.

Eccles, J. E., Adler, T. F., Futterman, R., Goff, S. B., Kaczala, C. M., Meece, J. I., & Midgley, L. C. (1983). Expectations, values, and academic behaviors. In J. T. Spence (Ed.), *Achievement and achievement motives* (pp. 75–145). San Francisco: W. H. Freeman.

Eccles, J., Adler, T., & Meece, J. L. (1984). Sex differences in achievement: A test of alternate theories. *Journal of Personality and Social Psychology, 46*, 26–43.

Eccles, J., & Hoffman, C. W. (1984). Sex roles, socialization, and occupational behavior. In H. W. Stevenson & A. E. Siegel (Eds.), *Research in child development and social policy: Vol. I* (pp. 367–420). Chicago: University of Chicago Press.

Eccles, J. S., & Jacobs, J. (1986). Social forces shape math participation. *Signs, 11*, 367–380.

Ehrhart, J. K., & Sandler, B. R. (1987). *Looking for more than a few good women in traditionally male fields.* Washington, DC: Project on the Status and Education of Women.

Epstein, C. F. (1973). Positive effects of the multiple negative. *American Journal of Sociology, 78*, 912–935.

Erikson, E. (1950). *Childhood and society.* New York: Norton.

Ernest, J. (1976). Mathematics and sex. *The American Mathematical Monthly, 83*, 595–614.

Espin, D. M. (1980). Perceptions of sexual discrimination among college women in Latin America and the United States. *Hispanic Journal of Behavioral Sciences, 2*, 1–19.

Etaugh, C., & Hall, P. (1980). Is preschool education more highly valued for boys than girls? *Sex Roles, 6*, 339–344.

Farmer, H. S. (1985). Model of career and achievement motivation for women and men. *Journal of Counseling Psychology, 32*, 363–390.

Fassinger, R. E. (1985). A causal model of career choice in college women. *Journal of Vocational Behavior, 27*, 123–153.

Fassinger, R. E. (1990). Causal models of career choice in two samples of college women. *Journal of Vocational Behavior, 36*, 225–248.

Ferraro, G. A. (1984). Bridging the wage gap: Pay equity and job evaluations. *American Psychologist, 39*, 1166–1170.

Ferree, M. M. (1976). The confused American housewife. *Psychology Today, 10*, 76–80.

Fine, M. (1985). Reflections on a feminist psychology of women: Paradoxes and prospects. *Psychology of Women Quarterly, 9*, 167–183.

Fiorentine, R. (1988). Increasing similarity in the values and life plans of male and female college students? Evidence and implications. *Sex Roles*, *18*, 143–158.

Fitzgerald, L. F. (1986). Career counseling women. In Z. Beibowitz & D. Lee (Eds.), *Adult career development*. Washington, DC: National Vocational Guidance Association.

Fitzgerald, L. F., & Crites, J. O. (1980). Toward a career psychology of women. *Journal of Counseling Psychology*, *27*, 44–62.

Fitzgerald, L. F., Fassinger, R. E., & Betz, N. E. (1989, August). *An individual differences model of vocational choice in college women*. Paper presented at the annual meeting of the American Psychological Association, New Orleans.

Fitzgerald, L., Shullman, S., Bailey, N., Richards, M., Swecker, J., Gold, Y., Ormerod, M., & Weitzman, L. (1988). The incidence and dimensions of sexual harassment in academia and the workplace. *Journal of Vocational Behavior*, *32*, 152–175.

Fitzgerald, L., Weitzman, L. M., Gold, Y., & Ormerod, M. (1988). Academic harassment: Sex and denial in scholarly garb. *Psychology of Women Quarterly*, *12*, 329–340.

Fitzpatrick, J. L., & Silverman, T. (1989). Women's selection of careers in engineering: Do traditional-nontraditional differences still exist? *Journal of Vocational Behavior*, *34*, 266–278.

Flanagan, J. C. (1971). *Project TALENT: Five years after high school and appendix II. Final Report*. Pittsburgh: University of Pittsburgh, American Institute for Research.

Fleming, J. (1986, September 13). Top schools pose problems for blacks. *Washington Post*, p. A6.

Fox, L. H., Brody, L., & Tobin, D. (1980). *Women and the mathematical mystique*. Baltimore: Johns Hopkins University Press.

Fox, L. H., Brody, L., & Tobin, D. (1985). Women and mathematics: The impact of early intervention programs upon course-taking and attitudes in high schools. In S. F. Chipman, L. R. Brush, & D. M. Wilson (Eds.), *Women and mathematics* (pp. 249–274). Hillsdale, NJ: Erlbaum.

Freeman, J. (1989). How to discriminate against women without really trying. In J. Freeman (Ed.), *Women: A feminist perspective* (4th ed.). Palo Alto, CA: Mayfield.

Freun, M. A., Rothman, A. I., & Steiner, J. W. (1974). Comparison of characteristics of male and female medical school applicants. *Journal of Medical Education*, *49*, 137–145.

Frieze, I. H., Parsons, J. E., Johnson, P. B., Ruble, D. N., & Zellman, G. L. (1978). *Women and sex roles: A social psychological perspective*. New York: W. W. Norton.

Gackenbach, J. (1978). The effect of race, sex, and career goal differences on sex-role attitudes at home and at work. *Journal of Vocational Behavior*, *12*, 93–101.

Gaddy, C. D., Glass, C. R., & Arnkoff, D. B. (1983). Career development of women in dual career families: The influence of sex-role identity. *Journal of Counseling Psychology*, *30*, 388–394.

Gerson, K. (1985). *Hard choices: How women decide about work, career, and motherhood*. Berkeley: University of California Press.

Gettys, L. D., & Cann, A. (1981). Children's perceptions of occupational sex stereotypes. *Sex Roles*, *7*, 301–308.

Gilbert, L. A. (1985). Measures of psychological masculinity and femininity: A comment on Gadd, Glass, and Arnkoff. *Journal of Counseling Psychology, 32*, 163–166.

Gilbert, L. A. (1988). *Sharing it all.* New York: Plenum.

Gilbert, L. A., & Rachlin, V. (1987). Mental health and psychological functioning of dual career couples. *Counseling Psychologist, 15*, 7–49.

Goldstein, E. (1979). Effects of same-sex and cross-sex role models on the subsequent academic productivity of scholars. *American Psychologist, 34*, 407–410.

Gonzales, J. T. (1988). Dilemmas of the high-achieving Chicano: The double-bind factor in male-female relationships. *Sex Roles, 18*, 367–380.

Goodale, J. G., & Hall, D. T. (1976). Inheriting a career: The influence of sex, value, and parents. *Journal of Vocational Behavior, 8*, 19–30.

Gottfredson, L. S. (1981). Circumscription and compromises: A developmental theory of occupational aspirations. *Journal of Counseling Psychology, 28*, 545–579.

Gove, W. R., & Tudor, J. F. (1973). Adult sex roles and mental illness. *American Journal of Sociology, 78*, 812–835.

Greenfield, S., Greiner, L., & Wood, M. M. (1980). The "Feminine Mystique" in male-dominated jobs: A comparison of attitudes and background factors of women in male-dominated versus female-dominated jobs. *Journal of Vocational Behavior, 17*, 291–309.

Greenglass, E. R., & Devins, R. (1982). Factors related to marriage and career plans in unmarried women. *Sex Roles, 8*, 57–72.

Gump, J., & Rivers, L. (1975). A consideration of race in efforts to end sex bias. In E. Diamond (Ed.), *Issues of sex bias and sex fairness in career interest measurement.* Washington, DC: National Institute of Education.

Gutek, B. A., & Larwood, L. (Eds.). (1987). *Women's career development.* Newburg Park, CA: Sage.

Gutek, B. A., Stromberg, A. H., & Larwood, L. (Eds.). (1988). *Women and work: An annual review, Vol. 3.* Newburg Park, CA: Sage.

Haber, S. (1980). Cognitive support for the career choices of college women. *Sex Roles, 6*, 129–138.

Hackett, G. (1985). The role of mathematics self-efficacy in the choice of math-related majors of college women and men: A path analysis. *Journal of Counseling Psychology, 32*, 47–56.

Hackett, G. (1992, August). *Career assessment and counseling for women.* Paper presented at the Annual Convention of the American Psychological Association, Washington, DC.

Hackett, G., & Betz, N. (1981). A self-efficacy approach to the career development of women. *Journal of Vocational Behavior, 18*, 326–339.

Hackett, G., Esposito, D., & O'Halloran, M. S. (1989). The relationship of role model influences to the career salience of educational and career plans of college women. *Journal of Vocational Behavior, 35*, 164–180.

Hall, R. M., & Sandler, B. R. (1982). *The classroom climate: A chilly one for women.* Washington, DC: PSEW, AAC.

Hall, R. M. & Sandler, B. R. (1984). *Out of the classroom: A chilly classroom climate for women?* Washington, DC: PSEW, AAC.

Hansen, R. D., & O'Leary, V. E. (1985). Sex-determined attributions. In V. E. O'Leary, R. K. Unger, & B. S. Wallston (Eds.), *Women, gender, and social psychology* (pp. 67–100). Hillsdale, NJ: Erlbaum.

Hansson, R. O., Chernovetz, M. E., & Jones, W. H. (1977). Maternal employment and androgyny. *Psychology of Women Quarterly*, 2, 76–78.

Hare-Mustin, R. T., Bennett, S. K., & Broderick, P. C. (1983). Attitude toward motherhood: Gender, generational, and religious comparisons. *Sex Roles*, 9, 643–660.

Harmon, L. W. (1980). Longitudinal changes in women's career aspirations: Development or historical? *Journal of Vocational Behavior*, 35, 46–63.

Harmon, L. W. (1981). Life and career plans of young adult college women: A follow-up study. *Journal of Counseling Psychology*, 28, 416–427.

Harmon, L. W. (1989). Longitudinal changes in women's career aspirations: Developmental or historical? *Journal of Vocational Behavior*, 35, 46–63.

Heilman, M. E. (1979). High school students' occupational interest as a function of projected sex ratios in male-dominated occupations. *Journal of Applied Psychology*, 64, 275–279.

Helmreich, R. L., Spence, J. T., Beane, W. E., Lucker, G. W., & Matthews, K. A. (1980). Making it in academic psychology: Demographic and personality correlates of attainment. *Journal of Personality and Social Psychology*, 39, 896–908.

Hendel, D. D. (1980). Experiential and effective correlates of math anxiety in adult women. *Psychology of Women Quarterly*, 5, 219–230.

Henry, M. D. (1985). Black reentry females: Their concerns and needs. *Journal of the National Association for Women Deans, Administrators, and Counselors*, 48, 8.

Hesse-Biber, S. (1985). Male and female students' perceptions of their academic environment and future career plans. *Human Relations*, 38 91–105.

Hewlett, S. A. (1985). *A lesser life*. New York: William Morrow.

Hilton, T. L., & Berglund, G. W. (1974). Sex differences in mathematical achievement: A longitudinal study. *Journal of Educational Research*, 67, 231–237.

Hoffman, L. W. (1977). Changes in family roles, socialization, and sex differences. *American Psychologist*, 32, 644–657.

Hoffman, L. W. (1984). Maternal employment and the young child. In M. Perlmutter (Ed.), *Mother/child interaction and parent/child relations in child development* (pp. 101–128). Hillsdale, NJ: Erlbaum.

Hoffman, L. W., & Nye, F. I. (1974). *Working mothers*. San Francisco: Jossey-Bass.

Hollingshead, A. (1949). *Elmtown's youth*. New York: Wiley.

Houseknecht, S. K., & Spanier, G. B. (1980). Marital disruption and higher education among women in the United States. *Sociological Quarterly*, 21, 375–389.

Houser, B. B., & Garvey, C. (1983). The impact of family, peers, and educational personnel upon career decision making. *Journal of Vocational Behavior*, 23, 35–44.

Houser, B. B., & Garvey, C. (1985). Factors that affect nontraditional vocational enrollment among women. *Psychology of Women Quarterly*, 9, 105–117.

Howe, F. (1979). Introduction: The first decade of women's studies. *Harvard Educational Review*, 49, 413–421.

Howe, L. K. (1977). *Pink-collar workers*. New York: Putnam.

Humphreys, S. M. (1982). *Women and minorities in science: Strategies for increasing participation*. Boulder, CO: Westview Press.

Huth, C. M. (1978). Married women's work status: The influence of parents and husbands. *Journal of Vocational Behavior*, 13, 255–262.

Hyde, J. S. (1985). *Half the human experience: The psychology of women* (3rd ed.). Lexington, MA: D. C. Heath.

Ilfeld, F., Jr. (1977). *Sex differences in psychiatric symptomatology*. Paper presented at the meeting of the American Psychological Association, San Francisco.

Jenkins, S. R. (1989). Longitudinal prediction of women's careers: Psychological, behavioral, and social-structural influences. *Journal of Vocational Behavior, 34*, 204–238.

Jones, J., & Welch, O. (1980). The black professional woman. *Journal of the National Association of Women Deans, Administrators, and Counselors, 43*, 29–32.

Key, M. R. (1975). Male and female in children's books. In R. K. Unger & F. L. Denmark (Eds.), *Woman: Dependent or independent variable* (pp. 55–70). New York: Psychological Dimensions.

Klein, S. S., & Simonson, J. (1984). Increasing sex equity in education: Roles for psychologists. *American Psychologist, 39*, 1187–1192.

Knapp, R. R., Knapp, L., & Knapp-Lee, L. (1985). Occupational interest measurement and subsequent career decisions. *Journal of Counseling Psychology, 32*, 348–354.

Knaub, P. K., & Eversoll, D. B. (1983). Is parenthood a desirable adult role? An assessment of attitudes held by contemporary women. *Sex Roles, 9*, 355–362.

Knell, S., & Winer, G. A. (1979). Effects of reading content on occupational sex-role stereotypes. *Journal of Vocational Behavior, 14*, 78–87.

Komarovsky, M. (1982). Female freshmen view their future: Career salience and its correlates. *Sex Roles, 8*, 299–314.

Krefting, L. A., & Berger, P. K. (1979). Masculinity-femininity perceptions of job requirements and their relationship to job sex types. *Journal of Vocational Behavior, 15*, 164–174.

Krefting, L. A., Berger, P. K., & Wallace, M. J. (1978). The contribution of sex-distribution, job content, and occupational classification to job sex typing: Two studies. *Journal of Vocational Behavior, 13*, 181–191.

Kriedberg, G., Butcher, A. L., & White, K. M. (1978). Vocational role choice in 2nd and 6th grade children. *Sex Roles, 4*, 175–182.

Kriger, S. F. (1972). Achievement and perceived parental childrearing attitudes of career women and homemakers. *Journal of Vocational Behavior, 2*, 419–432.

LaFromboise, T. (1986). *Bicultural competence for American Indian self-determination*. Paper presented at the Thirteenth Annual McDaniel Conference, Stanford, CA.

LaFromboise, T., & Plake, B. (1983). Toward meeting the educational research needs of American Indians. *Harvard Educational Review, 53*, 45–51.

Lantz, A. (1985). Strategies to increase mathematics enrollment. In S. F. Chipman, L. R. Brush, & D. M. Wilson (Eds.), *Women and mathematics: Balancing the equation* (pp. 329–354). Hillsdale, NJ: Erlbaum.

Larwood, L., Stromberg, A. H., & Gutek, B. A. (Eds.). (1985). *Women and work: An annual review, Vol. 1*. Newburg Park, CA: Sage.

Lemkau, J. P. (1979). Personality and background characteristics of women in male-dominated occupations: A review. *Psychology of Women Quarterly, 4*, 221–240.

Llabre, M. M., & Suarez, E. (1985). Predicting math anxiety and course performance in college women and men. *Journal of Counseling Psychology, 32*, 283–287.

Loo, C. M., & Rolison, G. (1986). Alienation of ethnic minority students at a predominantly white university. *Journal of Higher Education, 57*(1), 67.

Lott, B. (1985). The potential enrichment of social/personality psychology through feminist research and vice versa. *American Psychologist, 40*, 155–164.

Lyson, T. A., & Brown, S. S. (1982). Sex-role attitudes, curriculum choice, and career ambition: A comparison between women in typical and atypical college majors. *Journal of Vocational Behavior, 20*, 366–375.

Maccoby, E. E., & Jacklin, C. N. (1974). *The psychology of sex differences.* Stanford, CA: Stanford University Press.

MacKay, W. R., & Miller, C. A. (1982). Relations of socio-economic status and sex variables to the complexity of worker functions in the occupational choices of elementary school children. *Journal of Vocational Behavior, 20*, 31–37.

Marini, M. M. (1978). Sex differences in the determination of adolescent aspirations: A review of research. *Sex Roles, 4*, 723–754.

Marshall, S. J., & Wijting, J. P. (1980). Relationships of achievement motivation and sex-role identity to college women's career orientation. *Journal of Vocational Behavior, 16*, 299–311.

Martin, J. R. (1982). Excluding women from the educational realm. *Harvard Educational Review, 52*, 133–148.

Matthews, E., & Tiedeman, D. V. (1964). Attitudes toward career and marriage and the development of lifestyle in young women. *Journal of Counseling Psychology, 11*, 374–383.

McLure, G. T., & Piel, E. (1978). Career-bound girls and science careers: Perceptions of barriers and facilitating factors. *Journal of Vocational Behavior, 12*, 172–183.

Metzler-Brennan, E., Lewis, R. J., & Gerrard, M. (1985). Childhood antecedents of adult women's masculinity, femininity, and career role choices. *Psychology of Women Quarterly, 9*, 371–382.

Minnich, E. (1988). Education and the quest for equality. In C. Pearson, D. Shavlik, & J. Touchton (Eds.), *Educating the majority: How women are changing higher education* (pp. 112–120). Washington, DC: American Council on Education.

Moore, L. L. (1986). *Not as far as you think: The realities of working women.* Lexington, MA: D. C. Heath.

Murray, S. R., & Mednick, M.T.S. (1977). Black women's achievement orientation: Motivational and cognitive factors. *Psychology of Women Quarterly, 1*, 247–259.

Murray, S. R., & Scott, P. B. (Eds.). (1982). Special issue on black women. *Psychology of Women Quarterly, 6*(3).

National Project on Women in Education (1978). *Taking sexism out of education.* Washington, DC: U.S. Department of Health, Education, and Welfare.

National Science Foundation. (1990). *Women and minorities in science and engineering.* Washington, DC: Author.

Newman, D. K., Amidet, N. J., Carter, B. L., Day, D., Kruvant, W. J., & Russell, J. S. (1978). *Protest, politics, and prosperity: Black Americans and white institutions, 1940–1975.* New York: Pantheon.

Nieva, V. F., & Gutek, B. A. (1981). *Women and work: A psychological perspective.* New York: Praeger.

Nilsen, A. P. (1971). Women in children's literature. *College English, 32*, 918–926.

O'Connell, A. N. (1988). Synthesis and resynthesis: Profiles and patterns of achievement 2. In A. N. O'Connell & N. F. Russo (Eds.), *Models of achievement: Reflections of eminent women in psychology, Vol. II.* (pp. 317–366). Hillsdale, NJ: Erlbaum.

O'Connell, A. N., & Russo, N. F. (Eds.). (1983). *Models of achievement: Reflections of eminent women in psychology.* New York: Columbia University Press.

O'Connell, A. N., & Russo, N. F. (Eds.). (1988). *Models of achievement: Reflections of eminent women in psychology, Vol. II*. Hillsdale, NJ: Erlbaum.

O'Connell, L., Betz, M., & Kurth, S. (1989). Plans for balancing work and family life: Do women pursuing nontraditional and traditional occupations differ? *Sex Roles*, *20*, 35–46.

O'Donnell, J. A., & Anderson, D. G. (1978). Factors influencing choice of major and career of capable women. *Vocational Guidance Quarterly, 26*, 214–221.

Orcutt, M. A., & Walsh, W. B. (1979). Traditionality and congruence of career aspirations for college women. *Journal of Vocational Behavior, 14*, 1–11.

Orlofsky, J. L., & Stake, J. E. (1981). Psychological masculinity and femininity: Relationship to striving and self-concept in the achievement and interpersonal domains. *Psychology of Women Quarterly, 6*, 218–233.

Osipow, S. H. (1983). *Theories of career development* (3rd ed.). Englewood Cliffs, NJ: Prentice-Hall.

Paludi, M. A., & Fankell-Hauser, J. (1986). An idiographic approach to the study of women's achievement strivings. *Psychology of Women Quarterly, 10*, 89–100.

Panek, P. E., Rush, M. C., & Greenwalt, J. P. (1977). Current sex stereotypes of 25 occupations. *Psychological Reports, 40*, 212–214.

Parsons, F. (1909). *Choosing a vocation*. Boston: Houghton Mifflin.

Pearson, C., Shavlik, D., & Touchton, J. (Eds.). (1988). *Prospectus for educating the majority: How women are changing higher education*. Washington, DC: American Council on Education.

Pedro, J. D., Wolleat, P., Fennema, E., & Becker, A. D. (1981). Election of high school mathematics by females and males: Attributions and attitudes. *American Educational Research Journal, 18*, 207–218.

Perun, P. J., & Del Vento Bielby, D. (1981). Towards a model of female occupational behavior: A human development approach. *Psychology of Women Quarterly, 6*, 234–252.

Pfafflin, S. M. (1984). Women, science, and technology. *American Psychologist, 39*, 1183–1186.

Poole, M. E., & Clooney, G. H. (1985). Careers: Adolescent awareness and exploration of possibilities for self. *Journal of Vocational Behavior, 26*, 251–263.

Radloff, L. (1975). Sex differences in depression: The effects of occupation and marital status. *Sex Roles, 1*, 249–265.

Rand, L. M., & Miller, A. L. (1972). A developmental cross-sectioning of women's career and marriage attitude and life plans. *Journal of Vocational Behavior, 2*, 317–331.

Randour, M., Strasburg, G., & Lipman-Blumen, J. (1982). Women in higher education: Trends in enrollment and degrees earned. *Harvard Educational Review, 52*, 189–202.

Repetti, R. L., Matthews, K. A., & Waldron, I. (1989). Effects of paid employment on women's mental and physical health. *American Psychologist, 44*, 1394–1401.

Resnick, H., Viehe, J., & Segal, S. (1982). Is math anxiety a local phenomenon? A study of prevalence and dimensionality. *Journal of Counseling Psychology, 29*, 39–47.

Richardson, F. C., & Woolfolk, R. L. (1980). Mathematics anxiety. In I. G. Sarason (Ed.), *Test anxiety: Theory, research, and application* (pp. 275–288). Hillsdale, NJ: Erlbaum.

Richardson, M. S., & Johnson, M. (1984). Counseling women. In S. D. Brown & R. W. Lent (Eds.), *The handbook of counseling psychology* (pp. 832–877). New York: Wiley.

Rooney, G. S. (1983). Distinguishing characteristics of the life roles of worker, student, and homemaker for young adults. *Journal of Vocational Behavior*, 22, 324–342.

Rosenthal, D. A., & Chapman, D. C. (1982). The lady spaceman: Children's perceptions of sex-stereotyped occupations. *Sex Roles*, 8, 959–966.

Russo, N. F., & Denmark, F. L. (1984). Women, psychology and public policy: Selected issues. *American Psychologist*, 39, 1161–1165.

Russo, N. F., & O'Connell, A. N. (1980). Models from our past: Psychology's for mothers. *Psychology of Women Quarterly*, 5, 11–53.

Sadker, M. P., & Sadker, D. M. (1980). Sexism in teacher education texts. *Harvard Educational Review*, 50, 36–46.

Scott, K. P. (1981, April). Whatever happened to Jane and Dick? Sexism in texts re-examined. *Peabody Journal of Education*, 135–140.

Sears, P. S., & Barbie, A. H. (1977). Career and life satisfaction among Terman's gifted women. In J. C. Stanley, W. George, & C. Solano (Eds.), *The gifted and creative: Fifty year perspective* (pp. 154–172). Baltimore: Johns Hopkins University Press.

Sekaran, U. (1986). *Dual-career families*. San Francisco: Jossey-Bass.

Sells, L. (1973). High school mathematics as the critical filter in the job market. In *Developing opportunities for minorities in graduate education* (pp. 12–17). Proceedings of the Conference on Minority Graduate Education, University of California, Berkeley.

Sells, L. (1982). Leverage for equal opportunity through mastery of mathematics. In S. M. Humphreys (Ed.), *Women and minorities in science* (pp. 7–26). Boulder, CO: Westview Press.

Sewell, W. H., Haller, A. O., & Strauss, M. A. (1957). Social status and educational occupational aspiration. *American Sociological Review*, 22, 67–73.

Shann, M. H. (1983). Career plans of men and women in gender-dominant professions. *Journal of Vocational Behavior*, 22, 343–356.

Shepherd, D. M., & Barraclough, B. M. (1980). Work and suicide: An empirical investigation. *British Journal of Psychiatry*, 136, 469–478.

Sherman, J. (1981). Girls' and boys' enrollments in theoretical math courses: A longitudinal study. *Psychology of Women Quarterly*, 5, 681–689.

Sherman, J. (1982). Mathematics the critical filter: A look at some residues. *Psychology of Women Quarterly*, 7, 338–342.

Sherman, J. (1983). Girls talk about mathematics and their futures. *Psychology of Women Quarterly*, 7, 338–342.

Sherman, J., & Denmark, F. (Eds.). (1981). *Psychology of women: Future directions in research*. New York: Psychological Dimensions.

Sherman, J., & Fennema, E. (1977). The study of mathematics by high school girls and boys: Related variables. *American Educational Research Journal*, 14, 159–168.

Sherman, J., & Fennema, E. (1978). Sex-related differences in mathematics achievement and related factors: A further study. *Journal of Research in Mathematics Education*, 9, 189–203.

Shinar, E. H. (1975). Sexual stereotypes of occupations. *Journal of Vocational Behavior*, 7, 99–111.

Slevin, K. F., & Wingrove, C. R. (1983). Similarities and differences among three generations of women in attitudes toward the female role in contemporary society. *Sex Roles*, *9*, 609–624.

Smith, E. J. (1981). The working mother: A critique of the research. *Journal of Vocational Behavior*, *19*, 191–211.

Smith, E. J. (1982). The black female adolescent: A review of the educational, career, and psychological literature. *Psychology of Women Quarterly*, *6*, 261–288.

Smith, E. R. (1983). Issues in racial minorities' career behavior. In W. B. Walsh & S. H. Osipow (Eds.), *Handbook of Vocational Psychology* (pp. 161–222). Hillsdale, NJ: Erlbaum.

Spence, J. T. (Ed.). (1983). *Achievement and achievement motives*. San Francisco: W. H. Freeman.

Spence, J. T., & Helmreich, R. L. (1980). Masculine instrumentality and feminine expressiveness: Their relationships with sex role attitudes and behaviors. *Psychology of Women Quarterly*, *5*, 147–153.

Spence, J. T., & Helmreich, R. L. (1981). Androgyny versus gender schema: A comment on Bem's gender schema theory. *Psychological Review*, *88*, 365–368.

Spokane, A. R. (1991). *Career interventions*. Englewood Cliffs, NJ: Prentice Hall.

Stafford, I. P. (1984). Relation of attitudes toward women's roles and occupational behavior to women's self-esteem. *Journal of Counseling Psychology*, *31*, 332–338.

Stake, J. E. (1979). The ability/performance dimension of self-esteem: Implications for women's achievement behavior. *Psychology of Women Quarterly*, *3*, 365–377.

Standley, K., & Soule, B. (1974). Women in male-dominated professions: Contrasts in their personal and vocational histories. *Journal of Vocational Behavior*, *4*, 245–258.

Stephan, C. W., & Corder, J. (1985). The effects of dual career families on adolescents' sex-role attitudes, work and family plans, and choice of important others. *Journal of Marriage and the Family*, *47*, 921–929.

Stevens, G. (1986). Sex differentiated patterns of intergenerational occupational mobility. *Journal of Marriage and the Family*, *48*, 153–163.

Stewart, A. J. (1980). Personality and situation in the prediction of women's life patterns. *Psychology of Women Quarterly*, *5*, 195–206.

Stringer, D. M., & Duncan, E. (1985). Nontraditional occupations: A study of women who have made the choice. *Vocational Guidance Quarterly*, *33*, 241–248.

Stromberg, A. H., Larwood, L., & Gutek, B. A. (Eds.). (1987). *Women and work: An annual review, Vol. 2*. Newburg Park, CA: Sage.

Sutherland, E., & Veroff, J. (1985). Achievement motivation and sex roles. In V. E. O'Leary, R. K. Unger, & B. S. Wallston (Eds.), *Women, gender, and social psychology* (pp. 101–128). Hillsdale, NJ: Erlbaum.

Swaney, K., & Prediger, D. (1985). The relationship between interest-occupation congruence and job satisfaction. *Journal of Vocational Behavior*, *26*, 13–24.

Tangri, S. S. (1972). Determinants of occupational role innovation among college women. *Journal of Social Issues*, *28*, 177–199.

Tangri, S. S., & Jenkins, S. R. (1986). Stability and change in role innovation and life plans. *Sex Roles*, *14*, 647–662.

Teglasi, H. (1981). Children's choices of and value judgments about sex-typed toys and occupations. *Journal of Vocational Behavior*, *18*, 184–195.

Terman, L. M., & Oden, M. H. (1959). *Genetic studies of genius: V. The gifted group at midlife*. Stanford, CA: Stanford University Press.

Tidball, M. E. (1980). Women's colleges and women achievers revisited. *Signs, 5*, 504–517.

Tidball, M. E. (1985). Baccalaureate origins of entrants into American medical schools. *Journal of Higher Education, 56*, 394–399.

Tidball, M. E. (1986). Baccalaureate origins of recent natural science doctorates. *Journal of Higher Education, 57*, 606–620.

Tinsley, D. J., & Faunce, P. S. (1980). Enabling, facilitating, and precipitating factors associated with women's career orientation. *Journal of Vocational Behavior, 17*, 183–194.

Tobias, S. (1978). *Overcoming math anxiety*. New York: W. W. Norton.

Tremaine, L. S., & Schan, C. G. (1979). Sex role aspects in the development of children's vocational knowledge. *Journal of Vocational Behavior, 14*, 317–328.

Turner, B. F., & McCaffrey, J. H. (1974). Socialization and career orientation among Black and White college women. *Journal of Vocational Behavior, 5*, 307–319.

Tyler, L. E. (1978). *Individuality*. San Francisco: Jossey-Bass.

Umstot, M. E. (1980). Occupational sex-role liberality of third-, fifth-, and seventh-grade females. *Sex Roles, 6*, 611–618.

Unger, R. K., & Serbin, L. A. (Eds.). (1986). Sex, gender and social change [Special issue]. *Psychology of Women Quarterly, 14*, 11–12.

U.S. Bureau of Labor Statistics. (1985). *Women in the work force*. Washington, DC: Author.

U.S. Bureau of Labor Statistics. (1989). *Labor force statistics derived from the current population survey: A databook*. Washington, DC: Author.

U.S. Department of Labor. (1984). *Facts on women workers*. Washington, DC: Author.

U.S. Department of Labor, Bureau of Labor Statistics. (1988). *Employment and earnings*. Washington, DC: Author.

Vasquez, M. (1982). Confronting barriers to the participation of Mexican-American women in higher education. *Hispanic Journal of the Behavioral Sciences, 4*, 147–165.

Vetter, B. M. (1980). Working women scientists and engineers. *Science, 207*, 28–34.

Vetter, B. M. (1988). Women in engineering. *Bulletin of the American Association of Engineering Societies, 86* (Whole).

Vetter, B. M., & Babco, E. L. (1986). *Professional women and minorities: A manpower data resource service* (6th ed.). Washington, DC: Commission on Professionals in Science and Technology.

Voydanoff, P. (1988). Women, work, and family: Bernard's perspective on the past, present, and future. *Psychology of Women Quarterly, 12*, 269–280.

Wallston, B. S. (1981). What are the questions in psychology of women? A feminist approach to research. *Psychology of Women Quarterly, 5*, 597–617.

Walsh, M. R. (1979). The rediscovery of the need for a feminist medical education. *Harvard Educational Review, 49*, 447–466.

Walsh, W. B., & Osipow, S. H. (1993). *Advances in vocational psychology: Career counseling for women*. Hillsdale, NJ: Erlbaum.

Wampler, K. S. (1982). Counseling implications of the housewife role. *Counseling and Values, 26*, 125–132.

Ware, N. C., Steckler, N., & Leserman, J. (1985). The choice of a major among undergraduate women. *Journal of Higher Education, 56*, 73–84.

Warr, P., & Parry, G. (1982). Paid employment and women's psychological well-being. *Psychological Bulletin, 91*, 498–516.

Washburn, S. (1981). *Partners: How to have a loving relationship after liberation.* New York: Atheneum.

Watley, D. J., & Kaplan, R. (1971). Career or marriage? Aspirations and achievements of able and young college women. *Journal of Vocational Behavior, 1*, 29–43.

Weeks, M. O., & Botkin, D. R. (1987). A longitudinal study of the marriage role expectations of college women: 1961–1984. *Sex Roles, 17*, 49–58.

Weeks, M. O., & Gage, B. A. (1984). A comparison of the marriage-role expectations of college women enrolled in a functional marriage course in 1961, 1972, and 1978. *Sex Roles, 11*, 377–388.

Weishaar, M. E., Green, B. J., & Craighead, L. W. (1981). Primary influences of initial vocational choices for college women. *Journal of Vocational Behavior, 18*, 67–78.

Weitzman, L. J. (1979). *Sex role socialization.* Palo Alto, CA: Mayfield.

Wertheim, E. G., Widom, C. S., & Wortzel, L. H. (1978). Multivariate analyses of male and female professional career choice correlates. *Journal of Applied Psychology, 63*, 234–242.

White, M. J., Kruczek, T. A., Brown, M. T., & White, G. B. (1989). Occupational sex stereotypes among college students. *Journal of Vocational Behavior, 34*, 289–298.

Williams, J. (1977). *Psychology of women: Behavior in a biosocial context* (1st ed.). New York: W. W. Norton.

Williams, J. H. (1983). *Psychology of women: Behavior in a biosocial context* (2nd ed.). New York: Norton.

Williams, S. W., & McCullers, J. C. (1983). Personal factors related to typicalness of career and success in active professional women. *Psychology of Women Quarterly, 7*, 343–357.

Wirtenberg, T. J., & Nakamura, C. Y. (1976). Education: Barrier or boon to changing occupational roles of women. *Journal of Social Issues, 32*, 165–180.

Wise, L. L. (1985). Project TALENT: Mathematics course participation in the 1960's and its career consequences. In S. F. Chipman, L. R. Brush, & D. M. Wilson (Eds.), *Women and mathematics* (pp. 25–58). Hillsdale, NJ: Erlbaum.

Wolfe, L. K., & Betz, N. E. (1981). Traditionality of choice and sex-role identification as moderators of the congruence of occupational choice in college women. *Journal of Vocational Behavior, 18*, 43–55.

Wolfson, K. P. (1976). Career development patterns of college women. *Journal of Counseling Psychology, 23*, 119–125.

Wong, P. T. P., Kettlewell, G., & Sproule, C. F. (1985). On the importance of being masculine: Sex role, attribution and women's career achievement. *Sex Roles, 12*, 757–768.

Yanico, B. J. (1978). Sex-bias in career information: Effects of language on attitudes. *Journal of Vocational Behavior, 13*, 26–34.

Zappert, L., & Stansbury, K. (1984). *In the pipeline: A comparative analysis of men and women in graduate programs in science, engineering, and medicine at Stanford University.* Stanford, CA: Stanford University Press.

Zeff, S. B. (1982). A cross-cultural study of Mexican-American, black American, and white American women at a large urban university. *Hispanic Journal of the Behavioral Sciences*, *14*, 245–261.

Zuckerman, D. M. (1980). Self-esteem, personal traits, and college women's life goals. *Journal of Vocational Behavior*, *17*, 310–319.

Zuckerman, D. M. (1981). Family background, sex-role attitudes, and the goals of technical college and university students. *Sex Roles*, *7*, 1109–1126.

Zuckerman, D. M., & Sayre, D. H. (1982). Cultural sex role expectations and children's sex role concepts. *Sex Roles*, *8*, 853–862.

18

Work and Family Roles: Selected Issues

Beth L. Green and Nancy Felipe Russo

Multiple work and family roles have become the norm for the majority of American women. In 1988, 56% of all American women 16 years or older were in the labor force—54 million women. Fifty-five percent of these women combined the roles of worker and wife; 20% were divorced, widowed, or separated from their spouses (U.S. Bureau of the Census, 1990a).

The large proportion of women combining roles of wife and worker is a relatively recent development. Although the percentage of women in the labor force has risen for all marital status categories, the change has been especially dramatic for married women. From 1960 to 1988, the percentage of married women in the labor force increased by 78% (from 32% to 57%). In comparison, the percentage of divorced/widowed women in the labor force increased by 16% (from 37% to 43%); and never-married women, by 48% (from 44% to 65%).

Contemporary women are also combining the role of wife and worker with that of mother. In 1988, 55% of working wives had children under age 18. The child care responsibilities of these mothers were considerable—43% had children under age 6.

Working mothers are not necessarily wives, however. In 1988, 42% of divorced/separated working women were mothers, 33% with children under age 6. Interestingly, the table that provided these figures did not include this type of information for never-married working women who were also mothers (U.S. Bureau of the Census, 1990b, p. 385). From other sources, however, we know that in 1988 there were nearly 10 million children who lived with a never-married parent, and an estimated 9 of 10 of those children lived with their mothers (U.S. Bureau of the Census, 1989a).

These statistics provide a stark reminder that women's roles and circumstances have undergone major and rapid change. These changes involve new interrelationships among the roles of worker, wife, and mother that have implications for women's mental health and well-being. They underline the urgency for research on women's multiple roles and circumstances so that current realities of women's lives can be better understood.

Stereotyping and idealization of women's work and family roles must be replaced with an understanding of women's diverse realities. This chapter attempts a partial step toward constructing a more realistic understanding of the lives of women in the United States who work for pay. After presenting a brief profile of women at work and in the family, we summarize the recent literature on women's multiple roles, focusing on the implications of these roles for women's mental health. This focus on mental health is important for two reasons. First, women's mental health and well-being are important in their own right. Second—and the reason that this information is included in a chapter on women and work—"concern" about negative effects of employment on women's well-being can be used to undermine women's aspirations and to rationalize sex discrimination. We view women as actors, with the power to enact roles to their benefit. Accurate information about both benefits and problems associated with women's changing roles is a foundation for women's empowerment.

WOMEN'S EXPERIENCE AT WORK

A number of recent books discuss women's issues and experiences at work in greater depth (Anderson, 1988; Betz & Fitzgerald, 1987; Bose & Spitze, 1987; Crosby, 1987; Ferber, 1987; Gerson, 1985; Grossman & Chester, 1990; Gutek & Larwood, 1987; Hale & Kelly, 1989; Kelly & Bayes, 1988; Lee & Kanungo, 1984; Pleck, 1985; Rix, 1990; Rose & Larwood, 1988; Stromberg & Harkess, 1988; Statham, Miller & Mauksch, 1988). Here we focus on three interrelated issues—stereotyping and discrimination, sex segregation in the workplace, and employment rewards for women—that have particular implications for women's mental health and well-being.

Stereotyping and Discrimination

It is now illegal in the United States to assign most work roles by sex (although there are exceptions, e.g., actor and actress roles). Nonetheless, women still must take their feminine gender role, with its concomitant gender stereotypes, with them into the workplace (see chapter 11, this book, for a more complete discussion of the definitions of sex roles used here). Women continue to be stereotyped as caretakers and nurturers and are not taken seriously as providers despite the fact that women are single heads of households and the contributions of married women to their household incomes keep many families above the poverty line (Russo, Dantico & Meyer, 1986).

Although stereotyping and evaluation bias have become more subtle, they are nonetheless persistent (Swim, Borgida & Maruyama, 1989). Women have a different burden of proof for their competence. Men are assumed to be qualified unless evidence is provided to the contrary; women are doubted without evidence to the contrary (Lockheed & Hall, 1976). Equal performance does not bring equal rewards for women (Geis, Carter & Butler, 1982; Lott, 1985).

Stereotypes and subordinate status are mutually reinforcing. Women are seen as nurturing, submissive, dependent, and accommodating and thus are more likely to be seen (and see themselves) as suited to service tasks and subordinate positions. Occupying subordinate positions reinforces the impression of nurturance, dependence, and lack of leadership. The stereotype that women should be helpful to others leads to exploitation if they are helpful and to sanctions if they are not. When men accommodate others, the norm of reciprocity is engaged, and the others "owe" them favors in return. In contrast, accommodating women are taken for granted. Further, women's reasons for not accommodating are seen as less credible, and women are required to be more assertive to reach their goals than are men (Geis et al., 1982).

Gender stereotyping is thus linked to distinct employment issues for women (Barrett, 1984), who must deal with evaluation bias, greater pressure on their performance, exclusion from certain jobs and promotional opportunities, differential supervision, overprotection, unprofessional sexual remarks, unequal employment rewards, and sex segregation between and within occupations (Harlan & Weiss, 1981; Russo et al., 1986).

Sex Segregation

Although women are found in every occupation, sex segregation in the work force has not substantially changed. In 1980, 75% of women in the work force were in female occupations (i.e., where at least 50% of workers were women). In 1900, the figure was 60% (Fox & Hesse-Biber, 1984).

Sex segregation is both an outcome and a contributor to the persistence of sex discrimination in the workplace. Insofar as the roles of women at work require behaviors that fit gender and ethnic stereotypes, supervisors may be able to behave in discriminatory ways without feeling dissonance with other egalitarian attitudes. In consequence, people do not have to monitor their behaviors, nor are they able to recognize the discriminatory outcomes of carrying out their occupational roles (Kahn & Crosby, 1985).

Problems for women who enter traditionally male occupations include those associated with their token status.[1] Tokens are subjected to increased scrutiny and stereotyping. If the stereotypes are negative—as they are for women and minorities—they can be inhibiting and stress-producing (Izraeli, 1983; Lord & Saenz, 1985; Lord, Saenz & Godfrey, 1987; Ott, 1989; Spangler, Gordon & Pipkin, 1978).

Women must also deal with the responses of male peers to their entry into male-dominated occupations. While some men have been supportive, others have responded with hostility and harassment, including sexual harassment (Gruber & Bjorn, 1982; O'Farrell, 1982) and refusal to teach skills and knowledge essential to job performance (Deaux, 1984; Jurik, 1985). Evidence suggests that as the proportion of women increases in a traditionally male field, the attitudes of males toward women change from neutral to resistant. In contrast, as the proportion of males in traditionally female occupations increases, women's attitudes move from being favorable to neutral (Ott, 1989).

Sexual harassment appears to have a different function in male-dominated occupations compared with female-dominated occupations. In male-dominated occupations, coworkers are more likely to harass women in retaliation for perceived threats to male economic and social status. In traditionally female occupations, harassment is more likely to be conducted by supervisors who threaten the jobs of women who fail to comply with sexual demands. Legal protection is clearest and most effective for women who are harassed by their supervisors because differential power relationships are most clear and laws and policies specifically prohibit such harassment (Carothers & Crull, 1984). Such research underscores the importance of controlling for occupation in research on the experience of women at work.

O'Farrell and Harlan (1982) suggest that lack of job security underlies men's negative responses to "new women" in blue-collar occupations. However, even when economic status is not at issue, men may feel threatened by such women. Sex segregation is critical to male social status, and without it males must develop other accommodative strategies to maintain their belief in male superiority.

The report of a four-year, participant-observer study by Swerdlow (1989) of transit operatives provides a vivid description of the challenge women's entry into nontraditional occupations presents to the ideology of male supremacy. In her study, the males' job security was not at issue, and the most common attitudes were encouragement and support. However, women's competent performance in this nontraditional, blue-collar job setting challenged a "deeply held belief in male superiority" (p. 374). Men did not attempt to remove the women from the workplace to maintain that ideology. Instead they developed interpretations and practices that enabled them to reconcile women's competent performance with their chauvinistic beliefs. These practices included hostility directed at undermining feelings of competence and sexualization of the workplace and work relationships to objectify, demean, and dominate their fellow women workers.

These behaviors allowed men to simultaneously maintain their supremist ideology and to accept women in the workplace. When women made errors, they were spotlighted and remembered—and interpreted as evidence of women's incompetence in general. When women were competent, they received effusive praise as exceptions to the rule, and stereotypes could be safely maintained. Women were also perceived by men as not actually doing exactly the same work as men and as receiving preferential treatment.

For many men, sexualization of women was their major accommodation strategy. As Swerdlow (1989) so eloquently states, "By forcing sexual identities into high relief, men submerge the equality inherent in the work and superimpose traditional dominant and subordinate definitions of the sexes. Men have a stake in seeing women as sexual beings because in no arena is male domination less ambiguous for working-class men than sexuality" (p. 381).

Despite the fact that men persisted in regarding women as a group as sex objects, there is hope. Women did develop nonsexist, egalitarian relationships with their male work partners. Men's accommodative strategies enabled them to accept women coworkers and, over time, treat them individually as equals.

Although Swerdlow's (1989) research deals with blue-collar transit workers, her eloquent portrayal of attempts to maintain female subordination may apply across occupational categories and worker classes. It points to the need for researchers to examine strategies to maintain male gender-role supremacy in the presence of egalitarian changes in other roles in the workplace and in the family.

Employment Rewards

The dramatic changes in women's participation in the work force have not been matched by similar changes in employment rewards. A gender gap persists in the earnings of full-time wage and salary workers. In 1988, looking at median weekly earnings for that group, women earned $315 per week compared with $449 for men (i.e., they made 70¢ for every dollar earned by men).

This discussion focuses on salary inequities. It should be recognized that employee benefits, such as insurance, vacation and sick leave, and pensions, can constitute nearly 22% of the total compensation paid to employees (Hefferan, 1985). Women receive private pensions less often and in lower amounts than men, and many women do not receive survivor's benefits (Russo et al., 1986). Women also have less health insurance coverage than men (Perman & Stevens, 1989). A full analysis of factors influencing women's employment rewards would consider forms of compensation other than salaries.

The concentration of women in low-paying occupations is a major reason for the gender gap in wages (National Committee on Pay Equity, 1987). Overall, the larger the proportion of women in an occupation, the lower the earnings. The National Committee on Pay Equity (1987) reported that of all the "male" occupations, only "kitchen worker" fell into the bottom third of earnings, while no "female" occupation fell into the top third of earnings (p. 38).

Elimination of pay inequities will require analyses that go beyond occupational groupings to examine the employment settings of specific occupations. Women earn less than men in all major occupational groups, even those in which the majority of workers were women. One strategy to eliminate pay inequities has been to promote job evaluation strategies whereby a particular employer evaluates jobs in terms of job content—the skill and effort required, level of responsibility, and working conditions (National Committee on Pay Equity, 1987).

Ethnicity and Women's Work

The earnings gap in 1988 is greater when sex and race/ethnicity are taken into account and the standard of comparison is the group with the highest earnings: white males, at $465 per week. White women earned 68¢ for every dollar white men earned; black women, 62¢; Hispanic women, 56¢. In comparison, black men earned 75¢ and Hispanic men 66¢ for every dollar earned by white men. Addressing issues of racial/ethnic discrimination is essential for closing the earnings gap between the sexes.

Among these issues is the segregation of women of color into occupations that not only differ from white women, but differ from each other (National Committee on Pay Equity, 1987). For example, both black and Hispanic women are more likely to work in blue-collar jobs than Anglo women, but Hispanic women are more often found in manufacturing jobs than either black or Anglo women. Black women are more likely to work in service jobs than Hispanic women, particularly in health services (Russo et al., 1986). The higher the proportion of women of color in an occupation, the lower the earnings (National Committee on Pay Equity, 1987).

The forces that produce gender and ethnic pay differentials are complex. They are not explained by differences in education or training or in family responsibilities or by simple segregation (Treiman & Roos, 1983). Space precludes an in-depth discussion of differences in employment patterns by gender and ethnicity in this chapter (see National Committee on Pay Equity, 1987, and U.S. Commission on Civil Rights, 1990, for additional discussions). A key point here, however, is that researchers who seek to study how work-related psychological and social variables differ by gender and ethnicity must recognize that sex and race simultaneously affect the segregation that pervades the workplace. Comparisons across sex and racial groupings must be made with care.

It must be remembered that the behavior of individuals reflects the power and status of their position (Epstein, 1988; Snodgrass, 1985; Thompson, 1981; Kollock, Blumstein & Schwartz, 1985). Women's actions (and reactions to them) reflect their lower status and organizational powerlessness (Fox & Hesse-Biber, 1984). It is important to avoid the "fundamental attribution error" of assuming that deference, helpfulness, sensitivity, and other powerless behaviors are due to women's psychological traits, As Reid and Comas-Diaz (1990) have said so well, "Among the various characteristics which have been identified as contributors to status, gender and ethnicity are undoubtedly the most permanent, most noticeable, and have the most established attributional systems to accompany them" (p. 397).

The "Paradox of the Contented Female Worker"

The persistence of pay inequities and sex segregation contrasts with the widespread trends in the expression of egalitarian attitudes toward women in the work force (Kahn & Crosby, 1985). Sex discrimination is now recognized as a social problem by both men and women (Crosby & Herek, 1986; Kahn & Crosby, 1985). Employed women are aware of the existence of sex discrimination in the workplace and feel aggrieved and outraged about it (Crosby, 1982). Nonetheless, they continue to show similar levels of job satisfaction compared with men despite receiving lower employment rewards than men. This is not explained by different job values or preferences (Major, 1987).

Crosby (1982) has pointed out this "paradox of the contented female worker," positing a theory of relative deprivation to explain it. That is, relative deprivation occurs when people believe (1) their present condition is not as good as they want it to be and (2) their present condition is not as good as they believe they deserve it to be (Crosby, 1984a). Reference group is the key in this framework: women do not feel deprived when they earn less than men because they are comparing themselves with other women. Aspects of this theory have been investigated in research on factors contributing to gender differences in pay expectations, feelings of entitlement, and denial of disadvantage.

Pay Expectations

There are substantial differences in pay expectations: men expect to be paid more than women. For example, Major and Konar (1984) studied gender differences in expectations held by management interns for salaries at entry and at the peak of one's career. The gender differences were substantial for both figures: $2,600 at entry and nearly $20,000 at career peak. Men's expectations exceeded women's by 16.5% for entry salaries and by 46% for peak salaries.

Major and Konar explored the contribution of five factors hypothesized to contribute to these gender differences in pay expectations: career path factors, objective job inputs, perceived job inputs, job facet importance, and social comparisons. In other words, they explored the hypotheses that (1) sex differences in pay expectations may reflect differences in educational and occupational choices that lead to lower-paying occupations; (2) women may be less qualified or have poorer performance than men (at least this is the stereotype—as Major and Konar point out, there is little evidence for this factor); (3) women may have lower performance expectations, devalue their performance, and differ in their explanations for their performance compared with men; (4) women may value different facets of their job than men (and specifically may consider money less important); and (5) women may use different reference group comparisons than men—that is, since they are paid less than men, they may base their expectations on, and evaluate their outcomes against, a lower comparison standard.

Gender differences were found on only three of these factors: career path, job facet importance, and comparison standards. Thus, more than 50% of the women, compared with 10% of men, chose personnel as a career specialty. Women placed less importance on salary and more importance on interesting work than did men. Women also had different comparison salary expectations than men— women's estimate of the earnings of others entering their field was about $2,200 less than men's estimate. This was despite the fact that the supervisors of male and female interns did not differ in their estimates of what "typical others" would earn in the intern's field.

Regression analyses revealed that these three factors accounted for much (though not all) of the gender difference in pay expectations. Comparison pay estimates had the largest influence on pay expectations, accounting for 28% of their variance. Specialty area accounted for 15% of their variance; job facet importance, 5%. Number of years women planned to work and actual work performance as rated by supervisors did not help explain women's lower pay expectations.

Like Crosby (1982), Major and Konar (1984) suggested that one explanation for the gender difference in comparison standards is a tendency for men and women to compare themselves with others of the same sex, leading to a lower comparison standard for women. They also recognized, however, it could be that women use the same others for comparison, but estimate pay differently, due to differences in pay information.

Martin (1989) examined this latter possibility by investigating whether or not providing current and accurate salary information would eliminate the gender difference in comparison standards identified by Major and Konar (1984). She assessed preparedness for working in one's field, importance of job outcomes (friendly coworkers and supervisors, high salary, good promotional opportunity, chance to make decisions, job security, interest in the work, frequency of performance feedback, high status, and work importance), and salary expectation for the first year at work.

Women's salary expectations remained lower than men's, even when they were provided with the mean and the range of salary offers, but this varied with specialty area. Women also placed more importance on three job factors— friendly supervisors, interest in the work, and frequency of feedback. Interestingly, the gap in salary expectations between men and women was larger when specialty area and job facets were controlled. These variables appeared to suppress the relationship between gender and pay expectations.

Men had higher salary expectations than women in four of the five areas: accounting, finance/economic, marketing, and personnel. No difference was found for business administration. Martin suggests that the higher proportion of women in the specialty of business administration compared with the other four fields may have contributed to the lack of difference in pay expectations. These findings do differ from those of Major, McFarlin, and Gagnon (1984), who found that both sexes used the average amount taken by others as their comparison standard when given male and female standards for comparison. However, that research used college student samples working on a sex-neutral task in a laboratory. Future research on pay expectations thus should explore issues related to male dominance of occupations.

Such research needs to recognize that male dominance of occupations may relate to women's comparison standards in complex ways. One possibility is that the male dominance of an occupation lowers performance expectations for women, in turn leading to lowered feelings of entitlement and lower pay expectations if the woman enters such an occupation. Women have lower self-efficacy and performance expectations for traditionally male occupations, and a substantial amount of research has examined the relationship of those expectations to career choice (Betz & Hackett, 1981, 1983, 1987; Hackett & Betz, 1981; Lent, Brown & Larkin, 1986; Nevill & Schlecker, 1988).

Bridges's (1988) research confirmed that male dominance may adversely affect females' estimates of their aptitude for an occupation. In her study, which asked college students to estimate their aptitudes for various occupations, both sexes had higher estimates of their aptitudes for occupational fields dominated by their own sex compared with the fields dominated by the opposite sex. But the gender difference in estimations was greatest for the male-dominated occupations. For female-dominated occupations, there was only a 4.1 percentage point gap in the means of the estimated aptitudes for men and women; for male-dominated occupations, the gap was 12.7 points. The discrepancy was primarily due to the lower estimations women made for their aptitude for those occupations. This lowered estimation occurred despite the fact that the research participants were given bogus survey results purporting to prove that there were no differences by sex or race in the quality of performance in those occupations.

These results point to the importance of investigating the relationship of women's perceptions of male-dominated occupations to their expectations about their potential contributions and rewards in those occupations. However, whether or not low self-efficacy or self-estimations of aptitude merely lead to avoidance of male-dominated occupations by women (thereby perpetuating salary differentials through sex segregation) or whether or not they also affect salary expectations after career choices have been made is yet to be ascertained.

A comprehensive examination of inequities in the workplace would go beyond employment rewards to examine situations where women and men are paid equally, but where women are working harder and are more productive. Major et al. (1984) provide evidence that women not only expect to be paid less but pay themselves less than men do when given the same task to accomplish. Further, when given a fixed amount of money, women work longer and are more productive and more accurate than men, particularly when their work is monitored. The focus on pay inequities has led to a knowledge gap in this area. We need to know about performance inequities as well.

Although women's lower pay expectations are only one contributor to pay inequities, research by Major, Vanderslice, and McFarlin (1984) suggests their effect can be direct. Those researchers provide evidence that higher pay expectations on the part of job candidates directly lead to higher salary offers to equally qualified candidates without lowering the probability that the job will be offered. This suggests that while continuing to work for public policies to advance women's status in the workplace, an immediate strategy should be to raise women's expectations about what they can expect to earn. One way to do that is to expand their reference group to include the males in their professions.

Women's Reference Groups

Women do not necessarily compare themselves solely with other women, but when they do, it appears to be linked to their economic status. Zanna, Crosby, and Loewenstein (1987) explored the relationship between gender of reference group and feelings of dissatisfaction and deprivation. In their sample, in which the majority of women held professional positions (many in male-dominated occupations), 28% of the women used reference groups that were predominantly male, while 42% used reference groups that were predominantly female. Prestige ratings of jobs did not distinguish who used a male versus a female reference group, but salary level made a substantial difference. Women who compared themselves with males made substantially higher salaries than women who compared themselves with females, with women using mixed groups falling between the two.

Unfortunately, these researchers did not attempt to examine the effects of sex segregation within the occupations of the women studied. This would require going beyond occupational prestige (although that is correlated with proportion of males in an occupation) to examining the subfields of the occupations (e.g., one might expect an industrial psychologist to have a male referent group; a child psychologist, a female referent group).

Interesting differences in choice of reference group and marital and parental roles were discovered, however. Women who had female reference groups were more likely to be mothers, while women with male reference groups were likely to be married but have no children. Single women were more likely to use a mixed reference group (Zanna et al., 1987). These findings suggest that the mother role has a pervasive impact on women's identity at work as well as at home and that research that compares working women with housewives must control for maternal status.

The gender of one's reference group was found to relate to job attitudes. Women with male reference groups were more likely to perceive gaps between what they had and what they wished to have, felt entitled to have, or expected to have. Although these women had higher salaries than women with female reference groups, they were significantly more dissatisfied with their jobs than such women. Women with mixed reference groups resembled women in male reference groups in their job satisfaction.

In contrast, gender of reference group made no difference in women's attitudes toward the position of women generally or in their feelings about their domestic situation. As the authors point out, this suggests that women with male referents were not simply discontented no matter what the context.

The authors provide an excellent discussion of the many questions raised by these provocative findings. The important point here, however, is that strategies to address pay inequities must go beyond a focus on the objective qualities of women's jobs and include the attitudes and reference groups of women holding those jobs. More needs to be known about women's reference groups, which may differ for women of diverse ethnicity (Segura, 1989).

Research on the relationship of the subjective qualities of women's experience at work to job satisfaction should include investigation of the effects of attributions for success of coworkers in addition to self-attributions. In a study of gender differences in success-related attributions in a high-achieving, professional population, Russo, Kelly, and Deacon (1990) found that such women's job satisfaction was related to their belief that ability and hard work were important contributors to the success of their male colleagues. The less they considered such factors as important to male colleagues' success, the lower their job satisfaction (and vice versa). Russo and her colleagues suggest that a belief in what they termed "the Alger factor" (named after the Horatio Alger myth that with ability and hard work one will succeed) enabled the women in their sample to maintain their high levels of job satisfaction despite the fact that they earned less than their male colleagues. It may be that women's exaggerated estimations of male ability and effort are yet another contributor to the denial of individual disadvantage described below.

Future research also needs to go beyond salaries and include women's expectations regarding other forms of compensation, as well as access to training and promotional opportunities. For example, Segura (1989) found that working-class Chicanas perceived themselves as having occupational mobility in jobs with little or no advancement because they compared themselves with local working-class reference groups of similar ethnicity.

The Denial of Disadvantage

Crosby and her colleagues (Clayton & Crosby, 1986; Crosby & Clayton, 1986; Crosby, Pufall, Snyder, O'Connell, & Whalen, 1989) have suggested that women's failure to perceive the personal relevance of gender injustice in society contributes to the slow pace of change toward gender equality in the workplace. The "denial of individual disadvantage" (i.e., the failure to recognize that women we know face the same employment disadvantages as women in general) has been found in research in samples of heterosexual women (Crosby, 1982), lesbians (Crosby et al., 1989), blacks (Abeles, 1976), and French Canadians (Guimond & Dube-Simard, 1983). Sometimes that individual is ourselves, and the phenomenon is more aptly termed "denial of personal disadvantage" (Crosby et al., 1989, p. 81).

Overcoming denial of individual disadvantage will require having men in authority perceive discrimination against women at work. There is some evidence that husbands of employed women are more supportive of women's liberation than husbands of nonemployed women (Smith, 1985). However, Crosby and Herek (1986) found no relationship between men's concern with discrimination against women in general and their own wives' employment, occupational prestige, or educational level. However, men in high-prestige occupations were more concerned about sex discrimination than men in low-prestige occupations.

Why occupational prestige is associated with concern about the status of women is unclear. It may reflect effects of education. Crosby and Herek (1986) observe that it could have to do with a link between social class and authoritarianism, with lower-status men feeling threatened by any change to the status quo. It could also reflect the fact that high-prestige men feel relatively safe from female competition—fewer women are going to be competing with them. It may also be that high-prestige women in the workplace are less threatening to the ideology of male supremacy because they are more easily perceived as women who are "exceptions" to the norm of female inferiority. Certainly the strategies for maintaining women's subordination found in a blue-collar setting (Swerdlow, 1989) are found in high-prestige settings such as academe, including devaluation of female competence (Lott, 1985) and sexual harassment (Fitzgerald, Weitzman, Gold & Ormerod, 1988).

Crosby and her colleagues (1989) summarize emotional and cognitive mechanisms that help account for the denial of women's disadvantage on the part of both women and men, including self-protective cognitions. They point out the importance of identification with an oppressed group for discrimination to be perceived. They also document men and women's difficulty in perceiving discrimination when data are presented on a case-by-case basis, showing the need for information in aggregate form before discriminatory patterns can be revealed. They underscore that all people, whether sex-biased or not, have difficulty in perceiving sex bias in individual cases. They conclude that the need for social reform should not be measured by how concerned people are with their personal situation—people do not have a well-developed sense of their personal disadvantage. Their advice to employers: "Do not trust your own impressions any more than you trust the impressions of the women in your organization. Women may be motivated to deny their own disadvantage; but nobody . . . should trust conclusions based on unaggregated figures. Only by bringing all the data together can one see patterns" (p. 97).

Strategies for Changing Women's Status in the Workplace

The research on women's status referenced in this chapter suggests a variety of strategies for empowering women at work and eliminating inequalities in the workplace. Some of them focus on the women themselves. Workshops, networking groups, and other vehicles to help prepare women to deal with issues in the workplace, particularly when they are tokens, are one approach. Such workshops could help raise women's sense of entitlement and eliminate their denial of personal disadvantage by increasing their comparison standards and helping them understand how procedures and practices in the workplace promote gender bias in opportunities and outcomes.

Changing women's response to their treatment in the workplace is not sufficient, however. In addition to workshops designed to help women to deal with issues in the workplace, the persistence of evaluation bias suggests the need for workshops targeted toward (1) eliminating stereotyping and bias on the part of evaluators and (2) educating employers about the denial of individual disadvantage.

Blanchard and Crosby (1989) argue that, given that women and other disadvantaged groups minimize the level of their personal suffering from discrimination, affirmative action (which does not require members of disadvantaged groups to come forward on their own behalf) is critical for reform. Certainly effective change requires that strategies aimed at individuals must be complemented by a variety of institutional and policy-oriented efforts. Salary secrecy can be eliminated, and employers can be required to provide aggregate data on salaries and other forms of compensation so that bias in employment rewards can be monitored.

Public reminders about attitudes toward, and commitments to, affirmative action before each evaluation also help to reduce discriminatory behaviors (Snyder & Swann, 1976). Larwood, Szwajkowski, and Rose (1988) have pointed out that even well-intentioned managers "rationally" make discriminatory decisions in order to impress their higher-ups. Their research has shown that, in the absence of contrary evidence, managers will discriminate against women and ethnic minorities based on their beliefs about the preferences of those having power over them. Further, their work suggests that individuals holding power at the top of an organization will be perceived as preferring white males unless clear evidence to the contrary is provided. Larwood and her colleagues suggest such evidence might include appointing minorities and women to key positions, placing them in positions of authority that require others to work for them, and taking unusual steps to communicate a credible preference for equal opportunity that go beyond typical nondiscrimination pronouncements.

Rewards, accolades, and other indicators of quality also play an important role in eliminating evaluation bias and discriminatory behavior. If an authority "certifies" the quality of a product by a woman, it is less likely to be perceived as unequal (Pheterson, Kiesler & Goldberg, 1971). The purpose and criteria for rewards can be scrutinized, modified if necessary, and monitored.

Women's strategies to eliminate inequity have differed in different occupations (Sacks, 1983), and there is much to be learned from each of them. These strategies include individual and class action lawsuits; proposing legislation; lobbying; formation of unions; collective bargaining; strikes and sit-ins; stockholder proxy fights; consumer boycotts; changing professional ethics, accreditation, and licensing criteria to prohibit discriminatory behavior; forming women-oriented businesses to compete against sexist institutions; and public ridicule. Research that identifies what combinations of strategies are effective under what conditions is needed.

WOMEN'S STATUS IN THE FAMILY

Contemporary women make substantial economic contributions to their families, continue to have the major responsibility for housework and dependent care (including children and elderly parents), and disproportionately suffer the effects of violence and poverty (Russo et al., 1986; see also chapter 11, this book). Women's economic role in the family has continued to increase, even in the 1980s. In 1988, women were earners in 58% of families having earners; 16% of families with earners were maintained solely by women. In 1980, the comparable figures were 51% and 14%, respectively.

When women combine the role of wife and worker, their families have a substantial economic advantage over families where only the husband is an earner. In 1988, the median weekly income for husband-wife earner families was $773; it was $489 for husband-only earner families. The dual earner advantage is proportionately greater for ethnic minority families. For white families, the median weekly earnings for dual earners are 57% higher than for such families where the husband is the single earner; for dual earner black families, earnings are 62% higher; for Hispanic families, 68% higher.

Women's economic status in the workplace has both direct and indirect links to their mental health and well-being in their families (Belle, 1990). Income has been found to be positively associated with mental health for both white and black women (Baruch & Barnett, 1987; Ross & Huber, 1985). Although employment may create difficulties for women in caring for children, it may also provide a buffer for other types of stress, particularly for low-income women. Compared with housewives, employed married women with lower incomes appear more affected by stress due to childrearing but they are less affected by other life events. Thus, higher-income women's ability to purchase assistance to cope with time and work demands may mitigate stresses from childrearing that women with lower incomes cannot avoid (Cleary & Mechanic, 1983).

In addition, Ross, Mirowsky, and Huber (1983) found that the higher a woman's income, the more her husband was likely to share in home responsibilities (the correlation was with her income, not his). It may be that with money comes power to negotiate roles, with concomitant mental health benefits. However, women who make secondary or minimal contributions to family income may be "unable to redistribute obligations and thus will suffer continued difficulties and dissatisfaction" (Thoits, 1987b, p. 19).

Education is correlated with occupational status and income and varies across ethnic groups (Amaro & Russo, 1987). Kessler (1982) and Kessler and McRae (1982) reported that for women, whether or not they were employed, education was more important than earnings or family income in predicting psychological distress. Lower education and having young children have been related to level of depression for wives (Kessler, 1982). In one study, employment outside the home did not appear to protect a woman from depression independently of education (Warren & McEachren, 1983).

Education thus appears to be a significant preventive against psychological distress and depression (Warren & McEachren, 1983), perhaps because it may lead to an increased sense of mastery and sense of control, necessary conditions for the development of active problem-solving approaches. Education also widens "possibilities for new role bargains suggested through reading, travel, and lectures by 'experts' " (Thoits, 1987b, p. 18). It is a resource that leads to effectiveness in both homemaker and work roles, and it needs to be considered in research examining mental health effects of work and family resources and responsibilities.

Ethnic Minority Families

Racial and ethnic differences in psychological distress are enhanced among people with low incomes, particularly poor black women (Kessler & Neighbors, 1986). Social class is not sufficient to explain such differences; doing so will require simultaneously examining gender effects. Yet researchers continue to ignore the interactive effects of gender and ethnicity on mental health indicators, although these effects are clearly apparent in the use of mental health facilities (Russo, Amaro & Winter, 1987; Russo & Olmedo, 1983; Russo & Sobel, 1981).

Ethnic minority families have greater sources of stress as well as fewer resources to deal with that stress (cf. Amaro & Russo, 1987; Staples, 1987). For example, such families have lower incomes and larger family sizes. In married-couple families where husbands only are earners, whites have $14,600 to spend per child. In contrast, blacks have $8,900 and Hispanics have $8,000 per child in such families. For dual earner families, the figures are $30,663 per child for whites, and $17,700 and $15,500 for blacks and Hispanics, respectively. In general, the lower the education of the parents, the larger the family size (U.S. Bureau of the Census, 1989).

As Zinn (1989) has pointed out, different opportunity structures for the races have shaped family organization in numerous ways. The profound effect of location in the social structure on ethnic minority family organization can be seen in the large differences in proportion of never-married women by race. Black women are much more likely to be never married than either white or Hispanic women. For example, in 1988, 50% of black women 25–29 years of age were never married, compared with about 26% for white and for Hispanic women, respectively (Saluter, 1989).

Ethnic minority women are also more likely to be divorced and less likely to be remarried than white women. There are 146 divorced white women for every 1,000 white married women; for black women, the comparable number is 311; for Hispanic women, 167. Given ethnic minority women's greater likelihood of never marrying or divorcing if married, it is not surprising that such women are also more likely to be found in female-headed households than are white women, where stressors are more numerous and resources meager.

Female-Headed Households

Any discussion of women's multiple roles must recognize that a significant proportion of contemporary women are not married—that is, they are divorced, widowed, or never married—and a large proportion of these single women are mothers. In addition to the contribution of rising divorce rates to the numbers of single mothers, childbearing among unmarried women in the United States has now reached the highest levels ever recorded. In 1986, there were 34.3 births for every 1,000 unmarried women aged 15–44 years. The rates are highest among unmarried black women: 80.9, compared with 23.2 for white women (Saluter, 1989).

Thus, the number of one-parent families went from 3.8 million in 1970 to 9.4 million in 1988. Approximately 8.1 million of these families were maintained by women in 1988—87% of families. Over 33% of these mothers were never married; 57% were separated or divorced. Smaller proportions were widowed (7%) or had absent spouses for other reasons (3%).

The reasons women maintain one-parent families differ by ethnic group. White women are more likely to do so because of marital dissolution. In 1988, among whites, nearly 58% of female-headed families were maintained by women who were divorced or separated. For Hispanic women, the comparable figure was 47%; for black women, 33%. In contrast, black women are more likely to be never married. In 1988, 54% of black, female-headed families were maintained by women who were never married, compared with 17% of white women and 32% of Hispanic women. As Zinn (1989) observes, race and ethnicity create "different routes to female headship, but Whites, Blacks, and Latinos are all increasingly likely to end up in this family form" (p. 78).

The child care needs of such families are considerable, and lack of access to child care has a differential impact on ethnic minority children. In 1988, 24% of the 63.2 million children in the United States lived with a single parent, up from 12% in 1970. Most of such children are white (63%). However, the proportion of children living in such families was higher for ethnic minority families; 54% of black children and 30% of Hispanic children, compared with 19% of white children, lived with one parent in 1988. Among blacks, 61% of children under 6 years of age were living with one parent in 1988, compared with 17% of white children under age 6 (Saluter, 1989).

Rawlings (1989) points out that living in a one-parent family may not reflect one specific cause or be limited to one episode. At some point during childhood an estimated 60% of children will spend a significant number of years (six on the average) living with one parent (Rawlings, 1989).

Financial difficulties are greatest in female-headed households. In 1988, two-parent households with children under 18 present had a mean family income of $40,067. For woman-headed households, the figure was $11,989; 47% of those households had mean family incomes under $7,500.

This brief portrait of women's family resources and responsibilities points to the importance of examining the relationship of women's family roles to their roles in other social structures, such as the workplace and the community. The remainder of this chapter focuses on the interrelationships among women's work and family roles, with specific regard to one category of outcome: their impact on women's mental health and well-being.

MULTIPLE ROLES AND WOMEN'S MENTAL HEALTH: COMPLEX RELATIONSHIPS

Whether or not a combination of employment, marriage, and motherhood results in mental health costs or benefits depends on a variety of factors, including personality characteristics, family variables, and job variables. Women's roles as wife and worker, mother and caretaker, contribute to stress as well as well-being. Resources, stimulation, and social validation from one type of role may offset the strains of others. Although role conflict, overload, and strain are possible, many researchers have documented beneficial effects of multiple roles for women's physical and mental health (Aneshensel, 1986; Coleman, Antonucci & Adelmann, 1987; Gove & Zeiss, 1987; Helson, Elliot & Leigh, 1990; Pietromonaco, Manis & Frohardt-Lane, 1986; Thoits, 1986; Verbrugge, 1987).

Although marital status and satisfaction have long been an important predictor of psychological distress, researchers have just begun to examine the psychological functions of marriage for men and women in social, economic, and political contexts. Marriage is generally more likely to be associated with mental health for men than women. Further, the quality of marriage is more strongly related to home life satisfaction for women compared with men (Gove & Zeiss, 1987). This difference may reflect gender differences in the psychological functions of marriage. Males may have more instrumental gains from marriage (e.g., in the form of services, such as housekeeping). Females, who have fewer alternatives, may invest more emotionally in their marital roles (Gove, Hughes & Styles, 1983). The stronger impact of relationship quality for women compared with men may also reflect men's greater participation in employment roles that offer buffers to marital stress.

Thoits (1987a) has provided a succinct and lucid summary of theory and research on the relationship of women's multiple roles and mental health. She evaluated the proposition that multiple role occupancy is harmful to women, pointing out that this approach relies on an oversocialized, deterministic view of human beings. It fails to recognize that women are active agents who can construct their own realities and who may choose not to conform to role expectations. Further, role expectations held by women and significant others may be flexible, ambiguous, or inconsistent. Feminist researchers, who assume women are active agents and seek women's empowerment, have rebutted simplistic role overload/conflict approaches (Baruch, Biener & Barnett, 1987; Crosby, 1987).

In a review of 12 studies published between 1975 and 1983, Thoits (1987a) examined the relationship of multiple roles to measures of psychological distress, depression, or mental disorder. In the 8 studies that compared nonemployed wives with employed husbands, in all cases, nonemployed wives showed higher distress levels.

A beneficial effect of employment was not always found in the 12 studies that compared employed and nonemployed wives. Nonetheless, in the 5 studies in which significant differences were reported, employed wives were the group consistently found to be in better mental health.

A major problem with research that has examined the relationship between paid employment and mental health for wives is the failure to separate family responsibilities associated with the role of wife from those associated with the role of mother. In general, motherhood is associated with increased psychological distress for women whether or not they work outside the home (Barnett & Baruch, 1985; Gore & Mangione, 1983; Thoits, 1986). Distress appears higher when children are young (Thoits, 1986) and increases with the number of children living in the home (Brown, Bhrolchain & Harris, 1975; Pearlin & Johnson, 1977; Radloff, 1975). Unfortunately, whether or not the number, timing, and spacing of children were planned or even wanted is typically not ascertained. In any case, studies that compare employed wives with housewives must at minimum control for number and ages of children.

Role Quality

Understanding when multiple roles do and do not promote mental health requires consideration of the joint effects of the qualities of those roles. Research has only recently begun to consider joint effects of family and work roles (Amaro, Russo & Johnson, 1987). Research that does examine joint effects suggests that the independent effects of marital and occupational status are not sufficient to predict well-being for all role combinations. It is necessary to look at specific role combinations and to know whether or not each role is perceived as stressful.

Aneshensel (1986) found that women with multiple roles of wife and paid worker had the lowest rate of depression if marital and job strains were low. Depression scores among these women were significantly lower than among nonemployed wives with low marital strain. Further, employed wives with both high marital strain and high employment strain had lower rates of depression than wives with high marital strain but no employment. The latter group had the highest rates of depression. Thus, role quality was more important than role occupancy in predicting mental health, although employment per se also appeared to have positive mental health effects.

Similarly, in a study of women aged 35–55, Baruch and Barnett (1987) examined relationships of the quality of wife, mother, and paid worker roles to measures of self-esteem, pleasure (a combination of overall happiness, satisfaction, and optimism), and depressive symptomatology. They found that the more roles a woman occupied, the happier she was with each individual role. Once income was controlled, only occupancy of the employment role had significant effects on any measure of women's well-being: it was correlated with increased self-esteem. But the quality of the experiences of each of the three roles was significantly correlated with all three measures of well-being used in study: positively with self-esteem and pleasure, negatively with depressive symptomatology. They concluded: ''What really matters is the nature of the experiences within a role. Those concerned with women's mental health should now, therefore, turn their attention to understanding how to enhance the quality of women's experiences within each of their many roles'' (Baruch & Barnett, 1987, p. 72).

Achieving that understanding requires more complex paradigms. It will be necessary to assess both the advantages and the disadvantages of multiple roles, using a dynamic, psychosocial approach that focuses on relevant processes or mechanisms, and consider psychological, family, and job characteristics of both spouses (McBride, 1988, 1990).

Psychological Factors

The assumption that women are active agents implies that personality characteristics and other psychological variables should affect number, type, and quality of roles. Helson, Elliot, and Leigh (1990) analyzed data from a longitudinal study of Mills College graduates that assessed personality characteristics at age 21 and number of roles (partner, parent, and worker) at age 43. Personality variables were assessed by the California Psychological Inventory (Gough, 1987). A combination of higher independence, intellectual efficiency, social energy, and tolerance at age 21 predicted the number of these three roles women occupied 22 years later.

Examination of the differences among combinations of roles revealed that women with one role had greater unhappiness, discontent, alienation, and lack of organization than women with multiple roles. There was no evidence that the three-role group had more role conflict or overload than other groups. The only difference between the three-role group and two-role group was the greater communality (feelings of being similar to others) of the former group.

Those researchers affirmed that quality of roles was more important than number of roles in predicting women's psychological health. They first examined the relationship between number of multiple roles and psychological health at age 43 after antecedent personality characteristics were controlled. Measures of two dimensions of psychological health—well-being and effective functioning— were used. Number of roles was not correlated with psychological health at age 43 after controlling for such health at age 21.

Quality of roles (assessed through measures of marital satisfaction and status at work) did continue to predict psychological health even after controlling for previous psychological health, however. Regardless of previous psychological characteristics, marital satisfaction was associated with contentment, and status at work was associated with effective functioning. Status level of work was also associated with attributes of an enhanced self—autonomy, individuality, and complexity. Unfortunately, the joint effects of marital satisfaction and work status were not explored. Further, because the study is correlational, it is difficult to separate the effects of work status on personality versus the effects of personality on work status.

Autonomy and Mastery

The findings of Helson and her colleagues (1990) suggest an explanation for the psychological benefits of employment per se found by Aneshensel (1986) and Baruch and Barnett (1987); that is, employment—even when it is stressful—may contribute to a more autonomous sense of self, thus promoting mental health (Warren & McEachren, 1985).

Crohan, Antonucci, Adelman, and Coleman (1989) documented the importance of occupational status and income for women's feelings of control and efficacy. In their study, perceived control over one's life correlated positively with prestige of occupation (over and above its relationship to job satisfaction) for both black and white women. In addition, perceived control was correlated with income for black women.

Both job satisfaction and being married have been found to be related to life satisfaction for both black and white women (Crohan et al., 1989). Family roles may have different relationships to women's sense of identity than employment roles, however. For example, one study found that 35% of the women in the sample mentioned family-related roles as important to how they saw themselves, while 7% mentioned work roles (Kandel, Davies & Ravels, 1985). Few researchers have investigated the negative consequences of derived identity—a sense of self that reflects one's relationships with others rather than one's personal uniqueness. The derived identity of housewife may contribute to higher levels of psychological distress and undermine the autonomy necessary for high self-esteem. Married women report more derived identity than unmarried women (Warren & McEachren, 1985). Russo and Green (chapter 11, this volume) discuss in more detail the relationship between concepts such as autonomy, mastery, and instrumentality and women's mental health.

Agentic and Communal Qualities of Roles

A person-centered approach is not sufficient to explain the interrelationships among gender, the sex roles of wife and mother, and women's mental health and well-being. Psychological characteristics of autonomy and the associated concepts of mastery and agency may be necessary, but are not sufficient to achieve mental health. In examining aspects of the situation that influence women's mental health, there is evidence that the combination of agentic and communal qualities of roles affects mental health effects from stressful life changes (Stewart & Malley, 1987).

In a study of 103 divorcing mothers, Stewart and Malley (1987) found that women with no employment outside the home were likely to report lives with low agency and high communion (56%). Women with full-time employment, however, were more equally distributed across all four combinations: low agency/ low communion (35%); low agency/high communion (26%); high agency/low communion (22%); and high agency/high communion (17%). Although role combination was somewhat related to the agency-communion pattern, the agency-communion pattern was the better predictor of emotional and physical health. Lower depressive symptomatology was associated with balance in agency and communion (either high or low). Well-being was associated with balanced high agency and communion. Physical health was associated with communion alone, but appeared enhanced in combination with high agency. These findings with regard to role quality appear to differ from those found in research on androgyny (defined as a personality characteristic) and mental health, which suggest that the instrumentality dimension accounts for the greater mental health of androgynous individuals (Russo & Green, chapter 11, this volume).

Unfortunately, Stewart and Malley used an analysis of variance approach to ascertain the effects of agency and communion; a regression model, which would recognize that the two variables may not be independent, would have been preferable. It is also difficult to separate the contribution of role characteristics from the contribution of personality characteristics to variance in activities classified as agentic or communal. Further, the findings are inconsistent with other research that has found working women without children to be in better physical health than nonworking mothers (Coleman et al., 1987; Helson et al., 1990). Differences in income, education, and other health-related variables might explain that discrepancy in results, however. Verbrugge (1987) reported that the small association between family roles and health appeared curvilinear. In other words, high parenting demands (which would be classified as communal activities) were associated with poorer physical health. Despite the many problems with interpreting the findings, the approach is noteworthy. Research that investigates the relationship of the qualities of women's roles and circumstances to their mental health is a promising line of inquiry.

Marital Quality

The effects of women's employment on marital quality—that is, marital strain and marital satisfaction—appears to depend on a couple's attitudes toward the wife's employment. Perceived control over the choice to work is related to marital satisfaction in dual-career couples (Alvarez, 1985). Research on dual-worker married couples with preschool children has reported couples similar in attitudes toward women's roles to be higher in marital satisfaction levels (Cooper, Chassin & Zeiss, 1985).

The mix of the couple's attitudes and personality characteristics has been found to be important to marital satisfaction as well. Higher levels of marital satisfaction and lower conflict surrounding domestic tasks are associated with higher combined levels of instrumental and expressive personality characteristics

(Cooper et al., 1985; Gunter & Gunter, 1990). Individuals with such characteristics may have the best fit with the multiple agentic and communal qualities of work, marriage, and parenthood roles.

Ross et al. (1983) found that if a wife wanted to work, but had no help from her husband with home responsibilities, her distress level increased while his did not. Husbands' distress increased only in couples where the preference of both husband and wife was for the wife to stay at home. Lowest distress levels were found in dual-career couples who shared child care and and household responsibilities. It thus may be that difficulties in negotiation of child care tasks can explain the finding of Gove and Zeiss (1987) that the presence of children affected whether or not congruence between employment and wife's preference for working affected her happiness. Such findings point to the importance of research on marital power, multiple roles, and mental health.

Marital Power

Family roles are by definition reciprocal, that is, defined in terms of rights and responsibilities toward one another. Thus, they depend on shared expectations and agreements on trade-offs between employment and family responsibilities. How such trade-offs are negotiated in marriage clearly has mental health implications for women. A sense of power or influence in the relationship is related to relationship satisfaction for women in both heterosexual (Steil & Turetsky, 1987) and lesbian couples (Eldridge & Gilbert, 1990).

Employment may enhance a wife's ability to negotiate trade-offs to her satisfaction and mental health benefit. Employed wives have more influence over decision making in the home than nonemployed wives (Crosby, 1982). In a study of professional women, the amount a women earned relative to her husband (i.e., her income disparity) was more important than her absolute level of income in predicting her influence in family decision making. Influence was also correlated with how important a woman perceived her career to be (Steil & Turetsky, 1987).

Factors that contribute to equality in marital power appear to operate differently for women when they have children, at least among professional women. Steil and Turetsky (1987) found that for professional women without children, the women's perceived job importance was positively correlated with their influence in marital decision making. In addition, relative economic status—that is, a smaller income disparity for spouses—was associated with both greater influence in decision making and more freedom from household responsibilities for women.

For mothers, however, reduced income disparity did not affect either influence in decision making or responsibility for household or child care tasks. The only variable with an effect was psychological; the more a mother perceived her job as important, the less her responsibility for the household. Responsibility for child care was not affected by either variable.

Dominance of the husband in decision making per se did not relate to women's marital satisfaction. It was the outcome of the decision that was important. Women who had husbands who were "dominant" in decision making that resulted in shared responsibility for household tasks were satisfied as wives. The greater the sharing of household and child care tasks, the greater women's marital satisfaction.

Shared responsibility also enhanced women's psychological well-being, especially that of mothers. The more responsibility a woman had for child care, the higher her depressive symptomatology (dysphoric mood and somatic symptoms). For nonmothers, marital equality contributed to well-being through its association with marital satisfaction. For mothers, marital equality contributed to well-being even beyond its contribution to marital satisfaction, suggesting additional relief for direct stress from burdens of household tasks (Steil & Turetsky, 1987).

The burden of those tasks on women is considerable. It has been estimated that wives spend somewhere between 30 and 60 hours per week on household labor, compared with 10 to 20 hours per week spent by husbands (Berk, 1985; Berardo, Shehan & Leslie, 1987; Denmark, Shaw & Ciali, 1985). Further, women's household labor involves tasks that are more time-consuming and are of more immediate necessity (Gunter & Gunter, 1990).

Child Care

In 1987, 57% of employed mothers (single and married) had more than 105 million children under the age of 6 who required child care. These women use a substantial proportion of their income for child care, although the proportion differs by marital status: married women use 6% of their earnings for child care, while other women use 9%. Women below poverty level use 25% of their earnings for child care compared with 6% for women above poverty level (U.S. Bureau of the Census, 1990b).

Mental health benefits of mother's employment are increased when women are satisfied with their child care arrangements (Parry, 1986; VanMeter & Agronow, 1982). Ross and Mirowsky (1988) found number of children increased depression levels for nonemployed wives, but had no relationship to husbands' depression levels. For employed mothers, however, the relationship of number of children to depression depended both on accessibility of child care and on husband's support. If child care was accessible and husbands shared in it, depression levels were low. In contrast, employed mothers without accessible child care and with sole responsibility for it had extremely high depression levels.

Sharing of child care affects marital satisfaction for both men and women. In a study of parents of kindergarten and fourth-grade children in white, two-parent families, Barnett and Baruch (1987) found that mothers who worked outside the home spent significantly less time interacting with their children than nonemployed mothers, but the difference averaged only 7.16 hours (41.87 hours versus 49.03 hours), or a little more than an hour a day. Fathers' involvement with children average about 30 hours a week and did not significantly vary with wives' employment. They developed a measure of sharing of child care tasks, identifying the proportion of time child care was done by the mother alone (0–20% = 1, 20–40% = 2, and so forth). Sharing of child care also did not significantly vary with employment. Means for employed and nonemployed mothers were 3.47 and 3.60, respectively.

Employment did not greatly affect average level of role strain for these two groups of mothers. Out of 19 indicators of role strain, significant differences were found for only 4. Women who were not employed did report more dissatisfaction with the amount of time their husbands spent on household tasks. Women who were employed reported they did not have enough time for friends. They also perceived their husbands to be dissatisfied with both the amount of time the mothers spent with the children and the mother's overall time allocation. This perception was accurate: ratings by the fathers revealed that the more time the mother spent, relative to him, in child care tasks, the greater his satisfaction with her work schedule and her overall time allocation. This held even though fathers also perceived that lack of time they spent in child care was a source of dissatisfaction to their wives. Similarly, Benin and Agostinelli (1988) found husbands' perceptions of arguments over sharing tasks appeared to depend only on how satisfied they were with the division of tasks.

Thus, many men appear to be happy when they are not sharing in domestic tasks, and the fact that they know their wives are not happy about it does not lower their marital satisfaction. Perhaps research on male feelings of entitlement in the work setting (e.g., Major, 1987) may be helpful in understanding male feelings of entitlement in the family setting.

Interestingly, the lower the proportion of time working mothers assumed sole responsibility for child care tasks, the more they were likely to feel that they had too little time to spend with their family ($r = -.31$, $p < .01$). Barnett and Baruch (1987) suggest two possibilities to explain this finding. It could reflect working mothers' expectation that they would have sole responsibility for child care. Alternatively, it may be that it is easier to shoulder child care responsibilities than ask one's husband to take on tasks that he wishes to avoid. They also found that the more child care tasks a mother did alone, the more negative her view of the husband as a father and the more dissatisfied she was about the equity of the marriage.

The impact of husband's support on depressive symptomatology reported by Ross and Mirowsky (1988) has been found in other studies as well (Elman & Gilbert, 1984; Steil & Turetsky, 1987). In addition, children's support may also affect the relationship between employment and women's mental health (Schwartzberg & Dytell, 1988). A study of employed, married, rural women with adolescent children found that children's support for their mother's working was the only family-related variable related to women's satisfaction with her multiple roles. The other major predictors were all job-related: job performance, job progress, job duties, and reason for working (McKenry, Hamdorf, Walthers, & Murray, 1985).

Marital Equality and Ethnic Minority Women

The importance of examining issues of marital satisfaction and equality among diverse ethnic groups is underscored by the findings of Golding (1990). She used the National Institute of Mental Health's (NIMH) Epidemiological Catchment Area (ECA) data from Los Angeles to examine the relationship among division of housework, household strain, and depressive symptomatology among Hispanic and non-Hispanic white men and women 18 years of age and older (note that the men and women were not married to each other). Although she describes her study as examining consequences of housework, her measure is actually a measure of sharing of housework, not level of housework. Although her model rests on flawed assumptions, the data are quite interesting when they are cast with labels that more accurately represent what is being measured. We present them in some detail, as they document the need to conduct research that examines the interaction of gender and ethnicity in diverse ethnic groups.

Equity in sharing four household tasks—cooking the main meal, washing dishes, doing laundry, and cleaning the house—was ascertained, with 0 indicating responsibility of spouse, 1 indicating shared responsibility, and 2 indicating responsibility of respondent. These scores were summed into a scale that theoretically ranged from 0 to 8. The distribution of tasks was bimodal, with nearly 65% of women having sole responsibility for housework compared with 3% of men.

An interaction effect for ethnicity and gender was found in the division of household labor on these tasks. Mexican American women were most likely to have major responsibility for household tasks. Their mean rating was 7.4 on the 8-point scale, compared with non-Hispanic women, who had a mean rating of 6.4. In contrast, Mexican American men had a mean rating of 1.0, and non-Hispanic men had a mean rating of 2.2, both indicating little sharing of household tasks. Thus, Mexican American men were less likely to share housework than non-Hispanic men, and Mexican American women were less likely to share housework than non-Hispanic women.

The household strain measure included items assessing the presence or absence of having more household duties than one could do or should have to do, spending too many hours on housework, and housework's interference with other activities. These were summed to make a scale of 1 to 4. The level of household strain was low, but varied with gender and ethnicity. Mexican American women had the highest levels of household strain (1.3), followed by Mexican American men (.8), non-Hispanic women (.6), and non-Hispanic men (.3). Whether or not the perceived household strain of Mexican American men reflects a resistance to sharing housework tasks or reflects a larger overall level of household tasks for Mexican American families cannot be ascertained from this study.

Separate regression analyses for women and men were conducted to predict household strain. For women, being Mexican American and employed and having unequal sharing of housework predicted household strain. For men, being Mexican American predicted household strain. Lack of sharing of housework was associated with household strain for women, but not for men, perhaps because men rarely took on the responsibility for housework. The fact that inequities in housework were associated with household strain is consistent with research that inequities in division of household tasks are a source of grievance for women (Crosby, 1982) and is congruent with Steil and Turetsky's (1987) research described above.

Lack of sharing of housework was found to be associated with depressive symptomatology through its association with household strain for both Hispanic and non-Hispanic women. Household strain was associated with such symptomatology for both women and men, regardless of employment, age, and socioeconomic status. Unfortunately, the study provided no information about presence of children. Responsibility for child care was not distinguished from other forms of household responsibilities.

Lack of marital equality is associated with low education (Antill & Cotton, 1988; Rexroat & Shehan, 1987), but lack of education does not totally explain ethnic differences in marital equality. When Golding (1990) conducted her analyses on individuals with 12-grade education or above, the main effect for ethnicity that had been found for the entire sample disappeared, but the interaction effect for gender and ethnicity persisted.

Understanding Women's Inequality in the Family

The research reviewed in this chapter also shows that issues of women's equality in the family, as in the workplace, cross lines of ethnicity and class. We believe that understanding women's inequality in the family will require separating characteristics and behaviors mandated by masculine and feminine gender roles from those of family sex roles, particularly those of husband, wife, father, and mother. Masculine gender roles may change so that performing domestic tasks may not threaten masculine gender identity, but unless the sex roles of wife and mother change as well, inequalities in the family will persist, and women will continue to be responsible for household labor.

Evidence for this assertion is found in a study by Gunter and Gunter (1990). Those authors examined the relationship between gender role (masculinity versus femininity as measured by the Bem Sex Role Inventory) and sharing of domestic tasks in a white, middle-class population. They found that when husbands were androgynous or undifferentiated, both husbands and wives performed the domestic tasks that were frequent, repetitious, and pressing. When a husband was sex-typed, however, women performed most tasks and husbands the least. They suggest that the gender identity of masculine males "may be bound up not only in what they do, but equally in what they do not do. In other words, it may be as important to a sex-typed male *not* to dust or vacuum or change a diaper as it is to be able to change a tire or repair the plumbing" (p. 366).

Gunter and Gunter (1990) also found, however, that neither the husbands' nor the wives' gender-role orientation was related to the reasons given for performing household tasks. Women were more likely to report they did a task because it was their job or because it would not be done otherwise. Men, on the other hand, were more likely to report that domestic tasks were not their job.

In particular, factors contributing to inequities in the family appear to differ for women who are mothers, underscoring the importance of separating effects of the sex role of wife from that of mother. The sex role that has least changed for women is mother, who still is primarily responsible for child care, whether or not she is employed.

CONCLUSION

This brief portrait of women's roles and status at work and in the family suggests that although great changes have occurred in women's work and family roles, gender inequalities in rewards, resources, and status persist. These inequalities are magnified for women of color and have profound impact on the mental health and well-being of all women, particularly mothers. Factors contributing to women's disadvantaged status have been discussed, and some strategies for research and action to empower women have been identified.

In the final analysis, it may be naive to focus our attention on specific factors, such as sex segregation or husband-wife income disparity, that research identifies as currently contributing to gender-based inequities at work or in the family. As Reskin (1988), quoting Lieberson (1985), points out, "Dominant groups remain privileged because they write the rules, and the rules they write 'enable them to continue to write the rules' " (p. 60). She focused on sex segregation, reminding us that it is but a symptom of the basic cause of the earnings gap—that is, men's desire to preserve their advantaged position. The principle goes beyond the workplace. Attempts to eliminate inequitable outcomes that fail to recognize the dominant group's stake in maintaining its superior status are incomplete (Reskin, 1988). Unless we can forge strategies that promote human equality as a superordinate goal for both sexes and all races, women's disadvantaged status is unlikely to change.

NOTES

We would like to thank Allen Meyer, Laurie Chassen, Nancy Eisenberg, Jody Horn, and Teresa Levitan for feedback on the manuscript. Jan Lameroux, Carolyn Powers, Irina

Feier, and Sharu Kakar provided invaluable assistance in assembling materials and typing references.

1. Kanter (1977) defined women as tokens in a group unless they were more than 15 percent of the members.

REFERENCES

Abeles, R. P. (1976). Relative deprivation, rising expectations, and black militancy. *Journal of Social Issues*, *32*, 119–137.

Alvarez, W. F. (1985). The meaning of maternal employment for mothers and their perceptions of their three-year-old children. *Child Development*, *56*, 350–360.

Amaro, H., & Russo, N. F. (1987). Hispanic women and mental health: An overview of contemporary issues in research and practice. *Psychology of Women Quarterly*, *11*, 393–407.

Amaro, H., Russo, N. F., & Johnson, J. (1987). Family and work predictors of psychological well-being among Hispanic women professionals. *Psychology of Women Quarterly*, *11*, 505–521.

Anderson, M. (1988). *Thinking about women: Sociological prospectives on sex and gender*. New York: Macmillan.

Aneshensel, C. (1986). Marital and employment role-strain, social support, and depression among adult women. In S. Hobfoll (Ed.), *Stress, social support, and women* (pp. 99–114). Washington, DC: Hemisphere.

Antill, J. K., & Cotton, S. (1988). Factors affecting the division of labor in households. *Sex Roles*, *18*, 531–553.

Barnett, R. C., & Baruch, G. K. (1985). Women's involvement in social roles and psychological distress. *Journal of Personality and Social Psychology*, *49*, 135–145.

Barnett, R. C., & Baruch, G. K. (1987). Social roles, gender, and psychological distress. In R. C. Barnett, L. Biener, & G. K. Baruch (Eds.), *Gender and stress* (pp. 122–143). New York: Free Press.

Barrett, N. S. (1984). *Women as workers*. Paper presented at the National Conference on Women, the Economy, and Public Policy, Washington, DC.

Baruch, G. K., & Barnett, R. C. (1987). Role quality and psychological well-being. In F. Crosby (Ed.), *Spouse, parent, worker: On gender and multiple roles* (pp. 63–73). New Haven, CT: Yale University Press.

Baruch, G. K., Biener, L., & Barnett, R. C. (1987). Women and gender in research on work and family stress. *American Psychologist*, *42*, 130–136.

Belle, D. (1990). Poverty and women's mental health. *American Psychologist*, *49*, 384–389.

Benin, M. H., & Agostinelli, J. (1988). Husbands' and wives' satisfaction with the division of labor. *Journal of Marriage and the Family*, *50*, 349–361.

Berardo, D. H., Shehan, C. L., & Leslie, G. R. (1987). A residue of tradition: Jobs, careers and spouses' time in housework. *Journal of Marriage and the Family*, *49*, 381–390.

Berk, S. F. (1985). *The gender factory*. New York: Plenum.

Betz, N., & Fitzgerald, L. (1987). *The career psychology of women*. Orlando, FL: Academic Press.

Betz, N., & Hackett, G. (1981). The relationship of career-related self-efficacy expectations to perceived options in college women and men. *Journal of Counseling Psychology*, *28*, 399–410.

Betz, N., & Hackett, G. (1983). The relationship of mathematics self-efficacy expectations to the selection of science-based college majors. *Journal of Vocational Behavior*, *23*, 329–345.

Betz, N. E., & Hackett, G. (1987). Concept of agency in educational and career counseling. *Journal of Counseling Psychology*, *34*, 299–308.

Blanchard, F., & Crosby, F. (1989). *Affirmative action in perspective*. New York: Springer-Verlag.

Bose, C., & Spitze, G. (Eds.). (1987). *Ingredients for women's employment policy*. Albany: State University of New York Press.

Bridges, J. (1988). Sex differences in occupational performance expectations. *Psychology of Women Quarterly*, *12*, 75–90.

Brown, G. W., Bhrolchain, M. N., & Harris T. (1975). Social class and psychiatric disturbance among women in an urban population. *Sociology*, *9*, 225–254.

Carothers, S. C., & Crull, P. (1984). Contrasting sexual harassment in female- and male-dominated occupations. In K. B. Sacks & D. Remy (Eds.), *My troubles are going to have trouble with me* (pp. 209–228). New Brunswick, NJ: Yale University Press.

Clayton, S., & Crosby, F. J. (1986). Postscript: The nature of connections. *Journal of Social Issues*, *42*(2), 119–137.

Cleary, P. D., & Mechanic, D. (1983). Sex differences in psychological distress among married people. *Journal of Health and Social Behavior*, *24*, 111–121.

Coleman, L., Antonucci, T., & Adelman, P. (1987). Role involvement, gender, and well-being. In F. Crosby (Ed.), *Spouse, parent, worker: On gender and multiple roles* (pp. 138–154). New Haven, CT: Yale University Press.

Cooper, K., Chassin, L., & Zeiss, A. (1985). The relation of sex-role attitudes to the marital satisfaction and personal adjustment of dual-worker couples. *Sex Roles*, *12*, 227–241.

Crohan, S., Antonucci, T., Adelmann, P., & Coleman L. (1989). Job characteristics and well-being at midlife: Ethnic and gender comparisons. *Psychology of Women Quarterly*, *13*, 223–235.

Crosby, F. J. (1982). *Relative deprivation and working women*. New York: Oxford University Press.

Crosby, F. J. (1984a). The denial of personal discrimination. *American Behavioral Scientist*, *27*(3), 371–386.

Crosby, F. J. (1984b). Relative deprivation in organizational settings. *Research in Organizational Behavior*, *6*, 51–93.

Crosby, F. J. (Ed.). (1987). *Spouse, parent, worker: On gender and multiple roles*. New Haven, CT: Yale University Press.

Crosby, F. J., & Clayton, S. (1986). Introduction: The search for connections. *Journal of Social Issues*, *42*(2), 1–10.

Crosby, F. J., & Herek, G. M. (1986). Male sympathy with the situation of women: Does personal experience make a difference? *Journal of Social Issues*, *42*(2), 55–66.

Crosby, F. J., Pufall, A., Snyder, R. C., O'Connell, M., & Whalen, P. (1989). The denial of personal disadvantage among you, me, and all other ostriches. In M. Crawford & M. Gentry (Eds.), *Gender and thought: Psychological perspectives* (pp. 79–99). New York: Springer-Verlag.

Deaux, K. (1984). Blue-collar barriers. *American Behavioral Scientist*, *27*, 287–300.

Denmark, F. I., Shaw, J. S., & Ciali, S. D. (1985). The relationship between sex roles, living arrangements, and the division of household responsibilities. *Sex Roles*, *12*, 617–625.

Eldridge, N. S., & Gilbert, L. A. (1990). Correlates of relationship satisfaction in lesbian couples. *Psychology of Women Quarterly*, *14*, 43–62.

Elman, M. R., & Gilbert, L. A. (1984). Coping strategies for role conflict in married professional women with children. *Family Relations*, *33*, 317–327.

Epstein, C. F. (1988). *Deceptive distinctions: Sex, gender, and the social order*. New Haven, CT: Yale University Press.

Ferber, M. A. (1987). *Women and work, paid and unpaid: A selected, annotated bibliography*. New York: Garland.

Fitzgerald, L., Weitzman, L., Gold, Y., & Omerod, M. (1988). Academic harassment: Sex and denial in scholarly garb. *Psychology of Women Quarterly*, *12*, 223–235.

Fox, M. F., & Hesse-Biber, S. (1984). *Women at work*. New York: Mayfield.

Geis, F. L., Brown, V., Jennings, J., & Corrado-Taylor, D. (1984). Sex vs. status in sex associated stereotypes. *Sex Roles*, *11*, 771–785.

Geis, F. L., Carter, M. R., & Butler, D. J. (1982). *Research on seeing and evaluating people*. Newark, DE: University of Delaware.

Gerson, K. (1985). *Hard choices: How women decide about work, career, and motherhood*. Berkeley: University of California Press.

Golding, J. M. (1990). Division of household labor, strain, and depressive symptoms among Mexican Americans and non-Hispanic whites. *Psychology of Women Quarterly*, *14*, 103–117.

Gore, S., & Mangione, T. W. (1983). Social roles, sex roles, and psychological distress: Additive and interactive models of sex differences. *Journal of Health and Social Behavior*, *24*, 300–312.

Gough, H. C. (1957/1987). *Manual for the California Psychological Inventory*. Palo Alto, CA: Consulting Psychologists Press.

Gove, W. R., Hughes, M., & Styles, C. G. (1983). Does marriage have positive effects on the psychological well-being of the individual? *Journal of Health and Social Behavior*, *24*, 122–131.

Gove, W. R., & Zeiss, C. (1987). Multiple roles and happiness. In F. Crosby (Ed.), *Spouse, parent, worker: On gender and multiple roles* (pp. 125–137). New Haven, CT: Yale University Press.

Grossman, H., & Chester, N. (Eds.). (1990). *The experience and meaning of work in women's lives*. Hillsdsale, NJ: Erlbaum.

Gruber, J. E., & Bjorn, L. (1982). Blue-collar blues: The sexual harassment of women autoworkers. *Work and Occupations*, *9*, 271–298.

Guimond, S., & Dube-Simard, L. (1983). Relative deprivation and the Quebec nationalist movement: The cognition-emotion distinction and the personal-group deprivation issue. *Journal of Personality and Social Psychology*, *44*, 526–535.

Gunter, N. C., & Gunter, B. G. (1990). Domestic division of labor among working couples: Does androgyny make a difference? *Psychology of Women Quarterly*, *14*, 355–370.

Gutek, B., & Larwood, L. (Eds.). (1987). *Women's career development*. Newbury Park, CA: Sage.

Hackett, G., & Betz, N. E. (1981). A self-efficacy approach to the career development of women. *Journal of Vocational Behavior*, *18*, 326–339.

Hale, M., & Kelly, R. M. (Eds.). (1989). *Gender, bureaucracy, and democracy*. Westport, CT: Greenwood Press.

Harlan, A., & Weiss, C. (1981). *Moving up: Women in managerial careers*. Wellesley, MA: Wellesley College Center for Research on Women.

Hefferan, C. (1985). Employee benefits. *Family Economic Review, 1*, 6–14.

Helson, R., Elliot, T., & Leigh, J. (1990). Number and quality of roles: A longitudinal personality view. *Psychology of Women Quarterly, 14*, 83–101.

Izraeli, D. N. (1983). Sex effects or structural effects? An empirical test of Kanter's theory of proportions. *Social Forces, 62*, 153–165.

Jurik, N. (1985). An officer and a lady: Organizational barriers to women working as correctional officers in men's prisons. *Social Problems, 32*, 375–388.

Kahn, W. A., & Crosby, F. (1985). Change and status: Discriminating between attitudes and discriminatory behavior. In L. Larwood, B. A. Gutek, & A.H. Shromberg (Eds.), *Women and work: An annual review*, (Vol. 1, pp. 215–238). Beverly Hills: Sage.

Kandel, D. B., Davies, M., & Ravels, V. (1985). The stressfulness of daily social roles for women: Marital, occupational, and household roles. *Journal of Health and Social Behavior, 26*, 64–78.

Kanter, R. M. (1977). *Men and women of the corporation*. New York: Basic Books.

Kelly, R. M., & Bayes, J. (1988). *Comparable worth, pay equity, and public policy*. Westport, CT: Greenwood Press.

Kessler, R. C. (1982). A disaggregation of the relationships between socioeconomic status and psychological distress. *American Sociological Review, 47*, 752–764.

Kessler, R., & McRae, J. A., Jr. (1982). The effect of wives' employment on the mental health of married men and women. *American Sociological Review, 47*, 216–227.

Kessler, R., & Neighbors, H. (1986). A new perspective on the relationships among race, social class, and psychological distress. *Journal of Health and Social Behavior, 27*, 107–115.

Kollock, P., Blumstein, P., & Schwartz, P. (1985). Sex and power in interaction: Conversational privileges and duties. *American Sociological Review, 50*, 34–46.

Larwood, L., Szwajkowski, E., & Rose, S. (1988). Sex and race discrimination resulting from manager-client relationships: Applying the rational bias theory of managerial discrimination. *Sex Roles, 8*, 9–29.

Lee, M. D., & Kanungo, R. N. (Eds.). (1984). *Management of work and personal life: Problems and opportunities*. New York: Praeger.

Lent, R. W., Brown, S. D., & Larkin, K. C. (1986). Self-efficacy in the prediction of academic performance and perceived career options. *Journal of Counseling Psychology, 33*, 265–269.

Lieberson, S. (1985). *Making it count*. Berkeley: University of California Press.

Lockheed, M. E., & Hall, K. P. (1976). Conceptualizing sex as a status characteristic: Applications to leadership training strategies. *Journal of Social Issues, 32*, 111–124.

Lord, C. G., & Saenz, D. S. (1985). Memory deficits and memory surfeits: Differential cognitive consequences of tokenism for tokens and observers. *Journal of Personality and Social Psychology, 49*, 918–926.

Lord, C. G., Saenz, D. S., & Godfrey, D. K. (1987). Effects of perceived scrutiny on participant memory for social interactions. *Journal of Experimental Social Psychology, 23*, 498–517.

Lott, B. (1985). The devaluation of women's competence. *Journal of Social Issues, 41*, 43–60.

Major, B. (1987). Gender, justice and the psychology of entitlement. In P. Shaver & C. Hendrick (Eds.), *Sex and gender, Review of personality and social psychology* (pp. 124–148). Newbury Park, CA: Sage.

Major, B., & Konar, E. (1984). An investigation of sex differences in pay expectations and their possible causes. *Academy of Management Journal, 27*, 777–792.

Major, B., McFarlin, D., & Gagnon, D. (1984). Overworked and underpaid: On the nature of gender differences in personal entitlement. *Journal of Personality and Social Psychology, 47*, 1399–1412.

Major, B., Vanderslice, V., & McFarlin, D. B. (1984). Effects of pay expected on pay received: The confirmatory nature of initial expectations. *Journal of Applied Psychology, 14*, 399–412.

Martin, B. A. (1989). Gender differences in salary expectations when current salary information is provided. *Psychology of Women Quarterly, 13*, 87–96.

McBride, A. B. (1988). Mental effects of women's roles. *Image: Journal of Nursing Scholarship, 20*, 41–47.

McBride, A. B. (1990). Mental health effects of women's multiple roles. *American Psychologist, 45*, 381–384.

McKenry, M. C., Hamdorf, K. G., Walthers, C. M., & Murray, C. I. (1985). Family and job influence on role satisfaction of employed rural mothers. *Psychology of Women Quarterly, 9*, 242–257.

National Committee on Pay Equity. (1987). *Pay equity: An issue of race, ethnicity, and sex.* Washington, DC: U.S. Government Printing Office.

Nevill, D., & Schlecker, D. (1988). The relation of self-efficacy and assertiveness to willingness to engage in traditional/nontraditional career activities. *Psychology of Women Quarterly, 12*, 91–98.

O'Farrell, B. (1982). Women and non-traditional blue-collar jobs in the 1980's: An overview. In P. A. Wallace (Ed.), *Women in the workplace* (pp. 135–165). Boston: Auburn House.

O'Farrell, B., & Harlan, S. (1982). Craftsworkers and clerks: The effect of male co-worker hostility and women's satisfaction with non-traditional jobs. *Social Problems, 29*, 253–265.

Ott, M. E. (1989). Effects of the male-female ratio at work: Policewomen and male nurses. *Psychology of Women Quarterly, 13*, 41–57.

Parry, G. (1986). Paid employment, life events, social support, and mental health in working-class mothers. *Journal of Health and Social Behavior, 27*, 193–208.

Pearlin, L. I., & Johnson, J. (1977). Marital status, life-strains and depression. *American Sociological Review, 42*, 704–715.

Perman, L., & Stevens, L. (1989). Industrial segregation and the gender distribution of fringe benefits. *Gender and Society, 3*, 388–404.

Pheterson, G. L., Kiesler, S. B., & Goldberg, P. A. (1971). The evaluation of the performance of women as a function of their sex, achievement, and personal history. *Journal of Personality and Social Psychology, 19*, 114–118.

Pietromonaco, P. R., Manis, J., & Frohardt, L. K. (1986). Psychological consequences of multiple social roles. *Psychology of Women Quarterly, 10*, 373–381.

Pleck, J. H. (1985). *Working wives/working husbands.* Beverly Hills: Sage.

Radloff, L. S. (1975). Sex difference in depression: Occupational and marital status. *Sex Roles*, *1*, 249–265.

Rawlings, S. (1989). Single parents and their children. In U. S. Bureau of the Census, *Studies in marriage and the family* (Current population reports, series P-23, No. 162). Washington, DC: U.S. Government Printing Office.

Reid, P., & Comas-Diaz, L. (1990). Gender and ethnicity: Perspectives on dual status. *Sex Roles*, *22*, 397–407.

Reskin, B. (1988). Bringing the men back in: Sex differentiation and the devaluation of women's work. *Gender and Society*, *2*, 58–81.

Rexroat, C., & Shehan, C. (1987). The family life cycle and spouses' time in housework. *Journal of Marriage and the Family*, *49*, 737–750.

Rix, S. E. (Ed.). (1990). *The American woman 1990–91: A status report*. New York: W. W. Norton.

Rose, S., & Larwood, L. (Eds.). (1988). *Women's careers: Pathways and pitfalls*. New York: Praeger.

Ross, C. E., & Huber, J. (1985). Hardship and depression. *Journal of Health and Social Behavior*, *26*, 312–327.

Ross, C. E., & Mirowsky, J. (1988). Child care and emotional adjustment to wives' employment. *Journal of Health and Social Behavior*, *29*, 127–138.

Ross, C. E., Mirowsky, J., & Huber, J. (1983). Dividing work, sharing work, and in-between: Marriage patterns and depression. *American Sociological Review*, *48*, 809–823.

Russo, N. F., Amaro, H., & Winter, M. (1987). The use of inpatient mental health services by Hispanic women. *Psychology of Women Quarterly*, *11*, 427–442.

Russo, N. F., Dantico, M., & Meyer, D. A. (1986). American women and work: Current status and future prospects. In J. Monk & A. Schlegal (Eds.), *Women in the Arizona economy* (pp. 1–36). Tuscon, AZ: Southwest Institute for Research on Women.

Russo, N. F., Kelly, R. M., & Deacon, M. (1990). *Gender and success-related attributions: Beyond individualistic conceptions of achievement*. Unpublished manuscript.

Russo, N. F., & Olmedo, E. L. (1983). Women's utilization of outpatient psychiatric services: Some emerging priorities for rehabilitation psychologists. *Rehabilitation Psychology*, *28*(3), 141–155.

Russo, N. F., & Sobel, S. B. (1981). Sex differences in the utilization of mental health facilities. *Professional Psychology*, *12*, 7–19.

Sacks, K. (1983). In B. Haber (Ed.), *The woman's annual: 1982–1983* (pp. 263–283). Boston: G. K. Hall.

Saluter, A. (1989). Singleness in america. In U.S. Bureau of the Census, *Studies in marriage and the family* (Current population reports, series P-23, No. 162). Washington, DC: U.S. Government Printing Office.

Schwartzberg, N. S., & Dytell, R. S. (1988). Family stress and psychological well-being among employed and nonemployed mothers. In E. Goldsmith (Ed.), *Journal of Social Behavior and Personality* [Special issue: Work and family: Theory, research, and applications], *3*(4), 175–190.

Segura, D. (1989). Chicana and Mexican immigrant women at work: The impact of class, race, and gender on occupational mobility. *Gender and Society*, *3*(1), 37–52.

Smith, T. W. (1985). Working wives and women's rights: The connection between the employment status of wives and feminist attitudes of husbands. *Sex Roles, 12,* 501–508.

Snodgrass, S. E. (1985). Women's intuition: The effects of subordinate role on interpersonal sensitivity. *Journal of Personality and Social Psychology, 49,* 146–155.

Snyder, M., & Swann, W. B., Jr. (1976). When actions reflect attitudes: The politics of impression management. *Journal of Personality and Social Psychology, 34,* 1034–1042.

Spangler, E., Gordon, M. A., & Pipkin, R. M. (1978). Token women: An empirical test of Kanter's hypothesis. *American Journal of Sociology, 84,* 160–170.

Staples, R. (1987). Social structure in black female life. *Journal of Black Studies, 17,* 267–286.

Statham, A., Miller, E., & Mauksch, H. (Eds.). (1988). *The worth of women's work.* Albany: State University of New York Press.

Steil, J., & Turetsky, B. (1987). Marital influence levels and symptomatology among wives. In F. Crosby (Ed.), *Relative deprivation and working women* (pp. 74–90). New York: Oxford University Press.

Stewart, A. J., & Malley, J. E. (1987). Role combination in women: Mitigating agency and communion. In F. J. Crosby (Ed.), *Spouse, parent, worker: On gender and multiple roles* (pp. 44–62). New Haven, CT: Yale University Press.

Stromberg, A. H., & Harkess, S. (1988). *Women working.* Mountain View, CA: Mayfield.

Swerdlow, M. (1989). Men's accommodations to women entering a nontraditional occupation: A case of rapid transit operatives. *Gender and Society, 3,* 373–387.

Swim, J., Borgida, E., & Maruyama, G. (1989). Joan McKay versus John McKay: Do gender stereotypes bias evaluations? *Psychological Bulletin, 105,* 409–429.

Thoits, P. A. (1986). Multiple identities: Examining gender and marital status differences in distress. *American Sociological Review, 51,* 259–272.

Thoits, P. A. (1987a). Gender and marital status differences in control and distress: Common stress versus unique stress explanations. *Journal of Health and Social Behavior, 28,* 7–22.

Thoits, P. A. (1987b). Negotiating roles. In F. J. Crosby (Ed.), *Spouse, parent, worker: On gender and multiple roles* (pp. 11–22). New Haven, CT: Yale University Press.

Thompson, M. E. (1981). Sex differences: Differential access to power or sex role socialization? *Sex Roles, 7,* 413–424.

Treiman, D. J., & Roos, P. A. (1983). Sex and earnings in industrial society: A nine-nation comparison. *American Journal of Sociology, 89,* 612–650.

U.S. Bureau of the Census. (1989a). *Household and family characteristics: March 88* (Current population reports, series P-20, No. 162). Washington, DC: U.S. Government Printing Office.

U.S. Bureau of the Census. (1989b). *Studies in marriage and the family* (Current Population Reports, Series P-23, No. 162). Washington, DC: U.S. Government Printing Office.

U.S. Bureau of the Census. (1990a). *Statistical abstract of the United States: 1990* (110th ed.). Washington, DC: U.S. Government Printing Office.

U. S. Bureau of the Census. (1990b). *Who's minding the kids: Child care arrangements, 1986–87* (Household and Economic Studies, Current population reports, series P-70, No. 20). Washington, DC: U. S. Government Printing Office.

U.S. Commission on Civil Rights. (1990). *The economic status of black women: An exploratory investigation* (Staff Report). Washington, DC: U.S. Government Printing Office.

VanMeter, M. J., & Agronow, S. J. (1982). The stress of multiple roles: The case for role strain among married college women. *Family Relations, 33,* 131–138.

Verbrugge, L. M. (1987). Role responsibilities, role burdens and physical health. In F. J. Crosby (Ed.), *Spouse, parent, worker: On gender and multiple roles* (pp. 154–166). New Haven, CT: Yale University Press.

Warren, L. W., & McEachren, L. (1983). Psychosocial correlates of depressive symptomatology in adult women. *Journal of Abnormal Psychology, 92*(2), 151–160.

Warren, L. W., & McEachren, L. (1985). Derived identity and depressive symptomatology in women differing in marital and employment status. *Psychology of Women Quarterly, 9,* 133–144.

Zanna, M. P., Crosby, F., & Loewenstein, G. (1987). Male reference groups and discontent among female professionals. In B. Gutek & L. Larwood (Eds.), *Women's career development* (pp. 28–41). Newbury Park, CA: Sage.

Zinn, M. B. (1989). Family, feminism, and race in America. *Gender and Society, 4,* 68–82.

Epilogue

Bernice Lott

The theoretical and research literature on the psychology of women that continues to grow and enrich our discipline is a source of great pride to those of us who have participated in its development. Each year we publish a large number of papers in specialized journals like *The Psychology of Women Quarterly* and *Sex Roles*, as well as in journals dealing with such broad areas of concern as social psychology, personality, and child development. With this work, we have succeeded, like our counterparts in other fields of study, in making mainstream psychology sit up and take notice. We have raised cogent and sophisticated arguments in our critiques of traditional psychological assumptions, theories, questions, topics, and methods. We have been critical of previous work in psychology that either ignored women entirely and did not understand the potent influence of gender on human behavior, or trivialized important questions about gender by simply searching out ''sex differences.''

At the same time, we have presented an alternative agenda for research. Our feminist agenda asks new questions, proposes new relationships among personal and social variables, focuses on women's lives and experiences, is sensitive to the implications of our research for social policy and social change, and assumes that science is always done in a cultural/historical/political context.

This *Handbook* makes a valuable contribution to the advancement of the feminist agenda by providing students and professionals—teachers, researchers, and practitioners—with integrative summaries and analyses of the wide strands of theory and data that currently describe the psychology of women. It offers chapters on our history and research methods, on sexism and stereotypes, on developmental periods in women's lives, on health, relationships, victimization, achievement, and work. Readers of this volume have attended to the major issues studied and discussed by feminist psychologists during the past two or three decades.

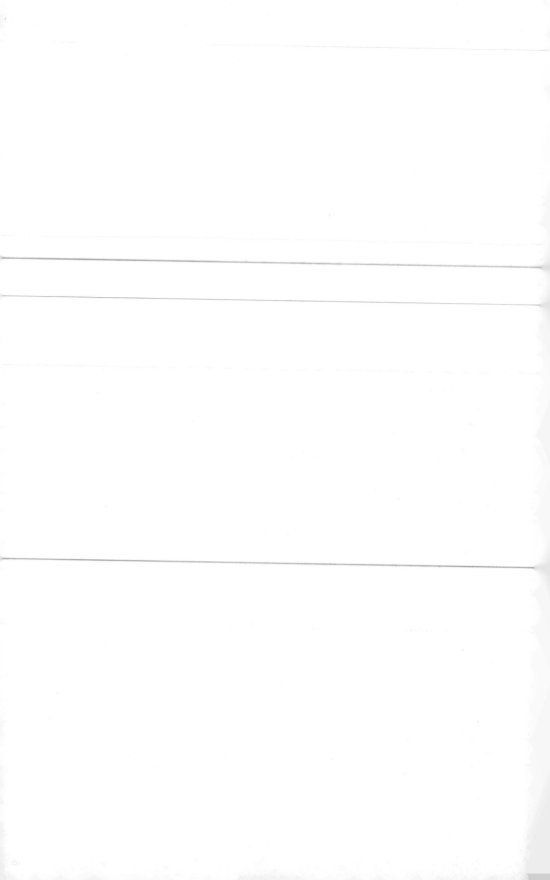

Bibliographical Essay

The following guide to literature on the psychology of women is not exhaustive. It is meant to direct the reader to some of the most useful sources of further information. Additional citations on more particular topics and studies are given in the extensive chapter references.

A sense of the history of the psychology of women can be gained by consulting several works. F. L. Denmark (1977), "The Psychology of Women: An Overview of an Emerging Field," *Personality and Social Psychology Bulletin, 3,* 356–367, offers a useful glance at the history of the field through the late 1970s. Other related surveys of the field include M. Mednick (1976), "Some Thoughts on the Psychology of Women: Selected Topics," *Annual Review of Psychology, 26,* 1–18; and J. Sherman and F. L. Denmark (1978), *The Psychology of Women: Future Directions of Research,* New York: Psychological Dimensions. More recent works include M. R. Walsh (Ed.), (1987), *The Psychology of Women: Ongoing Debates,* New Haven, CT: Yale University Press, which presents contrasting viewpoints on 14 significant issues; and A. Campbell (Ed.), (1989), *The Opposite Sex,* Topsfield, MA: Salem House, which offers a cross-cultural, interdisciplinary study of women and men from conception to adulthood. For a good introduction to the history of women in psychology, see A. N. O'Connell and N. F. Russo (Eds.), (1990), *Women in Psychology: A Bio-Bibliographic Sourcebook,* Westport, CT: Greenwood Press, which assesses the careers and contributions of some of the most influential women psychologists. Additional references with regard to the history of the psychology of women include N. F. Russo and F. L. Denmark (1987), "Contributions of Women to Psychology," *Annual Review of Psychology, 38,* 279–298; and A. N. O'Connell and N. F. Russo (Eds.), (1991), *Women's Heritage in Psychology: Origins, Development, & Future Directions,* New York: Cambridge University Press (Special centennial issue, *Psychology of Women Quarterly,* Whole No. 4).

Several works offer especially valuable insights on feminism and psychological research methods. F. Denmark, N. F. Russo, I. H. Frieze, and J. A. Sechzer (1988), "Guidelines for Avoiding Sexism in Psychological Research: A Report of the APA Ad Hoc Committee on Nonsexist Research," *American Psychologist, 43,* 582–585, briefly reflects the profession's interest in avoiding sexism in research methodology. S. Harding (Ed.), (1987), *Feminism and Methodology,* Bloomington: Indiana University Press; and J. Wirtenberg and B. L. Richardson (Eds.), (1983), *Methodological Issues in Sex Roles and Social Change,* New York: Praeger, are valuable collections of material on feminism and methodology. For a good overview of meta-analyses and the psychology of women, the reader should consult J. S. Hyde and M. C. Linn (Eds.), (1986), *The Psychology of Gender: Advances Through Meta-Analysis,* Baltimore: Johns Hopkins University Press.

Much information is available on society's view of women. A. H. Eagly (1987), *Sex Differences in Social Behavior: A Social-Role Interpretation,* Hillsdale, NJ: Erlbaum, is a good introduction to gender roles and stereotypes. For an international perspective on women and on gender roles, consult L. L. Adler (Ed.), (1991), *Women: In Cross-Cultural Perspective,* New York: Praeger; and L. L. Adler (Ed.), (in press), *International Handbook on Gender Roles,* Westport, CT: Greenwood Press. For a survey of the many instruments used to assess gender roles, the reader should consult C. A. Beere (1990), *Gender Roles: A Handbook of Tests and Measures,* Westport, CT: Greenwood Press. For an interesting cross-cultural study, see J. E. Williams and D. L. Best (1982), *Measuring Sex Stereotypes: A Thirty-Nation Study,* Beverly Hills, CA: Sage. For an introduction to sexism, see N. V. Benokraitis and J. R. Feagin (1986), *Modern Sexism: Blatant, Subtle, and Covert Discrimination,* Englewood Cliffs, NJ: Prentice-Hall. Also of interest is B. B. Hess and M. M. Ferree (Eds.), (1987), *Analyzing Gender,* Newbury Park, CA: Sage.

The development of women across the life span has also received a good deal of attention. For a useful introduction to the development of women from conception to adolescence, the reader should consult J. Gunn and A. Petersen (Eds.), (1984), *Girls at Puberty: Biological, Psychological, and Social Perspective,* New York: Plenum; J. Adelson (Ed.), (1980), *Handbook of Adolescent Psychology,* New York: Wiley; and P. Mussen, J. Conger, and J. Kagan (1963), *Child Development and Personality,* New York: Harper and Row. For an extensive overview of sources on women in later life, see J. M. Coyle (1989), *Women and Aging: A Selected, Annotated Bibliography,* Westport, CT: Greenwood Press. For a more detailed examination of older women, see J. E. Birren and K. W. Schaie (Eds.), (1985), *Handbook of the Psychology of Aging* (2nd ed.), New York: Van Nostrand Reinhold. For information on middle-aged women, see J. Giele (Ed.), (1982), *Women in the Middle Years: Current Knowledge and Directions for Research and Policy,* New York: Wiley-Interscience; and G. Baruch and J. Brooks-Gunn (Eds.), (1984), *Women in Mid-Life,* New York: Plenum.

There are many valuable works on the physical and mental health of women. Aside from the many journal articles, the reader should consult B. Ehrenreich and D. English (Eds.), (1977), *Seizing Our Bodies,* New York: Random House; E. Fee (Ed.), (1983), *Women and Health: The Politics of Sex in Medicine,* Farmingdale, New York: Baywood; C. B. Travis (1988), *Women and Health Psychology: Mental Health Issues,* and (1988), *Women and Health Psychology: Biomedical Issues,* Hillsdale, NJ: Erlbaum; and K. Weiss (Ed.), (1984), *Women's Health Care: A Guide to Alternatives,* Reston, VA: Reston, Prentice-Hall. For further information on women's mental health issues, see L. S. Brown and M. P. Root (Eds.), (1990), *Diversity and Complexity in Feminist Therapy*, New York: Harworth Press; and E. McGrath, G. P. Keita, B. R. Strickland, and N. F. Russo (1990), *Women and Depression: Risk Factors and Treatment Issues*, Washington, DC: American Psychological Association. For further information on menstruation, see S. Golub (Ed.), (1985), *Lifting the Curse of Menstruation*, New York: Harrington Park Press; D. Asso (1983), *Premenstrual Syndrome*, New York: Plenum; R. C. Friedman (Ed.), (1982), *Behavior and the Menstrual Cycle*, New York: Marcel Dekker; L. R. Gannon (1985), *Menstrual Disorders and Menopause: Biological, Psychological, and Cultural Research*, New York: Praeger; and P.M.S. O'Brien (1987), *Premenstrual Syndrome*, Oxford: Blackwell Scientific. For further reading on pregnancy, see J. W. Ballow (1978), *The Psychology of Pregnancy: Reconciliation and Resolution*, Lexington, MA: Lexington Books; A. D. Colman and L. L. Colman (1971), *Pregnancy: The Psychological Experience*, New York: Herder and Herder; R. P. Lederman (1984), *Psychosocial Adaptation in Pregnancy*, Englewood Cliffs, NJ: Prentice-Hall; and L. N. Sherwin (1987), *Psychosocial Dimensions of the Pregnant Family*, New York: Springer.

The victimization of women is an important area for further research. Among the many significant books on rape are S. S. Ageton (1983), *Sexual Assault Among Adolescents*, Lexington, MA: Lexington Books; A. W. Burgess (Ed.), (1988), *Rape and Sexual Assault*, New York: Garland; M. P. Koss and M. R. Harvey (1987), *The Rape Victim: Clinical and Community Approaches to Treatment*, Lexington, MA: Stephen Green Press; and D.E.H. Russell (1984), *Sexual Exploitation: Rape, Child Sexual Abuse, and Workplace Harassment*, Beverly Hills, CA: Sage. For more information on battered women, see K. Yllo and M. Bograd (Eds.), (1988), *Feminist Perspectives on Wife Abuse*, Beverly Hills, CA: Sage; A. R. Roberts (Ed.), (1984), *Battered Women and Their Families*, New York: Springer; D. Finkelhor, R. J. Gelles, G. T. Hotaling, and M. A. Straus (Eds.), (1983), *The Dark Side of Families: Current Family Violence Research*, Beverly Hills, CA: Sage; E. Gondolf and E. R. Fisher (1988), *Battered Women as Survivors: An Alternative to Treating Learned Helplessness*, Lexington, MA: Lexington Books; and M. D. Pagelow (1984), *Family Violence*, New York: Praeger. For more on sexual harassment in academia and the workplace, see N. E. Betz and L. F. Fitzgerald (1987), *The Career Psychology of Women*, New York: Academic Press; and B. Gutek (1985), *Sex and the Workplace*, San Francisco: Jossey-Bass.

Some of the most important issues related to the psychology of women concern the role of women in the workplace. Among the many valuable works on this topic are: M. T. Mednick, S. S. Tangri, and L. W. Hoffman (1975), *Women and Achievement: Social and Motivational Analyses*, New York: John Wiley & Sons; F. Crosby (Ed.), (1987), *Spouse, Parent, Worker: On Gender and Multiple Roles*, New Haven, CT: Yale University Press; N. Betz and L. Fitzgerald (1987), *The Career Psychology of Women*, New York: Academic Press; F. Blanchard and F. Crosby (1989), *Affirmative Action in Perspective*, New York: Springer; K. Gerson (1985), *Hard Choices: How Women Decide about Work, Career, and Motherhood*, Berkeley: University of California Press; H. Grossman and N. Chester (Eds.), (1990), *The Experience and Meaning of Work in Women's Lives*, Hillsdale, NJ: Erlbaum; B. Gutek and L. Larwood (Eds.), (1987), *Women's Career Development*, Newbury Park, CA: Sage; P. A. Wallace (Ed.), (1982), *Women in the Workplace*, Westport, CT: Auburn House; and S. Rose and L. Larwood (Eds.), (1988), *Women's Careers: Pathways and Pitfalls*, New York: Praeger.

RESOURCES ON TEACHING THE PSYCHOLOGY OF WOMEN COURSE

Bronstein, P., & Quina, K. (Eds.). (1988). *Teaching the psychology of people: Readings for gender and sociocultural awareness*. Washington, DC: American Psychological Association.

Brown, A., Goodwin, B. J., Hall, B. A., & Jackson-Lowman, H. (1985). A review of psychology of women textbooks: Focus on the Afro-American women. *Psychology of Women Quarterly, 9*, 29–38.

DeFour, D. C., & Paludi, M. A. (1991). Integrating the scholarship on ethnicity into the psychology of women course. *Teaching of Psychology, 18*, 85–90.

Denmark, F. L. (1983). Integrating the psychology of women into introductory psychology. In C. J. Scherere & A. R. Rogers (Eds.), *The G. Stanley Hall Lecture Series* (vol. 3, pp. 37–71). Washington, DC: American Psychological Association.

Golub, S., & Freedman, R. J. (1987). *Psychology of women: Resources for a core curriculum*. New York: Garland.

Lord, S. B. (1982). Teaching the psychology of women: Examination of a teaching-learning model. *Psychology of Women Quarterly, 7*, 71–80.

Matlin, M. (1989). Teaching psychology of women: A survey of instructors. *Psychology of Women Quarterly, 13*, 245–261.

Paludi, M. A. (1986). Teaching the psychology of gender roles: Some life-stage considerations. *Teaching of Psychology, 13*, 133–138.

Paludi, M. A. (1990). *Exploring/Teaching the psychology of women: A manual of resources*. Albany, NY: SUNY Press.

Paludi, M. A. (in press). Placing women psychologists in the psychology of women course. *Teaching of Psychology*.

Paludi, M. A. (in press). Teaching the psychology of women course from a life-cycle developmental perspective. *Teaching of Psychology*.

Richardson, M. S. (1982). Sources of tension in teaching the psychology of women. *Psychology of Women Quarterly, 7*, 45–54.

Riger, S. (1978). A technique for teaching the psychology of women: Content analysis. *Teaching of Psychology, 5*, 221–223.

Riger, S. (1979). On teaching the psychology of women. *Teaching of Psychology, 6*, 113–114.

Russo, N. F. (1982). Psychology of women: Analysis of the faculty and courses of an emerging field. *Psychology of Women Quarterly, 7*, 18–31.

Sargent, A. G. (1985). *Beyond sex roles*. New York: West.

Sholley, B. (1986). Value of book discussions in a psychology of women course. *Teaching of Psychology, 13*, 151–153.

Unger, R. K. (1982). Advocacy versus scholarship revisited: Issues in the psychology of women. *Psychology of Women Quarterly, 7*, 5–17.

Vedouato, S., & Vaughter, R. (1980). Psychology of women courses changing sexist and sex-typed attitudes. *Psychology of Women Quarterly, 4*, 587–591.

Walsh, M. R. (1985). The psychology of women course: A continuing catalyst for change. *Teaching of Psychology, 12*, 198–202.

RESOURCES ON THE PSYCHOLOGY OF WOMEN

Bardwick, J. (1970). *Feminine personality and conflict.* Belmont, CA: Brooks/Cole.

Bardwick, J. (1971). *Psychology of women: A study of biocultural conflicts.* New York: Harper & Row.

Bardwick, J. (Ed.). (1972). *Readings on the psychology of the woman.* New York: Harper & Row.

Cox, S. (Ed.). (1976). *Female psychology: The emerging self.* (2d ed.). Chicago: St. Martin's Press.

Cox, S. (Ed.). (1981). *Female psychology: The emerging self.* New York: St. Martin's Press.

Deaux, K. (1976). *The behavior of women and men.* Monterey, CA: Brooks/Cole.

Donelson, E., & Gullahorn, J. (1977). *Women: A psychological perspective.* New York: Wiley.

Freeman, J. (Ed.). (1975). *Women: A feminist perspective.* Palo Alto, CA: Mayfield.

Frieze, I., Parsons, J., Johnson, P., Ruble, D., & Zellman, G. (1978). *Women and sex roles: A social psychological perspective.* New York: Norton.

Gullahorn, J. E. (1979). *Psychology and women: In transition.* Washington, DC: Winston & Sons.

Hyde, J. S. (1985). *Half the human experience: The psychology of women* (3rd ed.). Lexington, MA: Heath.

Hyde, J. S. (1991). *Half the human experience.* (4th ed.). Lexington, MA: Heath.

Lott, B. (1987). *Women's lives: Themes and variations in gender learning.* Monterey, CA: Brooks/Cole.

Matlin, M. (1987). *The psychology of women.* New York: Holt.

Miller, J. B. (1976). *Toward a new psychology of women.* Boston: Beacon.

O'Leary, V. (1977). *Toward understanding women.* Monterey, CA: Brooks/Cole.

O'Leary, V., Wallston, B., & Unger, R. (Eds). (1985). *Women, gender, and social psychology.* Hillsdale, NJ: Erlbaum.

Paludi, M. A. (1992). *The psychology of women.* Dubuque, IA: Brown.

Sherman, J. (1971). *On the psychology of women: A survey of empirical studies.* Springfield, IL: Thomas.

Sherman, J., & Denmark, F. L. (Eds.). (1978). *The psychology of women: Future directions in research.* New York: Psychological Dimensions.

Tavris, C. (Ed.). (1973). *The female experience.* Del Mar, CA: Communications Research Machines.

Tavris, C., & Wade, C. (1984). *The longest war: Sex differences in perspective.* New York: Harcourt Brace Jovanovich.

Unger, R. K. (1979). *Female and male: Psychological perspectives.* New York: Harper and Row Publishers.

Unger, R. K., & Crawford, M. (1982). *Women & gender: A feminist psychology.* New York: McGraw-Hill.

Unger, R. K., & Denmark, F. L. (Eds.). (1975). *Woman: Dependent or independent variable?* New York: Psychological Dimensions.

Wainrib, B. R. (Ed.). (1992). *Gender issues across the life cycle.* New York: Springer.

Walsh, M. R. (Ed.). (1987). *The psychology of women: Ongoing debates.* New Haven, CT: Yale University Press.

Williams, J. (1987). *Psychology of women: Behavior in a biosocial context*. New York: Norton.

Williams, J. H. (Ed.). (1979). *Psychology of women: Selected readings*. New York: Norton.

Index

About the Editors and Contributors

LEONORE LOEB ADLER received her Ph.D. in Experimental Social Psychology from Adelphi University. She is the Director of the Institute for Cross-Cultural and Cross-Ethnic Studies and a Professor in the Department of Psychology at Molloy College, Rockville Centre, New York. Dr. Adler is active in many professional organizations, and most recently was elected to the American Psychological Association's Committee on International Relations in Psychology. She has received both the "Kurt Lewin Award" and the "Wilhelm Wundt Award" from different Divisions of the New York State Psychological Association, the "Distinguished Contributions of the Decade Award" from the International Organization for the Study of Group Tensions, and the "Certificate of Recognition" from the International Council of Psychologists, as well as the "President's Medal" from Molloy College. Dr. Adler has published over 70 professional papers and chapters, and is the author, editor, or co-editor of eleven books.

NANCY BETZ is a Professor in the Department of Psychology at the Ohio State University. She received her Ph.D. in Psychology from the University of Minnesota in 1976. She is the author of numerous articles and chapters on the topic of women's career development—her recent research has focused on applications of self-efficacy theory to women's career development, issues related to the underrepresentation of women and minorities in the sciences and engineering, and the career adjustment of academic women. She has authored two books, *Tests and Assessment* (with W. B. Walsh, 1987) and *The Career Psychology of*

Women (with Louise F. Fitzgerald, 1987). She recently finished a six-year term as Editor of the *Journal of Vocational Behavior*.

ANN BOGGIANO is currently Associate Professor of Psychology at the University of Colorado, Boulder. She obtained her Ph.D. from Princeton University for which she received the Outstanding Dissertation Award in Social Psychology. Her research focuses on factors influencing the development of maladaptive achievement behaviors. She is particularly interested in gender differences in achievement patterns.

ANGELA BROWNE is a social psychologist with particular expertise in the area of violence within families. Over the past 12 years, she has conducted research on patterns of physical assault and threat in couple relationships, the effects of witnessing family violence on children, and long-term effects of physical and sexual assault on women and child victims. During the 1980s, she conducted research on homicides in which battered women kill their abusers in self-defense, and authored the book *When Battered Women Kill* (1987). Dr. Browne is in the Public Sector Division of the Department of Psychiatry at the University of Massachusetts Medical Center. As a part of her work there, she spends one week each month on-grounds as Consulting Psychologist at Bedford Hills maximum security prison for women in New York State. She is also liaison to nine residential family shelters in the Worcester area. Angela recently prepared the American Medical Association's policy statement on ''Violence Against Women,'' and has testified for several committees of the U.S. Senate on related topics.

KAY DEAUX is Professor of Psychology and Women's Studies at the Graduate School and University Center of the City University of New York. Research topics include gender stereotypes, causal attributions for performance, and gender identity. She is the author of *The Behavior of Women and Men* and *Women of Steel*.

FLORENCE L. DENMARK received her Ph.D. in Social Psychology from the University of Pennsylvania. She was the President of the American Psychological Association, 1980–1981; the Eastern Psychological Association, 1985–1986; the New York State Psychological Association, 1972–1973; the International Council of Psychologists, 1989–1990; and Psi Chi, the National Honor Society in Psychology, 1978–1980. Dr. Denmark has been the Thomas Hunter Professor of Psychology at Hunter College of the City University of New York, and at present is the Robert Scott Pace Professor of Psychology at Pace University, where she is the Chair of the Department of Psychology. As one of the founding members of APA's Division of the Psychology of Women, Denmark's most significant research has focused on women and their contributions to psychology. Dr. Denmark is the recipient of numerous awards including the American Psychological

Association's Distinguished Contributions to Education and Training (1987) and, most recently, APA's Division 35's (Psychology of Women) Carolyn Wood Sherif Award (1991), and APA's Distinguished Contributions to Psychology in the Public Interest/Senior Career Award (1992).

CLAIRE ETAUGH is Professor of Psychology and Dean of the College of Liberal Arts and Sciences at Bradley University. She has published extensively on perceptions of women, effects of maternal employment on children, and attitudes toward employed mothers. Currently she is writing a textbook on child development.

LINDA C. FERNANDEZ is a recent graduate from Pace University's School/ Community psychology doctoral program. Her research interests include women's contributions to the history of psychology, stepfamilies, ethnic minority issues, and child psychotherapy. She is currently a psychologist with Federated Employment Guidance Service.

LOUISE F. FITZGERALD is Associate Professor of Educational Psychology and Psychology at the University of Illinois at Champaign-Urbana. She received her graduate degrees in Psychology from the Ohio State University and has published extensively on the career development of women. For the last 10 years she has been conducting research on sexual harassment in academia and the workplace, on which she has published numerous articles and chapters. She is the co-author with Nancy Betz of *The Career Psychology of Women*, and was recently named a Fellow of the Institute for the Study of Cultural Values and Ethics at the University of Illinois, where she also chairs the Chancellor's Committee on the Status of Women.

IRENE HANSON FRIEZE is Professor of Psychology and Women's Studies at the University of Pittsburgh. She has had a long-time interest in violence in marriage and is now studying violence in dating relationships. Other gender-related interests include professional women and achievement. In addition to many journal articles, she is co-author of *Women and Sex Roles: A Social-Psychological Perspective*.

LAURIE A. FROST is a doctoral candidate in Clinical Psychology at the University of Wisconsin–Madison. She received her B.A. in Psychology and Social Relations from Harvard University and her M.S. in Clinical Psychology from the University of Wisconsin–Madison. She has co-authored several papers on such diverse topics as psychosis proneness, the neuropsychological correlates of early adolescent psychopathology, and gender differences in mathematics performance, attitudes, and affect.

BETH L. GREEN is a graduate student in Social Psychology at Arizona State University and is interested in applications of social-psychological phenomena to health issues, including bulimia.

JANET SHIBLEY HYDE is Professor of Psychology and Women's Studies at the University of Wisconsin. Her research over the last decade has focused on meta-analyses of psychological gender differences. Her newest research is on psychological aspects of maternity leave. She is the author of *Half the Human Experience: The Psychology of Women* and *Understanding Human Sexuality*.

PHYLLIS A. KATZ is currently Director of the Institute for Research on Social Problems in Boulder, Colorado. Her research has focused on children's gender-role development and racial attitude acquisition. She is Founding Editor of *Sex Roles: A Journal of Research*, and Editor-Elect of the *Journal of Social Issues*. Her publications include many theoretical chapters and empirical papers on female identity, personality formation, how children develop race and gender stereotypes, and how to modify such behavior.

MARY KITE received her Ph.D. from Purdue University in 1987 and has been Assistant Professor of the Department of Psychological Science at Ball State University since that time. Her research focuses on stereotyping and prejudice; representative articles have appeared in *Journal of Personality and Social Psychology*, *Personality and Social Psychology Bulletin*, and *Psychology of Women Quarterly*.

MARY P. KOSS is Professor of Community and Family Medicine (with joint appointments in the Departments of Psychology and Psychiatry) at the University of Arizona. She received her A.B. degree from the University of Michigan and her Ph.D. in Clinical Psychology from the University of Minnesota. For more than 15 years she has studied rape, particularly among acquaintances, including its prevalence and impact. Her writings on the shortcomings of the National Crime Survey documentation of rape led to testimony before the U.S. Senate Committee on the Judiciary in 1990. Her national study of the prevalence of sexual victimization among college students is the subject of the book, *I Never Called It Rape: The Ms. Report on Recognizing, Fighting, and Surviving Date and Acquaintance Rape*, (authored by Robin Warshaw). In addition to many published papers, she is the co-author of the book, *The Rape Victim: Clinical and Community Interventions*, published in 1991. She is also associate editor of the *Psychology of Women Quarterly* and *Violence and Victims*. In 1989 she received the Stephen Schaefer Award for empirical contributions to the victim assistance field from the National Organization for Victim Assistance. Currently she is co-chair of the American Psychological Association's Task Force on Violence Against Women.

BERNICE LOTT did her undergraduate and graduate study in social psychology at UCLA and was awarded the Ph.D. at the age of 23. During the ensuing years Dr. Lott taught mentally retarded adolescents in a public junior high school, was a visiting faculty member in psychology at the University of Colorado, taught at Kentucky State College, worked for civil rights and social change during the 1960s, and went on to be a Dean and a faculty member at the University of Rhode Island, where she is now a Professor of Psychology and Women's Studies. Her scholarship is currently focused on the relationship between the social psychological and feminist perspectives; and her empirical research, for several years, has been concerned with the systematic investigation of interpersonal sexist discrimination as distancing behavior.

MAUREEN C. McHUGH is currently the Director of Women's Studies and Associate Professor of Psychology at Indiana University of Pennsylvania. She co-chaired a Division 35 (Psychology of Women) Task Force on Guidelines for Nonsexist Research in Psychology. She has presented and published on sex differences in attribution, expectancies, and intrinsic motivation. Her current research focuses on victimization of women, and victim blame/woman blame.

MARTHA T. MEDNICK is Professor of Psychology at Howard University in Washington, D.C. She has been a researcher and author in the field of psychology of women for the past twenty years. She is a past president of the Division of the Psychology of Women of the American Psychological Association, and has been awarded the APA Committee on Women in Psychology Leadership Award as well as the Carolyn Wood Sherif Memorial Award for feminist scholarship.

TAKAYO MUKAI, a graduate student at the University of Arizona, has research interests in developmental psychopathology of women, particularly risk factors for eating disorders in the United States and Japan. Currently, she is working on her dissertation, which compares eating attitudes and behaviors of girls in single-sex high schools and co-educational high schools.

ALAYNE J. ORMEROD is a doctoral candidate in Counseling Psychology at the University of Illinois at Urbana-Champaign where she holds the position of Course Coordinator. Her research interests include women's vocational behavior and sexual harassment. She is currently testing a model of women's vocational choice.

MICHELE A. PALUDI is Professor of Psychology at Hunter College, City University of New York. She is currently the Director of the Women's Studies Program at Hunter. In addition, she is the Coordinator of the Hunter College Sexual Harassment Panel. Dr. Paludi is the editor of *Ivory Power: Sexual Harassment on Campus* (1990) and co-author of *Academic and Workplace Sexual Harassment: A Resource Manual* (1991) and editor of the forthcoming *Working*

9 to 5: *Women, Men, Sex, and Power*. She is also the author of numerous scholarly papers on the topic of academic and workplace sexual harassment. Dr. Paludi received the 1988 Emerging Leader Award from the Committee on Women in Psychology.

MARY BROWN PARLEE is Professor of Psychology at the City University of New York Graduate Center. Her research interests include psychological aspects of menstruation and menopause, the social construction of scientific discourses about women's bodies, and general issues in feminist psychology; most of her teaching is in women's studies. In the past she has been director of CUNY's Center for the Study of Women and Society, a member of the Board of Directors of the National Council for Research on Women, a member of *Ms. Magazine*'s Advisory Board of Scholars, and an associate editor of *Psychology Today*. She is a past president of the Division of the Psychology of Women of the American Psychological Association and in 1977 received a Distinguished Publication Award from the Association for Women in Psychology.

VITA CARULLI RABINOWITZ received her Ph.D. in Social Psychology from Northwestern University. She is currently Associate Professor of Psychology at Hunter College and a member of the Social/Personality Doctoral Subprogram at the Graduate Center of the City University of New York. She has studied attributional processes in helping relationships and coping with victimization. Her recent research interests include the coping patterns of victims of sexual harassment. With Florence L. Denmark and Jeri A. Sechzer, she is currently investigating sex and gender bias across the spectrum of scientific research. In 1992, she received the Kurt Lewin Award from the New York State Psychological Association in recognition of outstanding achievement in social psychology.

PAMELA T. REID is Professor and Acting Head of Developmental Psychology in the Graduate School of the City University of New York. She is the current president of the Division of Psychology of Women. Her research interests have ranged from gender development and sex-typed behavior in children, to content analysis of television, and consideration of socio-historical explanations of racial behavior. Her recent research initiative focuses on family instability as instantiated by homelessness and the social and educational consequences for children.

NANCY FELIPE RUSSO is Professor of Psychology and Women's Studies at Arizona State University. Her more than 70 publications related to women's issues include *A Women's Mental Health Agenda*. Russo's current research focuses on the personal and social characteristics, coping resources, and mental health of women of diverse ethnicity.

SAUNDRA is currently Chairperson of the Psychology Department and Director of the African American Studies Program at Montclair State, New Jersey. Saundra has been recognized as the first African American and the first woman ever elected Chair of the Psychology Department since its establishment in 1967. She serves on the editorial board of the *Journal of Black Studies* and is a reviewer for *Black Books Bulletin*. Dr. Saundra received her Ph.D. in Social Psychology from the University of Maryland. She is interested in the socialization process and cultural stereotypes of women of color.

JERI A. SECHZER is Visiting Professor of Psychology at Pace University in New York. She received her Ph.D. in Physiological Psychology from the University of Pennsylvania. Professor Sechzer is active in many local, regional, and national scientific organizations concerned with sex and gender issues in research and education. Professor Sechzer is a Fellow and founding member of the Committee for Women in Science at the New York Academy of Sciences. She is a Fellow of the American Psychological Association, the American Psychological Society, and the New York Academy of Medicine. Dr. Sechzer has recently been elected to Fellowship status in the American Association for the Advancement of Science. With Vita C. Rabinowitz and Florence Denmark she is currently conducting a study of sex, gender, and values in behavioral and biological science. In addition to numerous scientific works, Professor Sechzer has written on sex and gender bias in psychological and biomedical research.

BONNIE SEEGMILLER, a Developmental Psychologist, is Associate Professor of Psychology at Hunter College in New York City. She holds a Ph.D. from New York University and has conducted research and published in a number of fields, including parent-child interactions, parenthood, cognitive and social development, the effects of maternal employment on children, advising, and gender-role development. She has long been interested in cross- and multi-cultural perspectives, and has lived and conducted research in a number of countries, such as Turkey and Mexico. She is currently studying gender and racial/ethnic/cultural differences attitudes toward parenting, and abuse.

LOUISE SILVERN is an Associate Professor at the University of Colorado, Boulder. She is a clinical psychologist who has published research concerning relationships between gender roles and mental health in children and adults. She is a consulting editor for *Sex Roles*.

VERONICA G. THOMAS is Acting Director, Institute for Urban Affairs and Research, and Associate Professor, Department of Human Development, Howard University. She is President of the Section on the Psychology of Black Women of the American Psychological Association. Dr. Thomas's areas of interests include the psychology of African-American women, well-being and coping in African-American families, and career aspirations and work values of women and minorities. Her work has appeared in such journals as *Sex Roles: A Journal of Research*, *Family Relations: Journal of Applied Family and Child Studies*,

Journal of Multicultural Counseling and Development, *Journal of Social Psychology*, and *Psychological Reports*.

CHERYL BROWN TRAVIS is a full professor at the University of Tennessee Psychology Department. A social psychologist, her emphasis has been on women and health psychology, especially where these are related to policy, planning, and decision making. Publications by Dr. Travis include two books on women's health: *Women and Health Psychology: Biomedical Issues* and *Women and Health Psychology: Mental Health Issues*.

RHODA UNGER is Professor of Psychology at Montclair State College and director of its all-college honors program. She is a past president of Division 35 of APA and an author/editor of numerous books on women and gender including *Woman: Dependent or Independent Variable?* (with Florence Denmark, 1975); *Female and Male* (1979); *Women, Gender, and Social Psychology* (with Virginia O'Leary and Barbara Wallston, 1985); *Representations: Social Constructions of Gender* (1989); and *Women and Gender: A Feminist Psychology* (with Mary Crawford, 1992). She was the first recipient of the Carolyn Wood Sherif Award from Division 35 and has been the recipient of two distinguished publication awards from the Association for Women in Psychology. In 1988–1989 she was a Fulbright scholar in Israel and a visiting professor at the University of Haifa in psychology/gender studies.